THE AMERICAN PHARMACEUTICAL ASSOCIATION'S

GUIDE TO PRESCRIPTION DRUGS

Donald Sullivan, Ph. D., R.Ph.

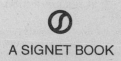

A SIGNET BOOK

SIGNET
Published by the Penguin Group
Penguin Putnam Inc., 375 Hudson Street,
New York, New York 10014, U.S.A.
Penguin Books Ltd, 27 Wrights Lane,
London W8 5TZ, England
Penguin Books Australia Ltd,
Ringwood, Victoria, Australia
Penguin Books Canada Ltd, 10 Alcorn Avenue,
Toronto, Ontario, Canada M4V 3B2
Penguin Books (N.Z.) Ltd, 182–190 Wairau Road,
Auckland 10, New Zealand

Penguin Books Ltd, Registered Offices:
Harmondsworth, Middlesex, England

First published by Signet, an imprint of Dutton NAL,
a member of Penguin Putnam Inc.

First Printing, October, 1998
10 9 8 7 6 5 4 3 2 1

To my parents, Jan and Donna Sullivan, my brother Jerry Sullivan, and a very special loved one, Amy Newman, for the love and support you gave me in writing this book. I could not have done it without you all.

CONTENTS

ACKNOWLEDGMENTS

I would like to thank Amy Newman. I could not have completed this book without all her help. Mere words cannot describe her contribution to this book. I would like to thank my family for all their help and support while writing this book. I am also grateful to the faculty of The Ohio State University College of Pharmacy, particularly Dr. Stephen W. Birdwell and the faculty in the Division of Pharmacy Practice and Administration. All these professors were instrumental in my undergraduate and graduate education. Without their commitment to providing the highest-quality pharmaceutical education, this book would not have been possible. I would like to thank the American Pharmaceutical Association for their commitment to the profession of pharmacy. Their contribution to the profession usually goes unnoticed, but they do more than most pharmacists will ever know. Finally, I would like to thank Deb Brody, Signet, and especially Rick Balkin for all their help and guidance during writing and editing of this book.

PREFACE

From the American Pharmaceutical Association
The National Professional Society of Pharmacists

Prescription medications are the most economical form of health care. They can save lives, improve the quality of one's life, and prevent more costly care such as hospitalization and surgery. But drugs work only if they are taken properly. This book is designed to help you do just that by providing up-to-date information about the most commonly prescribed drugs.

Consider the following:

- The Food and Drug Administration estimates that hospitalizations resulting from inappropriate prescription drug use cost the nation about $20 billion annually.
- 17 percent of hospitalizations of elderly Americans are the result of adverse drug events.
- Of the 2.3 billion prescriptions that are filled annually, approximately one half are not taken properly.
- Americans' failure to take their medications as instructed costs more than $100 billion a year in increased hospital and nursing home admissions, lost worker productivity, and premature death.

As you can see, billions in health care dollars can be saved each year if we can increase the proportion of patients who take their medicine correctly and reduce the incidence of preventable adverse effects of drugs. How can we confront this dual challenge?

The American Pharmaceutical Association believes that the pharmacist is the health professional best positioned in the community to bring about these improvements in drug use. No other health professional is as highly trained in the effects and use of pharmaceutical products.

Unfortunately, consumers often fail to take advantage of the pharmacist's expertise. Many Americans still hold a dated view of the pharmacist as a pill dispenser and seek little more in the pharmacy than fast service. Yet today's pharmacist does much more than fill prescriptions.

Pharmacists across America are changing the way they practice—often they're changing the layout of their pharmacies—so that patients, rather than drugs, are their focus. Many of today's pharmacists increase the likelihood of a patient's getting well when, at the time a drug product is dispensed, they review the patient's medication record to catch duplication or possible drug interactions and they provide instructions on how to properly take the medication. Some pharmacists work with the patient and physician to monitor the long-term effectiveness of the drug treatment.

Choosing a pharmacist is as important as choosing a physician. We advise you to use only one pharmacy so that all your medication records are at one location. Does your pharmacist talk to you about your medicine? Medication counseling is one of the pharmacist's most important roles, so choose a pharmacist who will answer all your questions, help you understand dosage instructions and potential adverse effects, and keep complete records on the drugs you take. The best way to avoid problems with medications is to make sure you understand clearly what your prescription instructions mean before you leave the pharmacy.

We all want to take charge of our own health care, and this book will help you do so when you are taking prescription drugs. It provides the information you need in clear and simple language. And it gives you information not found in other prescription drug guides, including side-effect percentages and price listings of brand name and generic drugs. But no book replaces the direct interaction you can have with a health professional. Don't hesitate to ask your pharmacist how to make the best use of your medications.

—John A. Gans, Pharm.D.
  Executive Vice President
  American Pharmaceutical Association

HOW TO USE THIS BOOK

BRAND NAME: This is the brand name or trade name of the drug given by the manufacturer and under which it is marketed. (Examples: Zantac, Premarin, and Prozac)

GENERIC NAME: This is the generic name or chemical name of the drug. If you know the generic name but do not know the brand name, look in the generic-to-brand-name cross reference to find the brand name.

GENERIC FORM AVAILABLE: This describes if a generic equivalent is available for the brand-name product.

THERAPEUTIC CLASS: This describes the therapeutic class the brand-name drug belongs to. The therapeutic class a drug belongs to is based primarily on how the drug works in the body.

DOSAGE FORMS: This describes the different types of dosage forms and strengths available. (Examples: cream, ointment, solution, capsule, liquid, suspension, tablet, sustained-release capsule, etc.)

MAIN USES: This describes which diseases or symptoms the drug is used to treat. Each individual disease or symptom the drug is used to treat must be approved by the Food and Drug Administration (FDA). There may, however, be other uses that are not approved by the FDA, but for which the drug is regularly prescribed. These so-called "unapproved uses" of the drug are commonly the result of testing and extensive use among physicians and other health care professionals. Even though formal approval for a particular unapproved use has not been obtained, strong evidence of its effectiveness may exist. Some unapproved, but scientifically supported, uses are included in this book. Unapproved uses for a drug are presented in brackets { }.

USUAL DOSE: This is the amount of the drug usually taken by adult patients. These adult doses have been approved by the FDA. Doses for children, the elderly, or those with kidney or liver disease may be less than those listed and are not included in this book. Doses may also be higher for more severe conditions.

AVERAGE PRICE: This is the average price of the drug based on pricing formulas used by pharmacies and actual price comparisons. The prices given are for 100 capsules or tablets unless otherwise stated. Prices for smaller quantities are provided only when large quantities of a particular drug are rarely prescribed. An example of this is an antibiotic, such as penicillin or amoxicillin, where only 30 or 40 tablets are typically prescribed.

Prices for quantities of 100 were chosen for a very simple reason: this allows the reader to easily calculate the price per tablet by dividing by 100 and then multiplying that number by the number of tablets prescribed by their physician. Also, if a (B) appears after a price, the price is for the brand name. If a (G) appears after a price, the price is for the generic. Price projections are based on data available at the beginning of 1997. These prices are only *averages* and should be used only as a general guide as to how expensive a particular drug may be. Other factors may affect prescription prices, such as size of the city, amount of pharmacy competition within a city, size of the pharmacy, and type of pharmacy (chain pharmacy [Revco, Rite Aid, Eckerd, and Walgreens], independently owned pharmacy [Jim's Pharmacy and Smith Brothers Drugs], and deep discounters [Phar-Mor and Drug Emporium]).

SIDE EFFECTS: The side effects included are based on the test results conducted by manufacturer that were submitted and approved by the FDA. Any side effect that occurred in more than 1% of patients during testing was included. For some drugs that are older and have been on the market for quite some time, percentages for each side effect were not available. Therefore, the side effects of these drugs were classified as "most common" and "less common" based on test results of the manufacturer and published experience in using the drug by health care professionals.

DRUG INTERACTIONS: When two drugs are taken together and produce some unwanted effect or side effects, a drug interaction is said to occur. Major drug interactions for each drug included in the book are described in this section. There may be other less significant interactions, but only the ones of major clinical significance that could be potentially harmful to the patient are listed. To avoid dangerous drug interactions, you should discuss all your current and any new medications with your doctor and pharmacist.

ALLERGIES: This section describes allergies to certain medications that may affect the decision whether or not you should take this drug.

PREGNANCY/BREAST-FEEDING: This section describes the effect or risk to an unborn child or infant for each prescription drug. The system used for ranking pregnancy risk was developed by the FDA to define the amount of risk to an unborn child. There are five levels in FDA's risk system: Category A, Category B, Category C, Category D, and Category X. The range of categories is from Category A (no risk to an unborn child during pregnancy) to Category X (definite risk of birth defects and possible death to an unborn child during pregnancy). Also, information is presented about whether the drug goes into the breast milk. Drugs that get into the breast milk may be dangerous to an infant who is breast-feeding. This is by no means an absolute guide. If you are pregnant or breast-feeding, talk to your doctor and pharmacist before taking any prescription or over-the-counter (nonprescription) drug.

OTHER BRAND NAMES: Some drugs are marketed under more than one brand name; in these cases, the pharmacist can dispense either brand. This section lists other brand names the drug is marketed under. You should ask the pharmacist for prices on the actual prescription drug and the brand names listed here and choose the one with the lowest price.

OTHER DRUGS IN THE SAME THERAPEUTIC CLASS: This section lists all other drugs in the same therapeutic class. This will allow you to compare prices, side effects, drug interactions, dosages, etc., with drugs similar to the one you were prescribed.

IMPORTANT INFORMATION TO REMEMBER: This is the most important part of the book. This section lists the most important information pharmacists think you should know about the drug. If you have any further questions, contact your pharmacist.

PRESCRIPTION DRUGS A–Z

BRAND NAME: **Accolate**

GENERIC NAME: zafirlukast

GENERIC FORM AVAILABLE: No

THERAPEUTIC CLASS: Asthma controller

DOSAGE FORMS: 20-mg tablets

MAIN USES: Asthma and {other breathing disorders}

USUAL DOSE: 20 mg twice daily

AVERAGE PRICE: $82.81 for 60 tablets

SIDE EFFECTS: headache 13%, infection 4%, nausea 3%, diarrhea 3%, general pain 2%, weakness 2%, stomach pain 2%, muscle pain 2%, dizziness 2%, fever 2%, back pain 2%, and vomiting 2%.

DRUG INTERACTIONS: The drug may increase the blood levels and effects of Coumadin. Allegra, erythromycin, Seldane, Seldane-D, Slo-bid, Theo-Dur, theophylline, Uni-Dur, and Uniphyl may decrease the blood levels of the drug. Aspirin may increase the blood levels of the drug.

ALLERGIES: Individuals allergic to zafirlukast or any of its derivatives should discuss this with their doctor or pharmacist before using this drug.

PREGNANCY/BREAST-FEEDING: Category B—No evidence of risk in humans. Either animal findings show risk, but human findings do not; or, if no adequate human studies have been done, animal findings show no risk. The drug is excreted in the breast milk; therefore, extreme caution should be used when breast-feeding.

OTHER BRAND NAMES: None

OTHER DRUGS IN THE SAME THERAPEUTIC CLASS: Zyflo

IMPORTANT INFORMATION TO REMEMBER: The drug should be taken on an empty stomach, one hour before meals or two hours after meals. The drug is not intended to provide immediately relief of a bronchospasm, shortness of breath, or an asthma attack; it is used only for prevention of attacks. To receive the full benefits of the drug, use it on a regular basis as a maintenance medication. The drug may take two to four weeks before noticeable benefits may be seen. Never exceed prescribed dosage unless directed to do so by a doctor.

BRAND NAME: Accupril

GENERIC NAME: quinapril

GENERIC FORM AVAILABLE: No

THERAPEUTIC CLASS: Ace inhibitor

DOSAGE FORMS: 5-mg, 10-mg, 20-mg, and 40-mg tablets

MAIN USES: High blood pressure and heart failure

USUAL DOSE: For high blood pressure: initially 10 mg daily, possibly increasing to 20 mg to 80 mg per day in one or two equally divided doses. For heart failure: initially 5 mg twice daily, possibly increasing to 20 mg to 40 mg per day in two equally divided doses.

AVERAGE PRICE: $127.27 for 5 mg and 10 mg; $135.87 for 20 mg; and $143.23 for 40 mg

SIDE EFFECTS: headache 6%, dizziness 4%, cough 4%, tiredness 3%, nausea and/or vomiting 2%, diarrhea 2%, stomach pain 1%, and back pain 1%.

DRUG INTERACTIONS: May decrease the absorption of the antibiotic Sumycin and other tetracyclines. High potassium levels may occur when used together with Dyrenium and Aldactone and potassium supplements such as Micro-K, K-Dur, Klor-Con, K-Lyte, and Slow-K. Patients on water pills, especially those recently started on a water pill, may experience low blood pressure. The drug may also increase the toxic effects of Eskalith and Lithobid, especially when taken with a water pill.

ALLERGIES: Individuals allergic to quinapril or other ACE inhibitors (such as those listed in "Other Drugs in the Same Therapeutic Class") should discuss this with their doctor or pharmacist before using this drug.

PREGNANCY/BREAST-FEEDING: Category C (first trimester)—Risk cannot be ruled out. Human studies are lacking, and animal studies are either positive for fetal risk or lacking as well. However, potential benefits may justify the potential risk in using the drug. Category D (second and third trimesters)—Positive evidence of risk. Human studies show risk to the fetus. Nevertheless, potential benefits may possibly outweigh the potential risk. This drug should not be taken by nursing mothers.

OTHER BRAND NAMES: None

OTHER DRUGS IN THE SAME THERAPEUTIC CLASS: Altace, Capoten, Lotensin, Mavik, Monopril, Prinivil, Univasc, Vasotec, and Zestril

IMPORTANT INFORMATION TO REMEMBER: Take this drug regularly and exactly as directed by your physician. Do not stop taking Accupril unless otherwise directed by your doctor. Avoid salt substitutes containing potassium. Before taking over-the-counter cold and allergy preparations, consult your doctor or pharmacist—these products may raise your blood pressure. If you experience swelling of the face, lips, or tongue or difficulty in breathing, contact your doctor immediately.

BRAND NAME: Accutane

GENERIC NAME: isotretinoin

GENERIC FORM AVAILABLE: No

THERAPEUTIC CLASS: Vitamin A derivative

DOSAGE FORMS: 10-mg, 20-mg, and 40-mg capsules

MAIN USES: Severe acne

USUAL DOSE: 10 mg to 40 mg twice a day for 15 to 20 weeks

AVERAGE PRICE: $95.19 for 10 mg (20 capsules); $112.56 for 20 mg (20 capsules); and 131.75 for 40 mg (20 capsules)

SIDE EFFECTS: scaling, burning, or redness of the lips 90%, dry skin or dry nose 80%, bloody nose 80%, eye irritation and/or redness 40%, joint pain 16%, skin disorders less than 10%, thinning of the hair less than 10%, sunburn more easily 5%, and stomach problems, tiredness, and headache less than 5%.

DRUG INTERACTIONS: The drug may decrease the effects of Tegretol. Doryx, Monocin, Monodox, Sumycin, and Vibramycin may increase incidence of pseudotumor cerebri (a dangerous increase in the blood pressure within the brain). Also, avoid vitamin A supplements or excess alcohol consumption.

ALLERGIES: Individuals allergic to isotretinoin, vitamin A, or any of its derivatives should discuss this with their doctor or pharmacist before taking this drug.

PREGNANCY/BREAST-FEEDING: Category X—Should not be used during pregnancy. Studies in animals and/or humans have shown fetal abnormalities and birth defects. The risks associated with using this drug clearly outweigh the benefits. This drug should never be used by someone who is pregnant or trying to become pregnant. Effective birth control should be used for at least one month before taking the drug and for at least one month after the drug has been discontinued. Also, women should never breast-feed while using this drug.

OTHER BRAND NAMES: None

OTHER DRUGS IN THE SAME THERAPEUTIC CLASS: Differin and Retin-A

IMPORTANT INFORMATION TO REMEMBER: Women should definitely use contraceptive measures while taking this drug to avoid becoming pregnant. Effective birth control should be used for at least one month before taking the drug and for at least one month after the drug has been discontinued. If a woman suspects she may be pregnant, she should stop taking the drug immediately. Individuals should also use a water-based sunscreen and avoid overexposure to the sun. The drug may increase the skin's sensitivity to sunlight, which may cause one to sunburn more easily. Headaches, visual disturbances, nausea, and vomiting may be symptoms of a condition called pseudotumor cerebri, which is a very serious disease of the brain. If these symptoms should occur, report them to a physician immediately. The drug should be taken with food or milk to increase absorption of the drug. Also, individuals taking the drug should not give blood until at least one month after the drug is discontinued.

BRAND NAME: Achromycin-V

GENERIC NAME: tetracycline

See entry for Sumycin

BRAND NAME: Aclovate

GENERIC NAME: alclometasone dipropionate

GENERIC FORM AVAILABLE: Yes

THERAPEUTIC CLASS: Topical corticosteroids

DOSAGE FORMS: 0.05% cream and ointment

MAIN USES: Skin rashes, swelling, and itching

USUAL DOSE: Apply a thin film two to three times per day.

AVERAGE PRICE: $15.99 (B) /$12.99 (G) for 15 g

SIDE EFFECTS: itching 2%, burning 1%, redness 1%, dry skin 1%, irritation 1%, and rash 1%.

DRUG INTERACTIONS: None of any clinical significance

ALLERGIES: Individuals allergic to alclometasone or any other topical corticosteroids (such as those listed in "Other Drugs in the Same Therapeutic Class") should discuss this with their doctor or pharmacist before using this drug.

PREGNANCY/BREAST-FEEDING: Category C—Risk cannot be ruled out. Human studies are lacking, and animal studies are either positive for fetal risk or lacking as well. However, potential benefits may justify the potential risk in using the drug. It is not known whether the drug is excreted in the breast milk; therefore, caution should be used when breast-feeding.

OTHER BRAND NAMES: None

OTHER DRUGS IN THE SAME THERAPEUTIC CLASS: Aristocort, Cordran, Cordran SP, Cutivate, Cyclocort, DesOwen, Diprolene, Elocon, Halog, Hytone, Kenalog, Lidex, Synalar, Temovate, Topicort, Tridesilon, Ultravate, Valisone, and Westcort

IMPORTANT INFORMATION TO REMEMBER: This drug is for external use only. Apply only a thin film of drug to skin and rub it in well. Never cover the skin after application with a bandage or wrapping unless directed to do so by a doctor. Never apply to damaged skin or open wounds unless directed to do so by a doctor. Discontinue use if irritation occurs.

BRAND NAME: Actigall

GENERIC NAME: ursodiol

GENERIC FORM AVAILABLE: No

THERAPEUTIC CLASS: Gallstone-dissolving agent

DOSAGE FORMS: 300-mg capsules

MAIN USES: Dissolving of some types of gallstones

USUAL DOSE: 300 mg to 900 mg per day in two or three divided doses

AVERAGE PRICE: $305.13

SIDE EFFECTS: mild diarrhea 6%, itching less than 1%, rash less than 1%, stomach pain less than 1%, gas less than 1%, and headache less than 1%.

DRUG INTERACTIONS: Some cholesterol-lowering drugs, such as Questran and Colestid, and some antacids containing aluminum, such as Maalox and Mylanta, may interfere with the absorption of this drug.

ALLERGIES: Individuals allergic to ursodiol, bile acids, or any of their derivatives should discuss this with their doctor or pharmacist before using this drug.

PREGNANCY/BREAST-FEEDING: Category B—No evidence of risk in humans. Either animal findings show risk, but human findings do not; or, if no adequate human studies have been done, animal findings show no risk. It is not known whether the drug is excreted in the breast milk; therefore, caution should be used when breast-feeding.

OTHER BRAND NAMES: None

OTHER DRUGS IN THE SAME THERAPEUTIC CLASS: None

IMPORTANT INFORMATION TO REMEMBER: This drug must be taken for several months in order for gallstones to dissolve. Gall-

stones do not dissolve completely in all patients and more gallstones may form. This therapy is not appropriate for everyone
with gallstones. Avoid antacids containing aluminum such as
Maalox and Mylanta; they may interfere with the absorption of
this drug.

BRAND NAME: Acular

GENERIC NAME: ketorolac tromethamine

GENERIC FORM AVAILABLE: No

THERAPEUTIC CLASS: Nonsteroidal anti-inflammatory eyedrop

DOSAGE FORMS: 0.5% eyedrop solution

MAIN USES: Itching due to seasonal eye allergies

USUAL DOSE: one drop four times daily for up to one week

AVERAGE PRICE: $41.17 for 5 mL

SIDE EFFECTS: short-term stinging and burning when administered
40%, eye irritation 3%, and allergic reactions 3%.

DRUG INTERACTIONS: The drug may increase the effects of
Coumadin.

ALLERGIES: Individuals allergic to ketorolac or any of its derivatives should discuss this with their doctor or pharmacist before using this drug.

PREGNANCY/BREAST-FEEDING: Category C—Risk cannot be ruled
out. Human studies are lacking, and animal studies are either positive for fetal risk or lacking as well. However, potential benefits
may justify the potential risk in using the drug. It is not known
whether the drug is excreted in the breast milk; therefore, caution
should be used when breast-feeding.

OTHER BRAND NAMES: None

OTHER DRUGS IN THE SAME THERAPEUTIC CLASS: Voltaren Oph-
thalmic Drops

IMPORTANT INFORMATION TO REMEMBER: Individuals should not
use the drug while wearing contact lenses. Keep the container
tightly closed and avoid touching the applicator tip to the eye—
this could contaminate the product over time. Also, only administer one drop at a time. After application, keep the eye open for at

least 30 seconds, roll the eyeball around, and avoid squinting. If a second drop is required, wait one to two minutes between drops. If another medication is to be used in the eye, wait at least 10 minutes before administering it.

BRAND NAME: Adalat and Adalat CC

GENERIC NAME: nifedipine

See entry for Procardia/Procardia XL

BRAND NAME: Adapin

GENERIC NAME: doxepin

See entry for Sinequan

BRAND NAME: Adderall

GENERIC NAME: Combination product containing: dextroamphetamine and amphetamine

GENERIC FORM AVAILABLE: No

THERAPEUTIC CLASS: Amphetamine stimulant

DOSAGE FORMS: 10-mg and 20-mg tablets

MAIN USES: Narcolepsy and attention deficit disorder (ADDH) with hyperactivity

USUAL DOSE: For narcolepsy: 5 mg to 60 mg per day in divided doses. For ADDH: 2.5 mg to 20 mg once or twice daily.

AVERAGE PRICE: $62.39

SIDE EFFECTS: Most common: irregular heartbeat, nervousness, irritability, false sense of well-being, restlessness, insomnia, and drowsiness after the drug wears off. Less common: blurred vision, changes in sex drive, diarrhea, nausea, vomiting, stomach pain, constipation, loss of appetite, weight loss, dizziness, lightheadedness, headache, dry mouth, unpleasant taste, pounding heartbeat, and increased sweating.

DRUG INTERACTIONS: Anafranil, Asendin, Elavil, Eldepryl, Endep, Nardil, Norpramin, Pamelor, Parnate, Sinequan, Surmontil,

Tofranil, or Vivactil and the drug may cause cardiovascular symptoms such as irregular heartbeat, high blood pressure, and fast heartbeat. Blocadren, Cartrol, Corgard, Inderal, Kerlone, Levatol, Lopressor, Normodyne, Sectral, Tenormin, Toprol-XL, Trandate, Visken, or Zebeta and the drug may cause high blood pressure, slow heart rate, and possibly heart block. The drug may increase the effects of Lanoxin. The analgesic effects of Demerol may be increased when used with this drug. Cytomel, Levoxyl, Levothroid, or Synthroid and this drug may increase the effects of both of these drugs when taken together.

ALLERGIES: Individuals allergic to dextroamphetamine, amphetamines, or any of their derivatives should discuss this with their doctor or pharmacist before using this drug.

PREGNANCY/BREAST-FEEDING: Category C—Risk cannot be ruled out. Human studies are lacking, and animal studies are either positive for fetal risk or lacking as well. However, potential benefits may justify the potential risk in using the drug. The drug is excreted in the breast milk; therefore, extreme caution should be used when breast-feeding.

OTHER BRAND NAMES: None

OTHER DRUGS IN THE SAME THERAPEUTIC CLASS: Adderall, Dexedrine, and Ritalin

IMPORTANT INFORMATION TO REMEMBER: The drug may cause dizziness. Caution should be used when performing activities that require coordination. Only take the drug exactly as directed by your physician. Do not discontinue the drug without first consulting your physician; also, do not increase the dose without first consulting with your physician. This prescription cannot be refilled—a new written prescription must be obtained each time. This medication is a controlled substance and may be habit-forming. The potential for abuse with this medication is high.

BRAND NAME: Adipex-P

GENERIC NAME: phentermine

GENERIC FORM AVAILABLE: No

THERAPEUTIC CLASS: Appetite suppressant

DOSAGE FORMS: 37.5-mg tablets

MAIN USES: Short-term use in weight loss

USUAL DOSE: 37.5 mg once daily

AVERAGE PRICE: $21.72 for 14 tablets

SIDE EFFECTS: Most common: increased blood pressure. Less common: heart palpitations, fast heartbeat, restlessness, insomnia, headache, dizziness, and dry mouth.

DRUG INTERACTIONS: Individuals who are currently taking Nardil or Parnate or who have taken either of these drugs within the past 14 days should not take Adipex-P.

ALLERGIES: Individuals allergic to phenteramine, amphetamines, or any of their derivatives should discuss this with their doctor or pharmacist before using this drug.

PREGNANCY/BREAST-FEEDING: Category C—Risk cannot be ruled out. Human studies are lacking, and animal studies are either positive for fetal risk or lacking as well. However, potential benefits may justify the potential risk in using the drug. It is not known whether the drug is excreted in the breast milk; therefore, caution should be used when breast-feeding.

OTHER BRAND NAMES: None

OTHER DRUGS IN THE SAME THERAPEUTIC CLASS: Didrex, Ionamin, Plegine, Pondimin, Redux, and Tenuate

IMPORTANT INFORMATION TO REMEMBER: Ideally the drug should be taken before breakfast or one to two hours after breakfast. Tolerance to the weight loss effect of this drug usually develops within a few weeks; therefore its effectiveness for weight loss is usually short-lived. Do not increase the dose if tolerance develops without first consulting with your physician. This medication is a controlled substance and may be habit-forming.

BRAND NAME: Aerobid and Aerobid-M

GENERIC NAME: flunisolide

GENERIC FORM AVAILABLE: No

THERAPEUTIC CLASS: Steroid inhaler

DOSAGE FORMS: 250 micrograms of drug per inhalation

MAIN USES: Asthma and {various other breathing disorders}

USUAL DOSE: two puffs twice daily

AVERAGE PRICE: $70.70

SIDE EFFECTS: headache 25%, sore throat 20%, nasal congestion 15%, diarrhea 10%, upset stomach 10%, nervousness 3%–9%, palpitations 3%–9%, chest pain 3%–9%, dizziness 3%–9%, cough 3%–9%, hoarseness 3%–9%, and runny nose 3%–9%.

DRUG INTERACTIONS: Caution should be used when taking this drug with oral corticosteroids such as Aristocort, Decadron, Deltasone, Medrol, and prednisone.

ALLERGIES: Individuals allergic to flunisolide and other inhaled steroids (such as those listed in "Other Drugs in the Same Therapeutic Class") should discuss this with their doctor or pharmacist before using this drug.

PREGNANCY/BREAST-FEEDING: Category C—Risk cannot be ruled out. Human studies are lacking, and animal studies are either positive for fetal risk or lacking as well. However, potential benefits may justify the potential risk in using the drug. It is not known whether the drug is excreted in the breast milk, therefore, caution should be used when breast-feeding.

OTHER BRAND NAMES: None

OTHER DRUGS IN THE SAME THERAPEUTIC CLASS: Azmacort, Beclovent, Flovent, and Vanceril

IMPORTANT INFORMATION TO REMEMBER: The drug is not intended to provide immediately relief of a bronchospasm, shortness of breath, or an asthma attack. To receive the full benefits of the drug, use it on a regular basis as a maintenance medication. The drug may take a few weeks before noticeable benefits may be seen. Never exceed prescribed dosage unless directed to do so by a doctor; excessive use beyond prescribed dosage can be dangerous. If another inhaler is also being used at the same time, use the other one a few minutes prior to using Aerobid. Some individuals complain about the bad taste of Aerobid; if this is the case, ask your doctor to prescribe Aerobid-M. Aerobid-M contains menthol, which masks the bad taste of the drug.

When using the inhaler, use the following procedure:

1) Shake the canister well.
2) Place the mouthpiece close to the mouth, but not touching the lips.

3) Exhale deeply.
4) Inhale slowly and deeply as you press the top of the canister to release the medication.
5) Hold your breath for a few seconds before exhaling.
6) Wait five minutes between puffs.
7) Rinse your mouth out with water after use; otherwise, this drug may cause a fungal infection in the mouth.
8) Be sure to wash the inhaler device (mouthpiece) regularly with warm soapy water to avoid bacterial contamination.

BRAND NAME: Akineton

GENERIC NAME: biperiden

GENERIC FORM AVAILABLE: No

THERAPEUTIC CLASS: Anticholinergic

DOSAGE FORMS: 2-mg tablets

MAIN USES: Parkinson's disease and drug-induced movement disorders

USUAL DOSE: 2 mg three to four times daily for Parkinson's and 2 mg one to three times daily for movement disorders

AVERAGE PRICE: $35.43

SIDE EFFECTS: Most common: nausea, vomiting, dry mouth, blurred vision, decreased sweating, painful urination, and constipation. Less common: drowsiness, dizziness, headache, loss of memory, numbness, false sense of well-being, and agitation.

DRUG INTERACTIONS: The drug should be used with caution when used with other drugs that have anticholinergic activity. These drugs include Anafranil, Asendin, Demerol, Elavil, Norpramin, Pamelor, Prolixin, Quinidex, Quinaglute, Serentil, Sinequan, Surmontil, Thorazine, Tofranil, Trilafon, Vivactil, and some antihistamines. Antacids may decrease the absorption of the drug.

ALLERGIES: Individuals allergic to biperiden or any of its derivatives should discuss this with their doctor or pharmacist before using this drug.

PREGNANCY/BREAST-FEEDING: Category C—Risk cannot be ruled out. Human studies are lacking, and animal studies are either positive for fetal risk or lacking as well. However, potential benefits

may justify the potential risk in using the drug. It is not known whether the drug is excreted in the breast milk; therefore, caution should be used when breast-feeding.

OTHER BRAND NAMES: None

OTHER DRUGS IN THE SAME THERAPEUTIC CLASS: Artane, Cogentin, and Kemadrin

IMPORTANT INFORMATION TO REMEMBER: Do not abruptly discontinue the medication if side effects occur. Gradual dose reduction may be necessary; check with your physician. Individuals should avoid using alcohol or depressants while taking this drug. This drug may cause some drowsiness. Caution should also be used when exercising and in hot weather while taking this drug. This drug may also cause a dry mouth; sugarless gum or hard candy will help take care of this problem. Individuals with glaucoma or prostate problems should only use the drug under the direct supervision of a doctor.

BRAND NAME: Aldactazide

GENERIC NAME: Combination drug containing: spironolactone and hydrochlorothiazide

GENERIC FORM AVAILABLE: No

THERAPEUTIC CLASS: potassium-sparing diuretic (water) + thiazide diuretic (water pill)

DOSAGE FORMS: 25-mg spironolactone/25-mg hydrochlorothiazide tablets and 50-mg spironolactone/50-mg hydrochlorothiazide tablets

MAIN USES: Swelling and water retention due to congestive heart failure, kidney or liver disease, and high blood pressure

USUAL DOSE: 25 mg to 200 mg of each component daily in a single or divided dose for water retention due to congestive heart failure or kidney or liver disease, and 50 mg to 100 mg of each component daily in single or divided dose for high blood pressure.

AVERAGE PRICE: $54.60 for 25-mg/25-mg tablets; $106.51 for 50-mg/50-mg tablets

SIDE EFFECTS: Most common: None. Less common: cramps, diarrhea, drowsiness, headache, enlarged breasts in men, itching, unsteady movement, increased sensitivity to sunlight (sunburn), gas, dizziness, and impotence.

DRUG INTERACTIONS: The drug may increase the toxic effects of Eskalith or Lithobid, and may also cause high blood sugar when used with Indocin. High potassium levels may occur when used together with Accupril, Altace, Capoten, Lotensin, Monopril, Prinivil, Univasc, or Vasotec, and potassium supplements such as Micro-K, K-Dur, Klor-Con, K-Lyte, and Slow-K. The drug may decrease the effects of Coumadin. Finally, individuals taking Lanoxin should inform their doctor of this before taking this drug.

ALLERGIES: Individuals allergic to Aldactone, Dyazide, Hydro-DIURIL, Maxzide, Moduretic, sulfa drugs, or any of their derivatives should discuss this with their doctor or pharmacist before using this drug.

PREGNANCY/BREAST-FEEDING: Category D—Positive evidence of risk. Human studies show risk to the fetus. Nevertheless, potential benefits may possibly outweigh the potential risk. This drug should not be taken by nursing mothers.

OTHER BRAND NAMES: None

OTHER DRUGS IN THE SAME THERAPEUTIC CLASS: Dyazide, Maxzide, and Moduretic

IMPORTANT INFORMATION TO REMEMBER: If the drug is to be taken once daily, take it in the morning due to increased urine output. Take the drug with food or milk if stomach upset occurs. This drug may also increase the sensitivity of the skin to sunburn in some individuals; therefore, a sunscreen is recommended during periods of prolonged exposure to the sun. Individuals with kidney disease should discuss this with their doctor before taking this drug. Before taking over-the-counter cold and allergy preparations, consult your doctor or pharmacist—these products may raise your blood pressure.

<u>BRAND NAME:</u> Aldactone

GENERIC NAME: spironolactone

GENERIC FORM AVAILABLE: Yes

THERAPEUTIC CLASS: Potassium-sparing diuretic (water pill)

DOSAGE FORMS: 25-mg, 50-mg, and 100-mg tablets

MAIN USES: Swelling and water retention due to congestive heart failure, kidney or liver disease, and high blood pressure

USUAL DOSE: 25 mg to 200 mg daily in a single or divided dose for edema due to congestive heart failure or kidney or liver disease, and 50 mg to 100 mg daily in single or divided dose for high blood pressure

AVERAGE PRICE: $60.13 (B)/$15.98 (G) for 25-mg tablets

SIDE EFFECTS: Most common: None. Less common: cramps, diarrhea, drowsiness, headache, enlarged breasts in men, itching, unsteady movement, gas, dizziness, and impotence.

DRUG INTERACTIONS: The drug may increase the toxic effects of Eskalith or Lithobid, and may also cause high blood sugar when used with Indocin. High potassium levels may occur when used together with Accupril, Altace, Capoten, Lotensin, Monopril, Prinivil, Univasc, or Vasotec, and potassium supplements such as Micro-K, K-Dur, Klor-Con, K-Lyte, and Slow K. The drug may decrease the effects of Coumadin. Finally, individuals taking Lanoxin should inform their doctor of this before taking this drug.

ALLERGIES: Individuals allergic to spironolactone or any of its derivatives should discuss this with their doctor or pharmacist before using this drug.

PREGNANCY/BREAST-FEEDING: Category D—Positive evidence of risk. Human studies show risk to the fetus. Nevertheless, potential benefits may possibly outweigh the potential risk. This drug should not be taken by nursing mothers.

OTHER BRAND NAMES: None

OTHER DRUGS IN THE SAME THERAPEUTIC CLASS: Dyrenium and Midamor

IMPORTANT INFORMATION TO REMEMBER: If the drug is to be taken once daily, take it in the morning due to increased urine output. If stomach upset occurs, take with food or milk. Individuals with kidney disease should discuss this with their doctor before taking this drug. Before taking over-the-counter cold and allergy preparations, consult your doctor or pharmacist—these products may raise your blood pressure.

BRAND NAME: **Aldoclor**

GENERIC NAME: Combination product containing: methyldopa and chlorothiazide

See individual entries for Aldomet and Diuril

BRAND NAME: **Aldomet**

GENERIC NAME: methyldopa

GENERIC FORM AVAILABLE: Yes

THERAPEUTIC CLASS: Centrally acting blood vessel dilator

DOSAGE FORMS: 125-mg, 250-mg, and 500-mg tablets; and 250 mg/5 mL suspension

MAIN USES: High blood pressure

USUAL DOSE: 125 mg to 500 mg two to four times daily

AVERAGE PRICE: $49.00 (B)/$22.40 (G) for 250 mg; $93.80 (B)/$54.60 (G) for 500 mg

SIDE EFFECTS: Most common: None. Less common: nausea, diarrhea, vomiting, weight gain, impotence, dry mouth, headache, drowsiness, depression, anxiety, fever, dizziness, Bell's palsy, and muscle pain.

DRUG INTERACTIONS: The chance for blood pressure becoming too low may occur when taken with other blood pressure medications. The drug may increase the toxic effects of Eskalith and Lithobid.

ALLERGIES: Individuals allergic to methyldopa or any of its derivatives should discuss this with their doctor or pharmacist before using this drug.

PREGNANCY/BREAST-FEEDING: Category B—No evidence of risk in humans. Either animal findings show risk, but human findings do not; or, if no adequate human studies have been done, animal findings show no risk. It is not known whether the drug is excreted in the breast milk; therefore, caution should be used when breast-feeding.

OTHER BRAND NAMES: None

OTHER DRUGS IN THE SAME THERAPEUTIC CLASS: Catapres

IMPORTANT INFORMATION TO REMEMBER: The drug may cause drowsiness, especially when treatment is begun or daily dosage is increased. To minimize this effect, start dosage increases in the evening. Drowsiness usually goes away once the body adjusts to the medication. Before taking over-the-counter cold and allergy preparations, consult your doctor or pharmacist—these products may raise your blood pressure. If stomach upset occurs, take with food or milk. This drug should be used with caution by individuals with liver disease.

BRAND NAME: Aldoril

GENERIC NAME: Combination product containing: methyldopa and hydrochlorothiazide

GENERIC FORM AVAILABLE: Yes

THERAPEUTIC CLASS: Centrally acting blood vessel dilator and diuretic (water pill)

DOSAGE FORMS: 250-mg methyldopa/15-mg hydrochlorothiazide tablets, 250-mg methyldopa/25-mg hydrochlorothiazide tablets, 500-mg methyldopa/30-mg hydrochlorothiazide tablets, and 500-mg methyldopa/50-mg hydrochlorothiazide tablets

MAIN USES: High blood pressure

USUAL DOSE: 250 mg methyldopa/15 mg hydrochlorothiazide to 500 mg methyldopa/50 mg hydrochlorothiazide two to four times daily

AVERAGE PRICE: $69.14 (B)/$24.58 (G) for 250 mg/15 mg tablets; and $79.61 (B)/$20.24 (G) for 250 mg/25 mg tablets

SIDE EFFECTS: Most common: None. Less common: nausea, diarrhea, vomiting, weight gain, dry mouth, headache, drowsiness, dizziness, Bell's palsy, muscle pain, nasal stuffiness, and impotence.

DRUG INTERACTIONS: The drug may increase the toxic effects of Eskalith and Lithobid. The chance for blood pressure becoming too low may occur when taken with other blood pressure medications.

ALLERGIES: Individuals allergic to methyldopa, Dyazide, Hydro-DIURIL, Maxzide, Moduretic, sulfa drugs, or any of their derivatives should discuss this with their doctor or pharmacist before using this drug.

PREGNANCY/BREAST-FEEDING: Category C—Risk cannot be ruled out. Human studies are lacking, and animal studies are either positive for fetal risk or lacking as well. However, potential benefits

may justify the potential risk in using the drug. It is not known whether the drug is excreted in the breast milk; therefore, caution should be used when breast-feeding.

OTHER BRAND NAMES: None

OTHER DRUGS IN THE SAME THERAPEUTIC CLASS: Aldoclor and Combipres

IMPORTANT INFORMATION TO REMEMBER: The drug may cause drowsiness, especially when treatment is begun or daily dosage is increased. To minimize this effect, start dosage increases in the evening. Drowsiness usually goes away once the body adjusts to the medication. Before taking over-the-counter cold and allergy preparations, consult your doctor or pharmacist—these products may raise your blood pressure. If stomach upset occurs, take with food or milk. If the drug is to be taken once daily, take it in the morning due to increased urine output caused by the hydrochlorothiazide component. Individuals with kidney or liver disease should discuss this with their doctor before taking this drug.

BRAND NAME: Alkeran

GENERIC NAME: melphalan

GENERIC FORM AVAILABLE: No

THERAPEUTIC CLASS: Alkylating anticancer agent

DOSAGE FORMS: 2-mg tablets

MAIN USES: Cancer

USUAL DOSE: 2 mg to 6 mg daily. The drug is usually taken for several days, followed by a "rest period" when no drug is taken.

AVERAGE PRICE: $227.14

SIDE EFFECTS: Most common: bone marrow suppression (white blood cells and platelets). Less common: nausea, vomiting, diarrhea, mouth sores, and liver toxicity.

DRUG INTERACTIONS: None of any clinical significance. However, the drug may increase bone marrow suppression when used with radiation or other cancer drugs.

ALLERGIES: Individuals allergic to melphalen or any of its derivatives should discuss this with their doctor or pharmacist before using this drug.

PREGNANCY/BREAST-FEEDING: Category D—Positive evidence of risk. Human studies show risk to the fetus. Nevertheless, potential benefits may possibly outweigh the potential risk. This drug should never be taken by nursing mothers or pregnant patients.

OTHER BRAND NAMES: None

OTHER DRUGS IN THE SAME THERAPEUTIC CLASS: Cytoxan and Leukeran

IMPORTANT INFORMATION TO REMEMBER: It is extremely important to follow the dosing schedule set by your physician. Do not deviate from this schedule. If unusual bleeding, bruising, black and tarry stools, blood in the urine, blood in the stool, or pinpoint red spots on the skin occur, contact your physician immediately. Nausea and vomiting may occur while taking this drug; if it is severe, notify your physician. Do not discontinue use unless directed by your physician. The drug may also lower the body's resistance to infection. At the first sign of infection—sore throat, fever, or chills—contact your physician immediately.

BRAND NAME: Allegra

GENERIC NAME: fexofenadine

GENERIC FORM AVAILABLE: No

THERAPEUTIC CLASS: Nonsedating antihistamine

DOSAGE FORMS: 60-mg capsules

MAIN USES: Allergies

USUAL DOSE: one tablet twice daily as needed

AVERAGE PRICE: $93.41

SIDE EFFECTS: cold or flu 3%, nausea 2%, abnormal menstrual periods 2%, drowsiness 1%, and tiredness 1%.

DRUG INTERACTIONS: Erythromycin and Nizoral may increase the blood levels of the drug.

ALLERGIES: Individuals allergic to fexofenadine, Seldane, Seldane-D, or any of their derivatives should discuss this with their doctor or pharmacist before using this drug.

PREGNANCY/BREAST-FEEDING: Category C—Risk cannot be ruled out. Human studies are lacking, and animal studies are either positive

for fetal risk or lacking as well. However, potential benefits may justify the potential risk in using the drug. It is not known whether the drug is excreted in the breast milk; therefore, caution should be used when breast-feeding.

OTHER BRAND NAMES: None

OTHER DRUGS IN THE SAME THERAPEUTIC CLASS: Claritin, Hismanal, Seldane, and Zyrtec

IMPORTANT INFORMATION TO REMEMBER: Do not take Allegra more frequently than every 12 hours. Unless otherwise directed by a physician, take only as needed for relief of allergies. This drug should be used cautiously when taken with E.E.S., ERYC, Ery-Tabs, erythromycin, Erythrocin, and Nizoral; these drugs may increase the blood levels of Allegra. If a pounding heartbeat or fainting occurs, report this to your physician immediately.

BRAND NAME: Allopurinol (various)

GENERIC NAME: allopurinol

See entry for Zyloprim

BRAND NAME: Alomide

GENERIC NAME: lodoxamide

GENERIC FORM AVAILABLE: No

THERAPEUTIC CLASS: Anti-allergy eyedrop

DOSAGE FORMS: 0.1% eyedrop solution

MAIN USES: Itching due to seasonal eye allergies

USUAL DOSE: one to two drops four times daily for up to three months

AVERAGE PRICE: $50.76 for 10 mL

SIDE EFFECTS: slight burning or stinging upon use in the eye 15%, itching 1%–5%, blurred vision 1%–5%, dry eye 1%–5%, headache 1.5%, scales on eyelid or eyelash less than 1%, and warm sensation in the eye less than 1%.

DRUG INTERACTIONS: None of any clinical significance

ALLERGIES: Individuals allergic to Iodoxamide or any of its derivatives should discuss this with their doctor or pharmacist before using this drug.

PREGNANCY/BREAST-FEEDING: Category B—No evidence of risk in humans. Either animal findings show risk, but human findings do not; or, if no adequate human studies have been done, animal findings show no risk. It is not known whether the drug is excreted in the breast milk; therefore, caution should be used when breast-feeding.

OTHER BRAND NAMES: None

OTHER DRUGS IN THE SAME THERAPEUTIC CLASS: Crolom

IMPORTANT INFORMATION TO REMEMBER: Individuals should not use the drug while wearing contact lenses unless otherwise directed by a physician. Keep the container tightly closed and avoid touching the applicator tip to the eye—this could contaminate the product over time. Also, only administer one drop at a time. After application, keep the eye open for at least 30 seconds, roll the eyeball around, and avoid squinting. If a second drop is required, wait one to two minutes between drops. If another medication is to be used in the eye, wait at least 10 minutes before administering it.

BRAND NAME: Alphagan

GENERIC NAME: brimonidine

GENERIC FORM AVAILABLE: No

THERAPEUTIC CLASS: Anti-glaucoma

DOSAGE FORMS: 0.2% solution

MAIN USES: Glaucoma

USUAL DOSE: one drop three times daily

AVERAGE PRICE: $27.19 for 5 mL

SIDE EFFECTS: dry mouth 10–30%, burning 10%–30%, stinging 10%–30%, headache 10%–30%, blurred vision 10%–30%, drowsiness 10%–30%, allergic reaction 10%–30%, feeling of something in the eye 10%–30%, eye itching 10%–30%, increased sensitivity of the eyes to sunlight 3%–9%, eyelid swelling and redness 3%–9%, dry eyes 3%–9%, tearing 3%–9%, dizziness 3%–9%, eye irritation 3%–9%, abnormal vision 3%–9%, muscle pain 3%–9%, eyelid crusting 1%–3%, abnormal taste 1%–3%, insomnia 1%–3%, depression 1%–3%, nervousness 1%–3%, pounding heartbeat 1%–3%, and dry nose 1%–3%.

DRUG INTERACTIONS: Alcohol, anxiety medications, and narcotic painkillers may intensify the drowsiness effect of the drug significantly.

ALLERGIES: Individuals allergic to brimonidine or any of its derivatives should discuss this with their doctor or pharmacist before using this drug.

PREGNANCY/BREAST-FEEDING: Category B—No evidence of risk in humans. Either animal findings show risk, but human findings do not; or, if no adequate human studies have been done, animal findings show no risk. It is not known whether the drug is excreted in the breast milk in significant quantities; therefore, caution should be used when breast-feeding.

OTHER BRAND NAMES: None

OTHER DRUGS IN THE SAME THERAPEUTIC CLASS: Iopidine

IMPORTANT INFORMATION TO REMEMBER: This drug may cause drowsiness. Individuals should use caution when driving, operating machinery, or any task where mental alertness is required. Alcohol, anxiety medications, and narcotic painkillers may intensify the drowsiness effect of the drug. Keep the container tightly closed and avoid touching the applicator tip to the eye—this could contaminate the product over time. Also, only administer one drop at a time. After application, keep the eye open for at least 30 seconds, roll the eyeball around, and avoid squinting. If a second drop is required, wait one to two minutes between drops. If another medication is to be used in the eye, wait at least 10 minutes before administering it. Only use the drug exactly as directed by your physician. Do not discontinue the drug without first consulting your physician.

BRAND NAME: Altace

GENERIC NAME: ramipril

GENERIC FORM AVAILABLE: No

THERAPEUTIC CLASS: ACE inhibitor

DOSAGE FORMS: 1.25-mg, 2.5-mg, 5-mg, and 10-mg capsules

MAIN USES: High blood pressure and {heart failure}

USUAL DOSE: 2.5 mg to 20 mg daily in one or two doses

AVERAGE PRICE: $97.79 for 2.5 mg; $105.67 for 5 mg; and $122.66 for 10 mg

SIDE EFFECTS: headache 5%, dizziness 2%, fatigue 2%, cough 1%, nausea 1%, and loss of taste 1%.

DRUG INTERACTIONS: May decrease the absorption of the antibiotic Sumycin and other tetracyclines. High potassium levels may occur when used together with Dyrenium and Aldactone and potassium supplements such as Micro-K, K-Dur, Klor-Con, K-Lyte, and Slow-K. Patients on water pills, especially those recently started on a water pill, may experience low blood pressure. The drug may also increase the toxic effects of Eskalith and Lithobid, especially when taken with a water pill.

ALLERGIES: Individuals allergic to ramipril or other ACE inhibitors (such as those listed in "Other Drugs in the Same Therapeutic Class") should discuss this with their doctor or pharmacist before using this drug.

PREGNANCY/BREAST-FEEDING: Category C (first trimester)—Risk cannot be ruled out. Human studies are lacking, and animal studies are either positive for fetal risk or lacking as well. However, potential benefits may justify the potential risk in using the drug. Category D (second and third trimesters)—Positive evidence of risk. Human studies show risk to the fetus. Nevertheless, potential benefits may possibly outweigh the potential risk. This drug should not be taken by nursing mothers.

OTHER BRAND NAMES: None

OTHER DRUGS IN THE SAME THERAPEUTIC CLASS: Accupril, Capoten, Lotensin, Mavik, Monopril, Prinivil, Univasc, Vasotec, and Zestril

IMPORTANT INFORMATION TO REMEMBER: Take this drug regularly and exactly as directed by your physician. Do not stop taking the drug unless otherwise directed by your doctor. Avoid salt substitutes containing potassium. Before taking over-the-counter cold and allergy preparations, consult your doctor or pharmacist—these products may raise your blood pressure. If you experience swelling of the face, lips, or tongue or difficulty in breathing, contact your doctor immediately.

BRAND NAME: Alupent

GENERIC NAME: metaproterenol

GENERIC FORM AVAILABLE: Yes for tablets and syrup

THERAPEUTIC CLASS: Beta-2-agonist bronchodilator

DOSAGE FORMS: 10-mg and 20-mg tablets; 10 mg/5 mL syrup; 5% inhalation solution; 0.4% and 0.6% unit-dose inhalation solution; and 0.65mg-per-inhalation metered-dose inhaler

MAIN USES: Asthma, chronic bronchitis, emphysema, and {other breathing disorders}

USUAL DOSE: 20 mg three to four times daily for the tablets; inhalation solution every four hours in an acute attack or three to four times daily regularly; and 2 to 3 puffs of the inhaler every three to four hours, with no more than 12 puffs per day for the inhaler.

AVERAGE PRICE: $50.60 (B)/29.90 (G) for 10 mg; $67.00 (B)/$28.56 (G) for 20 mg; $14.30 (B)/$8.78 (G) 120 mL syrup; and $41.93 for the inhaler

SIDE EFFECTS: Inhaler: nervousness 7%, headache 1%–4%, dizziness 1%–4%, pounding heartbeat 1%–4%, throat irritation 1%–4%, nausea 1%–4%, and fast heartbeat 1%. Solution: nervousness 14%, cough 3%, headache 3%, fast heartbeat 3%, and tremors 3%. Tablets: nervousness 20%, fast heartbeat 17%, tremors 17%, headache 7%, heart palpitations 4%, nausea 4%, and dizziness 3%.

DRUG INTERACTIONS: Anafranil, Asendin, Elavil, Nardil, Norpramin, Pamelor, Parnate, Sinequan, Surmontil, Tofranil, and Vivactil, and cough, cold, and allergy medications with decongestants may increase the toxicity of this medication. Blocadren, Cartrol, Corgard, Inderal, Levatol, Normodyne, Trandate, and Visken may decrease the effectiveness of the drug.

ALLERGIES: Individuals allergic to metaproterenol or any of its derivatives should discuss this with their doctor or pharmacist before using this drug.

PREGNANCY/BREAST-FEEDING: Category C—Risk cannot be ruled out. Human studies are lacking, and animal studies are either positive for fetal risk or lacking as well. However, potential benefits may justify the potential risk in using the drug. It is not known whether the drug is excreted in the breast milk; therefore, caution should be used when breast-feeding.

OTHER BRAND NAMES: Metaprel

OTHER DRUGS IN THE SAME THERAPEUTIC CLASS: Brethine, Bricanyl, Bronkometer, Maxair, Proventil, Serevent, Tornalate, Ventolin, and Volmax

IMPORTANT INFORMATION TO REMEMBER: Never exceed prescribed dosage unless directed to do so by a doctor; excessive use beyond prescribed dose is potentially dangerous and may even be fatal. Patients with irregular heartbeat or fast heartbeat should discuss this with their doctor before using this drug.

When using the inhaler, use the following procedure:

1) Shake the canister well.
2) Place the mouthpiece close to the mouth, but not touching the lips.
3) Exhale deeply.
4) Inhale slowly and deeply as you press the top of the canister to release the medication.
5) Hold your breath for a few seconds before exhaling.
6) Wait five minutes between puffs.
7) Be sure to wash the inhaler device (mouthpiece) regularly with warm soapy water to avoid bacterial contamination.

BRAND NAME: Ambien

GENERIC NAME: zolpidem

GENERIC FORM AVAILABLE: No

THERAPEUTIC CLASS: Imidazopyridine sedative

DOSAGE FORMS: 5-mg and 10-mg tablets

MAIN USES: Short-term treatment of insomnia

USUAL DOSE: 5 mg to 10 mg at bedtime

AVERAGE PRICE: $182.84 for 5 mg and $225.88 for 10 mg

SIDE EFFECTS: headache 7%, drowsiness 2%, nausea 2%, diarrhea 1%, dizziness 1%, and muscle pain 1%.

DRUG INTERACTIONS: Alcohol, anxiety medications, and narcotic painkillers may intensify the drowsiness effect of the drug significantly.

ALLERGIES: Individuals allergic to zolpidem or any of its derivatives should discuss this with their doctor or pharmacist before using this drug.

PREGNANCY/BREAST-FEEDING: Category B—No evidence of risk in humans. Either animal findings show risk, but human findings do not; or, if no adequate human studies have been done, animal findings show no risk. It is not known whether the drug is excreted in the breast milk in significant quantities; therefore, caution should be used when breast-feeding.

OTHER BRAND NAMES: None

OTHER DRUGS IN THE SAME THERAPEUTIC CLASS: None

IMPORTANT INFORMATION TO REMEMBER: This drug does cause drowsiness. Individuals should use caution when driving, operating machinery, or any task where mental alertness is required. Alcohol, anxiety medications, or narcotic painkillers may intensify the drowsiness effect of the drug. This medication is a controlled substance and may be habit-forming. Individuals who find the drug less effective over time should not increase their dose without first consulting their physician.

BRAND NAME: Amcill

GENERIC NAME: ampicillin

See entry for Omnipen

BRAND NAME: Amen

GENERIC NAME: medroxyprogesterone

See entry for Provera

BRAND NAME: Amoxicillin (various)

GENERIC NAME: amoxicillin

See entry for Amoxil

BRAND NAME: **Amoxil**

GENERIC NAME: amoxicillin

GENERIC FORM AVAILABLE: Yes

THERAPEUTIC CLASS: Broad-spectrum penicillin antibiotic

DOSAGE FORMS: 250-mg and 500-mg capsules; 125-mg and 250-mg chewable tablets; and 50 mg/mL, 125 mg/5 mL, and 250 mg/5 ml liquids

MAIN USES: Bacterial infections

USUAL DOSE: 250 mg to 500 mg every eight hours. Doses for small children may be lower.

AVERAGE PRICE: $18.68 (B)/$16.48 (G) for 250 mg; $30.78 (B)/$27.48 (G) for 500 mg; $29.68 (B)/$26.38 (G) for 250 mg chewables

SIDE EFFECTS: Most common: mild diarrhea, nausea, vomiting, and headache, yeast infections. Less common: allergic reactions, itching, and skin rash.

DRUG INTERACTIONS: The drug may decrease the effectiveness of birth control pills. The drug probenecid will decrease elimination of the drug by the kidneys.

ALLERGIES: Individuals allergic to amoxicillin or any of its derivatives, including other penicillins and cephalosporins, should discuss this with their doctor or pharmacist before taking this drug.

PREGNANCY/BREAST-FEEDING: Category B—No evidence of risk in humans. Either animal findings show risk, but human findings do not; or, if no adequate human studies have been done, animal findings show no risk. It is not known whether the drug is excreted in the breast milk; therefore, caution should be used when breast-feeding.

OTHER BRAND NAMES: Larotid, Polymox, Trimox, and Wymox

OTHER DRUGS IN THE SAME THERAPEUTIC CLASS: Omnipen, Spectrobid, and Veetids

IMPORTANT INFORMATION TO REMEMBER: Take the drug at even intervals around the clock (if three times a day, take every eight hours). Take the drug until all the medication prescribed is gone; otherwise, the infection may return. Women taking birth control pills should use another form of contraception while taking the drug and for the rest of the current menstrual cycle. Individuals taking the liquid form should shake it thoroughly before use, store the medication in the refrigerator, and discard any remaining medication after 14 days. Individuals taking the chewable tablets should drink a full glass of water after each dose.

BRAND NAME: Anafranil

GENERIC NAME: clomipramine

GENERIC FORM AVAILABLE: Yes

THERAPEUTIC CLASS: Tricyclic antidepressant

DOSAGE FORMS: 25-mg, 50-mg, and 75-mg capsules

MAIN USES: Obsessive-compulsive disorder

USUAL DOSE: Initially 25 mg per day at bedtime and increasing gradually to 100 mg in divided doses within the first two weeks.

AVERAGE PRICE: $113.44 for 25 mg; $152.96 for 50 mg; $201.36 for 75 mg

SIDE EFFECTS: dry mouth 84%, drowsiness 54%, tremor 54%, dizziness 54%, headache 52%, constipation 47%, ejaculation failure 42%, fatigue 39%, nausea 33%, increased sweating 29%, insomnia 25%, sex drive changes 21%, impotence 20%, nervousness 18%, weight increase 18%, abnormal vision 18%, urination disorders 14%, muscle pain 13%, diarrhea 13%, stomach pain 11%, increased appetite 11%, anxiety 9%, hot flashes 8%, and vomiting 7%.

DRUG INTERACTIONS: The drug should not be used with Nardil and Parnate. Haldol may increase the blood level of the drug. The drug may also increase the effects of certain drugs such as alcohol, anxiety medications, narcotic painkillers, cough and allergy products with decongestants, Coumadin, Lanoxin, and phenobarbital, and possibly Tagamet and Prozac. The drug may block the effects of Catapres, Dilantin, Ismelin, and Tegretol.

ALLERGIES: Individuals allergic to clomipramine, tricyclic antidepressants (those listed below in "Other Drugs in the Same Therapeutic Class"), or any of their derivatives should discuss this with their doctor or pharmacist before taking this drug.

PREGNANCY/BREAST-FEEDING: Category C—Risk cannot be ruled out. Human studies are lacking, and animal studies are either positive for fetal risk or lacking as well. However, potential benefits

may justify the potential risk in using the drug. It is not known whether the drug is excreted in the breast milk; therefore, caution should be used when breast-feeding.

OTHER BRAND NAMES: None

OTHER DRUGS IN THE SAME THERAPEUTIC CLASS: Asendin, Elavil, Endep, Norpramin, Pamelor, Sinequan, Surmontil, Tofranil, and Vivactil

IMPORTANT INFORMATION TO REMEMBER: The drug may require three to six weeks of use before improvement may be noticed. This drug does cause drowsiness. Individuals should use caution when driving, operating machinery, or any task where mental alertness is required. Alcohol, anxiety medications, or narcotic painkillers may intensify the drowsiness effect of the drug. The drug may cause a slight amount of dizziness or lightheadedness when rising from a sitting or lying-down position. Individuals should also use a sunscreen to avoid overexposure to the sun; the drug may increase the skin's sensitivity to sunlight, which may cause one to sunburn more easily. This drug may affect many other medical conditions, especially individuals with seizures. Discuss your complete medical history with your doctor before taking this drug.

BRAND NAME: Anaprox and Anaprox DS

GENERIC NAME: naproxen sodium

GENERIC FORM AVAILABLE: Yes

THERAPEUTIC CLASS: Nonsteroidal anti-inflammatory drug (NSAID)

DOSAGE FORMS: 275-mg and 550-mg tablets

MAIN USES: Arthritis, menstrual pain, general pain relief

USUAL DOSE: 275 mg to 550 mg two to four times daily

AVERAGE PRICE: $96.19 (B)/$58.94 (G) for 275 mg and $137.52 (B)/$85.56 (G) for 550 mg

SIDE EFFECTS: constipation 3%–9%, heartburn 3%–9%, stomach pain 3%–9%, nausea 3%–9%, headache 3%–9%, dizziness 3%–9%, ringing in the ears 3%–9%, and difficult breathing 3%–9%.

DRUG INTERACTIONS: Aspirin will decrease the concentration of this drug in the blood. This drug may also decrease the effects of Lasix, HydroDIURIL, Dyazide, Maxzide, and other water pills.

The drug may increase the blood levels of Eskalith, Lithobid, and Sandimmune. The drug may increase the toxic effects of the drug Rheumatrex. Caution should be used when taking the drug with Coumadin.

ALLERGIES: Individuals allergic to naproxen, Aleve, Naprosyn, or other NSAIDs (such as those listed in "Other Drugs in the Same Therapeutic Class") should discuss this with their doctor or pharmacist before taking this drug.

PREGNANCY/BREAST-FEEDING: Category B—No evidence of risk in humans. Either animal findings show risk, but human findings do not; or, if no adequate human studies have been done, animal findings show no risk. The drug should not, however, be used in late stages (last three months) of pregnancy. It is not known whether the drug is excreted in the breast milk; therefore, caution should be used when breast-feeding.

OTHER BRAND NAMES: Aleve (sold over-the-counter as a 200-mg tablet)

OTHER DRUGS IN THE SAME THERAPEUTIC CLASS: Ansaid, aspirin, Cataflam, Clinoril, Daypro, Disalcid, Dolobid, Easprin, Feldene, Indocin, Lodine, Lodine XL, Motrin, Nalfon, Naprosyn, Orudis, Oruvail, Relafen, Tolectin, Toradol, Voltaren, and Voltaren XR

IMPORTANT INFORMATION TO REMEMBER: This drug should be taken with food or milk to reduce the potential for injury to the stomach lining and stomach upset. This drug may take up to two weeks before a noticeable improvement in pain relief associated with arthritis is observed. Drinking alcohol while taking this drug may increase its potential to cause ulcers. This drug should only be used under the direct supervision of a doctor by individuals with a bleeding disorder or ulcer, or those who are currently taking Coumadin. Before taking over-the-counter pain relievers, consult your doctor or pharmacist. No more than one pain reliever should be taken at any one time unless otherwise directed by your doctor. This drug is now available over-the-counter (OTC) without a prescription in a 200-mg tablet under the brand name Aleve.

BRAND NAME: Anaspaz

GENERIC NAME: hyoscyamine

See entry for Levsin/Levsinex

BRAND NAME: Androderm

GENERIC NAME: testosterone

See entry for Testoderm Patch

BRAND NAME: Android, Android-10, and Android-25

GENERIC NAME: methyltestosterone

GENERIC FORM AVAILABLE: Yes

THERAPEUTIC CLASS: Androgen steroid

DOSAGE FORMS: 10-mg and 25-mg tablets, and 10-mg capsules

MAIN USES: Hypogonadism, delayed puberty in males, breast cancer, and {other male hormone disorders}

USUAL DOSE: The dosage must be strictly individualized based on age, sex, and diagnosis. For males, the usual dose is 10 mg to 50 mg daily; for breast cancer, the usual dose 50 mg to 200 mg daily.

AVERAGE PRICE: $200.29 for 10 mg and $500.69 for 25 mg

SIDE EFFECTS: Most common: bladder irritability in males, hair overgrowth in certain areas in females, enlargement of the breasts in males, male pattern baldness, acne, enlargement of penis, and frequent or persistent erections. Less common: diarrhea, changes in sex drive, insomnia, sores in the mouth, watery mouth, dizziness, swelling, vomiting, and nausea.

DRUG INTERACTIONS: The drug may increase the effects of Coumadin. The drug may also decrease blood sugar levels, which may decrease the amount of insulin needed.

FOOD INTERACTIONS: This drug should be taken with food or milk.

ALLERGIES: Individuals allergic to methyltestosterone, testosterone, or any of their derivatives should discuss this with their doctor or pharmacist before taking this drug.

PREGNANCY/BREAST-FEEDING: Category X—Should not be used during pregnancy. Studies in animals and/or humans have shown fetal abnormalities and birth defects. The risks associated with using this drug clearly outweigh the benefits. This drug should never be used by someone who is pregnant or trying to become pregnant. Also, women should never breast-feed while using this drug.

OTHER BRAND NAMES: None

OTHER DRUGS IN THE SAME THERAPEUTIC CLASS: Androderm, Halotestin, Metandren, Testoderm, Testred, and Winstrol

IMPORTANT INFORMATION TO REMEMBER: Only take the drug exactly as directed by your physician. Do not discontinue the drug without first consulting your physician. This drug should be taken with food or milk. Buccal tablets should not be chewed or swallowed—they should be dissolved under the tongue.

BRAND NAME: Anexsia 5/500

GENERIC NAME: Combination product containing: hydrocodone and acetaminophen

See entry for Vicodin/Vicodin ES/Vicodin HP

BRAND NAME: Anexsia 7.5/650

GENERIC NAME: Combination product containing: hydrocodone and acetaminophen

See entry for Lorcet Plus/Lorcet 10/650

BRAND NAME: Ansaid

GENERIC NAME: flurbiprofen

GENERIC FORM AVAILABLE: Yes

THERAPEUTIC CLASS: Nonsteroidal anti-inflammatory drug (NSAID)

DOSAGE FORMS: 50-mg and 100-mg tablets

MAIN USES: Arthritis and pain relief

USUAL DOSE: 200 mg to 300 mg per day, taken in two, three, or four divided doses

AVERAGE PRICE: $101.23 (B)/$96.34 (G) for 50 mg and $151.12 (B)/ $123.47 (G) for 100 mg

SIDE EFFECTS: stomach pain 3%–9%, diarrhea 3%–9%, nausea 3%–9%, headache 3%–9%, gas 1%–3%, vomiting 1%–3%, nervousness 1%–3%, dizziness 1%–3%, and blurred vision 1%–3%.

DRUG INTERACTIONS: Aspirin will decrease the concentration of this drug in the blood. This drug may also decrease the effects of Lasix, Dyazide, HydroDIURIL, Maxzide, and other water pills. The drug may increase the blood levels of Eskalith, Lithobid, and Sandimmune. The drug may increase the toxic effects of the drug Rheumatrex. Caution should be used when taking the drug with Coumadin.

ALLERGIES: Individuals allergic to flurbiprofen or other NSAIDs (such as those listed in "Other Drugs in the Same Therapeutic Class") should discuss this with their doctor or pharmacist before taking this drug.

PREGNANCY/BREAST-FEEDING: Category B—No evidence of risk in humans. Either animal findings show risk, but human findings do not; or, if no adequate human studies have been done, animal findings show no risk. The drug should not, however, be used in late stages (last three months) of pregnancy. It is not known whether the drug is excreted in the breast milk; therefore, caution should be used when breast-feeding.

OTHER BRAND NAMES: None

OTHER DRUGS IN THE SAME THERAPEUTIC CLASS: Anaprox, aspirin, Cataflam, Clinoril, Daypro, Disalcid, Dolobid, Easprin, Feldene, Indocin, Lodine, Lodine XL, Motrin, Nalfon, Naprosyn, Orudis, Oruvail, Relafen, Tolectin, Toradol, Voltaren, and Voltaren XR

IMPORTANT INFORMATION TO REMEMBER: This drug should be taken with food or milk to reduce the potential for injury to the stomach lining and stomach upset. This drug may take up to two weeks before a noticeable improvement in pain relief associated with arthritis is observed. Drinking alcohol while taking this drug may increase its potential to cause ulcers. This drug should only be used under the direct supervision of a doctor by individuals with a bleeding disorder or ulcer, or those who are currently taking Coumadin. Before taking over-the-counter pain relievers, consult your doctor or pharmacist. No more than one pain reliever should be taken at any one time unless otherwise directed by your doctor.

BRAND NAME: Antabuse

GENERIC NAME: disulfiram

GENERIC FORM AVAILABLE: Yes

THERAPEUTIC CLASS: Alcohol deterrent

DOSAGE FORMS: 250-mg and 500-mg tablets

MAIN USES: Deterrent for chronic alcoholics

USUAL DOSE: Initially 500 mg daily for one to two weeks, then reduce to 250 mg daily for maintenance.

AVERAGE PRICE: $82.26 (B)/$13.84 (G) for 250 mg

SIDE EFFECTS: Most common: drowsiness. Less common: blurred vision, unusual sensations (tingling, numbness, etc.), hepatitis, skin rash, tiredness, headache, mood changes, impotence, metallic or garlic-like aftertaste, and unusual tiredness.

DRUG INTERACTIONS: The drug should never be used with alcohol or with any medication that may contain alcohol. Even small amounts of alcohol will cause intense stomach pain, vomiting, flushing, dizziness, headache, sweating, chest pain, and difficulty breathing. The drug can increase the blood levels of the drug Dilantin. The drug should never be taken with Flagyl due to increased toxic effects when the two are combined. The drug may increase the effects of Coumadin.

ALLERGIES: Individuals allergic to disulfiram, sulfa, or any of their derivatives should discuss this with their doctor or pharmacist before taking this drug.

PREGNANCY/BREAST-FEEDING: Category C—Risk cannot be ruled out. Human studies are lacking, and animal studies are either positive for fetal risk or lacking as well. However, potential benefits may justify the potential risk in using the drug. It is not known whether the drug is excreted in the breast milk; therefore, caution should be used when breast-feeding.

OTHER BRAND NAMES: None

OTHER DRUGS IN THE SAME THERAPEUTIC CLASS: None

IMPORTANT INFORMATION TO REMEMBER: This medication should not be taken within 12 hours of using any alcohol. The blood alcohol level of an individual should be zero before therapy is begun. Once treatment has begun individuals should under no circumstance drink any alcohol. In fact, alcohol should not be used until at least 14 days after the last dose of the drug. Many cough and cold preparations contain alcohol. Individuals taking this drug should read all over-the-counter medication labels carefully. Consult your pharmacist before taking any of these preparations. Also, individuals should check with their physician before taking any anxiety medications or narcotic painkillers.

BRAND NAME: Antivert

GENERIC NAME: meclizine

GENERIC FORM AVAILABLE: Yes

THERAPEUTIC CLASS: Antihistamine

DOSAGE FORMS: 12.5-mg, 25-mg, and 50-mg tablets; and 25-mg chewable tablets

MAIN USES: Dizziness, motion sickness, and nausea

USUAL DOSE: 25 mg to 100 mg per day in divided doses for dizziness and nausea, and 25 mg to 50 mg one hour before exposure to motion for motion sickness.

AVERAGE PRICE: $41.78 (B)/$6.58 (G) for 12.5 mg; $81.40 (B)/ $10.98 (G) for 25 mg

SIDE EFFECTS: Most common: drowsiness. Less common: dry mouth and rarely blurred vision.

DRUG INTERACTIONS: Alcohol, anxiety medications, and narcotic painkillers may make the drowsiness caused by the drug much worse.

ALLERGIES: Individuals allergic to meclizine or any of its derivatives should consult their doctor or pharmacist before taking this drug.

PREGNANCY/BREAST-FEEDING: Category B—No evidence of risk in humans. Either animal findings show risk, but human findings do not; or, if no adequate human studies have been done, animal findings show no risk. It is not known whether the drug is excreted in the breast milk; therefore, caution should be used when breast-feeding.

OTHER BRAND NAMES: Bonine (sold over-the-counter as a 25-mg chewable tablet)

OTHER DRUGS IN THE SAME THERAPEUTIC CLASS: Benadryl and Dramamine

IMPORTANT INFORMATION TO REMEMBER: This drug may cause drowsiness. Individuals should use caution when driving, operating machinery, or any task where mental alertness is required. Alcohol, anxiety medications, or narcotic painkillers may increase the drowsiness effect of the drug. This drug should not be used by children under the age of 12. To prevent motion sickness, the drug should be taken one hour before exposure to motion.

BRAND NAME: Anusol-HC

GENERIC NAME: hydrocortisone

GENERIC FORM AVAILABLE: Suppository only

THERAPEUTIC CLASS: Steroid

DOSAGE FORMS: 25-mg suppositories and 2.5% cream

MAIN USES: Hemorrhoids and {other rectal irritations}

USUAL DOSE: one suppository or one application of the cream twice daily

AVERAGE PRICE: $31.58 (B)/$13.75 (G) for suppositories and $30.35 for 2.5% cream

SIDE EFFECTS: Most common: none. Less common: burning, itching, irritation, and dryness.

DRUG INTERACTIONS: None of any clinical significance

ALLERGIES: Individuals allergic to hydrocortisone, other topical steroids creams and ointments, or any of their derivatives should discuss this with their doctor or pharmacist before taking this drug.

PREGNANCY/BREAST-FEEDING: Category C—Risk cannot be ruled out. Human studies are lacking, and animal studies are either positive for fetal risk or lacking as well. However, potential benefits may justify the potential risk in using the drug. It is not known whether the drug is excreted in the breast milk; therefore, caution should be used when breast-feeding.

OTHER BRAND NAMES: None

OTHER DRUGS IN THE SAME THERAPEUTIC CLASS: Corticaine, Cortifoam, and Proctofoam-HC

IMPORTANT INFORMATION TO REMEMBER: Remove the foil wrapper before inserting the suppository. Store in a cool place to avoid melting, preferably the refrigerator. When inserting, lie on one side and bend the top leg slightly. Then insert suppository into rectum about one inch with one finger. Wash hands thoroughly before and after use. Individuals may want to use a finger cot to cover the finger when inserting a suppository.

BRAND NAME: Apresazide

GENERIC NAME: Combination product containing: hydralazine and hydrochlorothiazide

See individual entries for Apresoline and HydroDIURIL

BRAND NAME: Apresoline

GENERIC NAME: hydralazine

GENERIC FORM AVAILABLE: Yes

THERAPEUTIC CLASS: Vasodilator

DOSAGE FORMS: 10-mg, 25-mg, 50-mg, and 100-mg tablets

MAIN USES: High blood pressure and {congestive heart failure}

USUAL DOSE: Initially 10 mg four times daily for two to four days, then increase to 25 mg four times daily. Long-term doses are 40 mg to 200 mg per day in two to four divided doses. The maximum dose is 300 mg per day.

AVERAGE PRICE: $28.31 (B)/$8.78 (G) for 10 mg; $43.54 (B)/$12.74 (G) for 25 mg; $61.91 (B)/$16.48 (G) for 50 mg; $91.28 (B)/$20.88 (G) for 100 mg

SIDE EFFECTS: Most common: headache, anorexia, nausea, vomiting, diarrhea, heart palpitations, fast heartbeat, and angina. Less common: constipation, shortness of breath, low blood pressure, dizziness, numbness, tingling, muscle cramps, anxiety, flushing of the face, stuffy nose, watery eyes, and difficulty in urinating.

DRUG INTERACTIONS: Nardil and Parnate should be used with caution. Indocin may decrease the effects of the drug.

ALLERGIES: Individuals allergic to hydralazine or any of its derivatives should discuss this with their doctor or pharmacist before taking this drug.

PREGNANCY/BREAST-FEEDING: Category C—Risk cannot be ruled out. Human studies are lacking, and animal studies are either positive

for fetal risk or lacking as well. However, potential benefits may justify the potential risk in using the drug. It is not known whether the drug is excreted in the breast milk; therefore, caution should be used when breast-feeding.

OTHER BRAND NAMES: None

OTHER DRUGS IN THE SAME THERAPEUTIC CLASS: Loniten and Minipress

IMPORTANT INFORMATION TO REMEMBER: Do not stop taking the drug without first consulting with a doctor. The drug should be taken with food or milk to increase levels of the drug in the blood. The drug may cause drowsiness, headache, or heart palpitations during the first few days of therapy. Drowsiness may occur, but usually goes away once the body adjusts to the medication. Before taking over-the-counter cold and allergy preparations, consult your doctor or pharmacist—these products may raise your blood pressure.

BRAND NAME: Aralen

GENERIC NAME: chloroquine

GENERIC FORM AVAILABLE: Yes

THERAPEUTIC CLASS: Aminoquinolone antimalarial

DOSAGE FORMS: 500-mg tablets

MAIN USES: Prevention and treatment of malaria and amebic infections

USUAL DOSE: 500 mg every seven days for the prevention of malaria; initially 1000 mg, then 500 mg 6, 24, and 48 hours after the first dose to treat malaria; or 1000 mg daily for two days and 500 mg daily for two to three weeks to treat amebic infections.

AVERAGE PRICE: $84.53 (B)/$27.99 (G) for 14 tablets

SIDE EFFECTS: Most common: difficulty reading, vision disturbances, diarrhea, loss of appetite, stomach pain, vomiting, itching, and headache. Less common: bleaching of hair, hair loss, skin rash, and blue-black discoloration of the skin.

DRUG INTERACTIONS: Tagamet may increase the toxic effects of the drug.

ALLERGIES: Individuals allergic to chloroquine or any of its derivatives should discuss this with their doctor or pharmacist before taking this drug.

PREGNANCY/BREAST-FEEDING: Category C—Risk cannot be ruled out. Human studies are lacking, and animal studies are either positive for fetal risk or lacking as well. However, potential benefits may justify the potential risk in using the drug. It is not known whether the drug is excreted in the breast milk; therefore, caution should be used when breast-feeding.

OTHER BRAND NAMES: None

OTHER DRUGS IN THE SAME THERAPEUTIC CLASS: Lariam and Plaquenil

IMPORTANT INFORMATION TO REMEMBER: This drug should be taken with food or milk to reduce the potential for stomach upset. Use exactly as directed by your physician. Always complete the full course of therapy for both prevention and treatment uses. Individuals taking the drug for long periods of time should see their physician regularly for blood tests and eye exams. Vision problems should be reported to your physician immediately.

BRAND NAME: Arimidex

GENERIC NAME: anastrozole

GENERIC FORM AVAILABLE: No

THERAPEUTIC CLASS: Estrogen anticancer blocker

DOSAGE FORMS: 1-mg tablets

MAIN USES: Cancer (primarily advanced breast cancer)

USUAL DOSE: 1 mg once daily

AVERAGE PRICE: $189.90 (30 tablets)

SIDE EFFECTS: weakness 16%, nausea 16%, headache 13%, hot flashes 12%, general pain 11%, back pain 11%, trouble breathing 9%, vomiting 9%, cough 8%, diarrhea 8%, constipation 7%, stomach pain 7%, loss of appetite 7%, bone pain 7%, pharyngitis 6%, dizziness 6%, rash 6%, dry mouth 6%, swelling 5%, pelvic pain 5%, depression 5%, chest pain 5%, numbness 5%, vaginal bleeding 2%, weight gain 2%, vaginal dryness 2%, and sweating 2%.

DRUG INTERACTIONS: None of any clinical significance

ALLERGIES: Individuals allergic to anastrozole or any of its derivatives should discuss this with their doctor or pharmacist before using this drug.

PREGNANCY/BREAST-FEEDING: Category D—Positive evidence of risk. Human studies show risk to the fetus. Nevertheless, potential benefits may possibly outweigh the potential risks. This drug should not be given to nursing mothers.

OTHER BRAND NAMES: None

OTHER DRUGS IN THE SAME THERAPEUTIC CLASS: Nolvadex

IMPORTANT INFORMATION TO REMEMBER: It is extremely important to follow the dosing schedule set by your physician—do not deviate from this schedule. Nausea and vomiting may occur while taking this drug. Do not discontinue use unless directed by your physician. If stomach upset occurs, take the drug with food or milk.

BRAND NAME: Aristocort

GENERIC NAME: triamcinolone

GENERIC FORM AVAILABLE: Yes

THERAPEUTIC CLASS: Topical corticosteroid (cream and ointment) and glucocorticoid steroid (tablets)

DOSAGE FORMS: 0.025%, 0.1%, and 0.5% creams; 0.1% and 0.5% ointments; 1-mg, 2-mg, 4-mg, and 8-mg tablets; and 4-mg unit-of-use packs

MAIN USES: Skin rashes, swelling, and itching; endocrine disorders; and {multiple uses for its ability to reduce inflammation in various parts of the body, including asthma}

USUAL DOSE: For the tablets, 3 mg to 48 mg daily; for the cream and ointment, apply three to four times daily.

AVERAGE PRICE: $156.37 (B)/$15.67 (G) for 4-mg and 8-mg tablets; $12.79 (B)/$9.91 (G) for 15 g of 0.025% cream; $15.99 (B)/$12.04 (G) for 15 g of the 0.1% cream and ointment; and $34.25 (B)/$24.97 (G) for 15 g of 0.5% cream and ointment

SIDE EFFECTS: Short-term use of the tablets: Most common: none. Less common: diarrhea, nausea, dizziness, insomnia, nervousness, headache, and stomach pain. Long-term use of the tablets: high blood pressure, muscle weakness, peptic ulcer, hemorrhage, thin fragile skin, facial swelling, weight gain, menstrual irregularities, glaucoma, and many others. Long-term use of the tablets should be avoided if possible. Cream and ointment: Most common: none. Less common: burning, itching, irritation, and skin dryness.

DRUG INTERACTIONS: Amytal, Butisol, Dilantin, Mebaral, Mesantoin, Nembutal, Rifadin, Rifamate, Rifater, Seconal, and Tuinal may decrease the effects of the drug. The drug may increase blood glucose levels. Patients taking drugs for diabetes, including insulin, may need to adjust their dose. The drug may decrease the effects of water pills used to treat high blood pressure and potassium supplements such as K-Dur, Klor-Con, K-Lyte, K-Tab, Micro-K, and Slow-K.

ALLERGIES: Individuals allergic to triamcinolone or other steroids (such as those listed in "Other Drugs in the Same Therapeutic Class") should discuss this with their doctor or pharmacist before taking this drug.

PREGNANCY/BREAST-FEEDING: Category C—Risk cannot be ruled out. Human studies are lacking, and animal studies are either positive for fetal risk or lacking as well. However, potential benefits may justify the potential risk in using the drug. It is not known whether the drug is excreted in the breast milk; therefore, caution should be used when breast-feeding.

OTHER BRAND NAMES: Aristocort A Cream and Ointment

OTHER DRUGS IN THE SAME THERAPEUTIC CLASS: Cream and ointment: Aclovate, Cordran, Cordran SP, Cutivate, Cyclocort, Des-Owen, Diprolene, Elocon, Halog, Hytone, Kenalog, Lidex, Synalar, Temovate, Topicort, Tridesilon, Ultravate, Valisone, and Westcort. Tablets: Decadron, Deltasone, Medrol, and prednisone.

IMPORTANT INFORMATION TO REMEMBER: For the cream and ointment: this drug is for external use only. Apply only a thin film of drug to the skin and rub it in well. Never cover the skin after application with a bandage or wrapping unless directed to do so by a doctor. Never apply to damaged skin or open wounds unless directed to do so by a doctor. Discontinue use if irritation occurs. For the tablets: this drug should be taken with food or milk to reduce the potential for injury to the stomach lining and stomach upset. Drinking alcohol or taking aspirin while taking this drug may increase its potential to cause ulcers. Use exactly as directed by your physician. Never suddenly stop taking the drug without first consulting with your physician—this can be very dangerous. The drug may also cause some weight gain when used for long periods of time.

BRAND NAME: Armour Thyroid

GENERIC NAME: thyroid (dessicated) or thyroid extract

GENERIC FORM AVAILABLE: No

THERAPEUTIC CLASS: Thyroid replacement

DOSAGE FORMS: 15-mg, 30-mg, 60-mg, 90-mg, 120-mg, 180-mg, 240-mg, and 300-mg tablets

MAIN USES: Thyroid replacement therapy

USUAL DOSE: 15 mg to 180 mg per day

AVERAGE PRICE: $13.99 for 30 mg; $15.97 for 60 mg; $26.53 for 120 mg; and $42.14 for 180 mg

SIDE EFFECTS: The following side effects are rare: sensitivity to the heat, sweating, nervousness, fast heartbeat, pounding heartbeat, insomnia, stomach cramps, diarrhea, and weight loss. These are not normal side effects of the drug, but side effects associated with taking too much of the drug.

DRUG INTERACTIONS: The drug may increase the effects of Coumadin. The drug may also decrease the effects of diabetes drugs. Climara, Estrace, Estraderm, Ogen, Premarin, and Vivelle may decrease the effectiveness of the drug. Colestid and Questran may decrease the absorption of the drug in the stomach if taken with the drug.

ALLERGIES: Individuals allergic to dessicated thyroid extract, other thyroid preparations, or any of their derivatives should discuss this with their doctor or pharmacist before taking this drug.

PREGNANCY/BREAST-FEEDING: Category A—Controlled studies show no risk. Adequate well-controlled studies in pregnant women have failed to demonstrate risk to the fetus. Some caution should be used when breast-feeding while taking this drug.

OTHER BRAND NAMES: None

OTHER DRUGS IN THE SAME THERAPEUTIC CLASS: Levothroid, Levoxyl, and Synthroid

IMPORTANT INFORMATION TO REMEMBER: Do not stop taking the drug without first consulting with a doctor. It is important to take the drug at the same time every day for consistent effect. Before taking over-the-counter medications, consult with your doctor or pharmacist.

BRAND NAME: Artane

GENERIC NAME: trihexyphenidyl

GENERIC FORM AVAILABLE: Yes

THERAPEUTIC CLASS: Anticholinergic

DOSAGE FORMS: 2-mg and 5-mg tablets; 5-mg sequels (capsules); and 2 mg/5 mL elixir

MAIN USES: Parkinson's disease and drug-induced movement disorders

USUAL DOSE: 6 mg to 10 mg per day in two to four divided doses, or a single dose at bedtime; or 1 mg to 15 mg once or twice daily for drug-induced movement disorders

AVERAGE PRICE: $27.47 (B)/$18.67 (G) for 2 mg and $49.47 (B)/$21.98 (G) for 5 mg

SIDE EFFECTS: dry mouth 30%–50%, blurred vision 30%–50%, slight nausea 30%–50%, nervousness 30%–50%, drowsiness 30%–50%, slight risk of developing of narrow angle glaucoma; small percentage of individuals may experience constipation, vomiting, or decreased sweating.

DRUG INTERACTIONS: The drug may decrease the effects of Compazine, Haldol, Mellaril, Prolixin, Serentil, Stelazine, Thorazine, and Trilafon. The drug may also cause tardive dyskinesia (abnormal body movements) when used together with Haldol. Antacids may decrease the absorption of the drug.

ALLERGIES: Individuals allergic to trihexyphenidyl or any of its derivatives should discuss this with their doctor or pharmacist before taking this drug.

PREGNANCY/BREAST-FEEDING: Category C—Risk cannot be ruled out. Human studies are lacking, and animal studies are either positive

for fetal risk or lacking as well. However, potential benefits may justify the potential risk in using the drug. It is not known whether the drug is excreted in the breast milk; therefore, caution should be used when breast-feeding.

OTHER BRAND NAMES: None

OTHER DRUGS IN THE SAME THERAPEUTIC CLASS: Akineton, Cogentin, and Kemadrin

IMPORTANT INFORMATION TO REMEMBER: The drug should be taken with food or milk. Do not abruptly discontinue medication if side effects occur. Gradual dose reduction may be necessary; check with your physician. Individuals should avoid using alcohol or depressants while taking this drug. This drug may cause some drowsiness. Caution should also be used when exercising and in hot weather while taking this drug; the drug may increase an individual's sensitivity to hot weather. Individuals taking the drug should have a glaucoma exam at regular intervals. Individuals with glaucoma or prostate problems should only use the drug under the direct supervision of a doctor. This drug may also cause a dry mouth; sugarless gum or hard candy will help take care of this problem.

BRAND NAME: Asacol

GENERIC NAME: mesalamine

GENERIC FORM AVAILABLE: No

THERAPEUTIC CLASS: Salicylate

DOSAGE FORMS: 400-mg tablet

MAIN USES: Mildly to moderately active ulcerative colitis

USUAL DOSE: 800 mg three times a day for six weeks

AVERAGE PRICE: $85.17

SIDE EFFECTS: headache 35%, stomach pain 18%, belching 16%, pain 14%, nausea 13%, sore throat 11%, weakness 7%, dizziness 8%, diarrhea 7%, fever 7%, back pain 7%, vomiting 5%, and gas 3%.

DRUG INTERACTIONS: None of any clinical significance

ALLERGIES: Patients allergic to mesalamine, aspirin, or aspirin derivatives should consult their doctor or pharmacist before taking this drug.

PREGNANCY/BREAST-FEEDING: Category B—No evidence of risk in humans. Either animal findings show risk, but human findings do not; or, if no adequate human studies have been done, animal findings show no risk. It is not known whether the drug is excreted in the breast milk; therefore, caution should be used when breast-feeding.

OTHER BRAND NAMES: None

OTHER DRUGS IN THE SAME THERAPEUTIC CLASS: Azulfidine, Dipentum, Pentasa, and Rowasa

IMPORTANT INFORMATION TO REMEMBER: Do not crush or divide tablets—this will destroy the protective coating that ensures release of the drug in the intestines. Swallow the tablets whole. Colitis symptoms may become worse in 3% of those taking the drug.

BRAND NAME: Asendin

GENERIC NAME: amoxapine

GENERIC FORM AVAILABLE: Yes

THERAPEUTIC CLASS: Tricylic antidepressant

DOSAGE FORMS: 25-mg, 50-mg, 100-mg, and 150-mg tablets

MAIN USES: Depression

USUAL DOSE: Initially 50 mg two to three times daily; may be increased to 100 mg two to three times daily

AVERAGE PRICE: $150.70 (B)/$102.83 (G) for 25 mg; $184.34 (B)/$126.48 (G) for 50 mg; $244.73 (B)/$201.94 (G) for 100 mg; $342.87 (B)/$263.21 (G) for 150 mg

SIDE EFFECTS: drowsiness 14%, dry mouth 14%, constipation 12%, blurred vision 7%, nervousness 1%–5%, insomnia 1%–5%, nausea 1%–5%, dizziness 1%–5%, and headaches 1%–5%.

DRUG INTERACTIONS: The drug should not be taken with Nardil and Parnate; in fact, 14 days are needed between the time of the use of Nardil and Parnate and this drug. Alcohol, anxiety medications, and narcotic painkillers may make the drowsiness caused by the drug much worse. Compazine, Mellaril, Prolixin, Serentil, Stelazine, Thorazine, and Trilafon may increase the blood levels of the drug. Tagamet may increase the blood levels of the drug. The drug may decrease the effects of Catapres and Ismelin. The drug may increase the effects of decongestants found in cold and allergy products on the heart, possibly causing high blood pressure, fast heartbeat, or irregular heartbeat.

ALLERGIES: Individuals allergic to amoxapine or other tricylic antidepressants (such as those listed in "Other Drugs in the Same Therapeutic Class") should discuss this with their doctor or pharmacist before taking this drug.

PREGNANCY/BREAST-FEEDING: Category C—Risk cannot be ruled out. Human studies are lacking, and animal studies are either positive for fetal risk or lacking as well. However, potential benefits may justify the potential risk in using the drug. It is not known whether the drug is excreted in the breast milk; therefore, caution should be used when breast-feeding.

OTHER BRAND NAMES: None

OTHER DRUGS IN THE SAME THERAPEUTIC CLASS: Elavil, Endep, Norpramin, Pamelor, Sinequan, Surmontil, Tofranil, and Vivactil

IMPORTANT INFORMATION TO REMEMBER: Only take the drug exactly as directed by your physician. Do not discontinue the drug without first consulting your physician. The drug may require one to six weeks of use before improvement may be noticed. This drug does cause drowsiness. Individuals should use caution when driving, operating machinery, or any task where mental alertness is required. Alcohol, anxiety medications, and narcotic painkillers may intensify the drowsiness effect of the drug. The drug may cause a slight amount of dizziness or lightheadedness when rising from a sitting or lying-down position. Individuals should also use a sunscreen to avoid overexposure to the sun. The drug may increase the skin's sensitivity to sunlight, which may cause one to sunburn more easily.

BRAND NAME: Atarax

GENERIC NAME: hydroxyzine

GENERIC FORM AVAILABLE: Yes

THERAPEUTIC CLASS: Antihistamine

DOSAGE FORMS: 10-mg, 25-mg, 50-mg, 100-mg, and 10 mg/5 mL syrup

MAIN USES: Anxiety, allergic reactions, itching, and as a {sedative}

USUAL DOSE: 50 mg to 100 mg four times daily for anxiety, and 25 mg three to four times daily for allergic reactions and itching

AVERAGE PRICE: $68.17 (B)/$14.26 (G) for 10 mg; $91.57 (B)/$19.78 (G) for 25 mg; $122.44 (B)/$25.28 (G) for 50 mg; $164.12 (B)/$30.78 (G) for 100 mg

SIDE EFFECTS: Most common: drowsiness, thickening of mucus, and dry mouth. Less common: blurred vision, difficult or painful urination, dizziness, fast heartbeat, increased sweating, increased appetite, diarrhea, and nausea.

DRUG INTERACTIONS: Central nervous system (CNS) depression may be increased when used with alcohol, anxiety medications, or narcotic painkillers. The drug should not be taken with Nardil and Parnate. The drug should also not be used with Akineton, Artane, Cogentin, or Kemadrin.

ALLERGIES: Patients allergic to hydroxyzine, Vistaril, or any of their derivatives should consult their doctor or pharmacist before taking this drug.

PREGNANCY/BREAST-FEEDING: Category C—Risk cannot be ruled out. Human studies are lacking, and animal studies are either positive for fetal risk or lacking as well. However, potential benefits may justify the potential risk in using the drug. It is not known whether the drug is excreted in the breast milk; therefore, caution should be used when breast-feeding.

OTHER BRAND NAMES: None

OTHER DRUGS IN THE SAME THERAPEUTIC CLASS: Benadryl, PBZ, Periactin, Tavist, Temaril, and Vistaril

IMPORTANT INFORMATION TO REMEMBER: This drug may cause drowsiness. Individuals should use caution when driving, operating machinery, or any task where mental alertness is required. Alcohol, nerve medication, or narcotic painkillers may intensify the drowsiness effect of the drug. This drug may also cause a dry mouth; sugarless gum or hard candy will help take care of this problem. Patients with glaucoma or urinary or prostate problems should consult their doctor before taking this drug.

BRAND NAME: Ativan

GENERIC NAME: lorazepam

GENERIC FORM AVAILABLE: Yes

THERAPEUTIC CLASS: Benzodiazepine antianxiety

DOSAGE FORMS: 0.5-mg, 1-mg, and 2-mg tablets

MAIN USES: Anxiety and {sedation}

USUAL DOSE: 1 mg to 10 mg per day in divided doses

AVERAGE PRICE: $79.79 (B)/$14.26 (G) for 0.5 mg; $90.18 (B)/$20.55 (G) for 1 mg; $134.07 (B)/$23.08 (G) for 2 mg

SIDE EFFECTS: drowsiness 16%, dizziness 7%, weakness 4%, and unsteadiness 3%; others that occur less frequently: disorientation, depression, nausea, change in appetite, headache, and sleep disturbance.

DRUG INTERACTIONS: Central nervous system (CNS) depression may be increased when used with alcohol, narcotic painkillers, or other anxiety medications.

ALLERGIES: Individuals allergic to lorazepam or other benzodiazepines (such as those listed in "Other Drugs in the Same Therapeutic Class") should discuss this with their doctor or pharmacist before taking this drug.

PREGNANCY/BREAST-FEEDING: Category D—Positive evidence of risk. Human studies show risk to the fetus. Nevertheless, potential benefits may possibly outweigh the potential risk. This drug should not be taken by nursing mothers.

OTHER BRAND NAMES: None

OTHER DRUGS IN THE SAME THERAPEUTIC CLASS: Librium, Serax, Tranxene, Valium, and Xanax

IMPORTANT INFORMATION TO REMEMBER: This drug may cause drowsiness. Individuals should use caution when driving, operating machinery, or any task where mental alertness is required. The incidence of drowsiness and unsteadiness increases with age. Alcohol, anxiety medications, or narcotic painkillers may intensify the drowsiness effect of the drug. This medication is a controlled substance and may be habit-forming. Do not increase the dose of medication without consulting with your doctor; only take the amount prescribed by your doctor.

BRAND NAME: Atrofen

GENERIC NAME: baclofen

See entry for Lioresal

BRAND NAME: Atrohist Plus

GENERIC NAME: combination product containing: phenylephrine, phenylpropanolamine, chlorpheniramine, atropine, and scopolamine

See entry for Ru-Tuss/Ru-Tuss DE

BRAND NAME: Atromid-S

GENERIC NAME: clofibrate

GENERIC FORM AVAILABLE: Yes

THERAPEUTIC CLASS: Anti-lipidemic

DOSAGE FORMS: 500-mg capsules

MAIN USES: High triglycerides

USUAL DOSE: 2 gm per day in divided doses

AVERAGE PRICE: $98.87 (B)/$26.05 (G)

SIDE EFFECTS: Most common: nausea, vomiting, diarrhea, stomach pain, and gas. Less common: headache, dizziness, fatigue, muscle cramps, muscle aches, weakness, dry brittle hair, and hair loss.

DRUG INTERACTIONS: The drug may increase blood levels of Coumadin, Dilantin, and Orinase. The drug may also cause severe muscle disorders when used together with other cholesterol-lowering drugs such as Lescol, Lopid, Mevacor, Pravachol, and Zocor.

ALLERGIES: Individuals allergic to clofibrate or any of its derivatives should discuss this with their doctor or pharmacist before taking this drug.

PREGNANCY/BREAST-FEEDING: Category C—Risk cannot be ruled out. Human studies are lacking, and animal studies are either positive for fetal risk or lacking as well. However, potential benefits may justify the potential risk in using the drug. The drug does appear in breast milk; therefore, it should not be used by nursing mothers.

OTHER BRAND NAMES: None

OTHER DRUGS IN THE SAME THERAPEUTIC CLASS: Lopid

IMPORTANT INFORMATION TO REMEMBER: Take only the amount of medication prescribed by your doctor. In helping to reduce your cholesterol, drug therapy alone is usually not enough—it is important to also follow dietary restrictions. To avoid stomach upset, the drug should be taken with food or milk.

BRAND NAME: Atrovent

GENERIC NAME: ipratropium

GENERIC FORM AVAILABLE: No

THERAPEUTIC CLASS: Anticholinergic bronchodilator

DOSAGE FORMS: 0.02% inhalation solution in 2.5 mL unit-dose vials, 18-micrograms-per-inhalation metered-dose inhaler, 0.03% nasal spray, and 0.06% nasal spray

MAIN USES: Bronchospasms associated with chronic obstructive pulmonary disease (COPD) including chronic bronchitis, emphysema, nasal allergies, and relief of nasal symptoms caused by the common cold.

USUAL DOSE: two puffs of the inhaler or one unit-dose vial in a nebulizer three to four times daily; or two sprays of the nasal spray two to four times daily

AVERAGE PRICE: $40.76 for inhaler; $47.40 for 0.03% nasal spray; and $40.32 for 0.06% nasal spray

SIDE EFFECTS: Inhaler: cough 6%, nausea 3%, nervousness 3%, palpitations 2%, dizziness 2%, headache 2%, stomach distress 2%, dry mouth 2%, and blurred vision 1%. Nasal spray: headache 10%, upper respiratory infection 10%, slight nosebleed 9%, sore throat 8%, nasal dryness 5%, nausea 2%, nasal irritation 2%, dry mouth 1%, and nasal congestion 1%.

DRUG INTERACTIONS: None of any clinical significance

ALLERGIES: Individuals allergic to ipratropium or any of its derivatives, atropine or any of its derivatives, soya lecithin, soybeans, peanuts, or similar foods should consult their doctor or pharmacist before taking this drug.

PREGNANCY/BREAST-FEEDING: Category B—No evidence of risk in humans. Either animal findings show risk, but human findings do not; or, if no adequate human studies have been done, animal findings show no risk. It is not known whether the drug is excreted in the breast milk; therefore, caution should be used when breast-feeding.

OTHER BRAND NAMES: None

OTHER DRUGS IN THE SAME THERAPEUTIC CLASS: None

IMPORTANT INFORMATION TO REMEMBER: Inhaler and nasal spray: The drug is not intended for occasional use during shortness of breath episodes like some other inhaled products, or for acute allergy attacks. The drug should be used regularly as a maintenance medication and not for acute attacks. Never exceed prescribed dosage unless directed to do so by a doctor. Excessive use beyond prescribed dosage is potentially dangerous and may even be fatal. Patients with narrow-angle glaucoma, prostate problems, or bladder problems should discuss this with their doctor before using this drug. The unit-dose inhaled solution may be mixed with Proventil or Ventolin inhaled solutions if the mixture will be used within one hour.

When using the inhaler, use the following procedure:

1) Shake the canister well.
2) Place the mouthpiece close to the mouth, but not touching the lips.
3) Exhale deeply.
4) Inhale slowly and deeply as you press the top of the canister to release the medication.
5) Hold your breath for a few seconds before exhaling.
6) Wait five minutes between puffs.
7) Be sure to wash the inhaler device (mouthpiece) regularly with warm soapy water to avoid bacterial contamination.

When using the nasal spray, use the following procedure:

1) Blow your nose gently to clear your nostrils, if necessary.
2) Hold the spray bottle with your thumb at the bottom and your index and middle finger on the shoulder attached to the neck of the bottle.
3) With your other hand, gently place a finger against the side of your nose to close the opposite nostril.

4) Insert the tip of the bottle into the open nostril. Point the tip toward the back and outer side of the nostril once inside.

5) After releasing the spray, close your mouth, sniff deeply, hold your breath for a few seconds, then breathe out through your mouth.

6) Tilt your head back slightly for a few seconds to allow the drug to spread to the back of your nose.

7) Repeat the same procedure for the other nostril.

8) If using more than one spray in each nostril, wait five minutes between sprays.

BRAND NAME: A/T/S

GENERIC NAME: erythromycin

GENERIC FORM AVAILABLE: Yes (solution only)

THERAPEUTIC CLASS: Topical antibiotic

DOSAGE FORMS: 2% topical solution and 2% topical gel

MAIN USES: Acne

USUAL DOSE: Apply to acne areas twice daily.

AVERAGE PRICE: $23.57 (B) for 2% gel and $23.15 (B)/$10.48 (G) for 2% solution

SIDE EFFECTS: Most common: none. Less common: dry skin, scaly skin, itching, irritation, and burning sensation.

DRUG INTERACTIONS: None of any clinical significance

ALLERGIES: Individuals allergic to erythromycin or any of its derivatives should consult their doctor or pharmacist before taking this drug.

PREGNANCY/BREAST-FEEDING: Category C—Risk cannot be ruled out. Human studies are lacking, and animal studies are either positive for fetal risk or lacking as well. However, potential benefits may justify the potential risk in using the drug. It is not known whether the drug is excreted in the breast milk; therefore, caution should be used when breast-feeding.

OTHER BRAND NAMES: Erymax

OTHER DRUGS IN THE SAME THERAPEUTIC CLASS: Cleocin T, Emgel, Erygel, Erycette, and T-Stat

IMPORTANT INFORMATION TO REMEMBER: This drug is for external use only. It is important to use the medication continuously. It may take three to four weeks before a significant improvement may be seen. If no improvement is seen within this time period, contact your doctor. This medication contains alcohol, which may cause slight burning or stinging when first applied. Also, avoid contact with the eyes, nose, and mouth. Before applying, wash acne area thoroughly with warm soapy water to remove dirt and skin oils, pat skin dry, and then apply the drug. If you need to apply another medication for acne, wait at least one hour. Discontinue use if irritation occurs, and contact your doctor.

BRAND NAME: Augmentin

GENERIC NAME: Combination product containing: amoxicillin and clavulanate potassium

GENERIC FORM AVAILABLE: No

THERAPEUTIC CLASS: Broad-spectrum penicillin antibiotic + beta-lactamase inhibitor

DOSAGE FORMS: 250-mg, 500-mg, and 875-mg tablets; 125-mg, 200-mg, 250-mg, and 400-mg chewable tablets; 125 mg/5 mL, 200 mg/5 mL, 250 mg/5 mL, and 400 mg/5 mL suspension

MAIN USES: Bacterial infections

USUAL DOSE: 250 mg to 500 mg every 8 hours or 500 mg to 875 mg every 12 hours

AVERAGE PRICE: $80.71 for 250 mg (30 tablets); $121.03 for 500 mg (30 tablets); and $99.59 for 875 mg (20 tablets)

SIDE EFFECTS: diarrhea 9%, nausea 3%, skin rashes and itching 3%, vomiting 1%, and vaginal yeast infections 1%.

DRUG INTERACTIONS: The drug may decrease the effectiveness of oral contraceptives used for birth control. Women may become pregnant while taking Augmentin and oral contraceptives. The drug probenecid will decrease elimination of the drug by the kidneys.

FOOD INTERACTIONS: The drug should be taken with food or milk.

ALLERGIES: Individuals allergic to amoxicillin or any of its derivatives, including other penicillins and cephalosporins, should discuss this with their doctor or pharmacist before taking this drug.

PREGNANCY/BREAST-FEEDING: Category B—No evidence of risk in humans. Either animal findings show risk, but human findings do not; or, if no adequate human studies have been done, animal findings show no risk. It is not known whether the drug is excreted in the breast milk; therefore, caution should be used when breast-feeding.

OTHER BRAND NAMES: None

OTHER DRUGS IN THE SAME THERAPEUTIC CLASS: None

IMPORTANT INFORMATION TO REMEMBER: The drug should be taken with food or milk to reduce the potential for stomach upset. Also, take the drug at even intervals around the clock (if three times a day, take every eight hours). Take the drug until all the medication prescribed is gone; otherwise the infection may return. Women taking birth control pills should use another form of contraception while taking the drug and for the rest of the current menstrual cycle. Individuals taking the liquid form should shake it thoroughly before use, store the medication in the refrigerator, and discard any remaining medication after 14 days. Individuals taking the chewable tablets should drink a full glass of water after each dose.

BRAND NAME: Auralgan

GENERIC NAME: Combination product containing: antipyrine and benzocaine

GENERIC FORM AVAILABLE: Yes

THERAPEUTIC CLASS: Ear pain reliever

DOSAGE FORMS: 54 mg antipyrine and 14 mg benzocaine per 1 mL ear drops

MAIN USES: Ear pain and inflammation

USUAL DOSE: Apply enough drops until the ear canal is filled.

AVERAGE PRICE: $23.07 (B)/$13.84 (G)

SIDE EFFECTS: Most common: none. Less common: irritation and itching.

DRUG INTERACTIONS: None of any clinical significance

ALLERGIES: Individuals allergic to antipyrine, benzocaine, other local anesthetics, or any of their derivatives should consult their doctor or pharmacist before taking this drug.

PREGNANCY/BREAST-FEEDING: Category C—Risk cannot be ruled out. Human studies are lacking, and animal studies are either positive for fetal risk or lacking as well. However, potential benefits may justify the potential risk in using the drug. It is not known whether the drug is excreted in the breast milk; therefore, caution should be used when breast-feeding.

OTHER BRAND NAMES: Auroto

OTHER DRUGS IN THE SAME THERAPEUTIC CLASS: Tympagesic

IMPORTANT INFORMATION TO REMEMBER: Individuals may want to warm the medication to body temperature by holding the bottle in their hand for three to five minutes. When applying the drops, it is best to lie on one side with the affected ear facing up. Place the medication into the ear canal and lie still for several minutes. To be sure medication does not "run out," cotton may be placed in the ear. This drug should only be used when ear pain is present, and not on a regular basis unless instructed otherwise by your doctor. This medication should not be used if the individual has a perforated ear drum.

BRAND NAME: Auroto

GENERIC NAME: Combination product containing: antipyrine and benzocaine

See entry for Auralgan

BRAND NAME: Axid

GENERIC NAME: nizatidine

GENERIC FORM AVAILABLE: No

THERAPEUTIC CLASS: Stomach acid blocker

DOSAGE FORMS: 150-mg and 300-mg capsules

MAIN USES: Active stomach ulcers, active duodenal ulcers (ulcers of the upper part of the small intestine, sometimes called peptic ulcers), maintenance of healed duodenal ulcers, and the treatment of gastroesophageal reflux disease (GERD)

USUAL DOSE: 300 mg daily at bedtime or 150 mg twice daily for active stomach ulcers and active duodenal ulcers, 150 mg daily at bedtime for maintenance of healed duodenal ulcers, and 150 mg twice daily for gastroesophageal reflux disease

AVERAGE PRICE: $221.50 for 150 mg and $125.02 for 300 mg (30 capsules)

SIDE EFFECTS: headache 16%, diarrhea 7%, nausea 5%, gas 5%, dizziness 5%, vomiting 4%, upset stomach 4%, insomnia 3%, constipation 3%, drowsiness 2%, nervousness 1%, blurred vision 1%, and anemia 0.2%.

DRUG INTERACTIONS: The use of Axid and high doses of aspirin (3.9 g or more per day) together may increase aspirin in the blood to dangerous levels.

ALLERGIES: Individuals allergic to nizatidine or other stomach acid blockers (such as those listed in "Other Drugs in the Same Therapeutic Class") should discuss this with their doctor or pharmacist before taking this drug.

PREGNANCY/BREAST-FEEDING: Category C—Risk cannot be ruled out. Human studies are lacking, and animal studies are either positive for fetal risk or lacking as well. However, potential benefits may justify the potential risk in using the drug. The drug is excreted in the breast milk; therefore, extreme caution should be used when breast-feeding.

OTHER BRAND NAMES: Axid AR (over-the-counter)

OTHER DRUGS IN THE SAME THERAPEUTIC CLASS: Pepcid, Tagamet, and Zantac

IMPORTANT INFORMATION TO REMEMBER: Always complete the full course of therapy, and take Axid only as directed. Individuals taking high doses of aspirin (3.9 g or more per day) should make their doctor aware of this before taking Axid. Individuals may take antacids occasionally for heartburn or temporary flare-ups, but antacids must be taken one hour before or two hours after taking Axid. The drug is now available over-the-counter (OTC) without a prescription in a 75-mg tablet as Axid AR.

BRAND NAME: Aygestin

GENERIC NAME: norethindrone

GENERIC FORM AVAILABLE: No

THERAPEUTIC CLASS: Progestin

DOSAGE FORMS: 5-mg tablets

MAIN USES: Missed periods (secondary amenorrhea), endometriosis, and {abnormal uterine bleeding}

USUAL DOSE: 2.5 mg to 10 mg daily for 5 to 10 days for secondary amenorrhea, and 5 mg to 15 mg daily for endometriosis

AVERAGE PRICE: $24.30 for 14 tablets

SIDE EFFECTS: Most common: breakthrough bleeding, spotting, changes in menstrual flow, weight changes, changes in cervical secretions, swelling of the ankles and feet, changes in appetite, and tiredness. Less common: brown patches on the skin, headache, secretions from the breasts, skin rash, and depression.

DRUG INTERACTIONS: None of any clinical significance

ALLERGIES: Individuals allergic to norethindrone or other progesterones (such as those listed in "Other Drugs in the Same Therapeutic Class") should discuss this with their doctor or pharmacist before taking this drug.

PREGNANCY/BREAST-FEEDING: Category X—Should not be used during pregnancy. Studies in animals and/or humans have shown fetal abnormalities and birth defects. The risks associated with using this drug clearly outweigh the benefits. This drug should never be used by someone who is pregnant or trying to become pregnant. Also, women should never breast-feed while using this drug.

OTHER BRAND NAMES: None

OTHER DRUGS IN THE SAME THERAPEUTIC CLASS: Amen, Cycrin, and Provera

IMPORTANT INFORMATION TO REMEMBER: Stop using medication immediately if pregnancy is suspected. It is important to take the medication exactly as directed by your doctor. Do not stop taking the medication suddenly without consulting your doctor. It is best to take the medication at the same time every day. If migraines or vision problems occur, alert your doctor immediately.

BRAND NAME: Azmacort

GENERIC NAME: triamcinolone

GENERIC FORM AVAILABLE: No

THERAPEUTIC CLASS: Steroid inhaler

DOSAGE FORMS: 100-micrograms-per-inhalation metered-dose inhaler

MAIN USES: Asthma and {other diseases causing inflammation in the lungs}

USUAL DOSE: two puffs three to four times daily

AVERAGE PRICE: $63.45

SIDE EFFECTS: Most common: cough, dry mouth, hoarseness, and throat irritation. Less common: dry throat, headache, nausea, skin bruising, unpleasant taste, vaginal yeast infections, and thrush.

DRUG INTERACTIONS: Caution should be used when taking this drug with other oral corticosteroids such as Aristocort, Decadron, Deltasone, Medrol, and prednisone.

ALLERGIES: Individuals allergic to triamcinolone or other inhaled steroids (such as those listed in "Other Drugs in the Same Therapeutic Class") should discuss this with their doctor or pharmacist before taking this drug.

PREGNANCY/BREAST-FEEDING: Category C—Risk cannot be ruled out. Human studies are lacking, and animal studies are either positive for fetal risk or lacking as well. However, potential benefits may justify the potential risk in using the drug. It is not known whether the drug is excreted in the breast milk; therefore, caution should be used when breast-feeding.

OTHER BRAND NAMES: None

OTHER DRUGS IN THE SAME THERAPEUTIC CLASS: Aerobid, Beclovent, Flovent, and Vanceril

IMPORTANT INFORMATION TO REMEMBER: The drug is not intended to provide immediate relief of a bronchospasm, shortness of breath, or an asthma attack. To receive the full benefits of the drug, use it on a regular basis as a maintenance medication. The drug may take up to four weeks before noticeable benefits may be seen. Never exceed the prescribed dosage unless directed to do so by a doctor—excessive use beyond the prescribed dosage is potentially dangerous. If another inhaler is also being used at the same time, use the other one a few minutes prior to using Azmacort.

When using the inhaler use the following procedure:

1) Shake the canister well.
2) Place the mouthpiece close to the mouth, but not touching the lips.
3) Exhale deeply.
4) Inhale slowly and deeply as you press the top of the canister to release the medication.
5) Hold your breath for a few seconds before exhaling.
6) Wait five minutes between puffs.
7) Rinse your mouth out with water after use. Otherwise, this drug may cause a fungal infection in the mouth.
8) Be sure to wash the inhaler device (mouthpiece) regularly with warm soapy water to avoid bacterial contamination.

BRAND NAME: Azulfidine

GENERIC NAME: sulfasalazine

GENERIC FORM AVAILABLE: Yes for tablets, but not the EN-tabs

THERAPEUTIC CLASS: Salicylate-sulfonamide

DOSAGE FORMS: 500-mg tablets, 500-mg EN-tabs, and 250 mg/5 mL suspension

MAIN USES: Ulcerative colitis, arthritis, and {other inflammatory bowel disorders}

USUAL DOSE: Initially two to four grams in at least three divided doses per day. For maintenance, two grams daily in at least three divided doses.

AVERAGE PRICE: $28.58 (B)/$13.95 (G) 500 mg; $35.77 for 500-mg EN-tabs

SIDE EFFECTS: loss of appetite 33%, headache 33%, nausea 33%, stomach distress 33%, vomiting 33%, decreased sperm count (reversible if the drug is discontinued) 33%, skin rash 3%, itching 3%, fever 3%, anemia 3%, and urine discoloration 1%.

DRUG INTERACTIONS: The drug may reduce the absorption of folic acid and Lanoxin in the stomach and intestines. The drug may increase the blood levels of Coumadin, Dilantin, Mesantoin, Rheumatrex, and medications for diabetes.

ALLERGIES: Patients allergic to sulfa, mesalamine, aspirin, or aspirin derivatives should consult their doctor or pharmacist before taking this drug.

PREGNANCY/BREAST-FEEDING: Category B—No evidence of risk in humans. Either animal findings show risk, but human findings do not; or, if no adequate human studies have been done, animal findings show no risk. The drug, however, should not be used during the last three months of pregnancy. The drug is excreted in the breast milk; therefore, extreme caution should be used when breast-feeding.

OTHER BRAND NAMES: None

OTHER DRUGS IN THE SAME THERAPEUTIC CLASS: Asacol, Dipentum, Pentasa, and Rowasa

IMPORTANT INFORMATION TO REMEMBER: This drug should be taken with plenty of water (eight ounces is preferred). To avoid stomach upset, take the drug with food or milk. Also, take the drug at even intervals around the clock (if three times a day, take every eight hours). In some individuals the drug may discolor the urine and skin. This drug may also increase the sensitivity of the skin to sunburn in some individuals; therefore, a sunscreen is recommended during periods of prolonged exposure to the sun. Individuals taking the EN-tabs should not crush them—they must be swallowed whole.

BRAND NAME: Bactrim and Bactrim DS

GENERIC NAME: Combination product containing: sulfamethoxazole and trimethoprim

GENERIC FORM AVAILABLE: Yes

THERAPEUTIC CLASS: Sulfonamide + folic acid inhibitor antibiotic

DOSAGE FORMS: 80-mg trimethoprim/400-mg sulfamethoxazole tablets, 160-mg trimethoprim/800-mg sulfamethoxazole DS tablets, and 40-mg trimethoprim/200-mg sulfamethoxazole per 5 mL suspension

MAIN USES: Bacterial infections

USUAL DOSE: one tablet every 12 hours

AVERAGE PRICE: $32.55 (B)/$15.88 (G) for 20 tablets and $54.02 (B)/$24.51 (G) for 20 DS tablets

SIDE EFFECTS: Most common: fever, itching, skin rash, increased sensitivity of the skin to the sun, nausea, stomach pain, vomiting, and allergic skin reactions. Less common: Stevens-Johnson syndrome (aching joints and muscles, severe redness and blistering of the skin, and unusual tiredness or weakness), anemia, diarrhea, dizziness, headache, ringing in the ears, and nervousness.

DRUG INTERACTIONS: The drug may decrease the effects of Sandimmune. The drug may increase the blood levels of Dilantin, Mesantoin, Procan, and Rheumatrex. The drug may increase the effects of Coumadin and drugs for diabetes.

ALLERGIES: Individuals allergic to sulfamethoxazole, trimethoprim, other sulfa drugs, or any of their derivatives should discuss this with their doctor or pharmacist before using this drug.

PREGNANCY/BREAST-FEEDING: Category C—Risk cannot be ruled out. Human studies are lacking, and animal studies are either positive for fetal risk or lacking as well. However, potential benefits may justify the potential risk in using the drug. The drug is excreted in the breast milk; therefore, extreme caution should be used when breast-feeding.

OTHER BRAND NAMES: Septra and Septra DS

OTHER DRUGS IN THE SAME THERAPEUTIC CLASS: None

IMPORTANT INFORMATION TO REMEMBER: Take the drug at even intervals around the clock (if two times a day, take every 12 hours). Take the drug until all the medication prescribed is gone; otherwise the infection may return. Individuals should also use a sunscreen to avoid overexposure to the sun. The drug may increase the skin's sensitivity to sunlight, which may cause one sunburn more easily. This drug should be taken with plenty of water (eight ounces is preferred). For the suspension: Shake the bottle well before taking the drug. Also, the suspension tends to taste bad. Placing it in the refrigerator will help hide the bad taste. Otherwise, the drug does not have to be refrigerated.

BRAND NAME: **Bactroban**

GENERIC NAME: mupirocin

GENERIC FORM AVAILABLE: No

THERAPEUTIC CLASS: Topical antibacterial

DOSAGE FORMS: 2% ointment

MAIN USES: Bacterial skin infections and impetigo

USUAL DOSE: Apply three times daily.

AVERAGE PRICE: $22.12 for 15 g

SIDE EFFECTS: burning 1.5%, stinging 1.5%, pain 1.5%, redness 1%, dry skin 1%, and itching 1%.

DRUG INTERACTIONS: None of any clinical significance

ALLERGIES: Individuals allergic to mupirocin or any of its derivatives should discuss this with their doctor or pharmacist before using this drug.

PREGNANCY/BREAST-FEEDING: Category B—No evidence of risk in humans. Either animal findings show risk, but human findings do not; or, if no adequate human studies have been done, animal findings show no risk. It is not known whether the drug is excreted in the breast milk; therefore, caution should be used when breast-feeding.

OTHER BRAND NAMES: None

OTHER DRUGS IN THE SAME THERAPEUTIC CLASS: Garamycin

IMPORTANT INFORMATION TO REMEMBER: This drug is for external use only. Before applying, wash the affected area thoroughly with warm soapy water to remove dirt and skin oils, pat skin dry, and then apply only a thin film of drug to skin; do not rub it in. You may cover the skin after application with a bandage or wrapping. Discontinue use if irritation occurs. This drug is not for use in the eye.

BRAND NAME: Bancap-HC

GENERIC NAME: Combination product containing: hydrocodone and acetaminophen

See entry for Vicodin/Vicodin ES/Vicodin HP

BRAND NAME: Beclovent

GENERIC NAME: beclomethasone dipropionate

See entry for Vanceril

BRAND NAME: Beconase and Beconase AQ

GENERIC NAME: beclomethasone dipropionate

GENERIC FORM AVAILABLE: No

THERAPEUTIC CLASS: Steroid nasal spray

DOSAGE FORMS: 42-micrograms-per-inhalation aerosol and 0.042%-per-inhalation spray

MAIN USES: Nasal allergies, {nasal polyps}, and {nasal inflammation}

USUAL DOSE: one to two inhalations in each nostril twice daily for spray and one inhalation in each nostril two to four times daily for the aerosol

AVERAGE PRICE: $43.91 (Beconase) and $47.40 (Beconase AQ)

SIDE EFFECTS: For the aerosol: nasal irritation 11%, burning 11%, sneezing attacks 10%, nosebleeds 2%, and runny nose 1%. For the spray: nasal irritation 24%, sneezing attacks 4%, headache less than 5%, lightheadedness less than 5%, nausea less than 5%, nosebleeds less than 3%, stuffy nose less than 3%, and runny nose less than 3%.

DRUG INTERACTIONS: Caution should be used when taking this drug with other oral corticosteroids such as Aristocort, Decadron, Deltasone, Medrol, and prednisone.

ALLERGIES: Individuals allergic to beclomethasone dipropionate or other nasal steroids (such as those listed in "Other Drugs in the Same Therapeutic Class") should discuss this with their doctor or pharmacist before taking this drug.

PREGNANCY/BREAST-FEEDING: Category C—Risk cannot be ruled out. Human studies are lacking, and animal studies are either positive for fetal risk or lacking as well. However, potential benefits may justify the potential risk in using the drug. It is not known whether the drug is excreted in the breast milk; therefore, caution should be used when breast-feeding.

OTHER BRAND NAMES: Vancenase and Vancenase AQ

OTHER DRUGS IN THE SAME THERAPEUTIC CLASS: Dexacort, Flonase, Nasacort, Nasalide, and Rhinocort

IMPORTANT INFORMATION TO REMEMBER: The drug is not intended to provide immediate relief of nasal allergies. To receive the full benefits of the drug, use it on a regular basis as a maintenance medication. The drug may take up to three weeks before noticeable benefits may be seen. Never exceed the prescribed dosage unless directed to do so by a doctor—excessive use beyond the prescribed dosage is potentially dangerous. This drug should not be used by individuals with fungal, bacterial, systemic viral, or respiratory tract infections; unhealed wounds inside the nose; or tuberculosis.

When using the nasal spray or aerosol, use the following procedure:

1) Blow your nose gently to clear your nostrils, if necessary.
2) Hold the spray bottle with your thumb at the bottom and your index and middle finger on the shoulder attached to the neck of the bottle (top of the canister for the aerosol).
3) With your other hand, gently place a finger against the side of your nose to close the opposite nostril.
4) Insert the tip of the bottle or aerosol into the open nostril. Point the tip toward the back and outer side of the nostril once inside.
5) After releasing the spray, close your mouth, sniff deeply, hold your breath for a few seconds, then breathe out through your mouth.
6) Tilt your head back slightly for a few seconds to allow the drug to spread to the back of your nose.
7) Repeat the same procedure for the other nostril.
8) If using more than one spray in each nostril, wait five minutes between sprays.

BRAND NAME: Bellergal-S

GENERIC NAME: Combination product containing: phenobarbital, ergotamine, and levorotatory alkaloids of belladonna

GENERIC FORM AVAILABLE: Yes

THERAPEUTIC CLASS: Antispasmatic

DOSAGE FORMS: 40 mg phenobarbital/0.6 mg ergotamine tartrate/0.2 mg levorotatory alkaloids of belladonna combination tablets

MAIN USES: Stomach and intestinal disorders, menopausal disorders, {cluster headaches}, and {migraine headaches}

USUAL DOSE: one tablet twice daily

AVERAGE PRICE: $142.97 (B)/$73.67 (G)

SIDE EFFECTS: Most common: drowsiness. Less common: nausea, dry mouth, vomiting, diarrhea, tingling in the arms and legs, blurred vision, heart palpitations, decreased sweating, urine retention, fast heartbeat, and flushing.

DRUG INTERACTIONS: The drug may lower the blood levels and may decrease the effects of Coumadin. The drug may also increase the effect of Midrin. The drug may cause blood vessel constriction when used with Blocadren, Cartrol, Corgard, Inderal, Kerlone, Levatol, Lopressor, Normodyne, Sectral, Tenormin, Toprol-XL, Trandate, Visken, and Zebeta. The drug may affect the blood levels of Dilantin, Depakene, and Depakote.

ALLERGIES: Individuals allergic to phenobarbital, ergotamine, alkaloids of belladonna, or any of their derivatives should discuss this with their doctor or pharmacist before using this drug.

PREGNANCY/BREAST-FEEDING: Category X—Should not be used during pregnancy. Studies in animals and/or humans have shown fetal abnormalities and birth defects. The risks associated with using this drug clearly outweigh the benefits. This drug should never be used by someone who is pregnant or trying to become pregnant. Also, women should never breast-feed while using this drug.

OTHER BRAND NAMES: None

OTHER DRUGS IN THE SAME THERAPEUTIC CLASS: Donnatal

IMPORTANT INFORMATION TO REMEMBER: This drug does cause drowsiness. Individuals should use caution when driving, operating machinery, or any task where mental alertness is required. Alcohol, anxiety medications, or narcotic painkillers may intensify the drowsiness effect of the drug. Only take the drug exactly as direct by your physician. Do not discontinue the drug without first consulting your physician. Do not crush or divide the tablets; swallow the tablets whole. Caution should also be used when exercising and in hot weather while taking this drug—the drug may increase an individual's sensitivity to hot weather. The drug should be used cautiously by individuals with high blood pressure, heart disease, kidney disease, and liver disease.

BRAND NAME: Benadryl

GENERIC NAME: diphenhydramine

GENERIC FORM AVAILABLE: Yes

THERAPEUTIC CLASS: Antihistamine

DOSAGE FORMS: 25-mg and 50-mg capsules

MAIN USES: Allergies, allergic reactions, {motion sickness}, and {sedation}

USUAL DOSE: 25 mg to 50 mg three to four times a day

AVERAGE PRICE: $32.21 (B)/$11.93 (G) for 25 mg and $40.46 (B)/$15.38 (G) for 50 mg

SIDE EFFECTS: Most common: drowsiness, sleepiness, and dizziness. Less common: rash, dry mouth, headache, pounding heartbeat, restlessness, blurred vision, difficulty in urinating, diarrhea, and stuffy nose.

DRUG INTERACTIONS: Alcohol, anxiety medications, and narcotic painkillers may intensify the drowsiness effect of the drug. Individuals should not take Nardil or Parnate while taking this drug. The drug should also not be used with Akineton, Artane, Cogentin, and Kemadrin.

ALLERGIES: Individuals allergic to diphenhydramine or other antihistamines (such as those listed in "Other Drugs in the Same Therapeutic Class") should discuss this with their doctor or pharmacist before taking this drug.

PREGNANCY/BREAST-FEEDING: Category C—Risk cannot be ruled out. Human studies are lacking, and animal studies are either positive for fetal risk or lacking as well. However, potential benefits may justify the potential risk in using the drug. The drug is excreted in the breast milk and should not be used by women who are breast-feeding.

OTHER BRAND NAMES: None

OTHER DRUGS IN THE SAME THERAPEUTIC CLASS: Atarax, PBZ, Periactin, Tavist, Temaril, and Vistaril

IMPORTANT INFORMATION TO REMEMBER: This drug does cause drowsiness. Individuals should use caution when driving, operating machinery, or any task where mental alertness is required. Alcohol, anxiety medications, or narcotic painkillers may intensify the drowsiness effect of the drug. This drug may also cause a dry mouth; sugarless gum or hard candy will help take care of this problem. Patients with glaucoma or urinary or prostate problems should consult their doctor before taking this drug.

BRAND NAME: Benemid

GENERIC NAME: probenecid

GENERIC FORM AVAILABLE: Yes

THERAPEUTIC CLASS: Anti-gout

DOSAGE FORMS: 500-mg tablets

MAIN USES: Gout, {arthritis with gout-like symptoms}, and {to prolong the effects of antibiotics}

USUAL DOSE: 250 mg twice daily for one week, then 500 mg twice daily as a maintenance dose

AVERAGE PRICE: $58.50 (B)/$21.50 (G)

SIDE EFFECTS: Most common: none. Less common: headache, dizziness, vomiting, diarrhea, sore gums, weight loss, gas, increased urinary frequency, fever, itching, hair loss, and flushing.

DRUG INTERACTIONS: The drug may increase the blood levels of Lufyllin, penicillin, Indocin, Orudis, Oruvail, Ativan, heparin, Retrovir, Rheumatrex, rifampin, and many antibiotics. Aspirin may decrease the effectiveness of the drug.

ALLERGIES: Individuals allergic to probenecid or any of its derivatives should discuss this with their doctor or pharmacist before using this drug.

PREGNANCY/BREAST-FEEDING: Category B—No evidence of risk in humans. Either animal findings show risk, but human findings do not; or, if no adequate human studies have been done, animal findings show no risk. It is not known whether the drug is excreted in the breast milk; therefore, caution should be used when breast-feeding.

OTHER BRAND NAMES: Probalan

OTHER DRUGS IN THE SAME THERAPEUTIC CLASS: Anturane and ColBENEMID

IMPORTANT INFORMATION TO REMEMBER: This drug should be taken with plenty of water (eight ounces is preferred). This will help prevent kidney stones. If stomach upset occurs, the drug may be taken with food or milk. Only take the drug exactly as directed by your physician. Do not discontinue the drug without first consulting your physician. This drug is meant to prevent a gout attack; it will not help a gout attack once it has started. Individuals with a history of kidney stones, blood problems, or kidney disease should consult with their doctor before taking this drug.

BRAND NAME: Bentyl

GENERIC NAME: dicyclomine

GENERIC FORM AVAILABLE: Yes

THERAPEUTIC CLASS: Anticholinergic/antispasmatic

DOSAGE FORMS: 10-mg capsules, 20-mg tablets, 10 mg/5 mL syrup

MAIN USES: Irritable bowel syndrome and {other stomach and intestinal disorders}

USUAL DOSE: 20 mg to 40 mg three to four times daily, 30 minutes before meals

AVERAGE PRICE: $28.51 (B)/$17.56 (G) for 10 mg and $38.44 (B)/$24.17 (G) for 20 mg

SIDE EFFECTS: dry mouth 33%, dizziness 29%, blurred vision 27%, nausea 14%, lightheadedness 11%, drowsiness 9%, weakness 7%, constipation 6%, nervousness 6%, and fast heartbeat (rare).

DRUG INTERACTIONS: The drug may decrease the actions of Compazine, Haldol, Mellaril, Prolixin, Serentil, Stelazine, Thorazine, and Trilafon. Antacids and antidiarrheal drugs may decrease the absorption of the drug. The drug may decrease the absorption of Nizoral and Sporanox. The drug may increase the blood levels of Lanoxin.

ALLERGIES: Individuals allergic to dicyclomine or any of its derivatives should discuss this with their doctor or pharmacist before using this drug.

PREGNANCY/BREAST-FEEDING: Category C—Risk cannot be ruled out. Human studies are lacking, and animal studies are either positive for fetal risk or lacking as well. However, potential benefits may justify the potential risk in using the drug. It is not known whether the drug is excreted in the breast milk; therefore, caution should be used when breast-feeding.

OTHER BRAND NAMES: None

OTHER DRUGS IN THE SAME THERAPEUTIC CLASS: Cantil, Levsin, Pro-Banthīne, Robinul, and Spacol

IMPORTANT INFORMATION TO REMEMBER: This drug does cause drowsiness. Individuals should use caution when driving, operating machinery, or any task where mental alertness is required. Alcohol, anxiety medications, or narcotic painkillers may intensify the drowsiness effect of the drug. This drug may also cause a dry mouth; sugarless gum or hard candy will help take care of this problem. Patients with glaucoma, urinary or prostate problems, GI obstruction, or severe ulcerative colitis should consult their doctor before taking this drug. Caution should be used during hot weather due to decreased tolerance to the heat.

BRAND NAME: Benzac, Benzac AC, Benzac W

GENERIC NAME: benzoyl peroxide

GENERIC FORM AVAILABLE: Yes

THERAPEUTIC CLASS: Antibacterial/keratolytic

DOSAGE FORMS: 2.5%, 5%, and 10% water-based gels; 5% and 10% cleansing washes

MAIN USES: Acne

USUAL DOSE: Water-based gel: apply once daily; may increase to two to three times daily as tolerated. Cleansing wash: wash affected area one to two times daily.

AVERAGE PRICE: $17.85 (B)/$11.81 (G) for 2.5% gel; $18.55 (B)/$12.36 (G) for 5% gel; $19.06 (B)/$13.00 (G) for 10% gel; $24.31 (B)/$21.54 (G) for 5% wash; $27.46 (B)/$24.34 (G) for 10% wash

SIDE EFFECTS: Most common: none. Less common: itching, redness, stinging, and dry skin.

DRUG INTERACTIONS: Sunscreens containing PABA (paraaminobenzoic acid) may discolor the skin a yellowish-brown color when used with this drug.

ALLERGIES: Individuals allergic to benzoyl peroxide or any of its derivatives should discuss this with their doctor or pharmacist before using this drug.

PREGNANCY/BREAST-FEEDING: Category C—Risk cannot be ruled out. Human studies are lacking, and animal studies are either positive for fetal risk or lacking as well. However, potential benefits may justify the potential risk in using the drug. It is not known whether the drug is excreted in the breast milk; therefore, caution should be used when breast-feeding.

OTHER BRAND NAMES: None

OTHER DRUGS IN THE SAME THERAPEUTIC CLASS: Benzagel, Desquam-E, Desquam-X, and Persa-Gel

IMPORTANT INFORMATION TO REMEMBER: This drug is for external use only. Before applying, wash acne area thoroughly with warm soapy water to remove dirt and skin oils, pat skin dry, and then apply the drug. If you need to apply another medication for acne, wait at least one hour. When using the cleansing wash, be sure to rinse affected areas thoroughly with water. Avoid contact with eyes, mouth, and other mucous membranes with all Benzac products. These products may discolor fabric or hair. Do not apply the drug to irritated or damaged skin.

BRAND NAME: Benzagel

GENERIC NAME: benzoyl peroxide

See entry for Benzac

BRAND NAME: Benzamycin

GENERIC NAME: Combination product containing: erythromycin and benzoyl peroxide

GENERIC FORM AVAILABLE: No

THERAPEUTIC CLASS: Macrolide antibiotic + antibacterial/keratolytic

DOSAGE FORMS: 3% erythromycin and 5% benzoyl peroxide gel

MAIN USES: Acne

USUAL DOSE: Apply to infected area twice daily, morning and evening.

AVERAGE PRICE: $39.68 for 23.3 g

SIDE EFFECTS: dry skin 2%, itching 1%, and redness 1%.

DRUG INTERACTIONS: Sunscreens containing PABA (paraamino-benzoic acid) may discolor the skin a yellowish-brown color when used with this drug.

ALLERGIES: Individuals allergic to erythromycin, benzoyl peroxide, or any of their derivatives should discuss this with their doctor or pharmacist before using this drug.

PREGNANCY/BREAST-FEEDING: Category C—Risk cannot be ruled out. Human studies are lacking, and animal studies are either positive for fetal risk or lacking as well. However, potential benefits may justify the potential risk in using the drug. It is not known whether the drug is excreted in the breast milk; therefore, caution should be used when breast-feeding.

OTHER BRAND NAMES: None

OTHER DRUGS IN THE SAME THERAPEUTIC CLASS: None

IMPORTANT INFORMATION TO REMEMBER: This drug is for external use only. The drug must be stored in the refrigerator. Any unused drug should be discarded after three months. Before applying, wash acne area thoroughly with warm soapy water to remove dirt and skin oils, pat skin dry, and then apply the drug. If you need to apply another medication for acne, wait at least one hour. Avoid contact with eyes, mouth, and other mucous membranes. These products may discolor fabric or hair. Do not apply the drug to irritated or damaged skin.

BRAND NAME: Berocca and Berocca Plus

GENERIC NAME: B-C with folic acid

GENERIC FORM AVAILABLE: Yes

THERAPEUTIC CLASS: Multivitamins

DOSAGE FORMS: Multivitamin tablets

MAIN USES: Nutritional supplement

USUAL DOSE: one tablet daily

AVERAGE PRICE: $55.59 (Berocca) and $57.84 (B)/$18.02 (G) (Berocca Plus)

SIDE EFFECTS: Most common: none. Less common: diarrhea, gas, and stomach upset.

DRUG INTERACTIONS: The B vitamins in the drug may decrease the effect of Larodopa.

ALLERGIES: Individuals allergic to multivitamins or any of their derivatives should discuss this with their doctor or pharmacist before using this drug.

PREGNANCY/BREAST-FEEDING: Category B—No evidence of risk in humans. Either animal findings show risk, but human findings do not; or, if no adequate human studies have been done, animal findings show no risk. It is not known whether the drug is excreted in the breast milk; therefore, caution should be used when breast-feeding.

OTHER BRAND NAMES: None

OTHER DRUGS IN THE SAME THERAPEUTIC CLASS: Centrum, Cefol, Theragran, Theragran-M, and Vicon Forte

IMPORTANT INFORMATION TO REMEMBER: Only take the drug exactly as directly by your physician. Do not discontinue the drug without first consulting your physician. If stomach upset occurs, the drug may be taken with food or milk.

BRAND NAME: **Betagan**

GENERIC NAME: levobunolol

GENERIC FORM AVAILABLE: Yes

THERAPEUTIC CLASS: Noncardioselective beta-blocker

DOSAGE FORMS: 0.025% eyedrop solution and 0.5% eyedrop solution

MAIN USES: Glaucoma

USUAL DOSE: Initially one drop once daily, and a maintenance dose of one to two drops twice daily

AVERAGE PRICE: $25.76 (B)/$21.17 (G) for 0.5% (5 mL) and $21.54 (B)/$18.78 (G) for 0.25% (5 mL)

SIDE EFFECTS: Most common: slight discomfort upon use. Less common: burning, itching, eye pain, redness of the eyes, dryness of the eyes, headache, and dizziness.

DRUG INTERACTIONS: The drug may cause widening of the pupil when used with Epifrin. The drug may cause additive effects when used with Blocadren, Cartrol, Corgard, Inderal, Kerlone, Levatol, Lopressor, Normodyne, reserpine, Sectral, Tenormin, Toprol-XL, Trandate, Visken, and Zebeta.

ALLERGIES: Individuals allergic to levobunolol or any of its derivatives should discuss this with their doctor or pharmacist before using this drug.

PREGNANCY/BREAST-FEEDING: Category C—Risk cannot be ruled out. Human studies are lacking, and animal studies are either positive for fetal risk or lacking as well. However, potential benefits may justify the potential risk in using the drug. It is not known whether the drug is excreted in the breast milk; therefore, caution should be used when breast-feeding.

OTHER BRAND NAMES: None

OTHER DRUGS IN THE SAME THERAPEUTIC CLASS: Betimol, Ocupress, OptiPranolol, Timoptic, and Timoptic XE

IMPORTANT INFORMATION TO REMEMBER: Keep the container tightly closed and avoid touching the applicator tip to the eye—this could contaminate the product over time. Also, only administer one drop at a time. After application, keep the eye open for at least 30 seconds, roll the eyeball around, and avoid squinting. If a second drop is required, wait one to two minutes between drops. If another medication is to be used in the eye, wait at least 10 minutes before administering it. Only use the drug exactly as directly by your physician. Do not discontinue the drug without first consulting your physician.

BRAND NAME: Betimol

GENERIC NAME: timolol

Betimol is very similar to Timoptic. See entry for Timoptic/Timoptic-XE.

BRAND NAME: **Betoptic and Betoptic S**

GENERIC NAME: betaxolol

GENERIC FORM AVAILABLE: No

THERAPEUTIC CLASS: Cardioselective beta-blocker

DOSAGE FORMS: 0.5% eyedrop solution and 0.25% eyedrop suspension

MAIN USES: Glaucoma

USUAL DOSE: one to two drops in the affected eye(s) twice daily

AVERAGE PRICE: $75.68 for 15 mL of both

SIDE EFFECTS: Most common: slight discomfort upon use. Less common: burning, itching, eye pain, redness of the eyes, dryness of the eyes, headache, and dizziness.

DRUG INTERACTIONS: The drug may cause widening of the pupil when used with Epifrin. The drug may cause additive effects when used with Blocadren, Cartrol, Corgard, Inderal, Kerlone, Levatol, Lopressor, Normodyne, reserpine, Sectral, Tenormin, Toprol-XL, Trandate, Visken, and Zebeta.

ALLERGIES: Individuals allergic to betaxolol or any of its derivatives should discuss this with their doctor or pharmacist before using this drug.

PREGNANCY/BREAST-FEEDING: Category C—Risk cannot be ruled out. Human studies are lacking, and animal studies are either positive for fetal risk or lacking as well. However, potential benefits may justify the potential risk in using the drug. The drug is excreted in the breast milk; therefore, extreme caution should be used when breast-feeding.

OTHER BRAND NAMES: None

OTHER DRUGS IN THE SAME THERAPEUTIC CLASS: None

IMPORTANT INFORMATION TO REMEMBER: Keep the container tightly closed and avoid touching the applicator tip to the eye—this could contaminate the product over time. Also, only administer one drop at a time. After application, keep the eye open for at least 30 seconds, roll the eyeball around, and avoid squinting. If a second drop is required, wait one to two minutes between drops. If another medication is to be used in the eye, wait at least 10 minutes before administering it. Only take the drug exactly as directed by your physician. Do not discontinue the drug without first consulting your physician.

BRAND NAME: Biaxin

GENERIC NAME: clarithromycin

GENERIC FORM AVAILABLE: No

THERAPEUTIC CLASS: Macrolide antibiotic

DOSAGE FORMS: 250-mg and 500-mg tablets; 125 mg/5 mL and 250 mg/5 mL suspension

MAIN USES: Bacterial infections

USUAL DOSE: 250 mg to 500 mg every 12 hours

AVERAGE PRICE: $89.99 for 250 mg (20 tablets) and $99.87 for 500 mg (20 tablets)

SIDE EFFECTS: diarrhea 3%, nausea 3%, abnormal taste 3%, upset stomach 2%, stomach pain 2%, and headache 2%.

DRUG INTERACTIONS: **Warning:** This drug should not be used with Seldane, Seldane-D, or Hismanal; the drug may increase the blood levels of these drugs to extremely toxic and possibly life-threatening levels. Never take Biaxin with either Hismanal, Seldane, or Seldane-D. The drug may also increase the blood levels of Coumadin, Lanoxin, Retrovir, rifabutin, Slo-bid, Tegretol, Theo-Dur, theophylline, Uni-Dur, and Uniphyl. Propulsid or Orap and the drug may cause dangerous irregular heartbeats when taken together.

ALLERGIES: Individuals allergic to clarithromycin or other macrolide antibiotics (such as those listed in "Other Drugs in the Same Therapeutic Class") should discuss this with their doctor or pharmacist before taking this drug.

PREGNANCY/BREAST-FEEDING: Category C—Risk cannot be ruled out. Human studies are lacking, and animal studies are either positive for fetal risk or lacking as well. However, potential benefits may justify the potential risk in using the drug. The drug is excreted in the breast milk; therefore, extreme caution should be used when breast-feeding.

OTHER BRAND NAMES: None

OTHER DRUGS IN THE SAME THERAPEUTIC CLASS: Dynabac, E-Mycin, E.E.S., ERYC, EryPed, Ery-Tab, Ilosone, PCE, TAO, and Zithromax

IMPORTANT INFORMATION TO REMEMBER: If stomach upset occurs, take the drug with food or milk. Also, take the drug at even intervals around the clock (if twice a day, take every 12 hours). Take the drug until all the medication prescribed is gone; otherwise the infection may return. Individuals taking the liquid form should shake it thoroughly before use, store the medication in the refrigerator, and discard any remaining medication after 14 days. If severe diarrhea occurs while taking this drug, notify your doctor immediately. Never take the drug with Seldane, Seldane-D, or Hismanal (see "Drug Interactions").

BRAND NAME: Bleph-10

GENERIC NAME: sulfacetamide sodium

See entry for Sulamyd

BRAND NAME: Blocadren

GENERIC NAME: timolol maleate

GENERIC FORM AVAILABLE: Yes

THERAPEUTIC CLASS: Noncardioselective beta-blocker

DOSAGE FORMS: 5-mg, 10-mg, and 20-mg tablets

MAIN USES: High blood pressure, after heart attacks, and migraines

USUAL DOSE: 10 mg to 20 mg twice daily

AVERAGE PRICE: $56.40 (B)/$29.12 (G) for 5 mg; $69.76 (B)/$40.12 (G) for 10 mg; $128.66 (B)/$70.29 (G) for 20 mg

SIDE EFFECTS: slow heartbeat 9%, cold hands and feet 8%, dizziness 6%, tiredness 5%, low blood pressure 3%, headache 2%, difficulty breathing 2%, decreased sex drive 1%, chest pain 1%, irregular heartbeat 1%, nausea 1%, and upset stomach 1%.

DRUG INTERACTIONS: The drug may cause additive effects when used with reserpine. The drug may increase the effects of Calan, Cardene, Cardizem, Catapres, Dilacor XR, DynaCirc, Isoptin, Lanoxin, Norvasc, Plendil, Procardia, Sular, Tiazac, Verelan, and

Wytensin. Diabetic medications, insulin, Slo-bid, Theo-Dur, theophylline, Uni-Dur, and Uniphyl dosages may need to be adjusted when taking this drug. The drug may also interfere with glaucoma screening tests.

ALLERGIES: Individuals allergic to timolol or other beta-blockers (such as those listed in "Other Drugs in the Same Therapeutic Class") should discuss this with their doctor or pharmacist before taking this drug.

PREGNANCY/BREAST-FEEDING: Category C—Risk cannot be ruled out. Human studies are lacking, and animal studies are either positive for fetal risk or lacking as well. However, potential benefits may justify the potential risk in using the drug. The drug is excreted in the breast milk; therefore, extreme caution should be used when breast-feeding.

OTHER BRAND NAMES: None

OTHER DRUGS IN THE SAME THERAPEUTIC CLASS: Cartrol, Corgard, Inderal, Levatol, Normodyne, Trandate, and Visken

IMPORTANT INFORMATION TO REMEMBER: Only take the drug exactly as directed by your physician. Do not discontinue the drug without first consulting your physician. This drug may cause some tiredness, especially at first. Individuals should use caution when driving, operating machinery, or any task where mental alertness is required. Alcohol, anxiety medications, or narcotic painkillers may intensify the tiredness effect of the drug. Before taking over-the-counter cold and allergy preparations, consult your doctor or pharmacist. These products may raise your blood pressure. This drug may mask the symptoms of low blood sugar in diabetics.

BRAND NAME: Brethine and Brethaire

GENERIC NAME: terbutaline

GENERIC FORM AVAILABLE: No

THERAPEUTIC CLASS: Beta-2-agonist bronchodilator

DOSAGE FORMS: 2.5-mg and 5-mg tablets (Brethine); 0.20-mg inhaler (Brethaire)

MAIN USES: Asthma, chronic bronchitis, emphysema, and {other breathing disorders}

USUAL DOSE: 2.5 mg to 5 mg three times a day; two inhalations every four to six hours

AVERAGE PRICE: $40.65 for 2.5 mg; $53.22 for 5 mg; and $34.22 for the inhaler

SIDE EFFECTS: Most common: nervousness and tremor. Least common: headache, fast heartbeat, heart palpitations, drowsiness, nausea, vomiting, sweating, and muscle cramps. Other less common side effects for Brethaire inhaler: dry throat, wheezing, insomnia, unusual taste, irritated throat, and difficulty breathing.

DRUG INTERACTIONS: Decongestants in cough, cold, and allergy products, and Asendin, Endep, Elavil, Nardil, Norpramin, Pamelor, Parnate, Sinequan, Surmontil, Tofranil, and Vivactil may increase the toxicity of this drug. Blocadren, Cartrol, Corgard, Inderal, Levatol, Normodyne, reserpine, Trandate, and Visken may decrease the effects of the drug.

ALLERGIES: Individuals allergic to terbutaline or any of its derivatives should discuss this with their doctor or pharmacist before using this drug.

PREGNANCY/BREAST-FEEDING: Category B—No evidence of risk in humans. Either animal findings show risk, but human findings do not; or, if no adequate human studies have been done, animal findings show no risk. The drug is excreted in the breast milk; therefore, extreme caution should be used when breast-feeding.

OTHER BRAND NAMES: Bricanyl

OTHER DRUGS IN THE SAME THERAPEUTIC CLASS: Alupent, Bricanyl, Bronkometer, Maxair, Metaprel, Proventil, Serevent, Tornalate, Ventolin, and Volmax

IMPORTANT INFORMATION TO REMEMBER: Only take the drug exactly as directed by your physician. Never increase the dose of the drug without consulting with your physician. Prolonged use of the drug may cause tolerance to its effects to develop.

When using the inhaler, use the following procedure:

1) Shake the canister well.
2) Place the mouthpiece close to the mouth, but not touching the lips.
3) Exhale deeply.

4) Inhale slowly and deeply as you press the top of the canister to release the medication.
5) Hold your breath for a few seconds before exhaling.
6) Wait five minutes between puffs.
7) Be sure to wash the inhaler device (mouthpiece) regularly with warm soapy water to avoid bacterial contamination.

BRAND NAME: Bricanyl

GENERIC NAME: terbutaline

See entry for Brethine/Brethaire

BRAND NAME: Bromfed and Bromfed PD

GENERIC NAME: Combination product containing: brompheniramine and pseudoephedrine

GENERIC FORM AVAILABLE: Yes

THERAPEUTIC CLASS: Antihistamine + decongestant

DOSAGE FORMS: 12-mg brompheniramine/120-mg pseudoephedrine sustained-release capsules (Bromfed capsules); 6-mg brompheniramine/60-mg pseudoephedrine sustained-release capsules (Bromfed PD); 2 mg brompheniramine/30 mg pseudoephedrine per 5 mL liquid (Bromfed syrup); and 4 mg brompheniramine/60 mg pseudoephedrine (Bromfed tablets)

MAIN USES: Nasal allergies and congestion

USUAL DOSE: one capsule every 12 hours (Bromfed capsules), one to two capsules every 12 hours (Bromfed PD), two teaspoons every four to six hours (Bromfed syrup), and one tablet every four hours (Bromfed tablets)

AVERAGE PRICE: $101.17 (B)/$52.77 (G) Bromfed capsules; $107.77 (B)/$52.77 (G) for Bromfed PD

SIDE EFFECTS: Most common: none. Less common: drowsiness, nausea, giddiness, dry mouth, blurred vision, pounding heartbeat, flushing, and increased irritability or excitability (especially in children).

DRUG INTERACTIONS: Blocadren, Cartrol, Corgard, Inderal, Kerlone, Levatol, Lopressor, Normodyne, Sectral, Tenormin, Toprol-XL,

Trandate, Visken, and Zebeta may increase the effects of the drug. The drug may also reduce the effects of blood-pressure-lowering drugs.

ALLERGIES: Individuals allergic to brompheniramine, pseudoephedrine, or other antihistamine/decongestant combinations (such as those listed in "Other Drugs in the Same Therapeutic Class") should discuss this with their doctor or pharmacist before taking this drug.

PREGNANCY/BREAST-FEEDING: Category C—Risk cannot be ruled out. Human studies are lacking, and animal studies are either positive for fetal risk or lacking as well. However, potential benefits may justify the potential risk in using the drug. It is not known whether the drug is excreted in the breast milk; therefore, caution should be used when breast-feeding.

OTHER BRAND NAMES: None

OTHER DRUGS IN THE SAME THERAPEUTIC CLASS: Claritin-D, Comhist LA, Deconamine SR, Fedahist, Naldecon, Nolamine, Novafed-A, Ornade, Poly-Histine-D, Rynatan, Seldane-D, Semprex-D, Tavist-D, and Trinalin

IMPORTANT INFORMATION TO REMEMBER: This drug does cause drowsiness. Individuals should use caution when driving, operating machinery, or any task where mental alertness is required. Alcohol, anxiety medications, and narcotic painkillers may intensify the drowsiness effect of the drug. This drug may also cause a dry mouth; sugarless gum or hard candy will help take care of this problem. Patients with glaucoma, high blood pressure, heart conditions, or urinary or prostate problems should consult their doctor before taking this drug.

BRAND NAME: Bronkometer and Bronkosol

GENERIC NAME: isoetharine

GENERIC FORM AVAILABLE: Yes

THERAPEUTIC CLASS: Beta-2-agonist bronchodilator

DOSAGE FORMS: 340 micrograms isoetharine mesylate per inhalation (Bronkometer); and isoetharine 1% solution (Bronkosol)

MAIN USES: Asthma, chronic bronchitis, emphysema, and {other breathing disorders}

USUAL DOSE: one to two inhalations every four hours (Bronkometer) and three to seven inhalations by hand bulb nebulizer, up to every four hours (Bronkosol)

AVERAGE PRICE: $44.46 for 15 mL Bronkometer and $69.17 (B)/ $26.47 (G) for 30 mL Bronkosol

SIDE EFFECTS: Most common: fast heartbeat, pounding heartbeat, headache, nausea, changes in blood pressure, nervousness, trembling, insomnia, vomiting, weakness, and restlessness. Less common: tension, dizziness, and excitement.

DRUG INTERACTIONS: Decongestants in cough, cold, and allergy products may increase the toxicity of this drug. Blocadren, Cartrol, Corgard, Inderal, Levatol, Lopressor, Normodyne, reserpine, Trandate, and Visken may decrease the effect of the drug.

ALLERGIES: Individuals allergic to isoetharine or any of its derivatives should discuss this with their doctor or pharmacist before using this drug.

PREGNANCY/BREAST-FEEDING: Category C—Risk cannot be ruled out. Human studies are lacking, and animal studies are either positive for fetal risk or lacking as well. However, potential benefits may justify the potential risk in using the drug. It is not known whether the drug is excreted in the breast milk; therefore, caution should be used when breast-feeding.

OTHER BRAND NAMES: None

OTHER DRUGS IN THE SAME THERAPEUTIC CLASS: Alupent, Brethaire, Brethine, Maxair, Metaprel, Proventil, Serevent, Tornalate, and Ventolin

IMPORTANT INFORMATION TO REMEMBER: Only take the drug exactly as directed by your physician. Never take more of the drug without consulting with your physician. Due to its potential to cause insomnia, take the drug a few hours before bedtime if possible.

When using the inhaler, follow the following procedure:

1) Shake the canister well.
2) Place the mouthpiece close to the mouth, but not touching the lips.

3) Exhale deeply.
4) Inhale slowly and deeply as you press the top of the canister to release the medication.
5) Hold your breath for a few seconds before exhaling.
6) Wait five minutes between puffs.
7) Be sure to wash the inhaler device (mouthpiece) regularly with warm soapy water to avoid bacterial contamination.

BRAND NAME: Brontex

GENERIC NAME: Combination product containing: codeine and guaifenesin

GENERIC FORM AVAILABLE: No

THERAPEUTIC CLASS: Cough suppressant + expectorant

DOSAGE FORMS: 10-mg codeine/300-mg guaifenesin (tablets) and 10 mg codeine/300 mg guaifenesin per 20 mL (liquid)

MAIN USES: Cough

USUAL DOSE: one tablet every four hours as needed or four teaspoons every four hours

AVERAGE PRICE: $17.87 for 20 tablets and $19.99 for 120 mL of liquid

SIDE EFFECTS: Most common: drowsiness, dizziness, and upset stomach. Less common: headache, visual disturbances, disorientation, stomach pain, constipation, nausea, and vomiting.

DRUG INTERACTIONS: Alcohol, anxiety medications, narcotic painkillers, and medications used for depression may intensify the drowsiness effect of the drug. Nardil or Parnate should not be taken with this drug.

ALLERGIES: Individuals allergic to codeine, guaifenesin, or any of their derivatives should discuss this with their doctor or pharmacist before using this drug.

PREGNANCY/BREAST-FEEDING: Category C—Risk cannot be ruled out. Human studies are lacking, and animal studies are either positive for fetal risk or lacking as well. However, potential benefits may justify the potential risk in using the drug. Codeine is excreted in the breast milk; therefore, extreme caution should be used when breast-feeding.

OTHER BRAND NAMES: None

OTHER DRUGS IN THE SAME THERAPEUTIC CLASS: Hycotuss, Robitussin A-C, Tussi-Organidin NR, and Vicodin Tuss

IMPORTANT INFORMATION TO REMEMBER: This drug does cause drowsiness. Individuals should use caution when driving, operating machinery, or any task where mental alertness is required. Alcohol, anxiety medications, or narcotic painkillers may intensify the drowsiness effect of the drug. The drug should only be taken as needed to control a cough. This drug should not be used as a long-term therapy. This medication is a controlled substance and may be habit-forming. If stomach upset occurs, the drug may be taken with food or milk.

BRAND NAME: Bumex

GENERIC NAME: bumetanide

GENERIC FORM AVAILABLE: Yes

THERAPEUTIC CLASS: Loop diuretic (water pill)

DOSAGE FORMS: 0.5-mg, 1-mg, and 2-mg tablets

MAIN USES: Water retention (fluid retention due to congestive heart failure, kidney disease, or cirrhosis of the liver) and high blood pressure

USUAL DOSE: 0.5 mg to 2 mg daily

AVERAGE PRICE: $50.58 (B)/$38.26 (G) for 0.5 mg; $58.94 (B)/$40.68 (G) for 1 mg; and $84.35 (B)/$64.22 (G) for 2 mg

SIDE EFFECTS: high uric acid levels in the blood 18%, low levels of potassium and chloride in the blood 15%, high blood sugar 7%, muscle cramps 1%, dizziness 1%, low blood pressure 1%, headache 1%, and nausea 1%.

DRUG INTERACTIONS: The drug may increase the levels of Coumadin, Eskalith, and Lithobid in the blood. The drug may increase the chance of ototoxicity (hearing loss) when used with amphotericin B and cisplatin.

ALLERGIES: Individuals allergic to bumetanide or any of its derivatives should discuss this with their doctor or pharmacist before using this drug.

PREGNANCY/BREAST-FEEDING: Category C—Risk cannot be ruled out. Human studies are lacking, and animal studies are either positive for fetal risk or lacking as well. However, potential benefits may justify the potential risk in using the drug. It is not known whether the drug is excreted in the breast milk; therefore, caution should be used when breast-feeding.

OTHER BRAND NAMES: None

OTHER DRUGS IN THE SAME THERAPEUTIC CLASS: Demadex, Edecrin, and Lasix

IMPORTANT INFORMATION TO REMEMBER: If stomach upset occurs, the drug may be taken with food or milk. If the drug is to be taken once daily, take it in the morning due to increased urine output. Individuals with kidney disease should discuss this with their doctor before taking this drug. Before taking over-the-counter cold and allergy preparations, consult your doctor or pharmacist. These products may raise your blood pressure. The drug may cause the elimination of potassium from the body; it is therefore a good idea to eat a banana or drink orange, grapefruit, or apple juice every day to replace lost potassium.

BRAND NAME: BuSpar

GENERIC NAME: buspirone

GENERIC FORM AVAILABLE: No

THERAPEUTIC CLASS: Antianxiety

DOSAGE FORMS: 5-mg, 10-mg, and 15-mg tablets

MAIN USES: Anxiety

USUAL DOSE: 5 mg to 10 mg three times daily

AVERAGE PRICE: $83.32 for 5 mg, $145.36 for 10 mg, and $179.92 for 15 mg

SIDE EFFECTS: dizziness 12%, drowsiness 10%, nausea 8%, headache 6%, nervousness 5%, tiredness 4%, insomnia 3%, dry mouth 3%, lightheadedness 3%, excitement 2%, confusion 2%, diarrhea 2%, weakness 2%, and constipation 1%.

DRUG INTERACTIONS: Nardil and Parnate may increase blood pressure when used with this drug.

ALLERGIES: Individuals allergic to buspirone or any of its derivatives should discuss this with their doctor or pharmacist before using this drug.

PREGNANCY/BREAST-FEEDING: Category B—No evidence of risk in humans. Either animal findings show risk, but human findings do not; or, if no adequate human studies have been done, animal findings show no risk. The drug is excreted in the breast milk; therefore, extreme caution should be used when breast-feeding.

OTHER BRAND NAMES: None

OTHER DRUGS IN THE SAME THERAPEUTIC CLASS: None

IMPORTANT INFORMATION TO REMEMBER: This drug does cause drowsiness. Individuals should use caution when driving, operating machinery, or any task where mental alertness is required. Alcohol, anxiety medications, or narcotic painkillers may intensify the drowsiness effect of the drug. This drug, unlike the benzodiazepines (Ativan, Librium, Serax, Tranxene, Xanax, and Valium) is not habit-forming. It may take between 7 and 21 days before any improvement in symptoms is seen. Report any abnormal involuntary movements of the tongue or facial muscles to your doctor or pharmacist immediately.

BRAND NAME: Butisol Sodium

GENERIC NAME: butabarbital sodium

GENERIC FORM AVAILABLE: No

THERAPEUTIC CLASS: Barbiturate sedative

DOSAGE FORMS: 15-mg, 30-mg, 50-mg, and 100-mg tablets and 30 mg/mL elixir

MAIN USES: Sedation and insomnia

USUAL DOSE: 15 mg–30 mg three to four times daily for sedation and 50 mg–100 mg at bedtime for insomnia

AVERAGE PRICE: $62.34 for 5 mg; $82.81 for 30 mg; and $129.88 for 100 mg

SIDE EFFECTS: Most common: drowsiness, clumsiness, unsteadiness, dizziness, lightheadedness, and feeling of a hangover. Less common: nervousness, anxiety, constipation, feeling faint, headache, irritability, nausea, vomiting, nightmares, and insomnia.

DRUG INTERACTIONS: Alcohol, anxiety medications, and narcotic painkillers will intensify the drowsiness effect of the drug. The drug may decrease the blood levels of Aristocort, Coumadin, Decadron, Deltasone, Medrol, prednisone, and Tegretol. The drug may also decrease the effectiveness of birth control pills. Depakene and Depakote may increase the blood levels of the drug.

ALLERGIES: Individuals allergic to butabarbital sodium, Amytal, Mebaral, Nembutal, Seconal, Tuinal, or any of their derivatives should discuss this with their doctor or pharmacist before using this drug.

PREGNANCY/BREAST-FEEDING: Category D—Positive evidence of risk. Human studies show risk to the fetus. Nevertheless, potential benefits may possibly outweigh the potential risks. This drug should not be taken by nursing mothers or women who are pregnant.

OTHER BRAND NAMES: None

OTHER DRUGS IN THE SAME THERAPEUTIC CLASS: Amytal, Mebaral, Nembutal, Seconal, and Tuinal

IMPORTANT INFORMATION TO REMEMBER: This drug does cause drowsiness. Individuals should use caution when driving, operating machinery, or any task where mental alertness is required. Alcohol, anxiety medications, or narcotic painkillers may intensify the drowsiness effect of the drug. This medication is a controlled substance and may be habit-forming. Only take the drug exactly as directed by your physician. Do not increase the dose without first consulting with your physician. Women taking birth control pills should use another form of contraception while taking the drug and for the rest of the current menstrual cycle.

BRAND NAME: Cafergot

GENERIC NAME: Combination product containing: ergotamine and caffeine

GENERIC FORM AVAILABLE: No

THERAPEUTIC CLASS: Ergot alkaloid

DOSAGE FORMS: 2-mg ergotamine/100-mg caffeine suppositories

MAIN USES: Migraine headaches

USUAL DOSE: For the suppositories, use one suppository at the first sign of an attack, and one additional suppository one hour later as needed for full relief. Do NOT exceed two suppositories for any one attack or five suppositories in any seven-day period.

AVERAGE PRICE: $68.88 for 12 suppositories

SIDE EFFECTS: Most common: swelling of the face, fingers, lower legs, and feet; dizziness; drowsiness; dry mouth; diarrhea; nausea; vomiting; cold fingers or toes; and tingling in toes and fingers. Less common: chest pain, fast or slow heartbeat, blood pressure changes, nervousness, confusion, itching, weak or fast pulse, and vision changes.

DRUG INTERACTIONS: The drug may produce serious cardiovascular effects when used with Midrin, some local anesthetics, and cough and cold products that contain decongestants. Biaxin, Inderal, nicotine patches, and erythromycin may cause dangerous high blood pressure.

ALLERGIES: Individuals allergic to ergotamine, caffeine, or any of their derivatives should discuss this with their doctor or pharmacist before using this drug.

PREGNANCY/BREAST-FEEDING: Category X—Should not be used during pregnancy. Studies in animals and/or humans have shown fetal abnormalities and birth defects. The risks associated with using this drug clearly outweigh the benefits. This drug should never be used by someone who is pregnant or trying to become pregnant. Also, women should never breast-feed while using this drug.

OTHER BRAND NAMES: Ercaf and Wigraine

OTHER DRUGS IN THE SAME THERAPEUTIC CLASS: D.H.E. 45 and Sansert

IMPORTANT INFORMATION TO REMEMBER: Only take the drug exactly as directed by your physician. Do not increase the dose without first consulting with your physician. Do not use the drug for headaches other than migraine headaches. Individuals with high blood pressure, cardiovascular disease, or any heart condition should discuss this with their doctor before taking this drug. Individuals experiencing any signs of ergotism (headache, numbness and coldness of the feet and hands, and muscle pain) should contact their doctor immediately. Before taking over-the-counter cold, cough, and allergy preparations, consult your doctor or pharmacist.

These products may raise your blood pressure to very dangerous levels. This drug should be used cautiously by patients with heart disease.

For the suppository:

Store in a cool place to avoid melting, preferably the refrigerator. Remove the foil wrapper before inserting the suppository. When inserting, lie on one side and bend the top leg slightly. Then insert suppository into rectum about one inch with one finger. Wash hands thoroughly before and after use. Individuals may want to use a finger cot to cover finger when inserting a suppository.

BRAND NAME: Calan and Calan SR

GENERIC NAME: verapamil

GENERIC FORM AVAILABLE: Yes

THERAPEUTIC CLASS: Calcium channel blocker

DOSAGE FORMS: Calan: 40-mg, 80-mg, and 120-mg tablets. Calan SR: 120-mg, 180-mg, and 240-mg sustained-release tablets

MAIN USES: Angina and high blood pressure

USUAL DOSE: 80 mg to 120 mg of the tablets three times daily for angina and 120 mg to 240 mg of the sustained-release tablets once or twice daily for high blood pressure

AVERAGE PRICE: $43.97 (B)/$23.07 (G) for 40 mg; $61.20 (B)/ $14.28 (G) for 80 mg; $70.97 (B)/$17.58 (G) for 120 mg; $147.37 (B)/$105.57 (G) for Calan SR 180 mg; $158.29 (B)/ $124.27 (G) for Calan SR 240 mg

SIDE EFFECTS: constipation 7%, dizziness 3%, nausea 3%, low blood pressure 3%, headache 2%, swelling 2%, fluid build-up around the heart and lungs 2%, tiredness 2%, difficulty breathing 1%, slow heart rate 1%, and flushing 1%.

DRUG INTERACTIONS: The effects of Blocadren, Cartrol, Corgard, Inderal, Kerlone, Levatol, Lopressor, Minipress, Normodyne, Norpace, Sectral, Tenormin, Toprol-XL, Trandate, Visken, and Zebeta may be increased when taken with this drug. The drug may increase the blood levels of Tegretol, Sandimmune, Lanoxin, Quinidex, Quinaglute, and Procan.

ALLERGIES: Individuals allergic to verapamil or any of its derivatives should discuss this with their doctor or pharmacist before using this drug.

PREGNANCY/BREAST-FEEDING: Category C—Risk cannot be ruled out. Human studies are lacking, and animal studies are either positive for fetal risk or lacking as well. However, potential benefits may justify the potential risk in using the drug. The drug is excreted in the breast milk; therefore, extreme caution should be used when breast-feeding.

OTHER BRAND NAMES: Isoptin and Isoptin SR

OTHER DRUGS IN THE SAME THERAPEUTIC CLASS: Adalat, Adalat CC, Cardene, Cardene SR, Cardizem, Cardizem SR, Cardizem CD, Covera-HS, Dilacor XR, DynaCirc, Norvasc, Plendil, Procardia, Procardia XL, Sular, Vascor, and Verelan

IMPORTANT INFORMATION TO REMEMBER: This drug should be taken with food or milk. Only take the drug exactly as directed by your physician. Do not discontinue the drug without first consulting your physician. Before taking over-the-counter cold and allergy preparations, consult your doctor or pharmacist; these products may raise your blood pressure. Do not crush the sustained-release tablets. They can, however, be cut in half at the line in the center of the tablet. Swallow the tablets or half tablets whole. This drug may cause some tiredness at first—individuals should use caution when driving, operating machinery, or any task where mental alertness is required.

BRAND NAME: Capoten

GENERIC NAME: captopril

GENERIC FORM AVAILABLE: Yes

THERAPEUTIC CLASS: ACE inhibitor

DOSAGE FORMS: 12.5-mg, 25-mg, 50-mg, and 100-mg tablets

MAIN USES: High blood pressure, heart failure, and prevention of kidney failure in some diabetics

USUAL DOSE: 12.5 mg to 150 mg two or three times daily for high blood pressure, 50 mg to 100 mg three times daily for heart failure, and 25 mg three times daily to prevent kidney failure

AVERAGE PRICE: $93.92 (B)/$84.42 (G) for 12.5 mg; $101.54 (B)/ 91.28 (G) for 25 mg; $174.13 (B)/156.54 (G) for 50 mg; $231.88 (B)/208.46 (G) for 100 mg tablets

SIDE EFFECTS: rash 4%–7%, slight loss of taste 2%–4%, itching 2%, cough 1%–2%, nausea 1%–2%, diarrhea 1%–2%, headache 1%–2%, dizziness 1%–2%, tiredness 1%–2%, insomnia 1%–2%, chest pain 1%, fast heartbeat 1%, and palpitations 1%.

DRUG INTERACTIONS: May decrease the absorption of the anti- biotic Sumycin and other tetracyclines. High potassium levels may occur when used together with Dyrenium and Aldactone and potassium supplements such as Micro-K, K-Dur, Klor-Con, K-Lyte, and Slow-K. Patients on water pills, especially those re- cently started on a water pill, may experience low blood pres- sure. The drug may also increase the toxic effects of Eskalith and Lithobid, especially when taken with a water pill.

ALLERGIES: Individuals allergic to captopril or other ACE in- hibitors (such as those listed in "Other Drugs in the Same Thera- peutic Class") should discuss this with their doctor or pharmacist before using this drug.

PREGNANCY/BREAST-FEEDING: Category C (first trimester)—Risk cannot be ruled out. Human studies are lacking, and animal studies are either positive for fetal risk or lacking as well. However, po- tential benefits may justify the potential risk in using the drug. Category D (second and third trimesters)—Positive evidence of risk. Human studies show risk to the fetus. Nevertheless, potential benefits may possibly outweigh the potential risk. This drug should not be taken by nursing mothers.

OTHER BRAND NAMES: None

OTHER DRUGS IN THE SAME THERAPEUTIC CLASS: Accupril, Al- tace, Lotensin, Mavik, Monopril, Prinivil, Univasc, Vasotec, and Zestril

IMPORTANT INFORMATION TO REMEMBER: It's best to take the drug on an empty stomach—one hour before meals or two hours after meals—if possible. Take this drug regularly and exactly as directed by your physician. Do not stop taking the drug unless otherwise directed by your doctor. Avoid salt substitutes contain- ing potassium. Before taking over-the-counter cold and allergy preparations, consult your doctor or pharmacist—these products may raise your blood pressure. If you experience swelling of the face, lips, or tongue or difficulty in breathing, contact your doctor immediately.

BRAND NAME: Capozide

GENERIC NAME: Combination product containing: captopril and hydrochlorothiazide

See individual entries for Capoten and HydroDIURIL

BRAND NAME: Carafate

GENERIC NAME: sucralfate

GENERIC FORM AVAILABLE: Yes

THERAPEUTIC CLASS: Anti-ulcer stomach and intestine protectant

DOSAGE FORMS: 1-g tablets and 1 g/10 mL suspension

MAIN USES: Treatment and prevention of ulcers

USUAL DOSE: one tablet four times daily for treatment of an active ulcer and one tablet twice daily for prevention

AVERAGE PRICE: $103.169 (B)/$89.79 (G) for 1-g tablets

SIDE EFFECTS: constipation 2%; diarrhea, dry mouth, gas, headache, back pain, dizziness, nausea, vomiting, and stomach upset all occur in less than 1%.

DRUG INTERACTIONS: The drug may decrease the absorption of Cipro, Dilantin, Floxin, Lanoxin, Noroxin, Slo-bid, Sumycin, Synthroid, Tagamet, Theo-Dur, theophylline, Uni-Dur, Uniphyl, and Zantac. These drugs should be taken two hours before Carafate is taken. Antacids should not be taken within a half hour of taking this drug.

ALLERGIES: Individuals allergic to sucralfate or any of its derivatives should discuss this with their doctor or pharmacist before using this drug.

PREGNANCY/BREAST-FEEDING: Category B—No evidence of risk in humans. Either animal findings show risk, but human findings do not; or, if no adequate human studies have been done, animal findings show no risk. It is not known whether the drug is excreted in the breast milk; therefore, caution should be used when breast-feeding.

OTHER BRAND NAMES: None

OTHER DRUGS IN THE SAME THERAPEUTIC CLASS: None

IMPORTANT INFORMATION TO REMEMBER: It's best to take the drug on an empty stomach—one hour before meals or two hours after meals—if possible. Antacids should not be taken within a half hour of taking this drug. If using the suspension, shake the medication well.

BRAND NAME: Cardene

GENERIC NAME: nicardipine

GENERIC FORM AVAILABLE: Yes (capsules only)

THERAPEUTIC CLASS: Calcium channel blocker

DOSAGE FORMS: 20-mg and 30-mg capsules; 30-mg, 45-mg, and 60-mg sustained-release capsules

MAIN USES: Angina and high blood pressure

USUAL DOSE: 20 mg to 40 mg three times daily of regular capsules for angina and high blood pressure, and 30 mg to 60 mg twice daily of the sustained-release capsules for high blood pressure

AVERAGE PRICE: $61.05 (B)/$43.49 (G) for 20 mg; $97.09 (B)/$66.29 (G) for 30 mg; $95.36 for 30 mg SR; $151.91 for 45 mg SR; and $181.30 for 60 mg SR

SIDE EFFECTS: foot swelling 8%, headache 6%–8%, flushing 5%–9%, dizziness 4%–7%, weakness 4%–6%, pounding heartbeat 3%–4%, nausea 2%, fast heartbeat 1%–3%, upset stomach 1%–2%, nervousness 1%, and tiredness 1%.

DRUG INTERACTIONS: Tagamet may increase blood levels of the drug. The drug may increase the blood levels of Lanoxin and Sandimmune. Fentanyl and this drug may cause low blood pressure.

ALLERGIES: Individuals allergic to nicardipine or any of its derivatives should discuss this with their doctor or pharmacist before using this drug.

PREGNANCY/BREAST-FEEDING: Category C—Risk cannot be ruled out. Human studies are lacking, and animal studies are either positive for fetal risk or lacking as well. However, potential benefits may justify the potential risk in using the drug. It is not known

whether the drug is excreted in the breast milk; therefore, caution should be used when breast-feeding.

OTHER BRAND NAMES: None

OTHER DRUGS IN THE SAME THERAPEUTIC CLASS: Adalat, Adalat CC, Calan, Calan SR, Cardizem, Cardizem SR, Cardizem CD, Covera-HS, Dilacor XR, DynaCirc, Isoptin, Isoptin SR, Norvasc, Plendil, Procardia, Procardia XL, Sular, Vascor, and Verelan

IMPORTANT INFORMATION TO REMEMBER: Only take the drug exactly as directed by your physician. Do not discontinue the drug without first consulting your physician. Before taking over-the-counter cold and allergy preparations, consult your doctor or pharmacist—these products may raise your blood pressure. This drug may cause some tiredness at first. Individuals should use caution when driving, operating machinery, or any task where mental alertness is required.

BRAND NAME: Cardizem, Cardizem SR, and Cardizem CD

GENERIC NAME: diltiazem

GENERIC FORM AVAILABLE: Yes (not for Cardizem CD)

THERAPEUTIC CLASS: Calcium channel blocker

DOSAGE FORMS: Cardizem: 30-mg, 60-mg, 90-mg, and 120-mg tablets; Cardizem SR: 60-mg, 90-mg, and 120-mg sustained-release capsules; and Cardizem CD: 120-mg, 180-mg, 240-mg, and 300-mg sustained-release capsules

MAIN USES: Angina and high blood pressure

USUAL DOSE: 180 mg to 360 mg per day in three or four divided doses for angina, and 240 mg to 360 mg per day in one or two divided doses for high blood pressure

AVERAGE PRICE: $51.67 (B)/$28.57 (G) for 30 mg; $79.17 (B)/$35.17 (G) for 60 mg; $120.97 (B)/$49.47 (G) for 90 mg; $95.67 (B)/$80.27 (G) for Cardizem SR 60 mg; $116.57 (B)/$91.27 (G) for Cardizem SR 90 mg; $124.27 (B)/$102.94 (G) for Cardizem SR 120 mg; $142.80 for Cardizem CD 120 mg; $171.69 for Cardizem CD 180 mg; $244.02 for Cardizem CD 240 mg; $314.58 for Cardizem CD 300 mg

SIDE EFFECTS: headache 5%–12%, dizziness 3%–7%, slow heartbeat 3%–6%, first degree AV block 3%–8%, swelling 3%–6%, abnormal ECG 2%–4%, tiredness 2%–3%, constipation 2%, difficulty breathing 1%, palpitations 1%, and insomnia 1%.

DRUG INTERACTIONS: The effects of Blocadren, Cartrol, Corgard, Inderal, Kerlone, Levatol, Lopressor, Minipress, Normodyne, Norpace, Sectral, Tenormin, Toprol-XL, Trandate, Visken, and Zebeta may be increased when taken with this drug. The drug may increase the blood levels of Tegretol, Sandimmune, Lanoxin, Quinidez, Quinaglute, and Procan. Tagamet may increase the blood levels of the drug.

ALLERGIES: Individuals allergic to diltiazem or any of its derivatives should discuss this with their doctor or pharmacist before using this drug.

PREGNANCY/BREAST-FEEDING: Category C—Risk cannot be ruled out. Human studies are lacking, and animal studies are either positive for fetal risk or lacking as well. However, potential benefits may justify the potential risk in using the drug. The drug is excreted in the breast milk; therefore, extreme caution should be used when breast-feeding.

OTHER BRAND NAMES: None

OTHER DRUGS IN THE SAME THERAPEUTIC CLASS: Adalat, Adalat CC, Calan, Calan SR, Cardene, Cardene SR, Covera-HS, Dilacor XR, DynaCirc, Isoptin, Isoptin SR, Norvasc, Plendil, Procardia, Procardia XL, Sular, Vascor, and Verelan

IMPORTANT INFORMATION TO REMEMBER: Only take the drug exactly as directed by your physician. Do not discontinue the drug without first consulting your physician. Before taking over-the-counter cold and allergy preparations, consult your doctor or pharmacist—these products may raise your blood pressure. This drug may cause some tiredness at first. Individuals should use caution when driving, operating machinery, or any task where mental alertness is required.

BRAND NAME: Cardura

GENERIC NAME: doxazosin

GENERIC FORM AVAILABLE: No

THERAPEUTIC CLASS: Selective alpha-one-blood-vessel dilator

DOSAGE FORMS: 1-mg, 2-mg, 4-mg, and 8-mg tablets

MAIN USES: High blood pressure and benign prostatic hyperplasia (BPH)

USUAL DOSE: 1 mg to 16 mg once daily

AVERAGE PRICE: $128.49 for 1 mg and 2 mg; $139.89 for 4 mg; and $149.88 for 8 mg

SIDE EFFECTS: dizziness 19%, tiredness 12%, headache 14%, swelling 4%, nausea 3%, runny nose 3%, pounding heartbeat 2%, abnormal vision 2%, impotence 2%, nervousness 2%, diarrhea 2%, irregular heartbeat 1%, muscle pain, cramps or weakness 1%, and low blood pressure 1%.

DRUG INTERACTIONS: Caution should be used when this drug is taken with other drugs for high blood pressure; the combination may cause blood pressure to go too low.

ALLERGIES: Individuals allergic to doxazosin or any of its derivatives should discuss this with their doctor or pharmacist before using this drug.

PREGNANCY/BREAST-FEEDING: Category C—Risk cannot be ruled out. Human studies are lacking, and animal studies are either positive for fetal risk or lacking as well. However, potential benefits may justify the potential risk in using the drug. It is not known whether the drug is excreted in the breast milk; therefore, caution should be used when breast-feeding.

OTHER BRAND NAMES: None

OTHER DRUGS IN THE SAME THERAPEUTIC CLASS: Hytrin and Minipress

IMPORTANT INFORMATION TO REMEMBER: The first dose should be taken at bedtime to avoid dizziness and fainting. Only take the drug exactly as directed by your physician. Do not discontinue the drug without first consulting your physician. Before taking over-the-counter cold and allergy preparations, consult your doctor or pharmacist—these products may raise your blood pressure. This drug may cause some drowsiness at first. Individuals should use caution when driving, operating machinery, or any task where mental alertness is required. Individuals should get up slowly from a sitting or lying-down position, otherwise dizziness may occur.

BRAND NAME: Cartrol

GENERIC NAME: carteolol

GENERIC FORM AVAILABLE: No

THERAPEUTIC CLASS: Noncardioselective beta-blocker

DOSAGE FORMS: 2.5-mg and 5-mg tablets

MAIN USES: High blood pressure

USUAL DOSE: 2.5 mg to 10 mg once daily

AVERAGE PRICE: $143.05 for 2.5 mg and $162.47 for 5 mg

SIDE EFFECTS: tiredness 7%, muscle cramps 3%, chest pain 2%, insomnia 2%, tingling sensation 2%, back pain 2%, nausea 2%, and diarrhea 2%.

DRUG INTERACTIONS: The drug may increase the effects of reserpine. The drug may increase the effects of Calan, Cardene, Cardizem, Catapres, Dilacor XR, DynaCirc, Isoptin, Lanoxin, Norvasc, Plendil, Procardia, Sular, Tiazac, Verelan, and Wytensin. Diabetic medications, insulin, Slo-bid, Theo-Dur, theophylline, Uni-Dur, and Uniphyl dosages may need to be adjusted when taking this drug.

ALLERGIES: Individuals allergic to carteolol or other beta-blockers (such as those listed in "Other Drugs in the Same Therapeutic Class") should discuss this with their doctor or pharmacist before taking this drug.

PREGNANCY/BREAST-FEEDING: Category C—Risk cannot be ruled out. Human studies are lacking, and animal studies are either positive for fetal risk or lacking as well. However, potential benefits may justify the potential risk in using the drug. It is not known whether the drug is excreted in the breast milk; therefore, caution should be used when breast-feeding.

OTHER BRAND NAMES: None

OTHER DRUGS IN THE SAME THERAPEUTIC CLASS: Blocadren, Corgard, Inderal, Levatol, Normodyne, Trandate, and Visken

IMPORTANT INFORMATION TO REMEMBER: Only take the drug exactly as directed by your physician. Do not discontinue the drug without first consulting your physician. This drug may cause some tiredness, especially at first. Individuals should use caution when driving, operating machinery, or any task where mental alertness is required. Alcohol or central nervous system depressants may intensify the tiredness effect of the drug. Before taking over-the-counter cold and allergy preparations, consult your doctor or pharmacist—these products may raise your blood pressure. This drug may mask the symptoms of low blood sugar in diabetics.

BRAND NAME: Casodex

GENERIC NAME: bicalutamide

GENERIC FORM AVAILABLE: No

THERAPEUTIC CLASS: Anti-androgen, anticancer

DOSAGE FORMS: 50-mg tablets

MAIN USES: Prostate cancer

USUAL DOSE: 50 mg daily

AVERAGE PRICE: $430.50 for 30 tablets

SIDE EFFECTS: hot flashes 49%, breast pain 39%, enlarged breasts 38%, general pain 27%, constipation 17%, back pain 15%, weakness 15%, pelvic pain 13%, nausea 11%, and diarrhea 10%. Other less common side effects may include headache and swelling of the feet, legs, and ankles.

DRUG INTERACTIONS: The drug may increase the blood levels of Coumadin.

ALLERGIES: Individuals allergic to bicalutamide or any of its derivatives should discuss this with their doctor or pharmacist before using this drug.

PREGNANCY/BREAST-FEEDING: Category X—Should not be used during pregnancy. Studies in animals and/or humans have shown fetal abnormalities and birth defects. The risks associated with using this drug clearly outweigh the benefits. This drug should never be used by someone who is pregnant or trying to become pregnant. Also, women should never breast-feed while using this drug.

OTHER BRAND NAMES: None

OTHER DRUGS IN THE SAME THERAPEUTIC CLASS: Eulexin

IMPORTANT INFORMATION TO REMEMBER: Only take the drug exactly as directed by your physician. Do not discontinue the drug without first consulting with your physician. Also, take the drug at the same time every day. If stomach upset occurs, take the drug with food or milk.

BRAND NAME: Cataflam

GENERIC NAME: diclofenac potassium

GENERIC FORM AVAILABLE: No

THERAPEUTIC CLASS: Nonsteroidal anti-inflammatory drug (NSAID)

DOSAGE FORMS: 50 mg tablets

MAIN USES: Arthritis, pain relief, and menstrual pain

USUAL DOSE: 50 mg two to four times daily

AVERAGE PRICE: $198.75

SIDE EFFECTS: headache 7%, stomach pain 3%–9%, upset stomach 3%–9%, diarrhea 3%–9%, indigestion 3%–9%, constipation 3%–9%, peptic ulcer 1%–3%, stomach swelling 1%–3%, gas 1%–3%, rash 1%–3%, dizziness 3%, and ringing in the ears 1%–3%.

DRUG INTERACTIONS: Aspirin will decrease the concentration of this drug in the blood. This drug may also decrease the effects of Lasix, Dyazide, HydroDIURIL, Maxzide, and other water pills. The drug may increase the blood levels of Eskalith, Lithobid, and Sandimmune. The drug may increase the toxic effects of the drug Rheumatrex. Caution should be used when taking the drug with Coumadin.

ALLERGIES: Individuals allergic to diclofenac or other NSAIDs (such as those listed in "Other Drugs in the Same Therapeutic Class") should discuss this with their doctor or pharmacist before taking this drug.

PREGNANCY/BREAST-FEEDING: Category B—No evidence of risk in humans. Either animal findings show risk, but human findings do not; or, if no adequate human studies have been done, animal findings show no risk. The drug should not, however, be used in late stages (last three months) of pregnancy. The drug is excreted in the breast milk; therefore, extreme caution should be used when breast-feeding.

OTHER BRAND NAMES: None

OTHER DRUGS IN THE SAME THERAPEUTIC CLASS: Anaprox, Ansaid, aspirin, Clinoril, Daypro, Disalcid, Dolobid, Easprin, Feldene, Indocin, Lodine, Lodine XL, Motrin, Nalfon, Naprosyn, Orudis, Oruvail, Relafen, Tolectin, Toradol, Voltaren, and Voltaren XR

IMPORTANT INFORMATION TO REMEMBER: This drug should be taken with food or milk to reduce the potential for injury to the stomach lining and stomach upset. The tablets should not be crushed; they should be swallowed whole. This drug may take up to two weeks before a noticeable improvement in pain relief associated with arthritis is observed. Drinking alcohol while taking this drug may increase its potential to cause ulcers. This drug should only be used under the direct supervision of a doctor by individuals with a bleeding disorder or ulcer, or those who are currently taking Coumadin. Before taking over-the-counter pain relievers, consult your doctor or pharmacist. No more than one pain reliever should be taken at any one time unless otherwise directed by your doctor.

BRAND NAME: Catapres and Catapres TTS Patches

GENERIC NAME: clonidine

GENERIC FORM AVAILABLE: Yes for tablets

THERAPEUTIC CLASS: Central-acting blood vessel dilator

DOSAGE FORMS: 0.1-mg, 0.2-mg, and 0.3-mg tablets; and 0.1 mg/24 hr, 0.2 mg/24 hr, and 0.3 mg/24 hr skin patches

MAIN USES: High blood pressure and {attention deficit disorder (ADD)}

USUAL DOSE: Tablets: 0.1 mg–0.8 mg per day in divided doses. Transdermal patch: one 0.1 mg–0.3 mg patch weekly.

AVERAGE PRICE: $89.10 (B)/$26.36 (G) for 0.1-mg tablets; $130.90 (B)/$30.52 (G) for 0.2-mg tablets; $137.50 (B)/$40.60 (G) for 0.3-mg tablets; $47.02 for four 0.1-mg patches; $75.55 for four 0.2-mg patches; and $103.68 for four 0.3-mg patches

SIDE EFFECTS: For the tablets: dry mouth 40%, drowsiness 34%, dizziness 16%, constipation 10%, weakness 10%, nausea 5%, decreased sex drive 3%, impotence 3%, nervousness 3%, depression

1%, headache 1%, and rash 1%. For the patches: dry mouth 25%, drowsiness 12%, slight itching at the site of application 50%, skin redness at the site of application 25% (these two can be reduced by not using the adhesive overlay), tiredness 6%, headache 5%, insomnia 2%, dizziness 2%, and impotence 2%.

DRUG INTERACTIONS: Blood pressure control may be decreased when used with Elavil, Endep, Norpramin, Pamelor, Sinequan, Surmontil, Tofranil, or Vivactil. If the drug is used with a beta-blocker (Calan, Cardene, Cardizem, Catapres, Dilacor XR, DynaCirc, Isoptin, Norvasc, Plendil, Procardia, Sular, Tiazac, or Verelan) and one of the two is discontinued, dangerous increases in blood pressure may occur.

ALLERGIES: Individuals allergic to clonidine or any of its derivatives should discuss this with their doctor or pharmacist before using this drug.

PREGNANCY/BREAST-FEEDING: Category C—Risk cannot be ruled out. Human studies are lacking, and animal studies are either positive for fetal risk or lacking as well. However, potential benefits may justify the potential risk in using the drug. The drug is excreted in the breast milk; therefore, extreme caution should be used when breast-feeding.

OTHER BRAND NAMES: None

OTHER DRUGS IN THE SAME THERAPEUTIC CLASS: Aldomet

IMPORTANT INFORMATION TO REMEMBER: The drug may cause drowsiness, especially when treatment is begun or daily dosage is increased. To minimize this effect, start dosage increases in the evening. Drowsiness usually goes away once the body adjusts to the medication. Before taking over-the-counter cold and allergy preparations, consult your doctor or pharmacist—These products may raise your blood pressure. If stomach upset occurs, take with food or milk. Do not discontinue taking the drug without first consulting with your physician, due to potential for high blood pressure to reoccur.

When using the patches:

1) Do not cut or fold the patch in half. This may cause the medication inside to leak out.
2) Apply the patch to a clean, dry skin area on the upper arm or torso. This area should be free of hair, cuts, scars, or irritation.

3) Leave the patch on even during swimming, showering, and exercising. If the patch falls off, replace the patch with a new one.
4) When it's time to apply a new patch, use a different site on the skin. Rotate the sites where you apply the patches every time.
5) Get into the habit of applying the patch at the same time each week.
6) Dispose of used patches properly and keep out of reach of children.

BRAND NAME: Ceclor and Ceclor CD

GENERIC NAME: cefaclor

GENERIC FORM AVAILABLE: Yes (Ceclor only)

THERAPEUTIC CLASS: Cephalosporin antibiotic

DOSAGE FORMS: 250-mg and 500-mg capsules; 125 mg/5 mL, 187 mg/5 mL, 250 mg/5 mL, and 375 mg/5 mL oral suspensions; and 500-mg extended-release tablets

MAIN USES: Bacterial infections

USUAL DOSE: 250 mg to 500 mg every 8 hours; 500 mg every 12 hours (Ceclor CD)

AVERAGE PRICE: $80.28 (B)/$62.61 (G) for 250 mg (30 capsules); $148.95 (B)/$122.62 (G) for 500 mg (30 capsules); and $75.90 for 500 mg extended-release tablets (Ceclor CD)

SIDE EFFECTS: nausea 3%, diarrhea 3%, yeast infections 1%, and rash 1%.

DRUG INTERACTIONS: The drug may decrease the effectiveness of oral contraceptives used for birth control. Women may become pregnant while taking Ceclor and oral contraceptives. The drug probenecid will decrease elimination of the drug by the kidneys.

ALLERGIES: Individuals allergic to cefaclor, Amoxil, Omnipen, penicillin, or other cephalosporins (such as those listed in "Other Drugs in the Same Therapeutic Class") should discuss this with their doctor or pharmacist before taking this drug.

PREGNANCY/BREAST-FEEDING: Category B—No evidence of risk in humans. Either animal findings show risk, but human findings do not; or, if no adequate human studies have been done, animal findings show no risk. The drug is excreted in the breast milk; therefore, caution should be used when breast-feeding.

OTHER BRAND NAMES: None

OTHER DRUGS IN THE SAME THERAPEUTIC CLASS: Cedax, Ceftin, Cefzil, Duricef, Keflex, Keftab, Suprax, Ultracef, Vantin, and Velosef

IMPORTANT INFORMATION TO REMEMBER: If stomach upset occurs, take with food or milk. Also, take the drug at even intervals around the clock (if three times a day, take every eight hours). Take the drug until all the medication prescribed is gone; otherwise the infection may return. Women taking birth control pills should use another form of contraception while taking the drug and for the rest of the current menstrual cycle. Individuals taking the liquid form should shake it thoroughly before use, store the medication in the refrigerator, and discard any remaining medication after 14 days. The drug may produce a false positive for some glucose and protein urine tests.

BRAND NAME: Cedax

GENERIC NAME: ceftibuten

GENERIC FORM AVAILABLE: No

THERAPEUTIC CLASS: Cephalosporin antibiotic

DOSAGE FORMS: 400-mg capsules and 90 mg/5 mL and 180 mg/ 5 mL oral suspensions

MAIN USES: Bacterial infections

USUAL DOSE: 400 mg once daily

AVERAGE PRICE: $139.96 for 400 mg (20 capsules)

SIDE EFFECTS: nausea 4%, headache 3%, diarrhea 3%, dizziness 1%, stomach pain 1%, and vomiting 1%.

DRUG INTERACTIONS: The drug may decrease the effectiveness of oral contraceptives used for birth control. Women may become pregnant while taking Ceclor and oral contraceptives. The drug probenecid will decrease elimination of the drug by the kidneys.

ALLERGIES: Individuals allergic to ceftibuten, Amoxil, Omnipen, penicillin, or other cephalosporins (such as those listed in "Other Drugs in the Same Therapeutic Class") should discuss this with their doctor or pharmacist before taking this drug.

PREGNANCY/BREAST-FEEDING: Category B—No evidence of risk in humans. Either animal findings show risk, but human findings do not; or, if no adequate human studies have been done, animal findings show no risk. The drug is excreted in the breast milk; therefore, caution should be used when breast-feeding.

OTHER BRAND NAMES: None

OTHER DRUGS IN THE SAME THERAPEUTIC CLASS: Ceclor, Ceftin, Cefzil, Duricef, Keflex, Keftab, Suprax, Ultracef, Vantin, and Velosef

IMPORTANT INFORMATION TO REMEMBER: The tablets may be taken with or without food or milk. The suspension (oral liquid) must be taken at least two hours before a meal or one hour after a meal. Also, take the drug at approximately the same time every day. Take the drug until all the medication prescribed is gone; otherwise the infection may return. Women taking birth control pills should use another form of contraception while taking the drug and for the rest of the current menstrual cycle. Individuals taking the liquid form should shake it thoroughly before use, store the medication in the refrigerator, and discard any remaining medication after 14 days. The drug may produce a false positive for some glucose and protein urine tests.

BRAND NAME: Ceftin

GENERIC NAME: cefuroxime

GENERIC FORM AVAILABLE: No

THERAPEUTIC CLASS: Cephalosporin antibiotic

DOSAGE FORMS: 125-mg, 250-mg, and 500-mg tablets; and 125 mg/5 mL oral suspension

MAIN USES: Bacterial infections

USUAL DOSE: 125 mg to 500 mg every 12 hours

AVERAGE PRICE: $94.69 for 250 mg (20 tablets) and $179.66 for 500 mg (20 tablets)

SIDE EFFECTS: diarrhea 4%, nausea 3%, stomach pain 1%, gas 1%, and rash 1%.

DRUG INTERACTIONS: The drug may decrease the effectiveness of oral contraceptives used for birth control. Women may become pregnant while taking Ceftin and oral contraceptives. The drug probenecid will decrease elimination of the drug by the kidneys.

ALLERGIES: Individuals allergic to cefuroxime, Amoxil, Omnipen, penicillin, or other cephalosporins (such as those listed in "Other Drugs in the Same Therapeutic Class") should discuss this with their doctor or pharmacist before taking this drug.

PREGNANCY/BREAST-FEEDING: Category B—No evidence of risk in humans. Either animal findings show risk, but human findings do not; or, if no adequate human studies have been done, animal findings show no risk. The drug is excreted in the breast milk; therefore, caution should be used when breast-feeding.

OTHER BRAND NAMES: None

OTHER DRUGS IN THE SAME THERAPEUTIC CLASS: Ceclor, Cedax, Cefzil, Duricef, Keflex, Keftab, Suprax, Ultracef, Vantin, and Velosef

IMPORTANT INFORMATION TO REMEMBER: The drug should be taken with food or milk to increase the absorption of the drug. Also, take the drug at even intervals around the clock (if two times a day, take every 12 hours). Take the drug until all the medication prescribed is gone; otherwise the infection may return. Women taking birth control pills should use another form of contraception while taking the drug and for the rest of the current menstrual cycle. Individuals taking the liquid form should shake it thoroughly before use, store the medication in the refrigerator, and discard any remaining medication after 14 days. The drug may produce a false positive for some glucose and protein urine tests or a false negative for blood glucose in tests using ferricyanide.

BRAND NAME: Cefzil

GENERIC NAME: cefprozil

GENERIC FORM AVAILABLE: No

THERAPEUTIC CLASS: Cephalosporin antibiotic

DOSAGE FORMS: 250-mg and 500-mg tablets; 125 mg/5 mL and 250 mg/5 mL oral suspensions

MAIN USES: Bacterial infections

USUAL DOSE: 250 mg to 500 mg one to two times daily

AVERAGE PRICE: $80.51 for 250 mg (20 tablets) and $156.80 for 500 mg (20 tablets)

SIDE EFFECTS: nausea 4%, diarrhea 3%, diaper rash 2%, yeast infection 2%, vomiting 1%, stomach pain 1%, and rash 1%.

DRUG INTERACTIONS: The drug may decrease the effectiveness of oral contraceptives used for birth control. Women may become pregnant while taking Cefzil and oral contraceptives. The drug probenecid will decrease elimination of the drug by the kidneys.

ALLERGIES: Individuals allergic to cefprozil, Amoxil, Omnipen, penicillin, or other cephalosporins (such as those listed in "Other Drugs in the Same Therapeutic Class") should discuss this with their doctor or pharmacist before taking this drug.

PREGNANCY/BREAST-FEEDING: Category B—No evidence of risk in humans. Either animal findings show risk, but human findings do not; or, if no adequate human studies have been done, animal findings show no risk. The drug is excreted in the breast milk; therefore, caution should be used when breast-feeding.

OTHER BRAND NAMES: None

OTHER DRUGS IN THE SAME THERAPEUTIC CLASS: Ceclor, Ceftin, Cedax, Duricef, Keflex, Keftab, Suprax, Ultracef, Vantin, and Velosef

IMPORTANT INFORMATION TO REMEMBER: If stomach upset occurs, take with food or milk. Also, take the drug at even intervals around the clock (if two times a day, take every 12 hours). Take the drug until all the medication prescribed is gone; otherwise the infection may return. Women taking birth control pills should use another form of contraception while taking the drug and for the rest of the current menstrual cycle. Individuals taking the liquid form should shake it thoroughly before use, store the medication in the refrigerator, and discard any remaining medication after 14 days.

BRAND NAME: Cephulac

GENERIC NAME: lactulose

See entry for Chronulac

<u>BRAND NAME:</u> **Chibroxin**

GENERIC NAME: norfloxacin

GENERIC FORM AVAILABLE: No

THERAPEUTIC CLASS: Quinolone antibiotic

DOSAGE FORMS: 0.3% eyedrop solution

MAIN USES: Bacterial eye infections

USUAL DOSE: one to two drops four times daily

AVERAGE PRICE: $25.29 for 5 mL

SIDE EFFECTS: Most common: None. Less common: slight burning, stinging, itching, skin rash, and allergic reaction.

DRUG INTERACTIONS: None of any clinical significance

ALLERGIES: Individuals allergic to norfloxacin, Ciloxan, Noroxin, Ocuflox, or any of their derivatives should discuss this with their doctor or pharmacist before using this drug.

PREGNANCY/BREAST-FEEDING: Category C—Risk cannot be ruled out. Human studies are lacking, and animal studies are either positive for fetal risk or lacking as well. However, potential benefits may justify the potential risk in using the drug. It is not known whether the drug is excreted in the breast milk; therefore, caution should be used when breast-feeding.

OTHER BRAND NAMES: None

OTHER DRUGS IN THE SAME THERAPEUTIC CLASS: Ciloxan and Ocuflox

IMPORTANT INFORMATION TO REMEMBER: Use the drug for the full course of therapy, even if symptoms disappear; otherwise the infection may return. Use the drug at even intervals around the clock (if four times a day, use every six hours). Keep the container tightly closed and avoid touching the applicator tip to the eye—this could contaminate the product over time. Also, only administer one drop at a time. After application, keep the eye open for at least 30 seconds, roll the eyeball around, and avoid squinting. If a second drop is required, wait one to two minutes between drops. If another medication is to be used in the eye, wait at least 10 minutes before administering it.

BRAND NAME: **Choledyl and Choledyl SA**

GENERIC NAME: oxtriphylline

GENERIC FORM AVAILABLE: Yes (200-mg tablets only)

THERAPEUTIC CLASS: Xanthine bronchodilator

DOSAGE FORMS: 200-mg tablets, and 400-mg and 600-mg sustained-release tablets

MAIN USES: Asthma, chronic bronchitis, emphysema, and {other breathing disorders}

USUAL DOSE: 200 mg to 1200 mg daily in divided doses

AVERAGE PRICE: $50.24 for 400 mg and $61.26 for 600 mg

SIDE EFFECTS: Most common: nausea, nervousness, fast heartbeat, and restlessness. Less common: vomiting, diarrhea, stomach pain, headaches, irritability, insomnia, muscle twitching, pounding heartbeat, fast breathing, flushing, and low blood pressure.

DRUG INTERACTIONS: The drug may inhibit the effects of Blocadren, Cartrol, Corgard, Inderal, Kerlone, Levatol, Lopressor, Normodyne, Sectral, Tenormin, Toprol-XL, Trandate, Visken, and Zebeta. Dilantin, Tegretol, smoking, and nicotine patches may lower the blood levels of this drug. Cipro, Noroxin, Tagamet, Zantac, erythromycin, and TAO may increase blood levels of the drug. Individuals who stop smoking while taking the drug may have increased levels of the drug in the blood.

ALLERGIES: Individuals allergic to oxtriphylline, theophylline, or other xanthines (such as those listed in "Other Drugs in the Same Therapeutic Class") should discuss this with their doctor or pharmacist before taking this drug.

PREGNANCY/BREAST-FEEDING: Category C—Risk cannot be ruled out. Human studies are lacking, and animal studies are either positive for fetal risk or lacking as well. However, potential benefits may justify the potential risk in using the drug. The drug is excreted in the breast milk; therefore, extreme caution should be used when breast-feeding.

OTHER BRAND NAMES: None

OTHER DRUGS IN THE SAME THERAPEUTIC CLASS: aminophylline, Elixophyllin, Lufyllin, Quibron SR, Quibron T, Respbid, Slo-bid, Slo-Phyllin, Theo-24, Theo-Dur, Theo-X, Uni-Dur, and Uniphyl

IMPORTANT INFORMATION TO REMEMBER: Only take the drug exactly as directed by your physician. Do not discontinue the drug without first consulting your physician. Do not increase the dose without first consulting with your physician. This drug should be taken with plenty of water (eight ounces is preferred). Do not crush or divide the sustained-release (labeled SA) tablets—this will destroy the mechanism that slowly releases the drug into the bloodstream. Swallow the tablets whole. If stomach upset occurs, take with food or milk. Do not change between brand and generic once you are stabilized on one or the other.

BRAND NAME: Chronulac

GENERIC NAME: lactulose

GENERIC FORM AVAILABLE: Yes

THERAPEUTIC CLASS: Osmotic laxative

DOSAGE FORMS: 10 g/15 mL syrup

MAIN USES: Constipation, (prevention of bowel impactions), and (encephalopathy)

USUAL DOSE: 15 mL to 30 mL daily

AVERAGE PRICE: $29.04 (B)/$19.83 (G) for 240 mL

SIDE EFFECTS: Most common: none. Less common: gas, stomach cramps, nausea, and diarrhea.

DRUG INTERACTIONS: The effects of the drug may be decreased if taken with antacids.

ALLERGIES: Individuals allergic to lactulose or any of its derivatives should discuss this with their doctor or pharmacist before using this drug.

PREGNANCY/BREAST-FEEDING: Category B—No evidence of risk in humans. Either animal findings show risk, but human findings do not; or, if no adequate human studies have been done, animal findings show no risk. It is not known whether the drug is excreted in the breast milk; therefore, caution should be used when breast-feeding.

OTHER BRAND NAMES: Duphalac and Constilac

OTHER DRUGS IN THE SAME THERAPEUTIC CLASS: None

IMPORTANT INFORMATION TO REMEMBER: The syrup may be mixed with fruit juice, water, or milk. This drug should be taken with plenty of water (eight ounces is preferred). The drug may take 24–48 hours to work. Only take the drug exactly as directed by your physician. Do not increase the dose without first consulting with your physician. Due to galactose and lactose content, diabetics should use this drug with caution.

BRAND NAME: Ciloxan

GENERIC BRAND: ciprofloxacin

GENERIC FORM AVAILABLE: No

THERAPEUTIC CLASS: Quinolone antibiotic

DOSAGE FORMS: 0.3% eyedrop solution

MAIN USES: Bacterial eye infections and corneal ulcers

USUAL DOSE: Corneal ulcers: instill one to two drops in the affected eye every 15 minutes for the first six hours, then one to two drops every 30 minutes for the remainder of the first day. On the second day, instill one to two drops hourly. On the 3rd through the 14th days, instill one to two drops every four hours. Bacterial infections: one to two drops every two hours while awake for two days, then one to two drops every four hours while awake for the next five days.

AVERAGE PRICE: $30.64 for 5 mL

SIDE EFFECTS: slight burning and stinging 10%, crusty eyelids 1%–10%, itching 1%–10%, and feeling of foreign body in the eye 1%–10%.

DRUG INTERACTIONS: None of any clinical significance

ALLERGIES: Individuals allergic to ciprofloxacin, Cipro, Chibroxin, Ocuflox, or any of their derivatives should discuss this with their doctor or pharmacist before using this drug.

PREGNANCY/BREAST-FEEDING: Category C—Risk cannot be ruled out. Human studies are lacking, and animal studies are either positive for fetal risk or lacking as well. However, potential benefits may justify the potential risk in using the drug. It is not known whether the drug is excreted in the breast milk; therefore, caution should be used when breast-feeding.

OTHER BRAND NAMES: None

OTHER DRUGS IN THE SAME THERAPEUTIC CLASS: Chibroxin and Ocuflox

IMPORTANT INFORMATION TO REMEMBER: Use the drug for the full course of therapy, even if symptoms disappear; otherwise the infection may return. Keep the container tightly closed and avoid touching the applicator tip to the eye—this could contaminate the product over time. Also, only administer one drop at a time. After application, keep the eye open for at least 30 seconds, roll the eyeball around, and avoid squinting. If a second drop is required, wait one to two minutes between drops. If another medication is to be used in the eye, wait at least 10 minutes before administering it.

BRAND NAME: Cipro

GENERIC NAME: ciprofloxacin

GENERIC FORM AVAILABLE: No

THERAPEUTIC CLASS: Quinolone antibiotic

DOSAGE FORMS: 100-mg, 250-mg, 500-mg, and 750-mg tablets

MAIN USES: Bacterial infections

USUAL DOSE: 250 mg to 750 mg every 12 hours

AVERAGE PRICE: $63.68 for 100 mg (20 tablets); $78.40 for 250 mg (20 tablets); $90.72 for 500 mg (20 tablets); and $157.36 for 750 mg (20 tablets)

SIDE EFFECTS: nausea 5%, diarrhea 2%, vomiting 2%, stomach pains 2%, headache 1%, restlessness 1%, and rash 1%.

DRUG INTERACTIONS: Antacids, Videx, iron supplements, and Carafate may reduce the absorption of the drug. Choledy, Slo-bid, Theo-Dur, theophylline, Uni-Dur, Uniphyl, and aminophylline blood levels may be increased when used with this drug. The drug may also increase the effects of Coumadin.

ALLERGIES: Individuals allergic to ciprofloxacin or other quinolone antibiotics (such as those listed in "Other Drugs in the Same Therapeutic Class") should discuss this with their doctor or pharmacist before taking this drug.

PREGNANCY/BREAST-FEEDING: Category C—Risk cannot be ruled out. Human studies are lacking, and animal studies are either positive for fetal risk or lacking as well. However, potential benefits may justify the potential risk in using the drug. The drug is excreted in the breast milk; therefore, extreme caution should be used when breast-feeding.

OTHER BRAND NAMES: None

OTHER DRUGS IN THE SAME THERAPEUTIC CLASS: Floxin, Maxaquin, Noroxin, and Penetrex

IMPORTANT INFORMATION TO REMEMBER: Take the drug at even intervals around the clock (if twice a day, take every 12 hours). Take the drug until all the medication prescribed is gone; otherwise the infection may return. This drug should be taken with plenty of water (eight ounces is preferred). If stomach upset occurs, take with food. Do not take antacids, milk, or iron supplements within four hours of taking this drug. Individuals should also use a sunscreen to avoid overexposure to the sun. The drug may increase the skin's sensitivity to sunlight, which may cause one sunburn more easily. This drug may also cause a tear in the tendons of the lower leg. Report any soreness or pain of the lower legs to your physician immediately.

BRAND NAME: Claritin and Claritin-D

GENERIC NAME: loratadine (Claritin); loratadine and pseudoephedrine (Claritin D)

GENERIC FORM AVAILABLE: No

THERAPEUTIC CLASS: Nonsedating antihistamine

DOSAGE FORMS: 10-mg tablets (Claritin), 5-mg loratadine/120-mg pseudoephedrine tablets (Claritin-D 12-Hour), 10-mg loratadine/240-mg pseudoephedrine tablets (Claritin-D 24-Hour), and 1 mg/mL syrup

MAIN USES: Allergies

USUAL DOSE: one tablet daily as needed on an empty stomach (Claritin and Claritin-D 24-Hour) and one tablet twice daily as needed on an empty stomach (Claritin-D 12-Hour)

AVERAGE PRICE: $270.95 for Claritin; $152.68 for Claritin-D 12-Hour; and $232.99 for Claritin-D 24-Hour

SIDE EFFECTS: headache 12%, slight drowsiness 8%, slight fatigue 4%, and dry mouth 3%.

DRUG INTERACTIONS: Nizoral may increase the blood levels of the drug.

ALLERGIES: Individuals allergic to loratadine, antihistamines, or any of their derivatives should discuss this with their doctor or pharmacist before using this drug.

PREGNANCY/BREAST-FEEDING: Category B—No evidence of risk in humans. Either animal findings show risk, but human findings do not; or, if no adequate human studies have been done, animal findings show no risk. The drug is excreted in the breast milk; therefore, extreme caution should be used when breast-feeding.

OTHER BRAND NAMES: None

OTHER DRUGS IN THE SAME THERAPEUTIC CLASS: Allegra, Hismanal, Seldane, Seldane-D, and Zyrtec

IMPORTANT INFORMATION TO REMEMBER: It's best to take the drug on an empty stomach—one hour before meals or two hours after meals—if possible. Do not take Claritin more frequently than every 24 hours or Claritin D more frequently than every 12 hours. Take the drug only as needed for relief of allergies unless otherwise directed by a physician.

BRAND NAMES: Cleocin T

GENERIC NAME: clindamycin

GENERIC FORM AVAILABLE: Yes (solution only)

THERAPEUTIC CLASS: Topical antibiotic

DOSAGE FORMS: 1% gel, 1% solution, 1% lotion, and 2% vaginal cream

MAIN USES: Acne and vaginal bacterial infections

USUAL DOSE: Apply to the affected acne areas twice daily. For the vaginal cream: one applicatorful inserted into the vagina at bedtime for seven nights.

AVERAGE PRICE: $32.65 (B)/$27.92 (G) for 60-mL solution; $43.77 for 60-mL lotion; $31.49 for 30-g gel; and $35.09 for 2% vaginal cream

SIDE EFFECTS: Most common: none. Less common: skin dryness, itching, burning, peeling, and irritation.

DRUG INTERACTIONS: A/T/S, Benzamycin, Erycette, Erymax, and T-Stat may decrease the effectiveness of the drug.

ALLERGIES: Individuals allergic to clindamycin, Lincocin, or any of their derivatives should discuss this with their doctor or pharmacist before using this drug.

PREGNANCY/BREAST-FEEDING: Category B—No evidence of risk in humans. Either animal findings show risk, but human findings do not; or, if no adequate human studies have been done, animal findings show no risk. It is not known whether the drug is excreted in the breast milk; therefore, caution should be used when breast-feeding.

OTHER BRAND NAMES: None

OTHER DRUGS IN THE SAME THERAPEUTIC CLASS: A/T/S, Emgel, Erygel, Erycette, and T-Stat

IMPORTANT INFORMATION TO REMEMBER: For acne. This drug is for external use only. It is important to use the medication continuously. It may take three to four weeks before a significant improvement may be seen. If no improvement is seen within six weeks, contact your doctor. This medication contains alcohol, which may cause slight burning or stinging when first applied. Also, avoid contact with the eyes, nose, and mouth. Before applying, wash acne thoroughly with warm soapy water to remove dirt and skin oils, pat skin dry, and then apply the drug. If you need to apply another medication for acne, wait at least one hour. Before using the lotion, shake the bottle well. If using the gel, apply only a thin film of drug to skin. Discontinue use if irritation occurs. For the vaginal cream: use the drug for the full course of therapy, even if symptoms disappear; otherwise the infection may return. Continue using the drug even if your menstrual period begins. When using the vaginal cream, insert the applicator high into the vagina (two-thirds the length of the applicator) and push the plunger to release the cream. Do not use a tampon to hold the cream inside the vagina. It is recommended that your sexual partner use a condom until the infection clears up.

BRAND NAME: Climara

GENERIC NAME: estradiol

GENERIC FORM AVAILABLE: No

THERAPEUTIC CLASS: Estrogen replacement

DOSAGE FORMS: 0.05 mg/day and 0.1 mg/day patches

MAIN USES: Menopausal disorders

USUAL DOSE: one 0.05-mg or 0.1-mg patch applied weekly every week; or one patch applied weekly for three weeks, then off for one week

AVERAGE PRICE: $29.99 for four patches

SIDE EFFECTS: skin irritation at the site of application 31%, skin redness 9%; other possible side effects include: Most common: breast tenderness, breast pain, breast enlargement, swelling of feet and lower legs, stomach cramps, bloating, and nausea. Less common: changes in cervical secretions, yeast infections, headache, diarrhea, vomiting, migraine, depression, weight changes, dizziness, breakthrough bleeding, and changes in sex drive.

DRUG INTERACTIONS: The drug may interfere with the actions of Parlodel. The drug may increase the blood levels of Sandimmune. Liver toxicity may be increased when used with Dantrium.

ALLERGIES: Individuals allergic to estradiol, estrogens, other estrogen patches, or any of their derivatives should discuss this with their doctor or pharmacist before using this drug.

PREGNANCY/BREAST-FEEDING: Category X—Should not be used during pregnancy. Studies in animals and/or humans have shown fetal abnormalities and birth defects. The risks associated with using this drug clearly outweigh the benefits. This drug should never be used by someone who is pregnant or trying to become pregnant. Also, women should never breast-feed while using this drug.

OTHER BRAND NAMES: None

OTHER DRUGS IN THE SAME THERAPEUTIC CLASS: Estraderm and Vivelle

IMPORTANT INFORMATION TO REMEMBER: Use the drug exactly as directed by your physician. Do not discontinue the drug without first consulting your physician. Caution should be used by patients with previous or current episodes of cancer, high blood pressure, heart disease, or any other cardiovascular or blood vessel disease. This drug may increase the risk of uterine cancer in women who have been through menopause. Report any abnormal vaginal bleeding to your doctor immediately.

When using the patches:

1) Do not cut or fold the patch in half. This may cause the medication inside to leak out. Peel off the adhesive liner.
2) Apply the patch to a clean, dry skin area on the stomach. This area should be free of hair, cuts, scars, or irritation. Do not apply the patch to your breasts. Avoid the waistline since tight clothes may rub or remove the patch.
3) Leave the patch on even during swimming, showering, and exercising. If the patch falls off, replace the patch with a new one.
4) When it's time to apply a new patch, use a different site on the skin. Rotate the sites where you apply the patches every time.
5) Make it a habit to apply the patch at the same time each week.
6) Dispose of used patches properly and keep out of reach of children.

BRAND NAME: Clindex

GENERIC NAME: Combination product containing: chlordiazepoxide and clindium bromide

See entry for Librax

BRAND NAME: Clinoril

GENERIC NAME: sulindac

GENERIC FORM AVAILABLE: Yes

THERAPEUTIC CLASS: Nonsteroidal anti-inflammatory drug (NSAID)

DOSAGE FORMS: 150-mg and 200-mg tablets

MAIN USES: Arthritis, gouty arthritis, and pain relief

USUAL DOSE: 150 mg to 200 mg twice daily

AVERAGE PRICE: $105.47 (B)/$43.98 (G) for 150 mg and $114.49 (B)/$50.58 (G) for 200 mg

SIDE EFFECTS: stomach pain 10%, upset stomach 3%–9%, nausea 3%–9%, diarrhea 3%–9%, constipation 3%–9%, rash 3%–9%, dizziness 3%–9%, headache 3%–9%, gas 1%–3%, stomach cramps 1%–3%, itching 1%–3%, nervousness 1%–3%, and swelling 1%–3%.

DRUG INTERACTIONS: Aspirin will decrease the concentration of this drug in the blood. This drug may also decrease the effects of Lasix, Dyazide, HydroDIURIL, Maxzide, and other water pills. The drug may increase the blood levels of Eskalith, Lithobid, and Sandimmune. The drug may increase the toxic effects of the drug Rheumatrex. Caution should be used when taking the drug with Coumadin.

ALLERGIES: Individuals allergic to sulindac or other NSAIDs (such as those listed in "Other Drugs in the Same Therapeutic Class") should discuss this with their doctor or pharmacist before taking this drug.

PREGNANCY/BREAST-FEEDING: Category B—No evidence of risk in humans. Either animal findings show risk, but human findings do not; or, if no adequate human studies have been done, animal findings show no risk. The drug should not, however, be used in late stages (last three months) of pregnancy. The drug may be excreted in the breast milk; therefore, extreme caution should be used when breast-feeding.

OTHER BRAND NAMES: None

OTHER DRUGS IN THE SAME THERAPEUTIC CLASS: Anaprox, Ansaid, aspirin, Cataflam, Daypro, Disalcid, Dolobid, Easprin, Feldene, Indocin, Lodine, Lodine XL, Motrin, Nalfon, Naprosyn, Orudis, Oruvail, Relafen, Tolectin, Toradol, Voltaren, and Voltaren XL

IMPORTANT INFORMATION TO REMEMBER: This drug should be taken with food or milk to reduce the potential for injury to the stomach lining and stomach upset. This drug may take up to two weeks before a noticeable improvement in pain relief associated with arthritis is observed. Drinking alcohol while taking this drug may increase its potential to cause ulcers. This drug should only be used under the direct supervision of a doctor by individuals with a bleeding disorder or ulcer, or those who are currently taking Coumadin. Before taking over-the-counter pain relievers, consult your doctor or pharmacist. No more than one pain reliever should be taken at any one time unless otherwise directed by your doctor.

BRAND NAME: Clomid

GENERIC NAME: clomiphene citrate

See entry for Serophene

BRAND NAME: Clozaril

GENERIC NAME: clozapine

GENERIC FORM AVAILABLE: No

THERAPEUTIC CLASS: Antipsychotic

DOSAGE FORMS: 25-mg and 100-mg tablets

MAIN USES: Schizophrenia

USUAL DOSE: Initially 25 mg one to two times daily, increasing 25 mg–50 mg per day until 300 mg–450 mg daily in divided doses is reached.

AVERAGE PRICE: $53.50 for 25 mg (25 tablets) and $128.25 for 100 mg (25 tablets)

SIDE EFFECTS: drowsiness 39%, salivation 31%, fast heartbeat 25%, dizziness 19%, constipation 14%, low blood pressure 9%, headache 7%, tremors 6%, sweating 6%, dry mouth 6%, vision problems 5%, fever 5%, nausea 5%, stomach pain 4%, sleep disturbances 4%, nightmares 4%, restlessness 4%, vomiting 3%, confusion 3%, and insomnia 2%.

DRUG INTERACTIONS: Alcohol, anxiety medications, and narcotic painkillers intensify the drowsiness effect of the drug. The drug may cause bone marrow suppression and other blood disorders. Seizures and confused states may occur when this drug is used with Eskalith or Lithobid.

ALLERGIES: Individuals allergic to clozapine or any of its derivatives should discuss this with their doctor or pharmacist before using this drug.

PREGNANCY/BREAST-FEEDING: Category B—No evidence of risk in humans. Either animal findings show risk, but human findings do not; or, if no adequate human studies have been done, animal findings show no risk. The drug is excreted in the breast milk; therefore, extreme caution should be used when breast-feeding.

OTHER BRAND NAMES: None

OTHER DRUGS IN THE SAME THERAPEUTIC CLASS: None

IMPORTANT INFORMATION TO REMEMBER: This drug does cause drowsiness. Individuals should use caution when driving, operating machinery, or any task where mental alertness is required. Alcohol, anxiety medications, and narcotic painkillers may intensify the drowsiness effect of the drug. The drug may cause bone marrow suppression and other serious blood disorders. Regular blood tests should be conducted to avoid these problems. Some of the early symptoms of bone marrow suppression include fever, chills, and other flu-like symptoms. If these symptoms occur, contact your doctor immediately. Only take the drug exactly as directed by your physician. Do not discontinue the drug without first consulting your physician. Patients with glaucoma, prostate problems, or seizures should discuss this with their doctor before taking this drug.

BRAND NAME: Cogentin

GENERIC NAME: benztropine

GENERIC FORM AVAILABLE: Yes

THERAPEUTIC CLASS: Anticholinergic

DOSAGE FORMS: 0.5-mg, 1-mg, and 2-mg tablets

MAIN USES: Parkinson's disease and drug-induced movement disorders

USUAL DOSE: For Parkinson's disease: 0.5 mg to 6 mg daily in two to four equally divided doses or as a single dose at bedtime. For extrapyramidal disorders: 1 mg to 4 mg once or twice daily.

AVERAGE PRICE: $21.39 (B)/$10.98 (G) for 0.5 mg; $26.71 (B)/$11.97 (G) for 1 mg; $31.03 (B)/$14.28 (G) for 2 mg

SIDE EFFECTS: Most common: nausea, vomiting, dry mouth, blurred vision, decreased sweating, painful urination, and constipation. Less common: drowsiness, dizziness, headache, loss of memory, numbness, false sense of well-being, and agitation.

DRUG INTERACTIONS: The drug may decrease the effects of Compazine, Haldol, Mellaril, Prolixin, Serentil, Stelazine, Thorazine, and Trilafon. The drug may also cause abnormal body movements when used together with Haldol.

ALLERGIES: Individuals allergic to benztropine or any of its derivatives should discuss this with their doctor or pharmacist before using this drug.

PREGNANCY/BREAST-FEEDING: Category C—Risk cannot be ruled out. Human studies are lacking, and animal studies are either positive for fetal risk or lacking as well. However, potential benefits may justify the potential risk in using the drug. It is not known whether the drug is excreted in the breast milk; therefore, caution should be used when breast-feeding.

OTHER BRAND NAMES: None

OTHER DRUGS IN THE SAME THERAPEUTIC CLASS: Akineton, Artane, and Kemadrin

IMPORTANT INFORMATION TO REMEMBER: The drug should be taken with food or milk. Do not abruptly discontinue medication if side effects occur. Gradual dose reduction may be necessary; check with your physician. This drug may cause some limited drowsiness. Individuals should use caution when driving, operating machinery, or any task where mental alertness is required. Alcohol, anxiety medications, and narcotic painkillers may intensify the drowsiness effect of the drug. Caution should also be used when exercising and in hot weather while taking this drug; the drug may increase an individual's sensitivity to hot weather. Individuals taking the drug should have a glaucoma exam at regular intervals. Individuals with glaucoma or prostate problems should only use the drug under the direct supervision of a doctor.

BRAND NAME: Cognex

GENERIC NAME: tacrine

GENERIC FORM AVAILABLE: No

THERAPEUTIC CLASS: Anti-Alzheimer's

DOSAGE FORMS: 10-mg, 20-mg, 30-mg, and 40-mg capsules

MAIN USES: Mild to moderate dementia of Alzheimer's disease

USUAL DOSE: 10 mg four times daily for six weeks, then increase dosage 40 mg daily every six weeks as needed to a maximum of 160 mg per day

AVERAGE PRICE: $167.56 for 10 mg, 20 mg, 30 mg, or 40 mg

SIDE EFFECTS: elevated liver enzymes 29%, nausea 28%, diarrhea 16%, dizziness 12%, headache 11%, upset stomach 9%, loss of appetite 9%, runny nose 8%, stomach pain 8%, agitation 7%, insomnia 6%, tiredness 4%, nervousness 3%, and tremor 2%.

DRUG INTERACTIONS: Tagamet may increase the blood levels of the drug. Neuromuscular blockers and this drug may prolong or exaggerate muscle relaxation. The drug may increase the blood levels of Slo-bid, Theo-Dur, theophylline, Uni-Dur, and Uniphyl significantly. Smoking may lower the blood levels of the drug. This drug and one of the following—Anaprox, Ansaid, aspirin, Cataflam, Clinoril, Daypro, Disalcid, Dolobid, Easprin, Feldene, Indocin, Lodine, Motrin, Nalfon, Naprosyn, Orudis, Oruvail, Relafen, Tolectin, or Voltaren—when combined may increase the harmful effects and potential for injury to the stomach.

ALLERGIES: Individuals allergic to tacrine or any of its derivatives should discuss this with their doctor or pharmacist before using this drug.

PREGNANCY/BREAST-FEEDING: Category C—Risk cannot be ruled out. Human studies are lacking, and animal studies are either positive for fetal risk or lacking as well. However, potential benefits may justify the potential risk in using the drug. It is not known whether the drug is excreted in the breast milk; therefore, caution should be used when breast-feeding.

OTHER BRAND NAMES: None

OTHER DRUGS IN THE SAME THERAPEUTIC CLASS: None

IMPORTANT INFORMATION TO REMEMBER: It's best to take the drug on an empty stomach—one hour before meals or two hours after meals—if possible. Only take the drug exactly as directed by your physician. Do not discontinue the drug without first consulting your physician. Do not increase the dose without first consulting with your physician. The drug may affect liver function; liver enzyme tests should be performed regularly by your doctor. Individuals who experience yellowing of the skin or dark stools should report this to their doctor immediately.

BRAND NAME: ColBENEMID

GENERIC NAME: combination product containing: probenecid and colchicine

GENERIC FORM AVAILABLE: Yes

THERAPEUTIC CLASS: Anti-gout

DOSAGE FORMS: 500-mg probenecid/0.5-mg colchicine tablets

MAIN USES: Gout and chronic gouty arthritis

USUAL DOSE: one tablet one to two times daily

AVERAGE PRICE: $39.25 (B)/$19.67 (G)

SIDE EFFECTS: Most common: none. Less common: headache, dizziness, vomiting, diarrhea, sore gums, weight loss, gas, increased urinary frequency, fever, itching, hair loss, skin rash, back pain, pain in the ribs, and flushing.

DRUG INTERACTIONS: The drug may increase the blood levels of Lufyllin, Indocin, Orudis, Oruvail, Ativan, heparin, Retrovir, Rheumatrex, rifampin, and many antibiotics. Aspirin may decrease the effectiveness of the drug. Alcohol, in large amounts, may increase stomach and intestinal toxicity.

ALLERGIES: Individuals allergic to probenecid, colchicine, or any of their derivatives should discuss this with their doctor or pharmacist before using this drug.

PREGNANCY/BREAST-FEEDING: Category D—Positive evidence of risk. Human studies show risk to the fetus. Nevertheless, potential benefits may possibly outweigh the potential risk. This drug should not be taken by nursing mothers.

OTHER BRAND NAMES: None

OTHER DRUGS IN THE SAME THERAPEUTIC CLASS: Anturane and Benemid

IMPORTANT INFORMATION TO REMEMBER: This drug should be taken with plenty of water (eight ounces is preferred). This will help prevent kidney stones. If stomach upset occurs, the drug may be taken with food or milk. Only take the drug exactly as directed by your physician. Do not discontinue the drug without first consulting your physician. This drug is meant to prevent a gout attack; it will not help a gout attack once it has started. Individuals with a history of kidney stones, blood problems, or kidney disease should consult with their doctor before taking this drug. Alcohol, in large amounts, may increase the toxic effects to the stomach and intestines.

BRAND NAME: **Colchicine** (various brand-name manufacturers)

GENERIC NAME: colchicine

GENERIC FORM AVAILABLE: Yes

THERAPEUTIC CLASS: Anti-inflammatory

DOSAGE FORMS: 0.5-mg and 0.6-mg tablets

MAIN USES: Gout

USUAL DOSE: For prevention: 0.5 mg to 0.6 mg one to two times daily. For treatment of an acute attack: 0.5 mg to 0.6 mg initially, then 0.5 mg to 0.6 mg every one to two hours until pain is relieved (maximum 6 mg per attack)

AVERAGE PRICE: $15.99 for 0.6-mg tablets

SIDE EFFECTS: Most common: nausea, vomiting, diarrhea, and stomach pain. Less common: weight loss, hair loss, gas, itching, and flushing.

DRUG INTERACTIONS: The drug may decrease the absorption of vitamin B_{12} by the body. The drug may also increase bone marrow depression when used with drugs that depress the bone marrow, such as cancer drugs, over long periods of time.

ALLERGIES: Individuals allergic to colchicine or any of its derivatives should discuss this with their doctor or pharmacist before using this drug.

PREGNANCY/BREAST-FEEDING: Category D—Positive evidence of risk. Human studies show risk to the fetus. Nevertheless, potential benefits may possibly outweigh the potential risk. This drug should not be taken by nursing mothers.

OTHER BRAND NAMES: None

OTHER DRUGS IN THE SAME THERAPEUTIC CLASS: None

IMPORTANT INFORMATION TO REMEMBER: Only take the drug exactly as directed by your physician. When the drug is used for an acute attack, start taking the drug at the first sign of an attack, and stop taking the drug once the pain is gone. Individuals should also stop taking the drug at the first sign of nausea, diarrhea, vomiting, or stomach pain. It is important to continue taking other gout medications even during an acute attack. The drug cannot be used for prevention of another acute attack until three days after use for the first acute attack unless otherwise directed by your doctor.

BRAND NAME: Colestid

GENERIC NAME: colestipol

GENERIC FORM AVAILABLE: No

THERAPEUTIC CLASS: Cholesterol binder

DOSAGE FORMS: 5 g/packet or 5 g/scoop granules

MAIN USES: High cholesterol

USUAL DOSE: 5 g to 30 g daily in a single dose or in divided doses

AVERAGE PRICE: $55.66 for 30 packets and $69.62 for 450 g jar

SIDE EFFECTS: constipation 10%, stomach pain 1%–3%, belching 1%–3%, gas 1%–3%, nausea 1%–3%, vomiting 1%–3%, and diarrhea 1%–3%.

DRUG INTERACTIONS: The drug may affect the blood levels of Coumadin. This drug can interfere with the absorption of several drugs, some of which are: Lanoxin, diuretics (water pills), penicillin G, Inderal, Sumycin, Cytomel, Levothroid, Levoxyl, Synthroid, and Vancocin. Before taking any prescription drug, talk to your doctor or pharmacist.

ALLERGIES: Individuals allergic to colestipol or any of its derivatives should discuss this with their doctor or pharmacist before using this drug.

PREGNANCY/BREAST-FEEDING: Category C—Risk cannot be ruled out. Human studies are lacking, and animal studies are either positive for fetal risk or lacking as well. However, potential benefits may justify the potential risk in using the drug. It is not known whether the drug is excreted in the breast milk; therefore, caution should be used when breast-feeding.

OTHER BRAND NAMES: None

OTHER DRUGS IN THE SAME THERAPEUTIC CLASS: Questran and Questran Light

IMPORTANT INFORMATION TO REMEMBER: This drug may interfere with absorption of many prescription drug products; therefore, it's best to take the drug one to two hours before taking other medications or four hours after taking other medications. Only take the drug exactly as directed by your physician. Do not discontinue the drug without first consulting your physician.

How to mix the drug with liquid:

1) The drug needs to be mixed with liquid before it can be taken.
2) The drug may be mixed with water, milk, flavored drink, any fruit juice, cereals, soups (chicken noodle or tomato), and fruits. Most individuals prefer to mix the drug with heavy or pulpy fruit juices to improve taste.
3) Stir until the drug is completely mixed. The drug will not dissolve completely in the liquid.
4) Rinse the glass after drinking with a little more liquid and drink that as well. This ensures all the medication is taken.

BRAND NAME: Colyte

GENERIC NAME: Combination product containing: polyethylene glycol, sodium chloride, potassium chloride, sodium bicarbinate, and sodium sulfate

GENERIC FORM AVAILABLE: No

THERAPEUTIC CLASS: Isosmotic bowel laxative

DOSAGE FORMS: 60 g polyethlene glycol 3350/1.46 g sodium chloride/0.745 g potassium chloride/1.68 g sodium bicarbinate/5.68 g sodium sulfate per liter of solution

MAIN USES: Bowel cleanser before intestinal or colon examination

USUAL DOSE: Drink eight ounces every 10 minutes until three to four liters is consumed or as otherwise directed.

AVERAGE PRICE: $22.56

SIDE EFFECTS: Most common: nausea, stomach fullness, and bloating may occur in up to 50% of individuals taking the drug. Less common: stomach cramps, vomiting, and anal irritation.

DRUG INTERACTIONS: Other prescription medications should be taken one hour before using the drug or two hours after.

ALLERGIES: Individuals allergic to polyethylene glycol, sodium chloride, potassium chloride, sodium bicarbinate, sodium sulfate, or any of their derivatives should discuss this with their doctor or pharmacist before using this drug.

PREGNANCY/BREAST-FEEDING: Category C—Risk cannot be ruled out. Human studies are lacking, and animal studies are either positive for fetal risk or lacking as well. However, potential benefits may justify the potential risk in using the drug. It is not known whether the drug is excreted in the breast milk; therefore, caution should be used when breast-feeding.

OTHER BRAND NAMES: None

OTHER DRUGS IN THE SAME THERAPEUTIC CLASS: GoLYTELY and NuLYTELY

IMPORTANT INFORMATION TO REMEMBER: Other prescription medications should be taken one hour before drinking the solution or two hours after. Patients with intestinal disorders should discuss this with their doctor before taking this drug. No food should be eaten at least three hours before drinking the solution. Only clear liquids are allowed after drinking the solution. Individuals should drink one 8-ounce glass rapidly every 10 minutes; for best results, drink all of the solution prepared.

BRAND NAME: Combipres

GENERIC NAME: Combination product containing: clonidine and chlorthalidone. See individual entries for Catapres/Catapres TTS Patches and Hygroton

BRAND NAME: Comhist LA

GENERIC NAME: Combination product containing: chlorpheniramine, phenyltoloxamine, and phenylephrine

GENERIC FORM AVAILABLE: No

THERAPEUTIC CLASS: Antihistamine + decongestant

DOSAGE FORMS: 4 mg chlorpheniramine/50 mg phenyltoloxamine/20 mg phenylephrine in sustained-release capsules

MAIN USES: Nasal allergies and congestion

USUAL DOSE: one capsule every 8 to 12 hours

AVERAGE PRICE: $115.86

SIDE EFFECTS: Most common: drowsiness and dry mouth. Less common: nausea, giddiness, blurred vision, pounding heartbeat, flushing, increased irritability or excitability (especially in children), headache, dry throat, and insomnia.

DRUG INTERACTIONS: Blocadren, Cartrol, Corgard, Inderal, Kerlone, Levatol, Lopressor, Nardil, Normodyne, Parnate, Sectral, Tenormin, Toprol-XL, Trandate, Visken, or Zebeta may increase the effects of the drug. The drug may also reduce the effects of blood-pressure-lowering drugs.

ALLERGIES: Individuals allergic to chlorpheniramine, phenyltoloxamine, phenylephrine, or other antihistamine/decongestant combinations (such as those listed in "Other Drugs in the Same Therapeutic Class") should discuss this with their doctor or pharmacist before taking this drug.

PREGNANCY/BREAST-FEEDING: Category C—Risk cannot be ruled out. Human studies are lacking, and animal studies are either positive for fetal risk or lacking as well. However, potential benefits may justify the potential risk in using the drug. It is not known whether the drug is excreted in the breast milk; therefore, caution should be used when breast-feeding.

OTHER BRAND NAMES: None

OTHER DRUGS IN THE SAME THERAPEUTIC CLASS: Atrohist Plus, Bromfed, Bromfed PD, Claritin-D, Deconamine SR, Extendryl, Fedahist Gyrocaps, Naldecon, Nolamine, Novafed-A, Ornade, Poly-Histine-D, Rondec, Rynatan, Seldane-D, Semprex-D, Tavist-D, and Trinalin

IMPORTANT INFORMATION TO REMEMBER: This drug does cause drowsiness. Individuals should use caution when driving, operating machinery, or any task where mental alertness is required. Alcohol, anxiety medications, and narcotic painkillers may intensify the drowsiness effect of the drug. This drug may also cause a dry mouth; sugarless gum or hard candy will help take care of this problem. Patients with glaucoma, high blood pressure, heart conditions, or urinary or prostate problems should consult their doctor before taking this drug.

BRAND NAME: Compazine

GENERIC NAME: prochlorperazine

GENERIC FORM AVAILABLE: Yes (suppositories and tablets only)

THERAPEUTIC CLASS: Phenothiazine antipsychotic and antinausea

DOSAGE FORMS: 5-mg, 10-mg, and 25-mg tablets; 10-mg, 15-mg and 30-mg long-acting capsules; 5 mg/ 5 mL syrup; 2.5-mg, 5-mg, and 25-mg suppositories

MAIN USES: Nausea, vomiting, psychotic disorders, and (anxiety)

USUAL DOSE: For nausea, vomiting, and anxiety: 5-mg to 10-mg tablets three to four times daily; one 10-mg long-acting capsule every 12 hours; one 15-mg capsule upon arising; or one 25-mg suppository twice daily. For psychotic disorders: 15-mg to 150-mg daily in three or four divided doses.

AVERAGE PRICE: $87.49 (B)/$62.79 (G) for 5-mg tablets; $125.09 (B)/$89.69 (G) for 10-mg tablets; $132.89 for 10-mg capsules; $198.19 for 15-mg capsules; and $56.12 (B)/$34.15 (G) for 25 mg (12 suppositories)

SIDE EFFECTS: Most common: restlessness; blurred vision; muscle spasms of the face, neck, back, and other tic-like movements; weakness of arms and legs, fainting, lip smacking or puckering; constipation; decreased sweating; dizziness; drowsiness; dry mouth; and nasal congestion. Less common: nausea, vomiting, stomach pain, trembling hands, skin rash, difficulty in urinating, increased sensitivity of the skin to sunburn, changes in menstrual periods, decreased sexual ability, secretion of breast milk, and swelling or painful breasts.

DRUG INTERACTIONS: The drug may intensify the side effects of drugs used for depression, as well as increase their blood levels. Eskalith and Lithobid may decrease the absorption of the drug. Drugs used to treat high blood pressure may lower blood pressure too low when used with this drug. The drug may decrease the effectiveness of Larodopa. The drug may decrease the blood levels of Coumadin. Inderal and the drug may raise one another's blood levels.

ALLERGIES: Individuals allergic to prochlorprazine or any of its derivatives should discuss this with their doctor or pharmacist before using this drug.

PREGNANCY/BREAST-FEEDING: Category C—Risk cannot be ruled out. Human studies are lacking, and animal studies are either positive for fetal risk or lacking as well. However, potential benefits may justify the potential risk in using the drug. The drug is excreted in the breast milk; therefore, extreme caution should be used when breast-feeding.

OTHER BRAND NAMES: None

OTHER DRUGS IN THE SAME THERAPEUTIC CLASS: Mellaril, Phenergan, Prolixin, Serentil, Stelazine, Thorazine, Torecan, and Trilafon

IMPORTANT INFORMATION TO REMEMBER: This drug does cause drowsiness. Individuals should use caution when driving, operating machinery, or any task where mental alertness is required. Alcohol, anxiety medications, and narcotic painkillers may intensify the drowsiness effect of the drug. Individuals should also use a sunscreen to avoid overexposure to the sun. The drug may increase the skin's sensitivity to sunlight, which may cause one to sunburn more easily. Caution should also be used when exercising and in hot weather while taking this drug; the drug may increase an individual's sensitivity to hot weather. The eyes may also become sensitive to direct sunlight, and sunglasses may be needed.

BRAND NAME: Condylox

GENERIC NAME: podofilox

GENERIC FORM AVAILABLE: No

THERAPEUTIC CLASS: Antiviral

DOSAGE FORMS: 0.5% topical solution

MAIN USES: External genital warts

USUAL DOSE: Apply twice daily directly to the warts every 12 hours for three days, then do not use for four days. This one-week cycle may be repeated up to four times.

AVERAGE PRICE: $73.41

SIDE EFFECTS: skin eaten away 67%, burning 64%–78%, inflammation at the application site 63%–71%, pain 50%–72%, itching 50%–65%, chafing less than 5%, bleeding less than 5%, skin crusting and peeling less than 5%, and skin tenderness less than 5%.

DRUG INTERACTIONS: None of any clinical significance

ALLERGIES: Individuals allergic to podofilox or any of its derivatives should discuss this with their doctor or pharmacist before using this drug.

PREGNANCY/BREAST-FEEDING: Category C—Risk cannot be ruled out. Human studies are lacking, and animal studies are either positive for fetal risk or lacking as well. However, potential benefits may justify the potential risk in using the drug. It is not known whether the drug is excreted in the breast milk; therefore, caution should be used when breast-feeding.

OTHER BRAND NAMES: None

OTHER DRUGS IN THE SAME THERAPEUTIC CLASS: None

IMPORTANT INFORMATION TO REMEMBER: This drug is for external use only. The drug should only be applied directly to the warts—avoid contact with healthy skin. To avoid contact with healthy skin, place petroleum jelly on the healthy skin around the wart. Apply only a thin layer of drug to the wart. Never apply to damaged skin or open wounds unless directed to do so by a doctor. Discontinue use if irritation occurs. After application, let the area dry before placing clothing on the affected area. This drug should not be used for anal or mucous membrane warts. Sexual intercourse should be avoided while using the drug; your partner may experience skin irritation or an extreme burning sensation.

BRAND NAME: Cordarone

GENERIC NAME: amiodarone

GENERIC FORM AVAILABLE: No

THERAPEUTIC CLASS: Class III antiarrhythmic

DOSAGE FORMS: 200-mg tablets

MAIN USES: Irregular heartbeat

USUAL DOSE: 200 mg to 1600 mg daily in divided doses. Dosages are individualized for each person.

AVERAGE PRICE: $255.80 for 60 tablets

SIDE EFFECTS: nausea 10%–33%, vomiting 10%–33%, increased skin sensitivity to the sun 4%–9%, tiredness 4%–9%, tremors 4%–9%, dizziness 4%–9%, constipation 4%–9%, abnormal liver tests 4%–9%, vision problems 4%–9%, inflammation of the lungs 4%–9%, decreased sex drive 1%–3%, insomnia 1%–3%, headache 1%–3%, stomach pain 1%–3%, irregular heartbeat 1%–3%, flushing 1%–3%, and abnormal taste and smell 1%–3%.

DRUG INTERACTIONS: The drug may produce additive affects when used with other drugs for irregular heartbeat. The drug may increase the blood levels and effects of Coumadin, Dilantin, Lanoxin, Procan, Quinidex, and Quinaglute.

ALLERGIES: Individuals allergic to amiodarone or any of its derivatives should discuss this with their doctor or pharmacist before using this drug.

PREGNANCY/BREAST-FEEDING: Category D—Positive evidence of risk. Human studies show risk to the fetus. Nevertheless, potential benefits may possibly outweigh the potential risks. This drug should not be taken by nursing mothers.

OTHER BRAND NAMES: None

OTHER DRUGS IN THE SAME THERAPEUTIC CLASS: Betapace

IMPORTANT INFORMATION TO REMEMBER: Only take the drug exactly as directed by your physician. Do not discontinue the drug without first consulting your physician. This is a very dangerous drug if not taken exactly as directed; also, do not increase the dose without first consulting with your physician. Individuals should also use a sunscreen to avoid overexposure to the sun; the drug may increase the skin's sensitivity to sunlight, which may cause one to sunburn more easily. This sensitivity to sunlight can occur even months after treatment is stopped. Individuals undergoing any surgery (even dental and outpatient) or emergency treatment should inform the appropriate medical personnel that they are taking this drug. Individuals should notify their physician immediately if they experience a cough, painful breathing, or shortness of breath while taking this drug. Individuals taking the drug should have their thyroid function tested every six months.

BRAND NAME: Cordran and Cordran SP

GENERIC NAME: flurandrenolide

GENERIC FORM AVAILABLE: No

THERAPEUTIC CLASS: Topical corticosteroids

DOSAGE FORMS: 0.025% and 0.05% SP cream and ointment; 0.05% lotion; and 4 micrograms/cm^2 tape

MAIN USES: Skin rashes, swelling, and itching

USUAL DOSE: Apply thin film and massage into skin two to three times daily. The tape should be applied every 12 hours.

AVERAGE PRICE: $38.83 for large roll of tape; $18.76 for 0.025% (15 g); and $17.99 for 0.05% (15 g)

SIDE EFFECTS: Most common: none. Less common: burning, itching, irritation, dry skin, rash, and acne.

DRUG INTERACTIONS: None of any clinical significance

ALLERGIES: Individuals allergic to flurandrenolide or any of its derivatives should discuss this with their doctor or pharmacist before using this drug.

PREGNANCY/BREAST-FEEDING: Category C—Risk cannot be ruled out. Human studies are lacking, and animal studies are either positive for fetal risk or lacking as well. However, potential benefits may justify the potential risk in using the drug. It is not known whether the drug is excreted in the breast milk; therefore, caution should be used when breast-feeding.

OTHER BRAND NAMES: None

OTHER DRUGS IN THE SAME THERAPEUTIC CLASS: Aclovate, Aristocort, Cutivate, Cyclocort, DesOwen, Diprolene, Elocon, Halog, Hytone, Kenalog, Lidex, Synalar, Temovate, Topicort, Tridesilon, Ultravate, Valisone, and Westcort

IMPORTANT INFORMATION TO REMEMBER: This drug is for external use only. Apply only a thin film of drug to skin and rub it in well. Never cover the skin after application with a bandage or wrapping unless directed to do so by a doctor. Never apply to damaged skin or open wounds unless directed to do so by a doctor. Discontinue use if irritation occurs.

BRAND NAME: Corgard

GENERIC NAME: nadolol

GENERIC FORM AVAILABLE: Yes

THERAPEUTIC CLASS: Noncardioselective beta-blocker

DOSAGE FORMS: 20-mg, 40-mg, 80-mg, 120-mg, and 160-mg tablets

MAIN USES: High blood pressure and angina

USUAL DOSE: For high blood pressure: 80 mg to 320 mg once daily. For angina: 80 mg to 240 mg once daily.

AVERAGE PRICE: $98.69 (B)/$63.80 (G) for 20 mg; $115.69 (B)/ $79.51 (G) for 40 mg; $144.94 (B)/$99.75 (G) for 80 mg; $188.58 (B)/$137.70 (G) for 120 mg; $206.96 (B)/$166.52 (G) for 160 mg

SIDE EFFECTS: slow heart rate (common), dizziness 2%, tiredness 2%, low blood pressure 1%, heart failure 1%, decreased sexual ability 1%, constipation 1%, and irregular heartbeat 1%.

DRUG INTERACTIONS: The drug may cause additive effects when used with reserpine. The drug may increase the effects of Calan, Cardene, Cardizem, Catapres, Dilacor XR, DynaCirc, Isoptin, Lanoxin, Norvasc, Plendil, Procardia, Sular, Tiazac, Verelan, and Wytensin. Diabetic medications, insulin, Slo-bid, Theo-Dur, Uni-Dur, theophylline, and Uniphyl dosages may need to be adjusted when taking this drug. The drug may also interfere with glaucoma screening tests.

ALLERGIES: Individuals allergic to nadolol or other beta-blockers (such as those listed in "Other Drugs in the Same Therapeutic Class") should discuss this with their doctor or pharmacist before taking this drug.

PREGNANCY/BREAST-FEEDING: Category C—Risk cannot be ruled out. Human studies are lacking, and animal studies are either positive for fetal risk or lacking as well. However, potential benefits may justify the potential risk in using the drug. The drug is excreted in the breast milk; therefore, extreme caution should be used when breast-feeding.

OTHER BRAND NAMES: None

OTHER DRUGS IN THE SAME THERAPEUTIC CLASS: Blocadren, Cartrol, Inderal, Levatol, Normodyne, Trandate, and Visken

IMPORTANT INFORMATION TO REMEMBER: Only take the drug exactly as directed by your physician. Do not discontinue the drug without first consulting your physician. This drug may cause some tiredness, especially at first. Individuals should use caution when driving, operating machinery, or any task where mental alertness is required. Before taking over-the-counter cold and allergy preparations, consult your doctor or pharmacist; these products may raise your blood pressure. This drug may mask the symptoms of low blood sugar in diabetics.

BRAND NAME: Cormax

GENERIC NAME: clobètasol

See entry for Temovate

BRAND NAME: Cortisporin Otic

GENERIC NAME: Combination product containing: neomycin, polymyxin B, and hydrocortisone

GENERIC FORM AVAILABLE: Yes

THERAPEUTIC CLASS: Topical antibiotic + steroid

DOSAGE FORMS: Each milliliter (mL) contains 1% hydrocortisone/ 5 mg neomycin/10,000 units of polymyxin B in both solution and suspension forms

MAIN USES: Bacterial infections of the ear

USUAL DOSE: four drops in affected ear three to four times daily

AVERAGE PRICE: $24.47 (B)/$15.38 (G) for 10 mL

SIDE EFFECTS: Most common: none. Less common: local irritation, slight burning, itching, dry skin in ear canal, and crusty skin in the ear canal.

DRUG INTERACTIONS: None of any clinical significance

ALLERGIES: Individuals allergic to neomycin, polymyxin B, hydrocortisone, or any of their derivatives should discuss this with their doctor or pharmacist before using this drug.

PREGNANCY/BREAST-FEEDING: Category C—Risk cannot be ruled out. Human studies are lacking, and animal studies are either positive for fetal risk or lacking as well. However, potential benefits may justify the potential risk in using the drug. It is not known whether the drug is excreted in the breast milk; therefore, caution should be used when breast-feeding.

OTHER BRAND NAMES: None

OTHER DRUGS IN THE SAME THERAPEUTIC CLASS: Coly-Mycin S and Pediotic

IMPORTANT INFORMATION TO REMEMBER: Use the drug for the full course of therapy as directed by your doctor; otherwise the infection may return. If you are using the suspension, shake the bottle well.

Before inserting the drops, you may warm the medication bottle in your hands for three to five minutes. When inserting drops, lie down with affected ear facing up. Instill all the required drops at once. If you think you may have missed a drop or only inserted half a drop, it's OK to insert another one. Allow the medication to remain in the ear canal for at least five minutes. You may insert a piece of cotton to prevent the medication from running out of the ear.

BRAND NAME: Cotazym

GENERIC NAME: Combination product containing: lipase, protease, and amylase

Very similar to Creon. See entry for Creon 5/Creon 10/Creon 20.

BRAND NAME: Coumadin

GENERIC NAME: warfarin

GENERIC FORM AVAILABLE: Yes

THERAPEUTIC CLASS: Blood thinner

DOSAGE FORMS: 1-mg, 2-mg, 2.5-mg, 4-mg, 5-mg, 7.5-mg, and 10-mg tablets

MAIN USES: Thromboembolic disorders (blood thinner)

USUAL DOSE: 2 mg to 10 mg daily. The dosage for each individual patient needs to be carefully adjusted to achieve the maximum benefit.

AVERAGE PRICE: $76.44 for 2 mg; $79.96 for 5 mg; $120.70 for 7.5 mg; $124.32 for 10 mg

SIDE EFFECTS: Most common: bleeding, bruising, leukopenia (chills, fever, sore throat, unusual tiredness or weakness), diarrhea, nausea, vomiting, stomach pain, and hair loss. Less common: bloated stomach, gas, and blurred vision.

DRUG INTERACTIONS: Many drugs interact with Coumadin. Always inform your doctor or pharmacist about all medications—both prescription and over-the-counter—that you are currently taking before starting Coumadin therapy. The following drugs may enhance the effects of Coumadin: alcohol, Antabuse, aspirin,

Atromid-S, Bactrim, Bactrim DS, Cordarone, chloral hydrate, Cytomel, erythromycin, Flagyl, Glucagon, Levoxyl, Levothroid, Quinidex, Quinaglute, quinine, steroids, sulfinpyrazone, Synthroid, Tagamet, and Zyloprim. Some drugs decrease the effects of Coumadin; these include Amytal, Butisol, Dilantin, Fulvicin P/G, estrogens, Grifulvin V, Gris-PEG, Grisactin, Mebaral, Nembutal, Placidyl, rifampin, Seconal, Tegretol, Tuinal, and vitamin K.

ALLERGIES: Individuals allergic to warfarin or any of its derivatives should discuss this with their doctor or pharmacist before using this drug.

PREGNANCY/BREAST-FEEDING: Category X—Should not be used during pregnancy. Studies in animals and/or humans have shown fetal abnormalities and birth defects. The risks associated with using this drug clearly outweigh the benefits. This drug should never be used by someone who is pregnant or trying to become pregnant; also, women should never breast-feed while using this drug.

OTHER BRAND NAMES: None

OTHER DRUGS IN THE SAME THERAPEUTIC CLASS: heparin and Lovenox

IMPORTANT INFORMATION TO REMEMBER: Only take the drug exactly as directed by your physician. Do not discontinue the drug without first consulting your physician; also, do not increase the dose without first consulting with your physician. Individuals taking the drug should have regular physician visits to check their prothrombin time; this will ensure you are not receiving too little or too much drug. Before taking over-the-counter medications, consult your doctor or pharmacist. Avoid alcohol, aspirin, and other pain medications; these drugs can cause stomach bleeding when taken with Coumadin. Tylenol (acetaminophen) can be taken. Before any surgery or emergency treatment, inform the medical personnel you are taking Coumadin. Report any signs of abnormal bleeding to your physician immediately. It is also recommended that individuals use a soft toothbrush for brushing their teeth; this reduces the risk of gum bleeding.

BRAND NAME: Covera-HS

GENERIC NAME: verapamil

GENERIC FORM AVAILABLE: No

THERAPEUTIC CLASS: Calcium channel blocker

DOSAGE FORMS: 180-mg and 240-mg extended-release tablets with controlled onset

MAIN USES: Angina and high blood pressure

USUAL DOSE: 180 mg and 480 mg at bedtime

AVERAGE PRICE: $105.89 for 180 mg and $143.59 for 240 mg

SIDE EFFECTS: headache 7%, tiredness 4%, swelling 3%, dizziness 3%, constipation 3%, nausea 2%, and slow heartbeat 1%.

DRUG INTERACTIONS: The effects of Blocadren, Cartrol, Corgard, Inderal, Kerlone, Levatol, Lopressor, Minipress, Normodyne, Norpace, Sectral, Tenormin, Toprol-XL, Trandate, Visken, and Zebeta may be increased when taken with this drug. The drug may increase the blood levels of Tegretol, Sandimmune, Lanoxin, Quinidex, Quinaglute, and Procan.

ALLERGIES: Individuals allergic to verapamil or any of its derivatives should discuss this with their doctor or pharmacist before using this drug.

PREGNANCY/BREAST-FEEDING: Category C—Risk cannot be ruled out. Human studies are lacking, and animal studies are either positive for fetal risk or lacking as well. However, potential benefits may justify the potential risk in using the drug. The drug is excreted in the breast milk; therefore, extreme caution should be used when breast-feeding.

OTHER BRAND NAMES: None

OTHER DRUGS IN THE SAME THERAPEUTIC CLASS: Adalat, Adalat CC, Calan, Calan SR, Cardene, Cardene SR, Cardizem, Cardizem SR, Cardizem CD, Dilacor XR, DynaCirc, Norvasc, Plendil, Procardia, Procardia XL, Sular, Vascor, and Verelan

IMPORTANT INFORMATION TO REMEMBER: If stomach upset occurs, the drug should be taken with food or milk. Only take the drug exactly as directed by your physician. Do not discontinue the drug without first consulting your physician. Before taking over-the-counter cold and allergy preparations, consult your doctor or pharmacist; these products may raise your blood pressure. Do not crush, chew, or break the tablets; this will destroy the mechanism that ensures the sustained release of the medication.

BRAND NAME: Cozaar

GENERIC NAME: losartan

GENERIC FORM AVAILABLE: No

THERAPEUTIC CLASS: Angiotensin-II-receptor blocker

DOSAGE FORMS: 25-mg and 50-mg tablets

MAIN USES: High blood pressure

USUAL DOSE: 25 mg to 50 mg once daily

AVERAGE PRICE: $154.19 for 25 mg and $167.79 for 50 mg

SIDE EFFECTS: dizziness 4%, nasal congestion 2%, diarrhea 2%, upset stomach 1%, muscle cramps 1%, and tiredness 1%.

DRUG INTERACTIONS: Patients on diuretics (water pills), especially those recently started on a diuretic, may experience low blood pressure.

ALLERGIES: Individuals allergic to losartan or any of its derivatives should discuss this with their doctor or pharmacist before using this drug.

PREGNANCY/BREAST-FEEDING: Category C (first trimester)—Risk cannot be ruled out. Human studies are lacking, and animal studies are either positive for fetal risk or lacking as well. However, potential benefits may justify the potential risk in using the drug. Category D (second and third trimesters)—Positive evidence of risk. Human studies show risk to the fetus. Nevertheless, potential benefits may possibly outweigh the potential risk. This drug should not be taken by nursing mothers.

OTHER BRAND NAMES: None

OTHER DRUGS IN THE SAME THERAPEUTIC CLASS: None

IMPORTANT INFORMATION TO REMEMBER: Take this drug regularly and exactly as directed by your physician. Do not stop taking the drug unless otherwise directed by your doctor. Avoid salt substitutes containing potassium. Before taking over-the-counter cold and allergy preparations, consult your doctor or pharmacist; these products may raise your blood pressure.

BRAND NAME: Creon 5, Creon 10, and Creon 20

GENERIC NAME: Combination product containing the enzymes lipase, amylase, and protease

GENERIC FORM AVAILABLE: No

THERAPEUTIC CLASS: Pancreatic enzymes replacement

DOSAGE FORMS: 5,000 units lipase/16,600 units amylase/18,750 units protease in mini-microspheres in capsules (Creon 5); 10,000 units lipase/33,200 units amylase/37,500 units protease in mini-microspheres in capsules (Creon 10); and 20,000 units lipase/66,400 units amylase/75,000 units protease in mini-microspheres in capsules (Creon) 20

MAIN USES: Pancreatic enzyme replacement therapy

USUAL DOSE: one to four capsules with meals

AVERAGE PRICE: $51.67 (Creon 5), $66.67 (Creon 10), and $127.56 (Creon 20)

SIDE EFFECTS: Most common: none. Less common: nausea, vomiting, bloating, stomach cramps, diarrhea, and constipation.

DRUG INTERACTIONS: The drug should not be taken with antacids.

ALLERGIES: Individuals allergic to lipase, amylase, protease, or any of their derivatives should discuss this with their doctor or pharmacist before using this drug.

PREGNANCY/BREAST-FEEDING: Category C—Risk cannot be ruled out. Human studies are lacking, and animal studies are either positive for fetal risk or lacking as well. However, potential benefits may justify the potential risk in using the drug. It is not known whether the drug is excreted in the breast milk; therefore, caution should be used when breast-feeding.

OTHER BRAND NAMES: None

OTHER DRUGS IN THE SAME THERAPEUTIC CLASS: Cotazym, KU-ZYME, Pancrease MT, Viokase, and Zymase

IMPORTANT INFORMATION TO REMEMBER: This drug should be taken with food or milk. Only take the drug exactly as directed by your physician. Do not discontinue the drug without first consulting your physician; also, do not increase the dose without first consulting with your physician. Do not chew or crush the tiny spheres inside the capsules. Individuals can, however, sprinkle the capsule contents on cool, soft food (such as applesauce) and then swallow without chewing. This drug should be taken with plenty of water (eight ounces is preferred).

BRAND NAME: Crixivan

GENERIC NAME: indinavir

GENERIC FORM AVAILABLE: No

THERAPEUTIC CLASS: Protease inhibitor

DOSAGE FORMS: 200-mg and 400-mg capsules

MAIN USES: AIDS

USUAL DOSE: 800 mg every eight hours

AVERAGE PRICE: $145.25 for 200-mg and $284.51 for 400 mg

SIDE EFFECTS: nausea 12%, stomach pain 9%, headache 6%, diarrhea 5%, vomiting 4%, tiredness 4%, pain in the sides of the body 3%, insomnia 3%, taste changes 3%, back pain 2%, appetite changes 1%, dry mouth 1%, and dizziness 1%.

DRUG INTERACTIONS: Dilantin, Mycobutin, phenobarbital, Rifadin, Rimactine, and Tegretol may decrease the blood levels of the drug. The drug may increase the blood levels of Calan, Cardene, Cardizem, Catapres, Dilacor XR, DynaCirc, Halcion, Isoptin, Norvasc, Plendil, Procardia, Quinidex, Quinaglute, Sular, Tiazac, and Verelan. Nizoral may increase the blood levels of the drug. The drug should never be used with Hismanal, Seldane, or Seldane-D.

ALLERGIES: Individuals allergic to indinavir or any of its derivatives should discuss this with their doctor or pharmacist before using this drug.

PREGNANCY/BREAST-FEEDING: Category C—Risk cannot be ruled out. Human studies are lacking, and animal studies are either positive for fetal risk or lacking as well. However, potential benefits may justify the potential risk in using the drug. It is not known whether the drug is excreted in the breast milk; therefore, caution should be used when breast-feeding.

OTHER BRAND NAMES: None

OTHER DRUGS IN THE SAME THERAPEUTIC CLASS: Invirase and Norvir

IMPORTANT INFORMATION TO REMEMBER: The drug should always be taken one hour before or two hours after meals with a glassful of water (preferably eight ounces). The drug may be taken, however, with skim milk, juice, coffee, tea, or a light meal (such as dry toast with jelly; coffee with skim milk and sugar; or cornflakes with skim milk and sugar). Individuals should drink about 48 ounces of liquid per day while taking the drug. Also, take the drug at even intervals around the clock (if three times a day, take every eight hours). Only take the drug exactly as directed by your physician. Do not stop taking the drug without first consulting with your physician. It is important to have regular blood and liver function tests while taking this drug. Before taking any prescription or over-the-counter drugs, consult your physician or pharmacist.

BRAND NAME: Crolom

GENERIC NAME: cromolyn

GENERIC FORM AVAILABLE: No

THERAPEUTIC CLASS: Antiallergenic eyedrop

DOSAGE FORMS: 4% eyedrop solution

MAIN USES: Itching due to seasonal eye allergies

USUAL DOSE: one to two drops in each eye four to six times daily at regular intervals

AVERAGE PRICE: $49.91

SIDE EFFECTS: Most common: None. Less common: burning, stinging, itching, redness, and irritation.

DRUG INTERACTIONS: None of any clinical significance

ALLERGIES: Individuals allergic to cromolyn or any of its derivatives should discuss this with their doctor or pharmacist before using this drug.

PREGNANCY/BREAST-FEEDING: Category B—No evidence of risk in humans. Either animal findings show risk, but human findings do not; or, if no adequate human studies have been done, animal findings show no risk. It is not known whether the drug is excreted in the breast milk; therefore, caution should be used when breast-feeding.

OTHER BRAND NAMES: None

OTHER DRUGS IN THE SAME THERAPEUTIC CLASS: Alomide

IMPORTANT INFORMATION TO REMEMBER: Individuals should not use the drug while wearing contact lenses. Keep the container tightly closed and avoid touching the applicator tip to the eye—this could contaminate the product over time. Also, only administer one drop at a time. After application, keep the eye open for at least 30 seconds, roll the eyeball around, and avoid squinting. If a second drop is required, wait one to two minutes between drops. If another medication is to be used in the eye, wait at least 10 minutes before administering it.

BRAND NAME: Cutivate

GENERIC NAME: fluticasone

GENERIC FORM AVAILABLE: No

THERAPEUTIC CLASS: Topical corticosteroid

DOSAGE FORMS: 0.05% cream and 0.005% ointment

MAIN USES: Skin rashes, swelling, and itching

USUAL DOSE: Apply thin film twice daily.

AVERAGE PRICE: $18.49 for 15 g

SIDE EFFECTS: itching 1%–4%, slight burning 1%–4%, redness 1%–4%, slight irritation 1%–4%, lightheadedness 1%–4%, dry skin 1%–4%, and hives 1%–4%.

DRUG INTERACTIONS: None of any clinical significance

ALLERGIES: Individuals allergic to fluticasone or any of its derivatives should discuss this with their doctor or pharmacist before taking this drug.

PREGNANCY/BREAST-FEEDING: Category C—Risk cannot be ruled out. Human studies are lacking, and animal studies are either positive for fetal risk or lacking as well. However, potential benefits may justify the potential risk in using the drug. It is not known whether the drug is excreted in the breast milk; therefore, caution should be used when breast-feeding.

OTHER BRAND NAMES: None

OTHER DRUGS IN THE SAME THERAPEUTIC CLASS: Aclovate, Aristocort, Cordran, Cordran SP, Cyclocort, DesOwen, Diprolene, Elocon, Halog, Hytone, Kenalog, Lidex, Synalar, Temovate, Topicort, Tridesilon, Ultravate, Valisone, and Westcort

IMPORTANT INFORMATION TO REMEMBER: This drug is for external use only. Apply only a thin film of drug to skin and rub it in well. Never cover the skin after application with a bandage or wrapping unless directed to do so by a doctor. Never apply to damaged skin or open wounds unless directed to do so by a doctor. Discontinue use if irritation occurs.

BRAND NAME: Cyclocort

GENERIC NAME: amcinonide

GENERIC FORM AVAILABLE: No

THERAPEUTIC CLASS: Topical corticosteroid

DOSAGE FORMS: 0.1% cream, ointment, and lotion

MAIN USES: Skin rashes, swelling, and itching

USUAL DOSE: Apply thin film twice daily of the ointment; apply thin film two to three times daily of the cream; or apply twice daily for the lotion.

AVERAGE PRICE: $27.19 for 0.1% cream (15 g); $25.57 for 0.1% lotion (20 mL); $33.18 for 0.1% ointment (15 g)

SIDE EFFECTS: Most common: none. Less common: burning, itching, irritation, dry skin, rash, soreness of the skin, and acne.

DRUG INTERACTIONS: None of any clinical significance

ALLERGIES: Individuals allergic to amcinonide or any of its derivatives should discuss this with their doctor or pharmacist before using this drug.

PREGNANCY/BREAST-FEEDING: Category C—Risk cannot be ruled out. Human studies are lacking, and animal studies are either positive for fetal risk or lacking as well. However, potential benefits may justify the potential risk in using the drug. It is not known whether the drug is excreted in the breast milk; therefore, caution should be used when breast-feeding.

OTHER BRAND NAMES: None

OTHER DRUGS IN THE SAME THERAPEUTIC CLASS: Aclovate, Aristocort, Cordran, Cordran SP, Cutivate, DesOwen, Diprolene, Elocon, Halog, Hytone, Kenalog, Lidex, Synalar, Temovate, Topicort, Tridesilon, Ultravate, Valisone, and Westcort

IMPORTANT INFORMATION TO REMEMBER: This drug is for external use only. Apply only a thin film of drug to skin and rub it in well. Never cover the skin after application with a bandage or wrapping unless directed to do so by a doctor. Never apply to damaged skin or open wounds unless directed to do so by a doctor. Discontinue use if irritation occurs. If using the lotion, be sure to be shake it well.

BRAND NAME: Cycrin

GENERIC NAME: medroxyprogesterone

See entry for Provera

BRAND NAME: Cylert

GENERIC NAME: pemoline

GENERIC FORM AVAILABLE: No

THERAPEUTIC CLASS: Stimulant

DOSAGE FORMS: 18.75-mg, 37.5-mg, and 75-mg tablets, and 37.5-mg chewable tablets

MAIN USES: Attention deficit disorder with hyperactivity (ADDH)

USUAL DOSE: 37.5 mg daily in the morning. Depending on the patient, the dose may gradually be increased up to a maximum of 112.5 mg per day.

AVERAGE PRICE: $109.07 for 18.75 mg and $171.44 for 37.5 mg

SIDE EFFECTS: Most common: loss of appetite, insomnia, and weight loss. Less common: drowsiness; dizziness; irritability; depression; abnormal movements of tongue, lips, and face; stomach pain; nausea; headache; and possible growth suppression with long-term use.

DRUG INTERACTIONS: Increased risk of seizures when taken with other drugs used to treat epilepsy.

ALLERGIES: Individuals allergic to pemoline or any of its derivatives should discuss this with their doctor or pharmacist before using this drug.

PREGNANCY/BREAST-FEEDING: Category B—No evidence of risk in humans. Either animal findings show risk, but human findings do not; or, if no adequate human studies have been done, animal findings show no risk. It is not known whether the drug is excreted in the breast milk; therefore, caution should be used when breast-feeding.

OTHER BRAND NAMES: None

OTHER DRUGS IN THE SAME THERAPEUTIC CLASS: Adderall, Dexedrine, and Ritalin

IMPORTANT INFORMATION TO REMEMBER: This drug does cause some drowsiness in children and teens. Alcohol, anxiety medications, and narcotic painkillers may intensify the drowsiness effect of the drug. In adults, the drug causes stimulation, nervousness, and excitement. This medication is a controlled substance and may be habit-forming. The drug may require three to four weeks before noticeable improvement is seen. Do not stop taking the drug without first consulting your physician.

BRAND NAME: Cytomel

GENERIC NAME: liothyronine

GENERIC FORM AVAILABLE: No

THERAPEUTIC CLASS: Thyroid hormone

DOSAGE FORMS: 5-microgram, 25-microgram, and 50-microgram tablets

MAIN USES: Thyroid replacement therapy

USUAL DOSE: 25 micrograms to 75 micrograms daily

AVERAGE PRICE: $21.15 for 5 micrograms; $25.55 for 25 micrograms; and $39.61 for 50 micrograms

SIDE EFFECTS: The following side effects are rare: sensitivity to the heat, sweating, nervousness, fast heartbeat, heart palpitations, insomnia, stomach cramps, diarrhea, and weight loss.

DRUG INTERACTIONS: The drug may increase the effects of Coumadin. The drug may also decrease the effects of drugs used to treat diabetes. Estrogens may decrease the effectiveness of the drug. This drug may also enhance the effects of decongestants in cough and cold products. Colestid and Questran may decrease the absorption of the drug.

ALLERGIES: Individuals allergic to liothyronine or any of its derivatives should discuss this with their doctor or pharmacist before using this drug.

PREGNANCY/BREAST-FEEDING: Category A—Controlled studies show no risk. Adequate well-controlled studies in pregnant women did not show risk to the fetus. The drug is excreted in the breast milk; therefore, extreme caution should be used when breast-feeding.

OTHER BRAND NAMES: None

OTHER DRUGS IN THE SAME THERAPEUTIC CLASS: None

IMPORTANT INFORMATION TO REMEMBER: Do not stop taking the drug without first consulting with a doctor. It is important to the drug at the same time every day for consistent effect. Before taking over-the-counter medications, consult with your doctor or pharmacist.

BRAND NAME: Cytotec

GENERIC NAME: misoprostol

GENERIC FORM AVAILABLE: No

THERAPEUTIC CLASS: Stomach protectant

DOSAGE FORMS: 100-microgram and 200-microgram tablets

MAIN USES: Prevention of NSAID (drugs used for arthritis and pain relief) induced stomach ulcers

USUAL DOSE: 100 micrograms to 200 micrograms four times daily

AVERAGE PRICE: $74.11 for 100 micrograms and $102.84 for 200 micrograms

SIDE EFFECTS: diarrhea 13%, stomach pain 7%, nausea 3%, gas 3%, headache 2%, upset stomach 2%, vomiting 1%, constipation 1%, vaginal spotting 1%, and menstrual cramps 1%.

DRUG INTERACTIONS: Magnesium-containing antacids may make the diarrhea caused by the drug worse.

ALLERGIES: Individuals allergic to misoprostol or any of its derivatives should discuss this with their doctor or pharmacist before using this drug.

PREGNANCY/BREAST-FEEDING: Category X—Should not be used during pregnancy. Studies in animals and/or humans have shown fetal abnormalities and birth defects. The risks associated with using this drug clearly outweigh the benefits. This drug should never be used by someone who is pregnant or trying to become pregnant. Also, women should never breast-feed while using this drug.

OTHER BRAND NAMES: None

OTHER DRUGS IN THE SAME THERAPEUTIC CLASS: None

IMPORTANT INFORMATION TO REMEMBER: This drug should be taken with food or milk. The drug should never be taken by any woman who is pregnant or who is trying to become pregnant. If diarrhea develops and continues for more than one week, consult your physician. Only take the drug exactly as directed by your physician and do not increase the dose without first consulting with your physician.

BRAND NAME: Cytovene

GENERIC NAME: ganciclovir

GENERIC FORM AVAILABLE: No

THERAPEUTIC CLASS: Antiviral

DOSAGE FORMS: 250-mg capsules

MAIN USES: Viral infections

USUAL DOSE: 1 g three times daily or 500 mg six times daily

AVERAGE PRICE: $109.20 for 20 capsules

SIDE EFFECTS: diarrhea 41%, fever 38%, decrease in white blood cells 29%, nausea 28%, anemia 19%, stomach pain 17%, loss of appetite 15%, rash 15%, vomiting 13%, sweating 11%, infection 9%, numbness 8%, chills 7%, decrease in blood platelets 6%, pneumonia 6%, gas 6%, and itching 6%.

DRUG INTERACTIONS: Blood disorders have been associated with administration of this drug and Retrovir or bone marrow depressants such as cancer drugs.

ALLERGIES: Individuals allergic to ganciclovir, Zovirax, or any of their derivatives should discuss this with their doctor or pharmacist before using this drug.

PREGNANCY/BREAST-FEEDING: Category C—Risk cannot be ruled out. Human studies are lacking, and animal studies are either positive for fetal risk or lacking as well. However, potential benefits may justify the potential risk in using the drug. It is not known whether the drug is excreted in the breast milk; therefore, caution should be used when breast-feeding.

OTHER BRAND NAMES: None

OTHER DRUGS IN THE SAME THERAPEUTIC CLASS: Famvir, Valtrex, and Zovirax

IMPORTANT INFORMATION TO REMEMBER: This drug should be taken with food or milk. Blood tests, liver tests, and eye exams should be conducted by a physician on a regular basis. Also, take the drug at even intervals around the clock (if three times a day, take every eight hours). Take the drug until all the medication prescribed is gone unless directed otherwise by a physician. During periods of low blood counts, contact your doctor immediately if signs of an infection occur, such as fever, sore throat, or chills. Contraceptives, including barrier contraceptives (condoms) for men, should be used during treatment and for at least 90 days after treatment has stopped.

BRAND NAME: Cytoxan

GENERIC NAME: cyclophosphamide

GENERIC FORM AVAILABLE: No

THERAPEUTIC CLASS: Alkylating agent

DOSAGE FORMS: 25-mg and 50-mg tablets

MAIN USES: Cancer

USUAL DOSE: one to five mg per kg of body weight in divided doses over two to five days or three to five mg per kg of body weight twice weekly (1 kg = 2.2 pounds). Dosages are individualized based on body weight and type of cancer.

AVERAGE PRICE: $213.23 for 25 mg and $391.34 for 50 mg

SIDE EFFECTS: Most common: impairment of fertility, mouth sores, nausea, vomiting, hair loss, blood disorders, and anemia. Less common: urinary and kidney disorders, infections, stomach pain, and diarrhea.

DRUG INTERACTIONS: The drug may increase uric acid levels in the blood; therefore, probenecid and Anturane doses may have to be adjusted. The drug may increase bone marrow suppression when used with radiation or other cancer drugs. Caution should be used when combining this drug with other drugs that suppress the immune system such as Aristocort, Celestone, Decadron, Deltasone, and Imuran, Medrol, prednisone, and Sandiummune.

ALLERGIES: Individuals allergic to cyclophosphamide or any of its derivatives should discuss this with their doctor or pharmacist before using this drug.

PREGNANCY/BREAST-FEEDING: Category D—Positive evidence of risk. Human studies show risk to the fetus. Nevertheless, potential benefits may possibly outweigh the potential risk. This drug should not be taken by nursing mothers.

OTHER BRAND NAMES: None

OTHER DRUGS IN THE SAME THERAPEUTIC CLASS: Alkeran and Leukeran

IMPORTANT INFORMATION TO REMEMBER: If stomach upset occurs, take the drug with food or milk. It is extremely important to follow the dosing schedule set by your physician—do not deviate from this schedule. If unusual bleeding, bruising, black and tarry stools, blood in the urine, blood in the stool, or pinpoint red spots on the skin occur, contact your physician immediately. Nausea and vomiting may occur while taking this drug. Do not discontinue use unless directed by your physician. To prevent the bladder problems associated with taking this drug, drink plenty of water, preferably three quarts per day. You should also urinate as often as possible during the day and at least once during the night. If signs of an infection occur, such as fever, sore throat, or chills, contact your physician immediately.

BRAND NAME: Dalmane

GENERIC NAME: flurazepam

GENERIC FORM AVAILABLE: Yes

THERAPEUTIC CLASS: Benzodiazepine sedative

DOSAGE FORMS: 15-mg and 30-mg capsules

MAIN USES: Insomnia

USUAL DOSE: 15 mg to 30 mg at bedtime

AVERAGE PRICE: $68.71 (B)/$19.34 (G) for 15 mg and $83.47 (B)/$26.49 (G) for 30 mg

SIDE EFFECTS: Most common: drowsiness, dizziness, unsteadiness, disorientation, depression, and slurred speech. Less common: changes in appetite, changes in sex drive, depression, headache, diarrhea, nausea, heartburn, vision problems, weakness, pounding heartbeat, trouble urinating, staggering, and body pains.

DRUG INTERACTIONS: Central nervous system (CNS) depression may be increased when used with alcohol, narcotic painkillers, or other anxiety medications.

ALLERGIES: Individuals allergic to flurazepam, benzodiazepines, or other sleeping medications (such as those listed in "Other Drugs in the Same Therapeutic Class") should discuss this with their doctor or pharmacist before taking this drug.

PREGNANCY/BREAST-FEEDING: Category D—Positive evidence of risk. Human studies show risk to the fetus. Nevertheless, potential benefits may possibly outweigh the potential risk. This drug should not be taken by nursing mothers.

OTHER BRAND NAMES: None

OTHER DRUGS IN THE SAME THERAPEUTIC CLASS: Doral, Halcion, ProSom, and Restoril

IMPORTANT INFORMATION TO REMEMBER: This drug will cause drowsiness. Individuals should use caution when driving, operating machinery, or any task where mental alertness is required. The drug may take two to three days before maximum effect is seen. The incidence of drowsiness and unsteadiness increases with age. Alcohol, anxiety medications, and narcotic painkillers may intensify the drowsiness effect of the drug. This medication is a controlled substance and may be habit-forming. Do not increase the dose of medication without consulting with your doctor. Only take the amount prescribed by your doctor.

BRAND NAME: Danocrine

GENERIC NAME: danazol

GENERIC FORM AVAILABLE: Yes

THERAPEUTIC CLASS: Gonadotropin release inhibitor

DOSAGE FORMS: 50-mg and 100-mg, and 200-mg capsules

MAIN USES: Endometriosis and (fibrocystic breast disease)

USUAL DOSE: 100 mg to 400 mg twice daily for three to nine months

AVERAGE PRICE: $173.65 for 50 mg; $260.56 for 100 mg; $434.21 (B)/$224.05 (G) for 200 mg

SIDE EFFECTS: Most common: mssculinization (growth of facial hair, deep voice, decreasing breast size, and excessive growth of body hair), missed menstrual periods, breakthrough bleeding, heavy vaginal bleeding, irregular vaginal bleeding, vaginal spotting, decreased breast size, and weight gain. Less common: swelling of the feet and lower legs, muscle cramps, muscle spasms, unusual tiredness or weakness, acne, oily skin, oily hair, nervousness, mood changes, sweating, and flushing.

DRUG INTERACTIONS: The drug may increase the effects of Coumadin.

ALLERGIES: Individuals allergic to danazol or any of its derivatives should discuss this with their doctor or pharmacist before using this drug.

PREGNANCY/BREAST-FEEDING: Category X—Should not be used during pregnancy. Studies in animals and/or humans have shown fetal abnormalities and birth defects. The risks associated with using this drug clearly outweigh the benefits. This drug should never be used by someone who is pregnant or trying to become pregnant. Also, women should never breast-feed while using this drug.

OTHER BRAND NAMES: None

OTHER DRUGS IN THE SAME THERAPEUTIC CLASS: None

IMPORTANT INFORMATION TO REMEMBER: Only take the drug exactly as directed by your physician. Do not discontinue the drug without first consulting your physician. Individuals should also use a sunscreen to avoid overexposure to the sun; the drug may increase the skin's sensitivity to sunlight, which may cause one to sunburn more easily. Women who suspect they are pregnant should stop taking the drug immediately and contact their physician. Barrier birth control methods, such as condoms, should be used while taking the drug.

BRAND NAME: Darvocet-N

GENERIC NAME: Combination product containing: acetaminophen and propoxyphene

GENERIC FORM AVAILABLE: Yes

THERAPEUTIC CLASS: Narcotic analgesic + pain reliever

DOSAGE FORMS: 325-mg acetaminophen/50-mg propoxyphene tablets (Darvocet-N 50) and 650-mg acetaminophen/100-mg propoxyphene tablets (Darvocet-N 100)

MAIN USES: Mild to moderate pain

USUAL DOSE: two Darvocet-N 50 or one Darvocet-N 100 tablets every four hours as needed for pain

AVERAGE PRICE: $63.45 (B)/$20.88 (G)

SIDE EFFECTS: Most common: drowsiness, dizziness, tiredness, nausea, and vomiting. Less common: constipation, stomach pain, skin rash, headache, weakness, minor vision disturbances, feeling faint, and hallucinations.

DRUG INTERACTIONS: Alcohol, anxiety medications, and other narcotic painkillers may intensify the drowsiness effect of the drug. The drug may increase the blood levels of Tegretol. Liver toxicity may occur when used long-term with Anturane, Dilantin, and Mesantoin. This drug and Nardil or Parnate may cause severe and sometimes fatal reactions.

ALLERGIES: Individuals allergic to acetaminophen, propoxyphene, other pain relievers, or any of their derivatives should discuss this with their doctor or pharmacist before using this drug.

PREGNANCY/BREAST-FEEDING: Category C—Risk cannot be ruled out. Human studies are lacking, and animal studies are either positive for fetal risk or lacking as well. However, potential benefits may justify the potential risk in using the drug. The drug is excreted in the breast milk; therefore, extreme caution should be used when breast-feeding.

OTHER BRAND NAMES: None

OTHER DRUGS IN THE SAME THERAPEUTIC CLASS: Bancap-HC, DHCplus, Empirin #3, Empirin #4, Hydrocet, Lorcet 10/650, Lorcet Plus, Lortab, Percocet, Percodan, Phenaphen w/Codeine, Synalgos DC, Talacen, Tylenol #2, Tylenol #3, Tylenol #4, Tylox, Vicodin, and Zydone

IMPORTANT INFORMATION TO REMEMBER: This drug does cause drowsiness. Individuals should use caution when driving, operating machinery, or any task where mental alertness is required. Alcohol, anxiety medications, and other painkillers may intensify the drowsiness effect of the drug. Do not increase the dose without first consulting with your physician. This medication is a controlled substance and may be habit-forming.

BRAND NAME: Darvon and Darvon-N

GENERIC NAME: propoxyphene

See entry for Darvocet-N

BRAND NAME: Darvon Compound

GENERIC NAME: Combination product containing: propoxyphene, aspirin, and caffeine

Similar to Darvocet-N. See entry for Darvocet-N.

BRAND NAME: Daypro

GENERIC NAME: oxaprozin

GENERIC FORM AVAILABLE: No

THERAPEUTIC CLASS: Nonsteroidal anti-inflammatory drug (NSAID)

DOSAGE FORMS: 600-mg tablets

MAIN USES: Arthritis and (pain relief)

USUAL DOSE: 600 mg to 1800 mg once daily or in divided doses

AVERAGE PRICE: $176.41

SIDE EFFECTS: nausea 8%, upset stomach 8%, diarrhea 3%–9%, constipation 3%–9%, rash 3%–9%, dizziness 3%–9%, gas 1%–3%, vomiting 1%–3%, stomach pain 1%–3%, tiredness 1%–3%, depression 1%–3%, insomnia 1%–3%, ringing in the ears 1%–3%, and urinary problems 1%–3%.

DRUG INTERACTIONS: Aspirin will decrease the concentration of this drug in the blood. This drug may also decrease the effects of Lasix, Dyazide, HydroDIURIL, Maxzide, and other water pills. The drug may increase the blood levels of Eskalith, Lithobid, and Sandimmune. The drug may increase the toxic effects of the drug Rheumatrex. Caution should be used when taking the drug with Coumadin.

ALLERGIES: Individuals allergic to oxaprozin or other NSAIDs (such as those listed in"Other Drugs in the Same Therapeutic Class") should discuss this with their doctor or pharmacist before taking this drug.

PREGNANCY/BREAST-FEEDING: Category C—Risk cannot be ruled out. Human studies are lacking, and animal studies are either positive for fetal risk or lacking as well. However, potential benefits may justify the potential risk in using the drug. The drug should not, however, be used in late stages (last three months) of pregnancy. It is not known whether the drug is excreted in the breast milk; therefore, caution should be used when breast-feeding.

OTHER BRAND NAMES: None

OTHER DRUGS IN THE SAME THERAPEUTIC CLASS: Anaprox, Ansaid, aspirin, Cataflam, Clinoril, Disalcid, Dolobid, Easprin, Feldene, Indocin, Lodine, Lodine XL, Motrin, Nalfon, Naprosyn, Orudis, Oruvail, Relafen, Tolectin, Toradol, Voltaren, and Voltaren XR

IMPORTANT INFORMATION TO REMEMBER: This drug should be taken with food or milk to reduce the potential for injury to the stomach lining and stomach upset. This drug may take up to two weeks before a noticeable improvement in pain relief associated with arthritis is observed. Drinking alcohol while taking this drug may increase its potential to cause ulcers. This drug should only be used under the direct supervision of a doctor by individuals with a bleeding disorder or ulcer, or those who are currently taking Coumadin. Before taking over-the-counter pain relievers, consult your doctor or pharmacist. No more than one pain reliever should be taken at any one time unless otherwise directed by your doctor.

BRAND NAME: DDAVP

GENERIC NAME: desmopressin

GENERIC FORM AVAILABLE: No

THERAPEUTIC CLASS: Urinary controller

DOSAGE FORMS: 10 micrograms/spray nasal spray; 10 micrograms/0.1 mL intranasal solution; and 0.1-mg and 0.2-mg tablets

MAIN USES: Bedwetting and urinary problems in central cranial diabetes insipidus

USUAL DOSE: For bedwetting: one to four sprays of the nasal solution or spray at bedtime or 0.1 mg to 1.2 mg of the tablets per day in divided doses. For urinary problems in diabetics: 0.1 mL to 0.4 mL of the nasal spray or solution daily in single or divided doses.

AVERAGE PRICE: $124.63 for 0.1 mg (50 tablets); $254.63 for 0.2 mg (50 tablets); and $98.46 for 2.5 mL rhinal tube

SIDE EFFECTS: headache 5%, runny or stuffy nose 3%–8%, bloody nose 3%, dizziness 3%, stomach pain 2%, chills 2%, nostril pain 2%, upset stomach 2%, and watery and itchy eyes 2%.

DRUG INTERACTIONS: None of any clinical significance

ALLERGIES: Individuals allergic to desmopressin or any of its derivatives should discuss this with their doctor or pharmacist before using this drug.

PREGNANCY/BREAST-FEEDING: Category B—No evidence of risk in humans. Either animal findings show risk, but human findings do not; or, if no adequate human studies have been done, animal findings show no risk. It is not known whether the drug is excreted in the breast milk; therefore, caution should be used when breast-feeding.

OTHER BRAND NAMES: None

OTHER DRUGS IN THE SAME THERAPEUTIC CLASS: None

IMPORTANT INFORMATION TO REMEMBER: The nasal spray and nasal solution need to be kept in the refrigerator. Only take the drug exactly as directed by your physician. Do not discontinue the drug or increase the dose without first consulting your physician. When using the nasal spray or nasal solution, it is recommended that the dose should be split between each nostril. For example: if two sprays are to be used, instill one spray in each nostril.

BRAND NAME: Decadron

GENERIC NAME: dexamethasone

GENERIC FORM AVAILABLE: Yes

THERAPEUTIC CLASS: Glucocorticoid steroid

DOSAFE FORMS: 0.5-mg, 0.75-mg, 2-mg, 1.5-mg, 4-mg, and 6-mg tablets; 0.5 mg/5 mL elixir; 5–12 Dosepak; and 0.1% eye and ear drops

MAIN USES: Endocrine disorders, and multiple uses for its ability to reduce inflammation in various parts of the body, including for asthma

USUAL DOSE: 0.75 mg to 9 mg daily

AVERAGE PRICE: $72.60 (B)/$18.58 (G) for 0.5-mg tablets; $97.26 (B)/$20.78 (G) for 0.75-mg tablets; $186.84 (B)/$23.83 (G) for 1.5-mg tablets; and $13.42 for 5–12 Dosepak of 12 tablets

SIDE EFFECTS: Short-term use of the tablets: Most common: none. Less common: diarrhea, nausea, dizziness, insomnia, nervousness, headache, and stomach pain. Long-term use of the tablets: high blood pressure, muscle weakness, peptic ulcer, hemorrhage, thin fragile skin, facial swelling, weight gain, menstrual irregularities, glaucoma, and many others. Long-term use of the tablets should be avoided if possible.

DRUG INTERACTIONS: Antacids may decrease the absorption of the drug. Amytal, Butisol, Dilantin, Mebaral, Mesantoin, Nembutal, Rifadin, Rifamate, Rifater, Seconal, and Tuinal may decrease the effects of the drug. The drug may increase blood glucose levels. Patients taking drugs for diabetes, including insulin, may need to adjust their dose. The drug may decrease the effects of water pills used to treat high blood pressure and potassium supplements such as K-Dur, Klor-Con, K-Lyte, K-Tab, Micro-K, and Slow-K.

ALLERGIES: Individuals allergic to dexamethasone or other steroids (such as those listed in "Other Drugs in the Same Therapeutic Class") should discuss this with their doctor or pharmacist before taking this drug.

PREGNANCY/BREAST-FEEDING: Category C—Risk cannot be ruled out. Human studies are lacking, and animal studies are either positive for fetal risk or lacking as well. However, potential benefits may justify the potential risk in using the drug. It is not known whether the drug is excreted in the breast milk; therefore, caution should be used when breast-feeding.

OTHER BRAND NAMES: None

OTHER DRUGS IN THE SAME THERAPEUTIC CLASS: Aristocort, Celestone, Deltasone, Medrol, Pediapred, and Prelone

IMPORTANT INFORMATION TO REMEMBER: This drug should be taken with food or milk to reduce the potential for injury to the stomach lining and stomach upset. Drinking alcohol or taking aspirin while taking this drug may increase its potential to cause ulcers. Use exactly as directed by your physician. Never suddenly stop taking the drug without first consulting with your physician—this can be very dangerous. The drug may also cause some weight gain when used for long periods of time.

BRAND NAME: Deconamine and Deconamine SR

GENERIC FORM: Combination product containing: chlorpheniramine and pseudoephedrine

GENERIC FORM AVAILABLE: Yes

THERAPEUTIC CLASS: Antihistamine + decongestant

DOSAGE FORMS: 4-mg chlorpheniramine/60-mg pseudoephedrine tablets; 8-mg chlorpheniramine/120-mg pseudoephedrine sustained-release capsules; and 2 mg chlorpheniramine/30 mg pseudoephedrine per 5 mL syrup

MAIN USES: Nasal allergies and congestion

USUAL DOSE: one tablet of Deconamine three to four times daily as needed or one capsule of Deconamine SR every 12 hours as needed

AVERAGE PRICE: $51.38 Deconamine tablets; $79.95 (B)/ $26.38 (G) Deconamine SR capsules

SIDE EFFECTS: Most common: drowsiness. Less common: nausea, giddiness, dry mouth, blurred vision, pounding heartbeat, flushing, and increased irritability or excitability (especially in children).

DRUG INTERACTIONS: Blocadren, Cartrol, Corgard, Inderal, Kerlone, Levatol, Lopressor, Normodyne, Sectral, Tenormin, Toprol-XL, Trandate, Visken, and Zebeta may increase the effects of the drug. The drug may also reduce the effects of blood-pressure-lowering drugs. Nardil or Parnate may significantly raise blood pressure when taken with this drug.

PREGNANCY/BREAST-FEEDING: Category C—Risk cannot be ruled out. Human studies are lacking, and animal studies are either positive for fetal risk or lacking as well. However, potential benefits may justify the potential risk in using the drug. The drug is excreted in the breast milk; therefore, caution should be used when breast-feeding

OTHER BRAND NAMES: Novafed-A

OTHER DRUGS IN THE SAME THERAPEUTIC CLASS: Bromfed, Bromfed PD, Claritin-D, Comhist LA, Fedahist, Naldecon, Nolamine, Novafed-A, Ornade, Poly-Histine-D, Rondec, Rynatan, Seldane-D, Semprex-D, Tavist-D, and Trinalin

IMPORTANT INFORMATION TO REMEMBER: This drug does cause drowsiness. Individuals should use caution when driving, operating machinery, or any task where mental alertness is required. Alcohol, anxiety medications, and narcotic painkillers may intensify the drowsiness effect of the drug. This drug may also cause a dry mouth; sugarless gum or hard candy will help take care of this problem. Patients with glaucoma, high blood pressure, heart conditions, or urinary or prostate problems should consult their doctor before taking this drug.

BRAND NAME: Deconsal II

GENERIC NAME: Combination product containing: pseudoephedrine and guaifenesin

GENERIC FORM AVAILABLE: No

THERAPEUTIC CLASS: Decongestant + expectorant

DOSAGE FORMS: 60-mg pseudoephedrine/600-mg guaifenesin sustained-release tablets

MAIN USES: Nasal congestion and cough

USUAL DOSE: one to two tablets every 12 hours

AVERAGE PRICE: $81.90

SIDE EFFECTS: Most common: none. Less common: drowsiness, nausea, giddiness, dry mouth, blurred vision, pounding heartbeat, flushing, and increased irritability or excitability (especially in children).

DRUG INTERACTIONS: Blocadren, Cartrol, Corgard, Inderal, Kerlone, Levatol, Lopressor, Normodyne, Sectral, Tenormin, Toprol-XL, Trandate, Visken, and Zebeta may increase the effects of the drug. The drug may also reduce the effects of blood-pressure-lowering drugs. Nardil or Parnate may significantly raise blood pressure when taken with this drug.

ALLERGIES: Individuals allergic to pseudoephedrine, guaifenesin, or any of their derivatives should discuss this with their doctor or pharmacist before using this drug.

PREGNANCY/BREAST-FEEDING: Category C—Risk cannot be ruled out. Human studies are lacking, and animal studies are either positive for fetal risk or lacking as well. However, potential benefits may justify the potential risk in using the drug. Pseudoephedrine is excreted in the breast milk; therefore, caution should be used when breast-feeding.

OTHER BRAND NAMES: None

OTHER DRUGS IN THE SAME THERAPEUTIC CLASS: Duratuss, Entex, Entex LA, Entex PSE, Exgest LA, Guaifed, Guaifed-PD, and Zephrex LA

IMPORTANT INFORMATION TO REMEMBER: Patients with high blood pressure or heart conditions should consult their doctor before taking this drug. This drug should be taken with plenty of water (eight ounces is preferred). Do not crush or divide tablets—this will destroy the matrix that ensures the delayed release of the drug in the intestines. Swallow the tablets whole. The tablets may, however, be cut in half for easier swallowing. Do not increase the dose without first consulting with your physician.

BRAND NAME: **Deltasone**

GENERIC NAME: prednisone

GENERIC FORM AVAILABLE: Yes

THERAPEUTIC CLASS: Glucocorticoid steroid

DOSAGE FORMS: 2.5-mg, 5-mg, 10-mg, 20-mg, and 50-mg tablets; and 5-mg tablet Dosepak ·

MAIN USES: Endocrine disorders, and multiple uses for its ability to reduce inflammation in various parts of the body, including asthma

USUAL DOSE: normal doses range from 5 mg to 60 mg per day

AVERAGE PRICE: $6.90 (B)/$6.58 (G) for 2.5 mg; $8.78 (B)/ $6.91 (G) for 5 mg; $9.88 (B)/$7.57 (G) for 10 mg; $12.96 (B)/ $11.64 (G) for 20 mg; and $31.88 (B)/$24.95 (G) for 50 mg

SIDE EFFECTS: Short-term use of the tablets: Most common: none. Less common: diarrhea, nausea, dizziness, insomnia, nervousness, headache, and stomach pain. Long-term use of the tablets: high blood pressure, muscle weakness, peptic ulcer, hemorrhage, thin fragile skin, facial swelling, weight gain, menstrual irregularities, glaucoma, and many others. Long-term use of the tablets should be avoided if possible.

DRUG INTERACTIONS: Antacids may decrease the absorption of the drug. Amytal, Butisol, Dilantin, Mebaral, Mesantoin, Nembutal, Rifadin, Rifamate, Rifater, Seconal, and Tuinal may decrease the effects of the drug. The drug may increase blood glucose levels. Patients taking drugs for diabetes, including insulin, may need to adjust their dose. The drug may decrease the effects of water pills used to treat high blood pressure and potassium supplements, such as K-Dur, Klor-Con, K-Lyte, K-Tab, Micro-K, and Slow-K.

ALLERGIES: Individuals allergic to prednisone or other steroids (such as those listed in "Other Drugs in the Same Therapeutic Class") should discuss this with their doctor or pharmacist before taking this drug.

PREGNANCY/BREAST-FEEDING: Category C—Risk cannot be ruled out. Human studies are lacking, and animal studies are either positive for fetal risk or lacking as well. However, potential benefits may justify the potential risk in using the drug. The drug can be excreted in the breast milk; therefore, caution should be used when breast-feeding.

OTHER BRAND NAMES: Orasone

OTHER DRUGS IN THE SAME THERAPEUTIC CLASS: Aristocort, Celestone, Decadron, Medrol, Pediapred, and Prelone

IMPORTANT INFORMATION TO REMEMBER: This drug should be taken with food or milk to reduce the potential for injury to the stomach lining and stomach upset. Drinking alcohol while taking this drug may increase its potential to cause ulcers. Use exactly as directed by your physician. Never suddenly stop taking the drug without first consulting with your physician—this can be very dangerous. The drug may also cause some weight gain when used for long periods of time.

BRAND NAME: Demadex

GENERIC NAME: torsemide

GENERIC FORM AVAILABLE: No

THERAPEUTIC CLASS: Loop diuretic (water pill)

DOSAGE FORMS: 5-mg, 10-mg, 20-mg, and 100-mg tablets

MAIN USES: Water retention (fluid retention due to congestive heart failure, kidney disease, or cirrhosis of the liver) and high blood pressure

USUAL DOSE: 5 mg to 20 mg once daily

AVERAGE PRICE: $64.75 for 5 mg; $71.75 for 10 mg; $82.25 for 20 mg; $316.75 for 100 mg

SIDE EFFECTS: headache 7%, excessive urination 7%, dizziness 3%, runny nose 2%, weakness 2%, diarrhea 2%, ECG abnormality 2%, cough 2%, constipation 2%, nausea 2%, upset stomach 2%, sore throat 2%, chest pain 1%, insomnia 1%, and nervousness 1%.

DRUG INTERACTIONS: The drug may increase the levels of Coumadin, Eskalith, and Lithobid in the blood. Indocin and probenecid may make the drug less effective.

ALLERGIES: Individuals allergic to torsemide, sulfa drugs, or any of their derivatives should discuss this with their doctor or pharmacist before using this drug.

PREGNANCY/BREAST-FEEDING: Category B—No evidence of risk in humans. Either animal findings show risk, but human findings do not; or, if no adequate human studies have been done, animal findings show no risk. It is not known whether the drug is excreted in the breast milk; therefore, caution should be used when breast-feeding.

OTHER BRAND NAMES: None

OTHER DRUGS IN THE SAME THERAPEUTIC CLASS: Bumex, Edecrin, and Lasix

IMPORTANT INFORMATION TO REMEMBER: If stomach upset occurs, the drug may be taken with food or milk. If the drug is to be taken once daily, take it in the morning due to increased urine output. Individuals with kidney disease should discuss this with their doctor before taking this drug. Before taking over-the-counter cold and allergy preparations, consult your doctor or pharmacist—these products may raise your blood pressure. The drug may cause the elimination of potassium from the body. It is therefore a good idea to eat a banana or drink orange, grapefruit, or apple juice every day to replace lost potassium.

BRAND NAME: Demerol

GENERIC NAME: meperidine

GENERIC FORM AVAILABLE: No

THERAPEUTIC CLASS: Narcotic analgesic

DOSAGE FORMS: 50-mg and 100-mg tablets, and 50 mg/5 mL syrup

MAIN USES: Relief of moderate to severe pain

USUAL DOSE: 50 mg to 150 mg every three to four hours as needed

AVERAGE PRICE: $103.65 for 50 mg and $197.17 for 100 mg

SIDE EFFECTS: Most common: lightheadedness, dizziness, drowsiness, tiredness, low blood pressure, nausea, vomiting, and sweating. Less common: weakness, agitation, tremor, depressed breathing, hallucinations, dry mouth, constipation, disorientation, vision problems, muscle spasms, and slow heartbeat.

DRUG INTERACTIONS: The effects of the drug may be increased when used with Compazine, Mellaril, Prolixin, Serentil, Stelazine, Thorazine, or Trilafon. Alcohol, anxiety medications, or other narcotic painkillers may intensify the drowsiness and respiratory depression effects of the drug. This drug and Nardil or Parnate may cause severe and sometimes fatal reactions.

ALLERGIES: Individuals allergic to meperdine or any of its derivatives should discuss this with their doctor or pharmacist before using this drug.

PREGNANCY/BREAST-FEEDING: Category C—Risk cannot be ruled out. Human studies are lacking, and animal studies are either positive for fetal risk or lacking as well. However, potential benefits may justify the potential risk in using the drug. The drug is excreted in the breast milk; therefore, extreme caution should be used when breast-feeding.

OTHER BRAND NAMES: None

OTHER DRUGS IN THE SAME THERAPEUTIC CLASS: Dilaudid, Dolophine, Duragesic, Levo-Dromoran, MS Contin, MSIR, Oramorph SR, Roxanol, and Stadol.

IMPORTANT INFORMATION TO REMEMBER: This is a very potent drug and may cause a lot of drowsiness. Individuals should use extreme caution when driving, operating machinery, or any task where mental alertness is required. Alcohol, anxiety medications, and other narcotic painkillers will intensify the drowsiness effect of the drug. Do not increase the dose without first consulting with your physician—this could be very dangerous and possibly life-threatening. If stomach upset occurs, take the drug with food or milk. This medication is a controlled substance, may be habit-forming, and should only be used as needed for pain relief. This prescription cannot be refilled; a new written prescription must be obtained each time. The potential for abuse with this medication is high.

BRAND NAME: Demulen 1/35 and Demulen 1/50

GENERIC NAME: Combination product containing: ethinyl estradiol and ethynodiol diacetate

GENERIC FORM AVAILABLE: Yes

THERAPEUTIC CLASS: Progestin + estrogen contraceptive

DOSAGE FORMS: Demulen 1/35: each tablet contains 35 micrograms ethinyl estradiol/1 mg ethynodiol diacetate. Demulen 1/50: each tablet contains 50 micrograms ethinyl estradiol/1 mg ethynodiol diacetate.

MAIN USES: Birth control

USUAL DOSE: Take one tablet daily for 21 or 28 days, beginning on the fifth day of the cycle. Day One of the cycle is the first day of menstrual bleeding.

AVERAGE PRICE: $30.77 (B)/$16.47 (G) for both Demulen 1/35 and 1/50

SIDE EFFECTS: Most common: stomach cramps, bloating, acne, appetite changes, nausea, swelling of the feet and ankles, weight gain, swelling of the breasts, breast tenderness, and unusual tiredness or weakness. Less common: changes in vaginal bleeding, feeling faint, increased blood pressure, depression, stomach pain, vaginal itching, yeast infections, brown, blotchy spots on the skin, diarrhea, dizziness, headaches, migraines, increased body and facial hair, increased sensitivity of the skin to the sun, irritability, some hair loss from the scalp, vomiting, blood clots, weight loss, and changes in sexual desire.

DRUG INTERACTIONS: Antibiotics may decrease the effectiveness of the drug. The drug may interfere with the effectiveness of Parlodel. The drug may reduce the effects of Coumadin. The drug may increase the blood levels of Anafranil, Asendin, Elavil, Endep, Norpramin, Pamelor, Sinequan, Surmontil, Tofranil, and Vivactil when used for long periods of time. Smoking is not recommended while taking this drug due to the increased risk of heart disease, stroke, and high blood pressure.

ALLERGIES: Individuals allergic to ethinyl estradiol, ethynodiol diacetate, or any of their derivatives should discuss this with their doctor or pharmacist before using this drug.

PREGNANCY/BREAST-FEEDING: Category X—Should not be used during pregnancy. Studies in animals and/or humans have shown fetal abnormalities and birth defects. The risks associated with using this drug clearly outweigh the benefits. This drug should never be used by someone who is pregnant or trying to become pregnant. Also, women should never breast-feed while using this drug.

OTHER BRAND NAMES: None

OTHER DRUGS IN THE SAME THERAPEUTIC CLASS: Brevicon, Desogen, Levlen, Lo/Ovral, Loestrin, Modicon, Nordette, Norinyl, Ortho-Cept, Ortho-Cyclen, Ortho-Novum, Ovcon, and Ovral

IMPORTANT INFORMATION TO REMEMBER: Only take the drug exactly as directed by your physician. It is important to take the drug at the same time every day (bedtime). Do not discontinue the drug without first consulting your physician. The drug should not be used by women with a history of heart disease, stroke, high blood pressure, breast cancer, or other blood vessel disease. Breakthrough bleeding may occur during the first few months; if this persists, notify your doctor. This drug does not provide protection against the HIV (AIDS) virus. It is important to use a second method of birth control during the first week when treatment has just begun. It may be necessary to use a second form of birth control when antibiotics are being taken. Also, women who smoke run a higher risk of heart disease, stroke, and high blood pressure when taking this drug. If pregnancy is suspected, stop taking the drug immediately.

BRAND NAME: Denavir

GENERIC NAME: penciclovir

GENERIC FORM AVAILABLE: No

THERAPEUTIC CLASS: Topical antiviral

DOSAGE FORMS: 1% cream

MAIN USES: Cold sores

USUAL DOSE: Apply the drug every two hours while awake for four days.

AVERAGE PRICE: $34.91 for 2 g

SIDE EFFECTS: headache 5%, allergic reaction 1%, numbness in the lips or mouth 1%, taste changes 1%, rash 1%, and redness 1%

DRUG INTERACTIONS: None of any clinical significance

ALLERGIES: Individuals allergic to penciclovir, Zovirax, or any of their derivatives should discuss this with their doctor or pharmacist before using this drug.

PREGNANCY/BREAST-FEEDING: Category B—No evidence of risk in humans. Either animal findings show risk, but human findings do not; or, if no adequate human studies have been done, animal findings show no risk. It is not known whether the drug is excreted in the breast milk; therefore, caution should be used when breast-feeding.

OTHER BRAND NAMES: None

OTHER DRUGS IN THE SAME THERAPEUTIC CLASS: Zovirax

IMPORTANT INFORMATION TO REMEMBER: Only use the drug exactly as directed by your physician. It is important to use the drug every two hours while awake for maximum effectiveness. Use the drug for the full course of therapy; otherwise the infection may return. The drug should be started at the first sign of a cold sore in order to be most effective.

BRAND NAME: Depakene

GENERIC NAME: Valproic acid

Very similar to Depakote. See entry for Depakote.

BRAND NAME: Depakote

GENERIC NAME: divalproex sodium

GENERIC FORM AVAILABLE: No

THERAPEUTIC CLASS: Anticonvulsant and antiepileptic

DOSAGE FORMS: 125-mg, 250-mg, and 500-mg tablets and 125-mg capsules

MAIN USES: Seizures, mania, and migraine headaches

USUAL DOSE: Doses are very precise and are based on body weight. The normal dose is 15 mg to 60 mg per kg of body weight per day in single or divided doses. (1 kg = 2.2 pounds)

AVERAGE PRICE: $44.84 for 125 mg; $88.04 for 250 mg; $162.40 for 500 mg; and $45.09 for 125-mg capsules

SIDE EFFECTS: Most common: nausea, vomiting, indigestion, and drowsiness. Less common: diarrhea, stomach cramps, constipation, missed periods, weight changes, appetite changes, hallucinations, tremors, spots before the eyes, hair loss, behavioral changes, muscle weakness, depression, emotional upset, hyperactivity, and aggression.

DRUG INTERACTIONS: Alcohol, anxiety medications, and narcotic painkillers may intensify the drowsiness effect of the drug. The drug may increase the risk of bleeding in individuals taking Coumadin. The drug may increase the blood levels of Amytal, Butisol, Mebaral, Mysoline, Nembutal, phenobarbital, Seconal, and Tuinal. Lariam and Tegretol may decrease the blood levels of this drug. When Dilantin and Depakote are used together, this combination may decrease the blood levels of Depakote and increase the blood levels of Dilantin.

ALLERGIES: Individuals allergic to divalproex sodium, Depakene, or any of their derivatives should discuss this with their doctor or pharmacist before using this drug.

PREGNANCY/BREAST-FEEDING: Category D—Positive evidence of risk. Human studies show risk to the fetus. Nevertheless, potential benefits may possibly outweigh the potential risk. This drug should not be taken by nursing mothers.

OTHER BRAND NAME: None

OTHER DRUGS IN THE SAME THERAPEUTIC CLASS: Depakene

IMPORTANT INFORMATION TO REMEMBER: This drug does cause drowsiness. Individuals should use caution when driving, operating machinery, or any task where mental alertness is required. Alcohol, anxiety medications, and narcotic painkillers may intensify the drowsiness effect of the drug. Only take the drug exactly as directed by your physician. Do not discontinue the drug without first consulting your physician. Do not increase the dose without first consulting with your physician. If stomach upset occurs, take the drug with food or milk. The drug should not be used by patients with liver disease. Depakote capsules may be swallowed whole or the contents may be sprinkled over soft food (such as applesauce) and swallowed without chewing. Regular checkups with a doctor should be conducted to ensure proper therapeutic dosing.

BRAND NAME: Deponit

GENERIC NAME: nitroglycerin patch

See entry for Nitro-Dur

BRAND NAME: Depo-Provera

GENERIC NAME: medroxyprogesterone

GENERIC FORM AVAILABLE: No

THERAPEUTIC CLASS: Progestin

DOSAGE FORMS: 150 mg/mL intramuscular injection

MAIN USES: Birth control

USUAL DOSE: one 150-mg injection in the upper arm or buttocks every three months

AVERAGE PRICE: $55.53 per injection

SIDE EFFECTS: bleeding irregularities 5%–55%, weight changes more than 5%, headache more than 5%, nervousness more than 5%, stomach pain more than 5%, dizziness more than 5%, weakness more than 5%, decreased sex drive 1%–5%, backache 1%–5%, vaginal infection 1%–5%, pelvic pain 1%–5%, breast pain 1%–5%, leg cramps 1%–5%, depression 1%–5%, nausea 1%–5%, insomnia 1%–5%, acne 1%–5%, bloating 1%–5%, swelling 1%–5%, hot flashes 1%–5%, muscle pain 1%–5%, and no hair growth 1%–5%.

DRUG INTERACTIONS: None of any clinical significance

ALLERGIES: Individuals allergic to medroxyprogesterone or any of its derivatives should discuss this with their doctor or pharmacist before using this drug.

PREGNANCY/BREAST-FEEDING: Category X—Should not be used during pregnancy. Studies in animals and/or humans have shown fetal abnormalities and birth defects. The risks associated with using this drug clearly outweigh the benefits. This drug should never be used by someone who is pregnant or trying to become pregnant. Also, women should never breast-feed while using this drug.

OTHER BRAND NAMES: None

OTHER DRUGS IN THE SAME THERAPEUTIC CLASS: Micronor, Nor-QD, Norplant, and Ovrette

IMPORTANT INFORMATION TO REMEMBER: The drug should be used with caution by women with a history of heart disease, stroke, high blood pressure, breast cancer, or other blood vessel disease. Breakthrough bleeding may occur during the first few months. If this persists, notify your physician. This drug does not provide protection against the HIV (AIDS) virus. The first injection should be given sometime during the first five days after the start of a menstruation (period). Injections must be given every three months. If more than 14 weeks has passed since the last injection, a doctor should make sure the woman is not pregnant before giving her another injection. For women using the drug in clinical trials, only 0.3% became pregnant during the first year. According to clinical trials, 55% of women using the drug experienced abnormal or missed periods sometime during the first year of use and 68% after two years of use. Unlike other birth control medications (such as the pill), it may take nine months or longer to become pregnant after the drug is discontinued.

BRAND NAME: Desogen

GENERIC NAME: Combination product containing: desogestrel and ethinyl estradiol

See entry for Ortho-Cept

BRAND NAME: DesOwen

GENERIC NAME: desonide

GENERIC FORM AVAILABLE: Yes

THERAPEUTIC CLASS: Topical corticosteroid

DOSAGE FORMS: 0.05% cream, ointment, or lotion

MAIN USES: Skin rashes, swelling, and itching

USUAL DOSE: Apply a thin film two to three times daily.

AVERAGE PRICE: $18.11 (B)/$11.92 (G) for 0.05% cream and ointment

SIDE EFFECTS: Most common: none. Less common: burning, itching, irritation, dry skin, rash, soreness of the skin, and acne.

DRUG INTERACTIONS: None of any clinical significance

ALLERGIES: Individuals allergic to desonide or any of its derivatives should discuss this with their doctor or pharmacist before using this drug.

PREGNANCY/BREAST-FEEDING: Category C—Risk cannot be ruled out. Human studies are lacking, and animal studies are either positive for fetal risk or lacking as well. However, potential benefits may justify the potential risk in using the drug. It is not known whether the drug is excreted in the breast milk; therefore, caution should be used when breast-feeding.

OTHER BRAND NAMES: Tridesilon

OTHER DRUGS IN THE SAME THERAPEUTIC CLASS: Aclovate, Aristocort, Cordran, Cordran SP, Cutivate, Cyclocort, Diprolene, Elocon, Florone, Halog, Hytone, Kenalog, Lidex, Synalar, Temovate, Topicort, Tridesilon, Ultravate, Valisone, and Westcort

IMPORTANT INFORMATION TO REMEMBER: This drug is for external use only. Apply only a thin film of drug to skin and rub it in well. Never cover the skin after application with a bandage or wrapping unless directed to do so by a doctor. Never apply to damaged skin or open wounds unless directed to do so by a doctor. Discontinue use if irritation occurs. If using the lotion, be sure to shake it well.

BRAND NAME: Desquam-E and Desquam-X

GENERIC NAME: benzoyl peroxide

GENERIC FORM AVAILABLE: No

THERAPEUTIC CLASS: Antibacterial/keratolytic

DOSAGE FORMS: 2.5%, 5%, and 10% water-based gels; 2.5%, 5%, and 10% emollient gels; 5% and 10% washes; and 10% bar

MAIN USES: Acne

USUAL DOSE: Use one to two times daily for all products except the 10% bar, which may be used one to three times daily.

AVERAGE PRICE: $13.52 for 2.5% gel; $15.88 for 5% gel; $16.12 for 10% gel; $17.59 for 5% wash; and $21.83 for 10% wash

SIDE EFFECTS: excessively dry skin 4%, irritation 1%–10%, stinging 1%–10%, redness 1%–10%, and allergic reaction 1%–2%.

DRUG INTERACTIONS: Sunscreens containing PABA (paraamino-benzoic acid) may discolor the skin yellowish-brown when used with this drug.

ALLERGIES: Individuals allergic to benzoyl peroxide or any of its derivatives should discuss this with their doctor or pharmacist before using this drug.

PREGNANCY/BREAST-FEEDING: Category C—Risk cannot be ruled out. Human studies are lacking, and animal studies are either positive for fetal risk or lacking as well. However, potential benefits may justify the potential risk in using the drug. It is not known whether the drug is excreted in the breast milk; therefore, caution should be used when breast-feeding.

OTHER BRAND NAMES: None

OTHER DRUGS IN THE SAME THERAPEUTIC CLASS: Benzac, Benzagel, and Persa-Gel

IMPORTANT INFORMATION TO REMEMBER: This drug is for external use only. Before applying, wash acne thoroughly with warm soapy water to remove dirt and skin oils, pat skin dry, and then apply the drug. If you need to apply another medication for acne, wait at least one hour. When using the cleansing wash, be sure to rinse affected areas thoroughly with water. Avoid contact with eyes, mouth, and other mucous membranes with all Desquam products. These products may discolor fabric or hair. Do not apply the drug to irritated or damaged skin.

BRAND NAME: Desyrel

GENERIC NAME: trazodone

GENERIC FORM AVAILABLE: Yes

THERAPEUTIC CLASS: Triazolopyridine antidepressant

DOSAGE FORMS: 50-mg, 100-mg, 150-mg, and 300-mg tablets

MAIN USES: Depression and {insomnia}

USUAL DOSE: 50 mg to 300 mg per day given in single or divided doses

AVERAGE PRICE: $152.33 (B)/$21.54 (G) for 50 mg; $208.51 (B)/$30.67 (G) for 100 mg; $229.33 (B)/$65.98 (G) for 150 mg

SIDE EFFECTS: drowsiness 40%, dry mouth 34%, dizziness 28%, headache 20%, blurred vision 15%, nausea 13%, confusion 10%, constipation 8%, skin rash 7%, nasal congestion 6%, tiredness 6%, weight changes 5%, dizziness 5%, diarrhea 5%, muscle pains 5%, tremors 5%, low blood pressure 4%, bad taste in the mouth 2%, decreased concentration 1%, and decreased sex drive 1%.

DRUG INTERACTIONS: Alcohol, anxiety medications, and narcotic painkillers may intensify the drowsiness effect of the drug. Drugs used to treat high blood pressure may cause blood pressure to become too low when used with this drug. The drug may increase the blood levels of Dilantin.

ALLERGIES: Individuals allergic to trazodone or any of its derivatives should discuss this with their doctor or pharmacist before using this drug.

PREGNANCY/BREAST-FEEDING: Category C—Risk cannot be ruled out. Human studies are lacking, and animal studies are either positive for fetal risk or lacking as well. However, potential benefits may justify the potential risk in using the drug. The drug is excreted in the breast milk; therefore, extreme caution should be used when breast-feeding.

OTHER BRAND NAMES: None

OTHER DRUGS IN THE SAME THERAPEUTIC CLASS: None

IMPORTANT INFORMATION TO REMEMBER: The drug may require four weeks before improvement in symptoms of depression are seen; some individuals may see a difference within two weeks. This drug does cause drowsiness. Individuals should use caution when driving, operating machinery, or any task where mental alertness is required. Alcohol, anxiety medications, and narcotic painkillers may intensify the drowsiness effect of the drug. The drug may also cause dizziness when suddenly rising from a sitting or lying-down position. This drug may cause a permanent and many times painful erection of the penis in men. This side effect can be quite common and in many cases can only be corrected with surgery. Therefore, men may not want to use this drug. The drug should be taken with food or milk to increase the absorption of the drug.

BRAND NAME: **Dexacort** (nasal aerosol)

GENERIC NAME: dexamethasone

GENERIC FORM AVAILABLE: No

THERAPEUTIC CLASS: Steroid nasal inhaler

DOSAGE FORMS: 84 micrograms per inhalation delivered from a Turbinaire nasal aerosol

MAIN USES: Nasal allergies and nasal polyps

USUAL DOSE: two sprays in each nostril two to three times daily

AVERAGE PRICE: $61.23

SIDE EFFECTS: Most common: nasal irritation and dryness. Less common: sneezing, headache, lightheadedness, nausea, bloody nose, congestion, asthma, perforation of the nasal septum, and loss of smell.

DRUG INTERACTIONS: Caution should be used when taking this drug with other oral corticosteroids such as Aristocort, Deltasone, Decadron, Medrol, and prednisone.

ALLERGIES: Individuals allergic to dexamethasone or other nasal steroids (such as those listed in "Other Drugs in the Same Therapeutic Class") should discuss with their doctor or pharmacist before taking this drug.

PREGNANCY/BREAST-FEEDING: Category C—Risk cannot be ruled out. Human studies are lacking, and animal studies are either positive for fetal risk or lacking as well. However, potential benefits may justify the potential risk in using the drug. It is not known whether the drug is excreted in the breast milk; therefore, caution should be used when breast-feeding.

OTHER BRAND NAMES: None

OTHER DRUGS IN THE SAME THERAPEUTIC CLASS: Beconase, Beconase AQ, Flonase, Nasacort, Nasalide, Rhinocort, Vancenase, and Vancenase AQ

IMPORTANT INFORMATION TO REMEMBER: The drug is not intended to provide immediately relief of nasal allergies. To receive the full benefits of the drug, use it on a regular basis as a maintenance medication. If improvements are not seen in seven days, the individual needs to be reassessed by a doctor. The drug may take up to three weeks before the full benefits are seen. Never exceed prescribed dosage unless directed to do so by a doctor—excessive use beyond prescribed dosage is potentially dangerous. This drug should not be used by individuals with fungal, bacterial, systemic viral, or respiratory tract infections; unhealed wounds inside the nose; or tuberculosis.

When using the nasal spray or aerosol, use the following procedure:

1) Blow your nose gently to clear your nostrils, if necessary.
2) With your other hand, gently place a finger against the side of your nose to close the opposite nostril.
3) Insert the tip of the bottle or aerosol into the open nostril. Point the tip toward the back and outer side of the nostril once inside.
4) After releasing the spray, close your mouth, sniff deeply, hold your breath for a few seconds, then breathe out through your mouth.
5) Tilt your head back slightly for a few seconds to allow the drug to spread to the back of your nose.
6) Repeat the same procedure for the other nostril.
7) If using more than one spray in each nostril, wait five minutes between sprays.

BRAND NAME: Dexedrine

GENERIC NAME: dextroamphetamine

GENERIC FORM AVAILABLE: No

THERAPEUTIC CLASS: Amphetamine stimulant

DOSAGE FORMS: 5-mg, 10-mg, and 15-mg sustained-release capsules and 5-mg tablets

MAIN USES: Narcolepsy and attention deficit disorder with hyperactivity (ADDH)

USUAL DOSE: For narcolepsy: 5 mg to 60 mg per day in single or divided doses. For ADDH: 2.5 mg to 40 mg per day in single or divided doses.

AVERAGE PRICE: $62.02 for 5-mg sustained-release capsule; $77.28 for 10-mg sustained-release capsule; $99.35 for 15-mg sustained-release capsule; and $28.63 for 5-mg tablet

SIDE EFFECTS: Most common: irregular heartbeat, nervousness, irritability, false sense of well-being, restlessness, insomnia, and drowsiness after the drug wears off. Less common: blurred vision, changes in sex drive, diarrhea, nausea, vomiting, stomach pain, constipation, loss of appetite, weight loss, dizziness, lightheadedness, headache, dry mouth, unpleasant taste, pounding heartbeat, and increased sweating.

DRUG INTERACTIONS: Anafranil, Asendin, Elavil, Eldepryl, Endep, Nardil, Norpramin, Pamelor, Parnate, Sinequan, Surmontil, Tofranil, or Vivactil and the drug may cause cardiovascular symptoms such as irregular heartbeat, high blood pressure, and fast heartbeat. Blocadren, Cartrol, Corgard, Inderal, Kerlone, Levatol, Lopressor, Normodyne, Sectral, Tenormin, Toprol-XL, Trandate, Visken, or Zebeta and the drug may cause high blood pressure, slow heart rate, and possibly heart block. The drug may increase the effects of Lanoxin. The analgesic effects of Demerol may be increased when used with this drug. Cytomel, Levoxyl, Levothroid, or Synthroid and this drug may increase the effects of both when taken together.

ALLERGIES: Individuals allergic to dextroamphetamine, amphetamines, or any of their derivatives should discuss this with their doctor or pharmacist before using this drug.

PREGNANCY/BREAST-FEEDING: Category C—Risk cannot be ruled out. Human studies are lacking, and animal studies are either positive for fetal risk or lacking as well. However, potential benefits may justify the potential risk in using the drug. The drug is excreted in the breast milk; therefore, extreme caution should be used when breast-feeding.

OTHER BRAND NAMES: None

OTHER DRUGS IN THE SAME THERAPEUTIC CLASS: Adderall and Desoxyn

IMPORTANT INFORMATION TO REMEMBER: The drug may cause dizziness. Caution should be used when performing activities that require coordination. Only take the drug exactly as directed by your physician. Do not discontinue the drug without first consulting your physician; also, do not increase the dose without first consulting with your physician. This prescription cannot be refilled—a new written prescription must be obtained each time. This medication is a controlled substance and may be habit-forming. The potential for abuse with this medication is high.

BRAND NAME: Diabeta

GENERIC NAME: glyburide

See entry for Micronase

BRAND NAME: Diabinese

GENERIC NAME: chlorpropamide

GENERIC FORM AVAILABLE: Yes

THERAPEUTIC CLASS: First-generation sulfonylurea anti-diabetic

DOSAGE FORMS: 100-mg and 250-mg tablets

MAIN USES: Diabetes

USUAL DOSE: 100 mg to 500 mg daily in a single or divided doses

AVERAGE PRICE: $42.31 (B)/$8.34 (G) for 100 mg and $83.16 (B)/$16.15 (G) for 250 mg

SIDE EFFECTS: constipation 10%, nausea 2%–5%, itching 1%–3%, diarrhea 1%–2%, vomiting 1%–2%, dizziness 1%–2%, headache 1%–2%, and appetite changes 1%–2%.

DRUG INTERACTIONS: Alcohol may cause a severe stomach reaction (vomiting, pain, diarrhea, etc.) when used with this drug. The blood levels of both Coumadin and the drug, when combined, may initially increase, followed by a decrease in blood levels of both. Blocadren, Cartrol, Corgard, Inderal, Kerlone, Levatol, Lopressor, Normodyne, Sectral, Tenormin, Toprol-XL, Trandate, Visken, Zebeta, chloramphenicol, Esimil, Ismelin, Nardil, Parnate, high doses of aspirin, Bactrim, Gantanol, Gantrisin, and Septra may cause low blood sugar when used with this drug.

ALLERGIES: Individuals allergic to chlorpropamide, sulfa drugs, or any of their derivatives should discuss this with their doctor or pharmacist before using this drug.

PREGNANCY/BREAST-FEEDING: Category C—Risk cannot be ruled out. Human studies are lacking, and animal studies are either positive for fetal risk or lacking as well. However, potential benefits may justify the potential risk in using the drug. The drug is excreted in the breast milk; therefore, extreme caution should be used when breast-feeding.

OTHER BRAND NAMES: None

OTHER DRUGS IN THE SAME THERAPEUTIC CLASS: Orinase and Tolinase

IMPORTANT INFORMATION TO REMEMBER: If stomach upset occurs, take the drug with food or milk. To receive optimum effect, regular compliance with therapy is essential; this includes compliance with a prescribed diet. Avoid alcohol while taking this drug. Alcohol may cause severe stomach reactions (vomiting, pain, diarrhea, etc.). This drug lowers blood sugar. Individuals should be aware of the signs and symptoms of blood sugar that is too low: sweating, tremor, blurred vision, weakness, hunger, and confusion. If two or more of these symptoms are seen, treat with oral glucose (sugar) and/or contact your doctor. This drug may increase the risk of cardiovascular disease. Before taking over-the-counter cold and allergy preparations, consult your doctor or pharmacist—these products may affect your blood sugar.

BRAND NAME: Diamox

GENERIC NAME: acetazolamide

GENERIC FORM AVAILABLE: Yes

THERAPEUTIC CLASS: Carbonic anhydrase inhibitor

DOSAGE FORMS: 125-mg and 250-mg tablets and 500-mg Sequels (capsules)

MAIN USES: Glaucoma, seizures, and {altitude sickness}

USUAL DOSE: For glaucoma: 250 mg to 1 g daily in divided doses. For seizures: 375 mg to 1 g daily in divided doses.

AVERAGE PRICE: $41.32 (B)/$10.21 (G) for 125 mg; $46.13 (B)/$13.62 (G) for 250 mg; and $144.45 for 500 mg (brand-name only)

SIDE EFFECTS: More common: drowsiness; tiredness; diarrhea; increased urination; loss of appetite; nausea; vomiting; tingling feeling in the arms, legs, fingers, and toes; and weight loss. Less common: ringing in the ears, altered taste, confusion, and blurred vision.

DRUG INTERACTIONS: The effects of Desoxyn, Dexedrine, Quinidex, and Quinaglute may be increased. The effects of Urised may be reduced.

ALLERGIES: Individuals allergic to acetazolamide or any of its derivatives should discuss this with their doctor or pharmacist before using this drug.

PREGNANCY/BREAST-FEEDING: Category C—Risk cannot be ruled out. Human studies are lacking, and animal studies are either positive for fetal risk or lacking as well. However, potential benefits may justify the potential risk in using the drug. It is not known whether the drug is excreted in the breast milk; therefore, caution should be used when breast-feeding.

OTHER BRAND NAMES: None

OTHER DRUGS IN THE SAME THERAPEUTIC CLASS: Daranide and Neptazane

IMPORTANT INFORMATION TO REMEMBER: This drug does cause some drowsiness. Individuals should use caution when driving, operating machinery, or any task where mental alertness is required. Alcohol, anxiety medications, and narcotic painkillers may intensify the drowsiness effect of the drug. The drug may lower levels of potassium in the body; caution should be used by individuals with low potassium levels. Only take the drug exactly as directed by your physician. Do not discontinue the drug without first consulting your physician.

BRAND NAME: Dibenzyline

GENERIC NAME: phenoxybenzamine

GENERIC FORM AVAILABLE: No

THERAPEUTIC CLASS: Alpha-blocker

DOSAGE FORMS: 10-mg capsules

MAIN USES: Pheochromocytoma (high blood pressure and sweating associated with the disease)

USUAL DOSE: 20 mg to 40 mg two to three times a day

AVERAGE PRICE: $90.86

SIDE EFFECTS: Most common: pinpoint pupils, nausea, vomiting, diarrhea, nasal congestion, fast heartbeat, dizziness, and lightheadedness, especially when getting up from a sitting or lying-down position. Less common: confusion, drowsiness, dry mouth, headache, sexual impairments, and weakness.

DRUG INTERACTIONS: The drugs epinephrine and phenylephrine, which are contained in many cough, cold, and allergy medications, may produce low blood pressure and fast heartbeat.

ALLERGIES: Individuals allergic to phenoxybenzamine or any of its derivatives should discuss this with their doctor or pharmacist before using this drug.

PREGNANCY/BREAST-FEEDING: Category C—Risk cannot be ruled out. Human studies are lacking, and animal studies are either positive for fetal risk or lacking as well. However, potential benefits may justify the potential risk in using the drug. It is not known whether the drug is excreted in the breast milk; therefore, caution should be used when breast-feeding.

OTHER BRAND NAMES: None

OTHER DRUGS IN THE SAME THERAPEUTIC CLASS: None

IMPORTANT INFORMATION TO REMEMBER: Only take the drug exactly as directed by your physician. Do not discontinue the drug without first consulting your physician. Do not increase the dose without first consulting with your physician. Before taking over-the-counter cold, cough, and allergy preparations, consult your doctor or pharmacist—these products may raise your blood pressure. This drug does cause some drowsiness. Individuals should use caution when driving, operating machinery, or any task where mental alertness is required. Alcohol, anxiety medications, and narcotic painkillers may intensify the drowsiness effect of the drug. The drug may also cause dizziness when suddenly rising from a sitting or lying-down position.

BRAND NAME: Didronel

GENERIC NAME: etidronate disodium

GENERIC FORM AVAILABLE: No

THERAPEUTIC CLASS: Biphosphonate

DOSAGE FORMS: 200-mg and 400-mg tablets

MAIN USES: Paget's disease and bone diseases

USUAL DOSE: Doses are individualized based on the patient's weight. The usual dose is 5 mg to 10 mg per k of body weight per day for no more than six months at one time. (1 k = 2.2 pounds)

AVERAGE PRICE: $89.81 for 200 mg (30 tablets) and $169.40 for 400 mg (30 tablets)

SIDE EFFECTS: bone pain 10%–20%, diarrhea 8%–30%, nausea 8%–30%, fever 1%–10%, and convulsions 1%–10%.

DRUG INTERACTIONS: Antacids, milk, calcium supplements, iron supplements, and other mineral supplements may prevent the absorption of the drug by the body. The drug may alter the effectiveness of Coumadin.

ALLERGIES: Individuals allergic to etidronate disodium or any of its derivatives should discuss this with their doctor or pharmacist before using this drug.

PREGNANCY/BREAST-FEEDING: Category C—Risk cannot be ruled out. Human studies are lacking, and animal studies are either positive for fetal risk or lacking as well. However, potential benefits may justify the potential risk in using the drug. It is not known whether the drug is excreted in the breast milk; therefore, caution should be used when breast-feeding.

OTHER BRAND NAMES: None

OTHER DRUGS IN THE SAME THERAPEUTIC CLASS: None

IMPORTANT INFORMATION TO REMEMBER: It's best to take the drug on an empty stomach—two hours before meals or two hours after meals—if possible. This drug should be taken with plenty of water (eight ounces is preferred). It is important to maintain a well-balanced diet, including adequate amounts of vitamin D and calcium. However, do not take the drug within two hours of taking antacids, calcium supplements, iron supplements, or milk or other dairy products.

BRAND NAME: Differin

GENERIC NAME: adapalene

GENERIC FORM AVAILABLE: No

THERAPEUTIC CLASS: Vitamin A derivative

DOSAGE FORMS: 0.1% gel

MAIN USES: Acne

USUAL DOSE: Apply thin film to affected areas once daily at bedtime after washing.

AVERAGE PRICE: $28.07 (15 g)

SIDE EFFECTS: redness 10%–40%, scaling 10%–40%, dryness 10%–40%, itching 10%–40%, burning 10%–40%, skin irritation 1%, and sunburn 1%.

DRUG INTERACTIONS: Other acne drugs applied at the same time may increase the effects of the drug.

ALLERGIES: Individuals allergic to adapalene or any of its derivatives should discuss this with their doctor or pharmacist before using this drug.

PREGNANCY/BREAST-FEEDING: Category C—Risk cannot be ruled out. Human studies are lacking, and animal studies are either positive for fetal risk or lacking as well. However, potential benefits may justify the potential risk in using the drug. It is not known whether the drug is excreted in the breast milk; therefore, caution should be used when breast-feeding.

OTHER BRAND NAMES: None

OTHER DRUGS IN THE SAME THERAPEUTIC CLASS: Retin-A

IMPORTANT INFORMATION TO REMEMBER: The drug should be applied at bedtime 20–30 minutes after thoroughly washing and drying the skin. Keep the medication away from the corners of the nose, mouth, and any open wounds or sores. There may be some minor discomfort or peeling during the first few days of treatment. If these symptoms continue or become worse, contact your doctor. The drug should be stored below 80° F. This drug should not be used during the day or during suntanning due to the increased risk of severe sunburn. A water-based sunscreen should be used even if the medication is only used at bedtime. The drug may make the face more sensitive to wind and cold. After three to six weeks of therapy, some new areas of acne may appear. This is normal and only temporary; continue using the medication.

BRAND NAME: Diflucan

GENERIC NAME: fluconazole

GENERIC FORM AVAILABLE: No

THERAPEUTIC CLASS: Imidazole antifungal

DOSAGE FORMS: 50-mg, 100-mg, 150-mg, and 200-mg tablets

MAIN USES: Fungal infections and vaginal yeast infections

USUAL DOSE: For fungal infections: 50 mg to 200 mg daily. For vaginal yeast infections: one 150-mg tablet in one single dose.

AVERAGE PRICE: $288.54 for 100 mg (30 tablets); $472.50 for 200 mg (30 tablets); $21.51 for 150 mg (1 tablet)

SIDE EFFECTS: nausea 4%, headache 2%, skin rash 2%, vomiting 2%, stomach pain 2%, and diarrhea 2%.

DRUG INTERACTIONS: The drug and diabetic drugs may cause low blood sugar (hypoglycemia). The drug may increase the effects of Coumadin. The drug may increase the blood levels of Dilantin, Sandimmune, Slo-bid, Theo-Dur, theophylline, Uni-Dur, and Uniphyl; rifampin may decrease the blood levels of the drug. Individuals using Hismanal, Seldane, or Seldane-D and the drug should use caution due to the possibility of irregular heart rhythms. Propulsid and the drug may cause dangerous irregular heartbeats when taken together.

ALLERGIES: Individuals allergic to fluconazole, other antifungals, or any of their derivatives should discuss this with their doctor or pharmacist before using this drug.

PREGNANCY/BREAST-FEEDING: Category C—Risk cannot be ruled out. Human studies are lacking, and animal studies are either positive for fetal risk or lacking as well. However, potential benefits may justify the potential risk in using the drug. The drug is excreted in the breast milk; therefore, extreme caution should be used when breast-feeding.

OTHER BRAND NAMES: None

OTHER DRUGS IN THE SAME THERAPEUTIC CLASS: Sporanox and Nizoral

IMPORTANT INFORMATION TO REMEMBER: This drug should be taken with food or milk. Take the drug at the same time every day. Also, take the drug until all the medication prescribed is gone; otherwise, the infection may return. Patients with liver disease should discuss this with their doctor before taking this drug.

BRAND NAME: Dilacor XR

GENERIC NAME: diltiazem

GENERIC FORM AVAILABLE: No

THERAPEUTIC CLASS: Calcium channel blocker

DOSAGE FORMS: 120-mg, 180-mg, and 240-mg extended-release capsules

MAIN USES: Angina and high blood pressure

USUAL DOSE: 120 mg to 240 mg once daily

AVERAGE PRICE: $135.07 for 120 mg; $159.04 for 180 mg; $173.39 for 240 mg

SIDE EFFECTS: runny nose 10%, headache 9%, hoarse throat 6%, constipation 4%, cough 3%, flu-like symptoms 2%, swelling 2%, muscle pain 2%, diarrhea 2%, drowsiness 2%, vomiting 2%, nausea 2%, stomach pain 1%, insomnia 1%, and ringing in the ears 1%.

DRUG INTERACTIONS: The effects of Blocadren, Cartrol, Corgard, Inderal, Kerlone, Levatol, Lopressor, Minipress, Normodyne, Norpace, Sectral, Tenormin, Toprol-XL, Trandate, Visken, and Zebeta may be increased when taken with this drug. The drug may increase the blood levels of Tegretol, Sandimmune, Lanoxin, Quinidex, Quinaglute, and Procan.

ALLERGIES: Individuals allergic to diltiazem, Cardizem, or any of their derivatives should discuss this with their doctor or pharmacist before using this drug.

PREGNANCY/BREAST-FEEDING: Category C—Risk cannot be ruled out. Human studies are lacking, and animal studies are either positive for fetal risk or lacking as well. However, potential benefits may justify the potential risk in using the drug. The drug is excreted in the breast milk; therefore, extreme caution should be used when breast-feeding.

OTHER BRAND NAMES: None

OTHER DRUGS IN THE SAME THERAPEUTIC CLASS: Adalat, Adalat CC, Calan, Calan SR, Cardene, Cardene SR, Cardizem, Cardizem SR, Cardizem CD, Covera-HS, DynaCirc, Isoptin, Isoptin SR, Norvasc, Procardia, Procardia XL, Sular, Vascor, and Verelan

IMPORTANT INFORMATION TO REMEMBER: It's best to take the drug on an empty stomach—one hour before meals or two hours after meals—if possible. Only take the drug exactly as directed by your physician. Do not discontinue the drug without first consulting your physician. Before taking over-the-counter cold and allergy preparations, consult your doctor or pharmacist—these products may raise your blood pressure. This drug may cause some drowsiness at first. Individuals should use caution when driving, operating machinery, or any task where mental alertness is required. These capsules should be swallowed whole.

BRAND NAME: Dilantin

GENERIC NAME: phenytoin

GENERIC FORM AVAILABLE: Yes (but should not be used)

THERAPEUTIC CLASS: Hydantoin antiseizure

DOSAGE FORMS: 30-mg and 100 mg extended-release capsules; 50-mg chewable Infatabs; and 125 mg/5 mL liquid suspension.

MAIN USES: Epilepsy and seizures

USUAL DOSE: 100 mg to 300 mg daily in a single or divided dose. The dose for children may be lower.

AVERAGE PRICE: $27.60 for 30-mg capsules and $33.40 for 100-mg capsules

SIDE EFFECTS: Most common: central nervous system toxicity (mood changes, rolling eye movements, unsteadiness, nervousness, etc.), increase in gum tissue, bleeding or tender gums, constipation, mild dizziness, mild drowsiness, nausea, and vomiting. Less common: diarrhea, widening of nasal tip, thickening of the lips, swelling of the breasts, headache, unusual hair growth, insomnia, and muscle twitching.

DRUG INTERACTIONS: There are several drugs that interact with Dilantin; before taking any medication, consult with your doctor or pharmacist. Some of these drugs are: Antabuse, Bactrim, chloramphenicol, Cordarone, Diflucan, isoniazid, Coumadin, Septra, Gantrisin, Gantanol, Pediazole, Tagamet, and trimethoprim; these may increase the blood levels of the drug. Cancer drugs may decrease the effects of the drug. The drug may decrease the blood levels of Tegretol. Carafate, folic acid, rifampin, Slo-bid, Theo-Dur, theophylline, Uni-Dur, and Uniphyl may decrease blood levels of the drug. Depakene and Depakote may increase the effects of the drug. The drug itself, Dilantin, may decrease the blood levels of steroids (such as Aristocort, Deltasone, Decadron, Medrol, and prednisone), doxycycline, Mexitil, Norpace, Quinidex, Quinaglute, Slo-bid, Theo-Dur, theophylline, Uni-Dur, Uniphyl, and Vibramycin. The drug may decrease the effects of birth control pills, Larodopa, and some muscle relaxants. The drug may increase the blood levels of Mysoline.

ALLERGIES: Individuals allergic to phenytoin or any of its derivatives should discuss this with their doctor or pharmacist before using this drug.

PREGNANCY/BREAST-FEEDING; Category D—Positive evidence of risk. Human studies show risk to the fetus. Nevertheless, potential benefits may possibly outweigh the potential risks. This drug should not be taken by nursing mothers.

OTHER BRAND NAMES: None

OTHER DRUGS IN THE SAME THERAPEUTIC CLASS: Mesantoin

IMPORTANT INFORMATION TO REMEMBER: This drug does cause some drowsiness. Individuals should use caution when driving, operating machinery, or any task where mental alertness is required. Alcohol, anxiety medications, and narcotic painkillers may intensify the drowsiness effect of the drug. Avoid drinking alcohol while taking this drug. Only take the drug exactly as directed by your physician. Do not discontinue the drug without first consulting your physician. Also do not increase the dose without first consulting with your physician. Before taking over-the-counter medications, consult your doctor or pharmacist. Birth control pills may be ineffective while taking this drug; another method of birth control is recommended. Practice good oral hygiene to help prevent gum disease associated with taking this drug. Diabetics should monitor their blood sugar frequently while taking this drug.

BRAND NAME: Dilatrate-SR

GENERIC NAME: isosorbide dinitrate

GENERIC FORM AVAILABLE: No

THERAPEUTIC CLASS: Anti-anginal

DOSAGE FORMS: 40-mg sustained-release capsules

MAIN USES: Prevention of angina

USUAL DOSE: 40 mg to 80 mg every 8 to 12 hours

AVERAGE PRICE: $76.44

SIDE EFFECTS: headache 25% and low blood pressure 2%–36% are the most common. Less common: flushing, restlessness, dizziness, weakness, nausea, vomiting, and sweating.

DRUG INTERACTIONS: Alcohol and the drug may produce low blood pressure. Apresoline, Loniten, or Vasodilan and the drug may also produce low blood pressure.

ALLERGIES: Individuals allergic to isosorbide dinitrate or other nitrates (such as those listed in "Other Drugs in the Same Therapeutic Class") should discuss this with their doctor or pharmacist before taking this drug.

PREGNANCY/BREAST-FEEDING: Category C—Risk cannot be ruled out. Human studies are lacking, and animal studies are either positive for fetal risk or lacking as well. However, potential benefits may justify the potential risk in using the drug. It is not known whether the drug is excreted in the breast milk; therefore, caution should be used when breast-feeding.

OTHER BRAND NAMES: None

OTHER DRUGS IN THE SAME THERAPEUTIC CLASS: Imdur, Ismo, Isordil, Monoket, and Sorbitrate

IMPORTANT INFORMATION TO REMEMBER: This drug does not relieve angina attacks, it only prevents them. Only take the drug exactly as directed by your physician. Do not discontinue the drug or increase the dose without first consulting your physician. Do not crush, chew, or divide capsules—this will destroy the matrix that delays the release of the medication. Swallow the capsules whole. Do not drink alcohol while taking the drug. The headache that is common with this drug usually goes away with continued use. If it does not, contact your doctor. Before taking over-the-counter cold and allergy preparations, consult your doctor or pharmacist.

BRAND NAME: Dilaudid

GENERIC NAME: hydromorphone

GENERIC FORM AVAILABLE: Yes, for some strengths

THERAPEUTIC CLASS: Narcotic analgesic

DOSAGE FORMS: 2-mg, 4-mg, and 8-mg tablets; 5 mg/5 mL liquid; and 3-mg suppositories

MAIN USES: Moderate to severe pain

USUAL DOSE: Tablets: 2 mg to 4 mg every four to six hours. Suppositories: one suppository every six to eight hours.

AVERAGE PRICE: $68.43 (B)/$39.36 (G) for 2 mg; $88.35 (B)/$63.63 (G) for 4 mg; $160.79 for 8 mg; and $140.35 for 3 mg (30 suppositories)

SIDE EFFECTS: Most common: lightheadedness, dizziness, drowsiness, tiredness, nausea, vomiting, constipation, and sweating. Less common: weakness, agitation, tremor, depressed breathing, hallucinations, dry mouth, low blood pressure, disorientation, vision problems, muscle spasms, and slow heartbeat.

DRUG INTERACTIONS: The effects of the drug may be increased when used with Compazine, Mellaril, Prolixin, Serentil, Stelazine, Thorazine, or Trilafon. Alcohol, anxiety medications, and narcotic painkillers may intensify the drowsiness and respiratory depression effects of the drug. This drug and Nardil or Parnate may cause severe and possibly fatal reactions.

ALLERGIES: Individuals allergic to hydromorphone or any of its derivatives should discuss this with their doctor or pharmacist before using this drug.

PREGNANCY/BREAST-FEEDING: Category C—Risk cannot be ruled out. Human studies are lacking, and animal studies are either positive for fetal risk or lacking as well. However, potential benefits may justify the potential risk in using the drug. It is not known whether the drug is excreted in the breast milk; therefore, caution should be used when breast-feeding.

OTHER BRAND NAMES: None

OTHER DRUGS IN THE SAME THERAPEUTIC CLASS: Demerol, Dolophine, Duragesic, Levo-Dromoran, MS Contin, MSIR, Oramorph SR, Roxanol, and Stadol

IMPORTANT INFORMATION TO REMEMBER: This is a very potent drug and may cause a lot of drowsiness. Individuals should use extreme caution when driving, operating machinery, or any task where mental alertness is required. Alcohol, anxiety medications, and narcotic painkillers may intensify the drowsiness effect of the drug. Do not increase the dose without first consulting with your physician—this could be very dangerous and possibly life-threatening. If stomach upset occurs, take the drug with food or milk. This medication is a controlled substance, may be habit-forming, and should only be used as needed for pain relief. This prescription cannot be refilled; a new written prescription must be obtained each time. The potential for abuse with this medication is high.

For the suppository:

Store in a cool place to avoid melting, preferably the refrigerator. Remove the foil wrapper before inserting the suppository. When inserting, lie on one side and bend the top leg slightly. Then insert suppository into rectum about one inch with one finger. Wash hands thoroughly before and after use. Individuals may want to use a finger cot to cover finger when inserting a suppository.

BRAND NAME: Dipentum

GENERIC NAME: olsalazine

GENERIC FORM AVAILABLE: No

THERAPEUTIC CLASS: Salicylate

DOSAGE FORMS: 250-mg capsules

MAIN USES: Ulcerative colitis

USUAL DOSE: 500 mg twice daily with meals

AVERAGE PRICE: $90.09

SIDE EFFECTS: diarrhea 11%, stomach pain 10%, nausea 5%, headache 5%, muscle and joint pain 4%, bloating 2%, depression 2%, skin rash 2%, dizziness 1%, and appetite changes 1%.

DRUG INTERACTIONS: The drug may increase the effects of Coumadin.

ALLERGIES: Individuals allergic to olsalazine, Asacol, Pentasa, Rowasa, aspirin, or any of their derivatives should discuss this with their doctor or pharmacist before using this drug.

PREGNANCY/BREAST-FEEDING: Category C—Risk cannot be ruled out. Human studies are lacking, and animal studies are either positive for fetal risk or lacking as well. However, potential benefits may justify the potential risk in using the drug. It is not known whether the drug is excreted in the breast milk; therefore, caution should be used when breast-feeding.

OTHER BRAND NAMES: None

OTHER DRUGS IN THE SAME THERAPEUTIC CLASS: Asacol, Azulfidine, Pentasa, and Rowasa.

IMPORTANT INFORMATION TO REMEMBER: Only take the drug exactly as directed by your physician. Do not discontinue the drug without first consulting your physician. This drug should be taken with food or milk to reduce the potential for injury to the stomach lining and stomach upset.

BRAND NAME: Diprolene and Diprolene AF

GENERIC NAME: betamethasone diproprionate

GENERIC FORM AVAILABLE: No

THERAPEUTIC CLASS: Topical corticosteroid

DOSAGE FORMS: 0.05% ointment, lotion, AF cream, and gel

MAIN USES: Skin rashes, redness, and itching

USUAL DOSE: For AF cream, gel, and ointment: apply thin film one to two times daily. For the lotion: apply a few drops one to two times daily.

AVERAGE PRICE: $34.16 for 15 g

SIDE EFFECTS: burning, itching, irritation, dry skin, rash, soreness of the skin, and acne, approximately 1% for each. The same side effects for the lotion were slightly higher, approximately 1%–5%.

DRUG INTERACTIONS: None of any clinical significance

ALLERGIES: Individuals allergic to betamethasone or any of its derivatives should discuss this with their doctor or pharmacist before using this drug.

PREGNANCY/BREAST-FEEDING: Category C—Risk cannot be ruled out. Human studies are lacking, and animal studies are either positive for fetal risk or lacking as well. However, potential benefits may justify the potential risk in using the drug. It is not known whether the drug is excreted in the breast milk; therefore, caution should be used when breast-feeding.

OTHER BRAND NAMES: None

OTHER DRUGS IN THE SAME THERAPEUTIC CLASS: Aclovate, Aristocort, Cordran, Cordran SP, Cutivate, Cyclocort, DesOwen, Elocon, Florone, Halog, Hytone, Kenalog, Lidex, Synalar, Temovate, Topicort, Tridesilon, Ultravate, Valisone, and Westcort

IMPORTANT INFORMATION TO REMEMBER: This drug is for external use only. Apply only a thin film of drug to skin and rub it in well. Never cover the skin after application with a bandage or wrapping unless directed to do so by a physician. Never apply to damaged skin or open wounds unless directed to do so by a doctor. Discontinue use if irritation occurs. If using the lotion, be sure to shake it well.

BRAND NAME: Diprosone

GENERIC NAME: betamethasone

See entry for Diprolene/Diprolene AF

BRAND NAME: Disalcid

GENERIC NAME: salsalate

GENERIC FORM AVAILABLE: Yes

THERAPEUTIC CLASS: Nonsteroidal anti-inflammatory drug (NSAID)

DOSAGE FORMS: 500-mg and 750-mg tablets, and 500-mg capsules

MAIN USES: Arthritis and pain relief

USUAL DOSE: 3000 mg daily in two to three divided doses

AVERAGE PRICE: $52.23 (B)/$13.07 (G) for 500 mg and $67.30 (B)/$21.76 (G) for 750 mg

SIDE EFFECTS: Most common: ringing in the ears, nausea, heartburn, hearing difficulties, rash, and dizziness. Less common: stomach pain, diarrhea, low blood pressure, skin rash, and itching.

DRUG INTERACTIONS: Other NSAIDS (such as Anaprox, Ansaid, Aleve, aspirin, Cataflam, Clinoril, Daypro, Dolobid, Easprin, Feldene, Indocin, Lodine, Motrin, Nalfon, Naprosyn, Orudis, Oruvail, Relafen, Tolectin, and Voltaren) may decrease the concentration of the drug in the blood. This drug may also decrease the effects of Lasix, Dyazide, HydroDIURIL, Maxzide, and other water pills. The drug may increase the blood levels of Eskalith, Lithobid, and Sandimmune. The drug, when used with Depakene, may increase the occurrence of stomach bleeding and ulcers. The drug may increase the toxic effects of the drug Rheumatrex. Caution should be used when taking the drug with Coumadin.

ALLERGIES: Individuals allergic to aspirin, salsalate, or any of their derivatives should discuss this with their doctor or pharmacist before using this drug.

PREGNANCY/BREAST-FEEDING: Category C—Risk cannot be ruled out. Human studies are lacking, and animal studies are either positive for fetal risk or lacking as well. However, potential benefits may justify the potential risk in using the drug. The drug should not, however, be used during the late stages (last three months) of pregnancy. It is not known whether the drug is excreted in the breast milk; therefore, caution should be used when breast-feeding.

OTHER BRAND NAMES: Salflex

OTHER DRUGS IN THE SAME THERAPEUTIC CLASS: Anaprox, Ansaid, aspirin, Cataflam, Clinoril, Daypro, Dolobid, Easprin, Feldene, Indocin, Lodine, Lodine XL, Motrin, Nalfon, Naprosyn, Orudis, Oruvail, Relafen, Tolectin, Toradol, Voltaren, and Voltaren XR

OTHER INFORMATION TO REMEMBER: This drug should be taken with food or milk to reduce the potential for injury to the stomach lining and stomach upset. This drug may take up to two weeks before a noticeable improvement in pain relief associated with arthritis is observed. Drinking alcohol while taking this drug may increase its potential to cause ulcers. This drug should only be used under the direct supervision of a doctor by individuals with a bleeding disorder or ulcer, or those who are currently taking Coumadin. Before taking over-the-counter pain relievers, consult your doctor or pharmacist. Hearing problems may be a symptom of too high a dose. If ringing in the ears or hearing problems occur, contact your doctor immediately. Most of the time these hearing problems disappear once the dose of the drug is reduced. No more than one pain reliever should be taken at any time unless otherwise directed by your doctor.

BRAND NAME: Ditropan

GENERIC NAME: oxybutynin

GENERIC FORM AVAILABLE: Yes

THERAPEUTIC CLASS: Urinary antispasmatic

DOSAGE FORMS: 5-mg tablets and 5 mg/5 mL syrup

MAIN USES: Urinary problems

USUAL DOSE: 5 mg two to three times daily

AVERAGE PRICE: $53.33 (B)/$24.62 (G) for 5-mg tablets

SIDE EFFECTS: Most common: drowsiness, decreased sweating, constipation, and dry mouth. Less common: pounding heartbeat, fast heartbeat, insomnia, restlessness, headache, nausea, vomiting, diarrhea, and impotence.

DRUG INTERACTIONS: The drug may decrease the effects of Compazine, Haldol, Mellaril, Prolixin, Serentil, Stelazine, Thorazine, and Trilafon. The drug may cause tardive dyskinesia (abnormal body movements) when used with Haldol.

ALLERGIES: Individuals allergic to oxybutynin or any of its derivatives should discuss this with their doctor or pharmacist before using this drug.

PREGNANCY/BREAST-FEEDING: Category B—No evidence of risk in humans. Either animal findings show risk, but human findings do not; or, if no adequate human studies have been done, animal findings show no risk. It is not known whether the drug is excreted in the breast milk; therefore, caution should be used when breast-feeding.

OTHER BRAND NAMES: None

OTHER DRUGS IN THE SAME THERAPEUTIC CLASS: None

IMPORTANT INFORMATION TO REMEMBER: This drug may cause some drowsiness. Individuals should use caution when driving, operating machinery, or any task where mental alertness is required. Alcohol, anxiety medications, and narcotic painkillers may intensify the drowsiness effect of the drug. Only take the drug exactly as directed by your physician. Caution should also be used when exercising and in hot weather while taking this drug; the drug may increase an individual's sensitivity to hot weather. Individuals with glaucoma or prostate problems should consult with their doctor before taking this drug.

BRAND NAME: Diulo

GENERAL NAME: metolazone

See entry for Zaroxolyn

BRAND NAME: Diuril

GENERIC NAME: chlorothiazide

GENERIC FORM AVAILABLE: Yes

THERAPEUTIC CLASS: Thiazide diuretic (water pill)

DOSAGE FORMS: 250-mg and 500-mg tablets

MAIN USES: High blood pressure and water retention (fluid retention due to congestive heart failure, kidney disease, or cirrhosis of the liver)

USUAL DOSE: 500 mg to 1000 mg daily as a single or divided dose

AVERAGE PRICE: $19.78 (B)/$9.11 (G) for 250 mg and $28.52 (B)/$13.73 (G) for 500 mg

SIDE EFFECTS: Most common: none. Less common: low potassium, weakness, dizziness, irritability, muscle cramps, low blood pressure, headache, restlessness, increased thirst, diarrhea, stomach pain, vomiting, dry mouth, increased sensitivity to sunburn, and muscle spasms.

DRUG INTERACTIONS: The drug may require dosage adjustments to diabetic and gout medications. Colestid and Questran may decrease the absorption of the drug. The drug may increase the blood levels of Eskalith and Lithobid.

ALLERGIES: Individuals allergic to chlorothiazide, sulfa drugs, or any of their derivatives should discuss this with their doctor or pharmacist before using this drug.

PREGNANCY/BREAST-FEEDING: Category C—Risk cannot be ruled out. Human studies are lacking, and animal studies are either positive for fetal risk or lacking as well. However, potential benefits may justify the potential risk in using the drug. It is not known whether the drug is excreted in the breast milk; therefore, caution should be used when breast-feeding.

OTHER BRAND NAMES: None

OTHER DRUGS IN THE SAME THERAPEUTIC CLASS: Enduron, Esidrix, HydroDIURIL, Hydromox, Hygroton, and Oretic

IMPORTANT INFORMATION TO REMEMBER: If the drug is to be taken once daily, take it in the morning due to increased urine output. Before taking over-the-counter cold and allergy preparations, consult your doctor or pharmacist—these products may raise your blood pressure. The drug may cause the elimination of potassium from the body. It is therefore a good idea to eat a banana or drink orange, grapefruit, or apple juice every day to replace lost potassium. This drug may also increase the sensitivity of the skin to sunburn in some individuals; therefore, a sunscreen is recommended during periods of prolonged exposure to the sun.

BRAND NAME: Dolobid

GENERIC NAME: diflunisal

GENERIC FORM AVAILABLE: Yes

THERAPEUTIC CLASS: Nonsteroidal anti-inflammatory drug (NSAID)

DOSAGE FORMS: 250-mg and 500-mg tablets

MAIN USES: Arthritis and pain relief

USUAL DOSE: 250 mg to 500 mg every 8 to 12 hours

AVERAGE PRICE: $139.69 for 250 mg (brand-name only) and $166.68 (B)/$76.32 (G) for 500 mg

SIDE EFFECTS: Most common: nausea, vomiting, stomach pain, diarrhea, headache, and rash. Less common: constipation, gas, insomnia, dizziness, ringing in the ears, and tiredness.

DRUG INTERACTIONS: Aspirin will decrease the concentration of this drug in the blood. This drug may also decrease the effects of Lasix, Dyazide, HydroDIURIL, Maxzide, and other water pills. The drug may increase the blood levels of Eskalith, Lithobid, and

Sandimmune. The drug may increase the toxic effects of the drug Rheumatrex. Caution should be used when taking the drug with Coumadin.

ALLERGIES: Individuals allergic to diflunisal or any of its derivatives should discuss this with their doctor or pharmacist before using this drug.

PREGNANCY/BREAST-FEEDING: Category C—Risk cannot be ruled out. Human studies are lacking, and animal studies are either positive for fetal risk or lacking as well. However, potential benefits may justify the potential risk in using the drug. The drug should not, however, be used during the late stages (last three months) of pregnancy. The drug is excreted in the breast milk; therefore, extreme caution should be used when breast-feeding.

OTHER BRAND NAMES: None

OTHER DRUGS IN THE SAME THERAPEUTIC CLASS: Anaprox, Ansaid, aspirin, Cataflam, Clinoril, Daypro, Disalcid, Easprin, Feldene, Indocin, Lodine, Lodine XL, Motrin, Nalfon, Naprosyn, Orudis, Oruvail, Relafen, Tolectin, Toradol, Voltaren, and Voltaren XR

IMPORTANT INFORMATION TO REMEMBER: This drug should be taken with food or milk to reduce the potential for injury to the stomach lining and stomach upset. This drug may take up to two weeks before a noticeable improvement in pain relief associated with arthritis is observed. Drinking alcohol while taking this drug may increase its potential to cause ulcers. This drug should only be used under the direct supervision of a doctor by individuals with a bleeding disorder or ulcer, or those who are currently taking Coumadin. Before taking over-the-counter pain relievers, consult your doctor or pharmacist. No more than one pain reliever should be taken at any one time unless otherwise directed by your doctor. This drug may also cause a dry mouth; sugarless gum or hard candy will help take care of this problem.

BRAND NAME: Donnatal and Donnatal Extentabs

GENERIC NAME: belladonna alkaloids.

GENERIC FORM AVAILABLE: Yes

THERAPEUTIC CLASS: Barbiturate/anticholinergic antispasmatic

DOSAGE FORMS: 0.0194-mg atropine sulfate/0.1037-mg hyoscyamine/0.0065-mg scopolamine/16.2-mg phenobarbital tablets, capsules, and per 5 mL elixir. Sustained-release tablets (Donnatal Extentabs) contain the equivalent of three Donnatal tablets in a dosage form intended to provide activity over a 12-hour period.

MAIN USES: Irritable bowel syndrome and duodenal ulcers

USUAL DOSE: one to two tablets/capsules three to four times daily; one to two teaspoons of the elixir three to four times daily; and one Extentab tablet every 8 to 12 hours

AVERAGE PRICE: $19.01 (B)/$7.24 (G) for the tablets and capsules; and $65.71 for the Extentabs

SIDE EFFECTS: Most common: drowsiness; constipation; dizziness; decreased sweating; and dry mouth, nose, and throat. Less common: bloated feeling, decreased saliva, difficulty in swallowing, headache, loss of memory, blurred vision, increased sensitivity of the eyes to sunlight, nausea, vomiting, and unusual tiredness or weakness.

DRUG INTERACTIONS: Alcohol, anxiety medications, and narcotic painkillers may intensify the drowsiness effect of the drug. The drug may decrease effectiveness of Compazine, Haldol, Mellaril, Prolixin, Serentil, Stelazine, Thorazine, and Trilafon. The drug may cause Coumadin to become less effective.

FOOD INTERACTIONS: The drug should be taken 30 minutes before meals.

ALLERGIES: Individuals allergic to belladonna alkaloids, phenobarbital, or any of their derivatives should discuss this with their doctor or pharmacist before using this drug.

PREGNANCY/BREAST-FEEDING: Category C—Risk cannot be ruled out. Human studies are lacking, and animal studies are either positive for fetal risk or lacking as well. However, potential benefits may justify the potential risk in using the drug. It is not known whether the drug is excreted in the breast milk; therefore, caution should be used when breast-feeding.

OTHER BRAND NAMES: None

OTHER DRUGS IN THE SAME THERAPEUTIC CLASS: Butibel

IMPORTANT INFORMATION TO REMEMBER: This drug does cause drowsiness. Individuals should use caution when driving, operating machinery, or any task where mental alertness is required. Alcohol, anxiety medications, and narcotic painkillers may intensify the drowsiness effect of the drug. The drug should be taken 30 minutes before meals. Do not increase the dose without first consulting with your physician. Caution should also be used when exercising and in hot weather while taking this drug; the drug may increase an individual's sensitivity to hot weather. Individuals with glaucoma, or prostate or urinary problems should discuss this with their doctor before taking this drug.

BRAND NAME: Doral

GENERIC NAME: quazepam

GENERIC FORM AVAILABLE: No

THERAPEUTIC CLASS: Benzodiazepine sedative

DOSAGE FORMS: 7.5-mg and 15-mg tablets

MAIN USES: Insomnia

USUAL DOSE: 15 mg at bedtime initially; may reduce to 7.5 mg nightly

AVERAGE PRICE: $175.50 for 7.5 mg and $191.80 for 15 mg

SIDE EFFECTS: daytime drowsiness 12%, headache 5%, tiredness 2%, dizziness 2%, dry mouth 2%, and upset stomach 1%.

DRUG INTERACTIONS: Central nervous system (CNS) depression may be increased when used with alcohol, narcotic painkillers, or other anxiety medications.

ALLERGIES: Individuals allergic to flurazepam, benzodiazepines, or other sleeping medications (such as those listed in "Other Drugs in the Same Therapeutic Class") should discuss this with their doctor or pharmacist before taking this drug.

PREGNANCY/BREAST-FEEDING: Category X—Should not be used during pregnancy. Studies in animals and/or humans have shown fetal abnormalities and birth defects. The risks associated with using this drug clearly outweigh the benefits. This drug should never be used by someone who is pregnant or trying to become pregnant. Also, women should never breast-feed while using this drug.

OTHER BRAND NAMES: None

OTHER DRUGS IN THE SAME THERAPEUTIC CLASS: Dalmane, Halcion, ProSom, and Restoril

IMPORTANT INFORMATION TO REMEMBER: This drug will cause drowsiness. Individuals should use caution when driving, operating machinery, or any task where mental alertness is required. The drug may take two to three days before maximum effect is seen. The incidence of drowsiness and unsteadiness increases with age. Alcohol, anxiety medications, and narcotic painkillers may intensify the drowsiness effect of the drug. This medication is a controlled substance and may be habit-forming. Do not increase the dose of medication without consulting with your doctor; only take the amount prescribed by your doctor.

BRAND NAME: Doryx

GENERIC NAME: doxycycline hyclate

GENERIC FORM AVAILABLE: No

THERAPEUTIC CLASS: Tetracycline antibiotic

DOSAGE FORMS: 100 mg doxycycline coated pellets in a capsule

MAIN USES: Bacterial infections and severe acne

USUAL DOSE: 100 mg every 12 hours for one day, then 100 mg daily

AVERAGE PRICE: $115.24 (30 capsules)

SIDE EFFECTS: Most common: discoloration on infants and children's teeth, increased sensitivity to sunburn, dizziness, diarrhea, nausea, vomiting, stomach pain, and burning stomach. Less common: sore or darkened tongue, discoloration of the skin and mucous membranes, and fungal overgrowth.

DRUG INTERACTIONS: Antacids, calcium supplements, iron supplements, magnesium laxatives, and other mineral supplements may bind to the drug in the stomach and intestines and prevent its absorption by the body. The drug may decrease the effectiveness of birth control pills.

ALLERGIES: Individuals allergic to doxycycline or other tetracyclines (such as those listed in "Other Drugs in the Same Therapeutic Class") should discuss this with their doctor or pharmacist before taking this drug.

PREGNANCY/BREAST-FEEDING: Category D—Positive evidence of risk. Human studies show risk to the fetus. Nevertheless, potential benefits may possibly outweigh the potential risks. This drug should not be taken by nursing mothers.

OTHER BRAND NAMES: None

OTHER DRUGS IN THE SAME THERAPEUTIC CLASS: Achromycin V, Minocin, Monodox, Sumycin, Vibramycin, and Vibra-Tabs

IMPORTANT INFORMATION TO REMEMBER: If stomach upset occurs, take the drug with food. Take the drug at the same time every day. Also, take the drug until all the medication prescribed is gone; otherwise the infection may return. This drug should be taken with plenty of water (eight ounces is preferred) and the capsules should be swallowed whole. Avoid taking antacids, calcium supplements, iron supplements, magnesium laxatives, and other mineral supplements within two hours of taking the drug. Women taking birth control pills should use another form of contraception while taking the drug and for the rest of the current menstrual cycle. Individuals should also use a sunscreen to avoid overexposure to the sun; the drug may increase the skin's sensitivity to sunlight, which may cause one to sunburn more easily. The drug should not be used by children under eight years of age due to the potential of permanent tooth staining.

BRAND NAME: **Dovonex**

GENERIC NAME: calcipotriene

GENERIC FORM AVAILABLE: No

THERAPEUTIC CLASS: Vitamin D derivative

DOSAGE FORMS: 0.005% cream and ointment

MAIN USES: Psoriasis and {scaly skin}

USUAL DOSE: Apply a thin layer twice daily.

AVERAGE PRICE: $51.26 for 30 g

SIDE EFFECTS: burning 10%–15%, itching 10%–15%, skin irritation 10%–15%, red skin 1%–10%, peeling 1%–10%, dry skin 1%–10%, rash 1%–10%, and worsening of psoriasis 1%–10%.

DRUG INTERACTIONS: None of any clinical significance

ALLERGIES: Individuals allergic to calcipotriene, vitamin D, or any of their derivatives should discuss this with their doctor or pharmacist before using this drug.

PREGNANCY/BREAST-FEEDING: Category C—Risk cannot be ruled out. Human studies are lacking, and animal studies are either positive for fetal risk or lacking as well. However, potential benefits may justify the potential risk in using the drug. It is not known whether the drug is excreted in the breast milk; therefore, caution should be used when breast-feeding.

OTHER BRAND NAMES: None

OTHER DRUGS IN THE SAME THERAPEUTIC CLASS: None

IMPORTANT INFORMATION TO REMEMBER: This drug is for external use only. Gently rub a thin film of drug completely into skin. Never cover the skin after application with a bandage or wrapping unless directed to do so by a doctor. Never apply to open wounds or sores unless directed to do so by a doctor. Discontinue use if irritation occurs.

BRAND NAME: Duphalac

GENERIC NAME: lactulose

See entry for Chronulac

BRAND NAME: Duragesic

GENERIC NAME: fentanyl transdermal system

GENERIC FORM AVAILABLE: No

THERAPEUTIC CLASS: Narcotic analgesic

DOSAGE FORMS: 25 micrograms/hr, 50 micrograms/hr, 75 micrograms/hr, and 100 micrograms/hr patches

MAIN USES: Chronic pain

USUAL DOSE: Apply one patch every 72 hours.

AVERAGE PRICE: $72.67 for 25 micrograms/hr (five patches); $108.96 for 50 micrograms/hr (five patches); $166.43 for 75 micrograms/hr (five patches); $207.36 for 100 micrograms/hr (five patches)

SIDE EFFECTS: nausea 10% or more, constipation 10% or more, vomiting 10% or more, dry mouth 10% or more, drowsiness 10% or more, confusion 3%–10%, stomach pain 3%–10%, headache 3%–10%, dizziness 3%–10%, nervousness 3%–10%, hallucinations 3%–10%, appetite changes 3%–10%, diarrhea 3%–10%, difficulty urinating 3%–10%, difficulty breathing 3%–10%, depression 3%–10%, euphoria 3%, low blood pressure 3%, respiratory depression 2%–4%, and high blood pressure 1%.

DRUG INTERACTIONS: Alcohol, anxiety medications, or other narcotic painkillers may intensify the drowsiness and respiratory depression effects of the drug.

ALLERGIES: Individuals allergic to fentanyl or any of its derivatives should discuss this with their doctor or pharmacist before using this drug.

PREGNANCY/BREAST-FEEDING: Category C—Risk cannot be ruled out. Human studies are lacking, and animal studies are either positive for fetal risk or lacking as well. However, potential benefits may justify the potential risk in using the drug. The drug is excreted in the breast milk; therefore, extreme caution should be used when breast-feeding.

OTHER BRAND NAMES: None

OTHER DRUGS IN THE SAME THERAPEUTIC CLASS: Demerol, Dilaudid, Dolophine, Levo-Dromoran, MS Contin, MSIR, Oramorph SR, Roxanol, and Stadol

IMPORTANT INFORMATION TO REMEMBER: This is a very potent drug and may cause a lot of drowsiness. Individuals should use extreme caution when driving, operating machinery, or any task where mental alertness is required. Alcohol, anxiety medications, and other narcotic painkillers may intensify the drowsiness effect of the drug. Do not increase the dose without first consulting with your physician—this could be very dangerous and possibly life-threatening. This medication is a controlled substance, may be habit-forming, and should only be used as needed for pain relief. This drug should only be used for chronic pain under the close supervision of a physician. This prescription cannot be refilled; a new written prescription must be obtained each time. External sources of heat (heating pads, electric blankets, water beds, etc.) may accelerate the absorption of the drug, causing a toxic dose.

When using the patches:

1) Do not cut or fold the patch in half. This may cause the medication inside to leak out.

2) Apply the patch to a clean, dry skin area on the upper arm or torso. This area should be free of hair, cuts, scars, or irritation.

3) Leave the patch on even during showering, bathing, and exercising. If the patch falls off, replace the patch with a new one.

4) When it's time to apply a new patch, use a different site on the skin. Rotate the sites where you apply the patches every time.

5) Dispose of used patches properly and keep out of reach of children.

BRAND NAME: Duricef

GENERIC NAME: cefadroxil

GENERIC FORM AVAILABLE: Yes

THERAPEUTIC CLASS: Cephalosporin antibiotic

DOSAGE FORMS: 500-mg capsules, 1000 mg tablets; or 125 mg/ 5 mL, 250 mg/5 mL, and 500 mg/5 mL oral suspension

MAIN USES: Bacterial infections

USUAL DOSE: 1000 mg to 2000 mg daily in two divided doses

AVERAGE PRICE: $96.20 (B)/$70.00 (G) for 500 mg (20 capsules) and $177.40 for 1000 mg (20 tablets)

SIDE EFFECTS: Most common: none. Less common: nausea, vomiting, diarrhea, rash, vaginal yeast infections, and stomach pain.

DRUG INTERACTIONS: The drug may decrease the effectiveness of oral contraceptives used for birth control. Women may become pregnant while taking Duricef and oral contraceptives. The drug probenecid will decrease elimination of the drug by the kidneys.

ALLERGIES: Individuals allergic to cefadroxil or other cephalosporins (such as those listed in "Other Drugs in the Same Therapeutic Class") should discuss this with their doctor or pharmacist before taking this drug.

PREGNANCY/BREAST-FEEDING: Category B—No evidence of risk in humans. Either animal findings show risk, but human findings do not; or, if no adequate human studies have been done, animal findings show no risk. It is not known whether the drug is excreted in the breast milk; therefore, caution should be used when breast-feeding.

OTHER BRAND NAMES: Ultracef

OTHER DRUGS IN THE SAME THERAPEUTIC CLASS: Ceclor, Cedax, Ceftin, Cefzil, Keflex, Keftab, Suprax, Vantin, and Velosef

IMPORTANT INFORMATION TO REMEMBER: If stomach upset occurs, take with food or milk. Also, take the drug at even intervals around the clock (if two times a day, take every 12 hours). Take the drug until all the medication prescribed is gone; otherwise the infection may return. Women taking birth control pills should use another form of contraception while taking the drug and for the rest of the current menstrual cycle. Individuals taking the liquid form should shake it thoroughly before use, store the medication in the refrigerator, and discard any remaining medication after 14 days. The drug may produce a false positive for some glucose and protein urine tests.

BRAND NAME: Dyazide

GENERIC NAME: Combination product containing: triamterene and hydrochlorothiazide

GENERIC FORM AVAILABLE: Yes

THERAPEUTIC CLASS: Potassium-sparing diuretic (water pill) + thiazide diuretic (water pill)

DOSAGE FORMS: 37.5-mg triamterene/25-mg hydrochlorothiazide capsules

MAIN USES: Swelling and water retention due to congestive heart failure, kidney or liver disease, and high blood pressure.

USUAL DOSE: one to two capsules once or twice daily

AVERAGE PRICE: $43.97 (B)/$35.17 (G)

SIDE EFFECTS: Most common: none. Less common: dizziness, nausea, vomiting, stomach pain, diarrhea, high potassium, muscle cramps, headache, increased sensitivity to sunlight (sunburn), dry mouth, and skin rash.

DRUG INTERACTIONS: The drug may increase the toxic effects of Eskalith or Lithobid. High potassium levels may occur when used together with Accupril, Altace, Capoten, Lotensin, Monopril, Prinivil, Univasc, Vasotec, and potassium supplements such as Micro-K, K-Dur, Klor-Con, K-Lyte, K-Tab, and Slow-K. The drug may decrease the effects of Coumadin. Individuals taking Lanoxin should inform their doctor of this before taking this drug.

ALLERGIES: Individuals allergic to triamterene, hydrochlorothiazide, Dyrenium, HydroDIURIL, Maxzide, Moduretic, sulfa drugs, or any of their derivatives should discuss this with their doctor or pharmacist before using this drug.

PREGNANCY/BREAST-FEEDING: Category C—Risk cannot be ruled out. Human studies are lacking, and animal studies are either positive for fetal risk or lacking as well. However, potential benefits may justify the potential risk in using the drug. It is not known whether the drug is excreted in the breast milk; therefore, caution should be used when breast-feeding.

OTHER BRAND NAMES: None

OTHER DRUGS IN THE SAME THERAPEUTIC CLASS: Aldactazide, Maxzide, and Moduretic

IMPORTANT INFORMATION TO REMEMBER: If the drug is to be taken once daily, take it in the morning due to increased urine output. If stomach upset occurs, take the drug with food or milk. This drug may also increase the sensitivity of the skin to sunburn in some individuals; therefore, a sunscreen is recommended during periods of prolonged exposure to the sun. Individuals with kidney disease should discuss this with their doctor before taking this drug. Before taking over-the-counter cold and allergy preparations, consult your doctor or pharmacist—these products may raise your blood pressure.

BRAND NAME: Dynabac

GENERIC NAME: dirithromycin

GENERIC FORM AVAILABLE: No

THERAPEUTIC CLASS: Macrolide antibiotic

DOSAGE FORMS: 250-mg enteric coated tablets

MAIN USES: Bacterial infections

USUAL DOSE: two tablets daily

AVERAGE PRICE: $61.50 (20 tablets)

SIDE EFFECTS: stomach pain 10%, headache 9%, nausea 8%, diarrhea 8%, vomiting 3%, dizziness 2%, pain 2%, gas 2%, rash 1%, itching 1%, and insomnia 1%.

DRUG INTERACTIONS: It is recommended that this drug should not be used with Seldane, Seldane-D, or Hismanal; the drug may potentially increase the blood levels of these drugs to extremely toxic and possibly life-threatening levels. The drug may also increase the blood levels of Coumadin, Retrovir, rifabutin, Slo-bid, Theo-Dur, Uni-Dur, Uniphyl, and Tegretol. Antacids may increase the absorption of the drug. Propulsid and the drug may cause dangerous irregular heartbeats when taken together.

ALLERGIES: Individuals allergic to dirithromycin or other macrolide antibiotics (such as those listed in "Other Drugs in the Same Therapeutic Class") should discuss this with their doctor or pharmacist before taking this drug.

PREGNANCY/BREAST-FEEDING: Category C—Risk cannot be ruled out. Human studies are lacking, and animal studies are either positive for fetal risk or lacking as well. However, potential benefits may justify the potential risk in using the drug. The drug is excreted in the breast milk; therefore, extreme caution should be used when breast-feeding.

OTHER BRAND NAMES: None

OTHER DRUGS IN THE SAME THERAPEUTIC CLASS: Biaxin, E-Mycin, E.E.S., ERY-TAB, ERYC, EryPed, Ilosone, PCE, TAO, and Zithromax

IMPORTANT INFORMATION TO REMEMBER: This drug should be taken with food or milk to reduce the potential for stomach upset. Also, take the drug at even intervals around the clock (if twice a day, take every 12 hours). Take the drug until all the medication prescribed is gone; otherwise the infection may return. Do not crush or divide tablets—this will destroy the protective coating that ensures release of the drug in the intestines. Swallow the tablets whole. If severe diarrhea occurs while taking this drug, notify your doctor immediately. The drug should be used with extreme caution in combination with Seldane, Seldane-D, or Hismanal (see "Drug Interactions").

BRAND NAME: DynaCirc and DynaCirc SR

GENERIC NAME: isradipine

GENERIC FORM AVAILABLE: No

THERAPEUTIC CLASS: Calcium channel blocker

DOSAGE FORMS: 2.5-mg and 5-mg capsules; and 5-mg and 10-mg controlled-release capsules

MAIN USES: High blood pressure

USUAL DOSE: 2.5 mg to 5 mg twice daily for DynaCirc or 5 mg to 10 mg once daily for DynaCirc SR

AVERAGE PRICE: $78.45 for 2.5 mg and $115.08 for 5 mg

SIDE EFFECTS: headache 14%, dizziness 7%, swelling 7%, pounding heartbeat 4%, tiredness 4%, flushing 3%, chest pain 2%, nausea 2%, difficulty breathing 2%, stomach discomfort 2%, fast heartbeat 2%, rash 2%, weakness 1%, vomiting 1%, and diarrhea 1%.

DRUG INTERACTIONS: The effects of Blocadren, Cartrol, Corgard, Inderal, Kerlone, Levatol, Lopressor, Minipress, Normodyne, Norpace, Sectral, Tenormin, Toprol-XL, Trandate, Visken, and Zebeta may be increased when taken with this drug. The drug may increase the blood levels of Tegretol, Sandimmune, Lanoxin, Quinidex, Quinaglute, and Procan. Tagamet may increase the blood levels of the drug.

ALLERGIES: Individuals allergic to isradipine or any of its derivatives should discuss this with their doctor or pharmacist before using this drug.

PREGNANCY/BREAST-FEEDING: Category C—Risk cannot be ruled out. Human studies are lacking, and animal studies are either positive for fetal risk or lacking as well. However, potential benefits may justify the potential risk in using the drug. It is not known whether the drug is excreted in the breast milk; therefore, caution should be used when breast-feeding.

OTHER BRAND NAMES: None

OTHER DRUGS IN THE SAME THERAPEUTIC CLASS: Adalat, Adalat CC, Calan, Calan SR, Cardene, Cardene SR, Cardizem, Cardizem SR, Cardizem CD, Covera-HS, Dilacor XR, Isoptin, Isoptin SR, Norvasc, Procardia, Procardia XL, Sular, Vascor, and Verelan

IMPORTANT INFORMATION TO REMEMBER: If stomach upset occurs, take the drug with food or milk. Only take the drug exactly as directed by your physician. Do not discontinue the drug without first consulting your physician. Before taking over-the-counter cold and allergy preparations, consult your doctor or pharmacist—these products may raise your blood pressure. This drug may cause some drowsiness at first. Individuals should use caution when driving, operating machinery, or any task where mental alertness is required.

BRAND NAME: Dyrenium

GENERIC NAME: triamterene

GENERIC FORM AVAILABLE: No

THERAPEUTIC CLASS: Potassium-sparing diuretic (water pill)

DOSAGE FORMS: 50 mg and 100 mg capsules

MAIN USES: Swelling and water retention due to congestive heart failure, kidney or liver disease, and high blood pressure

USUAL DOSE: 100 mg twice daily

AVERAGE PRICE: $49.70 for 50 mg and $62.44 for 100 mg

SIDE EFFECTS: Most common: none. Less common: dizziness, nausea, vomiting, stomach pain, diarrhea, high potassium, muscle cramps, headache, increased sensitivity to sunlight (sunburn), dry mouth, and skin rash.

DRUG INTERACTIONS: The drug may increase the toxic effects of Eskalith or Lithobid. High potassium levels may occur when used together with Accupril, Altace, Capoten, Lotensin, Monopril, Prinivil, Univasc, and Vasotec, and potassium supplements such as Micro-K, K-Dur, Klor-Con, K-Lyte, K-Tab, and Slow-K. The drug may decrease the effects of Coumadin.

ALLERGIES: Individuals allergic to triamterene or any of its derivatives should discuss this with their doctor or pharmacist before using this drug.

PREGNANCY/BREAST FEEDING: Category B—No evidence of risk in humans. Either animal findings show risk, but human findings do not; or, if no adequate human studies have been done, animal findings show no risk. It is not known whether the drug is excreted in the breast milk; therefore, caution should be used when breast-feeding.

OTHER BRAND NAMES: None

OTHER DRUGS IN THE SAME THERAPEUTIC CLASS: Aldactone and Midamor

IMPORTANT INFORMATION TO REMEMBER: If the drug is to be taken once daily, take it in the morning due to increased urine output. This drug should be taken with food or milk to reduce the potential for stomach upset. This drug may also increase the sensitivity of the skin to sunburn in some individuals; therefore, a sunscreen is recommended during periods of prolonged exposure to the sun. Individuals with kidney disease should discuss this with their doctor before taking this drug. Before taking over-the-counter cold and allergy preparations, consult your doctor or pharmacist—these products may raise your blood pressure.

BRAND NAME: Easprin

GENERIC NAME: aspirin

GENERIC FORM AVAILABLE: No

THERAPEUTIC CLASS: Nonsteroidal anti-inflammatory drug (NSAID)

DOSAGE FORMS: 975-mg enteric coated tablets

MAIN USES: Arthritis and pain relief

USUAL DOSE: 975 mg three to four times daily

AVERAGE PRICE: $51.29

SIDE EFFECTS: Most common: ringing in the ears, nausea, hearing impairment, rash, and dizziness. Less common: stomach pain, diarrhea, headache, and drowsiness.

DRUG INTERACTIONS: Other NSAIDs (such as Anaprox, Ansaid, Aleve, aspirin, Cataflam, Clinoril, Daypro, Disalcid, Dolobid, Feldene, Indocin, Lodine, Motrin, Nalfon, Naprosyn, Orudis, Oruvail, Relafen, Tolectin, and Voltaren) may decrease the concentration of the drug in the blood. This drug may also decrease the effects of Lasix, Dyazide, HydroDIURIL, Maxzide, and other water pills. The drug may increase the blood levels of Dilantin, Eskalith, Lithobid, and Sandimmune. The drug may increase the blood levels of Depakene and Depakote, as well as potentially cause other blood disorders. The drug may increase the toxic effects of the drug Rheumatrex. Extreme caution should be used when taking the drug with Coumadin.

ALLERGIES: Individuals allergic to aspirin or any of its derivatives should discuss this with their doctor or pharmacist before using this drug.

PREGNANCY/BREAST-FEEDING: Category C—Risk cannot be ruled out. Human studies are lacking, and animal studies are either positive for fetal risk or lacking as well. However, potential benefits may justify the potential risk in using the drug. The drug should not, however, be used during the late stages (last three months) of pregnancy. The drug is excreted in the breast milk; therefore, extreme caution should be used when breast-feeding.

OTHER BRAND NAMES: None

OTHER DRUGS IN THE SAME THERAPEUTIC CLASS: Anaprox, Ansaid, aspirin, Cataflam, Clinoril, Daypro, Dolobid, Disalcid, Feldene, Indocin, Lodine, Lodine XL, Motrin, Nalfon, Naprosyn, Orudis, Oruvail, Relafen, Tolectin, Toradol, Voltaren, and Voltaren XR

IMPORTANT INFORMATION TO REMEMBER: This drug should be taken with food or milk to reduce the potential for injury to the stomach lining and stomach upset. The drug should not be taken with antacids; antacids will affect the enteric coating on the Easprin tablets. This drug may take up to two weeks before a noticeable improvement in pain relief associated with arthritis is observed. Drinking alcohol while taking this drug may increase its potential to cause ulcers. This drug should only be used under the direct supervision of a doctor by individuals with a bleeding disorder or ulcer, or those who are currently taking Coumadin. Before taking over-the-counter pain relievers, consult your doctor or pharmacist. Hearing problems may be a symptom of too high a dose; if ringing in the ears or hearing problems occur, contact your doctor immediately. Most of the time these hearing problems disappear once the dose of the drug is reduced. No more than one pain reliever should be taken at any one time unless otherwise directed by your doctor.

BRAND NAME: EC-Naprosyn

GENERIC NAME: naproxen

See entry for Naprosyn/Naprosyn-EC

BRAND NAME: **E.E.S.**

GENERIC NAME: erythromycin ethylsuccinate

GENERIC FORM AVAILABLE: Yes

THERAPEUTIC CLASS: Macrolide antibiotic

DOSAGE FORMS: 400-mg tablets; 200 mg/5 mL and 400 mg/5 mL suspension

MAIN USES: Bacterial infections

USUAL DOSES: 400 mg every six hours. Doses for children may be less.

AVERAGE PRICE: $26.71 (B)/$18.79 (G) for 400-mg tablets

SIDE EFFECTS: Most common: nausea, vomiting, stomach pain, diarrhea, and appetite changes. Less common: dizziness, headache, abnormal taste, and confusion.

DRUG INTERACTIONS: **Warning:** This drug should not be used with Seldane, Seldane-D, or Hismanal. The drug may increase the blood levels of these drugs to extremely toxic and possibly life-threatening levels. The drug may also increase the blood levels of Coumadin, Retrovir, rifabutin, Sandimmune, Slo-bid, Theo-Dur, theophylline, Uni-Dur, Uniphyl, and Tegretol. Propulsid and the drug may cause dangerous irregular heartbeats when taken together.

ALLERGIES: Individuals allergic to erythromycin or other macrolide antibiotics (such as those listed in "Other Drugs in the Same Therapeutic Class") should discuss this with their doctor or pharmacist before taking this drug.

PREGNANCY/BREAST-FEEDING: Category B—No evidence of risk in humans. Either animal findings show risk, but human findings do not; or, if no adequate human studies have been done, animal findings show no risk. The drug is excreted in the breast milk; therefore, extreme caution should be used when breast-feeding.

OTHER BRAND NAMES: EryPed (oral suspension only)

OTHER DRUGS IN THE SAME THERAPEUTIC CLASS: Biaxin, Dynabac, E-Mycin, ERY-TAB, ERYC, EryPed, Erythrocin, Ilosone, PCE, TAO, and Zithromax

IMPORTANT INFORMATION TO REMEMBER: If stomach upset occurs, take the drug with food or milk. Also, take the drug at even intervals around the clock (if four times a day, take every six hours). Take the drug until all the medication prescribed is gone; otherwise the infection may return. Individuals taking the liquid form should shake it thoroughly before use, and store the medication in the refrigerator. If severe diarrhea occurs while taking this drug, notify your doctor immediately. Never take the drug with Seldane, Seldane-D, or Hismanal (see "Drug Interactions").

BRAND NAME: Effexor

GENERIC NAME: venlafaxine

GENERIC FORM AVAILABLE: No

THERAPEUTIC CLASS: Neurotransmitter reuptake inhibitor antidepressant

DOSAGE FORMS: 25-mg, 37.5-mg, 50-mg, 75-mg, and 100-mg tablets

MAIN USES: Depression

USUAL DOSE: 75 mg to 150 mg daily in two to three divided doses

AVERAGE PRICE: $133.63 for 25 mg; $137.63 for 37.5 mg; $141.75 for 50 mg; $150.27 for 75 mg; $159.29 for 100 mg

SIDE EFFECTS: nausea 37%, headache 25%, drowsiness 23%, dry mouth 22%, dizziness 19%, insomnia 18%, constipation 15%, nervousness 13%, sweating 12%, weakness 12%, abnormal ejaculation/orgasm 12%, loss of appetite 11%, diarrhea 8%, vomiting 6%, blurred vision 6%, impotence 6%, tremors 5%, gas 3%, rash 3%, chills 3%, chest pain 2%, high blood pressure 2%, fast heartbeat 2%, decreased sex drive 2%, abnormal taste 2%, and ringing in the ears 2%.

DRUG INTERACTIONS: Tagamet may increase the blood levels of the drug. Alcohol, anxiety medications, and narcotic painkillers may intensify the drowsiness effect of the drug. The drug should not be used until 14 days after Nardil or Parnate have been discontinued. Nardil and Parnate should not be taken until seven days after Effexor has been stopped.

ALLERGIES: Individuals allergic to venlafaxine or any of its derivatives should discuss this with their doctor or pharmacist before using this drug.

PREGNANCY/BREAST-FEEDING: Category C—Risk cannot be ruled out. Human studies are lacking, and animal studies are either positive for fetal risk or lacking as well. However, potential benefits may justify the potential risk in using the drug. It is not known whether the drug is excreted in the breast milk; therefore, caution should be used when breast-feeding.

OTHER BRAND NAMES: None

OTHER DRUGS IN THE SAME THERAPEUTIC CLASS: Serzone

IMPORTANT INFORMATION TO REMEMBER: Only take the drug exactly as directed by your physician. Do not discontinue the drug without first consulting your physician. This drug does cause drowsiness. Individuals should use caution when driving, operating machinery, or any task where mental alertness is required. Alcohol, anxiety medications, and narcotic painkillers may intensify the drowsiness effect of the drug. This drug should be taken with food or milk to reduce the potential for stomach upset.

BRAND NAME: Elavil

GENERIC NAME: amitriptyline

GENERIC FORM AVAILABLE: Yes

THERAPEUTIC CLASS: Tricyclic antidepressant

DOSAGE FORMS: 10-mg, 25-mg, 50-mg, 75-mg, 100-mg, and 150-mg tablets

MAIN USES: Depression and {insomnia}

USUAL DOSE: 40 mg to 150 mg daily in divided doses or at bedtime

AVERAGE PRICE: $23.52 (B)/$9.88 (G) for 10 mg; $52.77 (B)/ $13.14 (G) for 25 mg; $92.37 (B)/$14.79 (G) for 50 mg; $106.02 (B)/$17.06 (G) for 75 mg; $133.96 (B)/$19.78 (G) for 100 mg; $190.30 (B)/$27.48 (G) for 150 mg

SIDE EFFECTS: Most common: drowsiness, dizziness, dry mouth, headache, increased appetite, nausea, tiredness, weight gain, and unpleasant taste. Less common: diarrhea, excessive sweating, heartburn, insomnia, vomiting, irregular heartbeat, muscle tremors, urinary difficulties, and impotence.

DRUG INTERACTIONS: The drug should not be taken with Nardil or Parnate; in fact, 14 days are needed between the time of the use of

Nardil or Parnate and this drug. Alcohol, anxiety medications, and narcotic painkillers may make the drowsiness caused by the drug much worse. Compazine, Mellaril, Prolixin, Serentil, Stelazine, Thorazine, and Trilafon may increase the blood levels of the drug. Tagamet may increase the blood levels of the drug. The drug may decrease the effects of Catapres and Ismelin. The drug may increase the effects of decongestants found in cough, cold, and allergy products on the heart, possibly causing high blood pressure, fast heartbeat, or irregular heartbeats.

ALLERGIES: Individuals allergic to amitriptyline or other tricylic antidepressants (such as those listed in "Other Drugs in the Same Therapeutic Class") should discuss this with their doctor or pharmacist before taking this drug.

PREGNANCY/BREAST-FEEDING: Category D—Positive evidence of risk. Human studies show risk to the fetus. Nevertheless, potential benefits may possibly outweigh the potential risk. This drug should not be taken by nursing mothers.

OTHER BRAND NAMES: Endep

OTHER DRUGS IN THE SAME THERAPEUTIC CLASS: Asendin, Endep, Norpramin, Pamelor, Sinequan, Surmontil, Tofranil, and Vivactil

IMPORTANT INFORMATION TO REMEMBER: Only take the drug exactly as directed by your physician. Do not discontinue the drug without first consulting your physician. The drug may require one to six weeks of use before improvement may be noticed. This drug does cause drowsiness. Individuals should use caution when driving, operating machinery, or any task where mental alertness is required. Alcohol, anxiety medications, and narcotic painkillers may intensify the drowsiness effect of the drug. The drug may cause a slight amount of dizziness or lightheadedness when rising from a sitting or lying-down position. Individuals should also use a sunscreen to avoid overexposure to the sun; the drug may increase the skin's sensitivity to sunlight, which may cause one to sunburn more easily.

BRAND NAME: Eldepryl

GENERIC NAME: selegiline

GENERIC FORM AVAILABLE: No

THERAPEUTIC CLASS: Anti-Parkinson's agent

DOSAGE FORMS: 5-mg capsules

MAIN USES: Parkinson's disease

USUAL DOSE: 5 mg at breakfast and lunch

AVERAGE PRICE: $255.98

SIDE EFFECTS: nausea 20%, dizziness 14%, stomach pain 8%, confusion 6%, hallucinations 6%, dry mouth 6%, vivid dreams 4%, headache 4%, unusual movements of the body 4%, nervousness 2%, diarrhea 2%, pounding heartbeat 2%, and muscle aches 2%.

DRUG INTERACTIONS: This drug and Luvox, Prozac, Paxil, or Zoloft, when taken together, may cause serotonin syndrome (mental status changes, restlessness, shivering, tremor, incoordination, etc.). Demerol and possibly other narcotic painkillers may cause a severe reaction when taken with this drug.

ALLERGIES: Individuals allergic to selegiline or any of its derivatives should discuss this with their doctor or pharmacist before using this drug.

PREGNANCY/BREAST-FEEDING: Category C—Risk cannot be ruled out. Human studies are lacking, and animal studies are either positive for fetal risk or lacking as well. However, potential benefits may justify the potential risk in using the drug. It is not known whether the drug is excreted in the breast milk; therefore, caution should be used when breast-feeding.

OTHER BRAND NAMES: None

OTHER DRUGS IN THE SAME THERAPEUTIC CLASS: None

IMPORTANT INFORMATION TO REMEMBER: This drug should be taken with food or milk to reduce the potential for stomach upset. This drug does cause drowsiness. Individuals should use caution when driving, operating machinery, or any task where mental alertness is required. Alcohol, anxiety medications, and narcotic painkillers may intensify the drowsiness effect of the drug. The drug may also cause dizziness when suddenly rising from a sitting or lying-down position. Individuals taking more than 10 mg per day should avoid tyramine-containing foods (wines, sherry, liquors, aged cheese, smoked or pickled meats, sauerkraut, beer, and overripe fruits), alcoholic beverages, large quantities of caffeine-containing beverages, and over-the-counter cold and allergy preparations. If not avoided, these may cause a severe high-blood-pressure reaction.

BRAND NAME: Elixophyllin and Elixophyllin XR

GENERIC NAME: theophylline

See entry for Theo-Dur (same drug but different dosage forms)

BRAND NAME: Elocon

GENERIC NAME: mometasone

GENERIC FORM AVAILABLE: No

THERAPEUTIC CLASS: Topical corticosteroid

DOSAGE FORMS: 0.1% ointment, lotion, and cream

MAIN USES: Skin rashes, swelling, and itching

USUAL DOSE: For the cream and ointment: apply a thin film to the affected area once daily. For the lotion: apply a few drops to affected area once daily.

AVERAGE PRICE: $23.79 for 0.1% cream and ointment (15 g); and $26.29 for 0.1% lotion (30 mL)

SIDE EFFECTS: burning 1%–2%, itching 1%, stinging 1%, skin changes 1%, and irritation 1%.

DRUG INTERACTIONS: None of any clinical significance

ALLERGIES: Individuals allergic to mometasone or any of its derivatives should discuss this with their doctor or pharmacist before using this drug.

PREGNANCY/BREAST-FEEDING: Category C—Risk cannot be ruled out. Human studies are lacking, and animal studies are either positive for fetal risk or lacking as well. However, potential benefits may justify the potential risk in using the drug. It is not known whether the drug is excreted in the breast milk; therefore, caution should be used when breast-feeding.

OTHER BRAND NAMES: None

OTHER DRUGS IN THE SAME THERAPEUTIC CLASS: Aclovate, Aristocort, Cordran, Cordran SP, Cutivate, Cyclocort, DesOwen, Diprolene, Diprolene AF, Florone, Florone E, Halog, Hytone, Kenalog, Lidex, Synalar, Temovate, Topicort, Tridesilon, Ultravate, Valisone, and Westcort

IMPORTANT INFORMATION TO REMEMBER: This drug is for external use only. Apply only a thin film of drug to skin and rub it in well. Never cover the skin after application with a bandage or wrapping unless directed to do so by a doctor. Never apply to damaged skin or open wounds unless directed to do so by a doctor. Discontinue use if irritation occurs. If using the lotion, be sure to shake it well.

BRAND NAME: Emgel

GENERIC NAME: erythromycin

GENERIC FORM AVAILABLE: No

THERAPEUTIC CLASS: Topical antibiotic

DOSAGE FORMS: 2% topical gel

MAIN USES: Acne

USUAL DOSE: Apply sparingly as thin layer twice daily.

AVERAGE PRICE: $25.31

SIDE EFFECTS: Most common: burning. Less common: peeling, dryness, itching, redness, oiliness, and tender skin.

DRUG INTERACTIONS: None of any clinical significance

ALLERGIES: Individuals allergic to erythromycin or any of its derivatives should consult their doctor or pharmacist before taking this drug.

PREGNANCY/BREAST FEEDING: Category B—No evidence of risk in humans. Either animal findings show risk, but human findings do not; or, if no adequate human studies have been done, animal findings show no risk. It is not known whether the drug is excreted in the breast milk; therefore, caution should be used when breast-feeding.

OTHER BRAND NAMES: None

OTHER DRUGS IN THE SAME THERAPEUTIC CLASS: A/T/S, Cleocin T, Erygel, Erycette, and T-Stat

IMPORTANT INFORMATION TO REMEMBER: This drug is for external use only. It is important to use the medication continuously. It may take three to four weeks before a significant improvement may be seen. If no improvement is seen within this time period, contact your doctor. This medication contains alcohol, which may cause slight burning or stinging when first applied. Also, avoid contact with the eyes, nose, and mouth. Before applying, wash acne area thoroughly with warm soapy water to remove dirt and skin oils, pat skin dry, and then apply the drug. If you need to apply another medication for acne, wait at least one hour. Discontinue use if irritation occurs.

BRAND NAME: Empirin with Codeine

GENERIC NAME: Combination product containing: aspirin and codeine

GENERIC FORM AVAILABLE: Yes

THERAPEUTIC CLASS: Narcotic analgesic + pain reliever

DOSAGE FORMS: Empirin #3: 325 mg aspirin/30 mg codeine. Empirin #4: 325 mg aspirin/60 mg codeine.

MAIN USES: Mild to moderate pain

USUAL DOSE: one to two tablets every four to six hours as needed

AVERAGE PRICE: $51.42 (B)/$21.98 (G) for Empirin #3 and $120.12 (B)/$23.04 (G) for Empirin #4

SIDE EFFECTS: Most common: drowsiness, lightheadedness, dizziness, nausea, vomiting, constipation, and respiratory depression. Less common: itching, skin rashes, euphoria, sweating, thirst, headache, ringing in the ears, and difficulty hearing.

DRUG INTERACTIONS: Alcohol, anxiety medications, and other narcotic painkillers may intensify the drowsiness effect of the drug. Other NSAIDs (such as Anaprox, Ansaid, Aleve, aspirin, Cataflam, Clinoril, Daypro, Disalcid, Dolobid, Easprin, Feldene, Indocin, Lodine, Motrin, Nalfon, Naprosyn, Orudis, Oruvail, Relafen, Tolectin, and Voltaren) may decrease the concentration of the drug in the blood. This drug may also decrease the effects of Lasix, Dyazide, HydroDIURIL, Maxzide, and other water pills. The drug may increase the blood levels of Eskalith, Lithobid, and Sandimmune. The drug may increase the blood levels of Depakene and Depakote, as well as potentially cause other blood disorders. The drug may increase the toxic effects of the drug Rheumatrex. Caution should be used when taking the drug with Coumadin. This drug and Nardil or Parnate may cause severe and sometimes fatal reactions.

ALLERGIES: Individuals allergic to aspirin, codeine, or any of their derivatives should discuss this with their doctor or pharmacist before using this drug.

PREGNANCY/BREAST-FEEDING: Category C—Risk cannot be ruled out. Human studies are lacking, and animal studies are either positive for fetal risk or lacking as well. However, potential benefits may justify the potential risk in using the drug. The drug is excreted in the breast milk; therefore, extreme caution should be used when breast-feeding.

OTHER BRAND NAMES: None

OTHER DRUGS IN THE SAME THERAPEUTIC CLASS: Bancap-HC, Darvocet, Darvon, Darvon Compound, DHCplus, Hydrocet, Lorcet 10/650, Lorcet Plus, Lortab, Percocet, Percodan, Phenaphen w/Codeine, Synalgos DC, Talacen, Tylenol #2, Tylenol #3, Tylenol #4, Tylox, Vicodin, and Zydone

IMPORTANT INFORMATION TO REMEMBER: This drug does cause drowsiness. Individuals should use caution when driving, operating machinery, or any task where mental alertness is required. Alcohol, anxiety medications, and other narcotic painkillers may intensify the drowsiness effect of the drug. Do not increase the dose without first consulting with your physician. This medication is a controlled substance and may be habit-forming. If stomach upset occurs, take the drug with food or milk. This drug should only be used under the direct supervision of a doctor by individuals with a bleeding disorder or ulcer, or those who are currently taking Coumadin. Before taking over-the-counter pain relievers, consult your doctor or pharmacist.

BRAND NAME: E-Mycin

GENERIC NAME: erythromycin

See entry for ERY-TAB

BRAND NAME: **Endep**

GENERIC NAME: amitriptyline

See entry for Elavil

BRAND NAME: **Enduron**

GENERIC NAME: methyclothiazide

GENERIC FORM AVAILABLE: Yes

THERAPEUTIC CLASS: Thiazide diuretic (water pill)

DOSAGE FORMS: 2.5-mg and 5-mg tablets

MAIN USES: High blood pressure and water retention (fluid retention due to congestive heart failure, kidney disease, or cirrhosis of the liver)

USUAL DOSE: 2.5 mg to 5 mg daily

AVERAGE PRICE: $64.11 (B)/$15.71 (G) for 5 mg

SIDE EFFECTS: Most common: none. Less common: low potassium, weakness, dizziness, irritability, muscle cramps, low blood pressure, headache, restlessness, increased thirst, diarrhea, stomach pain, vomiting, dry mouth, increased sensitivity to sunburn, and muscle spasms.

DRUG INTERACTIONS: The drug may require dosage adjustments to diabetic and gout medications. Colestid and Questran may decrease the absorption of the drug. The drug may increase the blood levels of Eskalith and Lithobid.

ALLERGIES: Individuals allergic to methyclothiazide, sulfa drugs, or any of their derivatives should discuss this with their doctor or pharmacist before using this drug.

PREGNANCY/BREAST-FEEDING: Category B—No evidence of risk in humans. Either animal findings show risk, but human findings do not; or, if no adequate human studies have been done, animal findings show no risk. The drug is expected in the breast milk; therefore, extreme caution should be used when breast-feeding.

OTHER BRAND NAMES: None

OTHER DRUGS IN THE SAME THERAPEUTIC CLASS: Aldactone, Diuril, Esidrix, HydroDIURIL, Hydromox, Hygroton, and Oretic

IMPORTANT INFORMATION TO REMEMBER: If the drug is to be taken once daily, take it in the morning due to increased urine output. Before taking over-the-counter cold and allergy preparations, consult your doctor or pharmacist—these products may raise your blood pressure. The drug may cause the elimination of potassium from the body. It is therefore a good idea to eat a banana or drink orange, grapefruit, or apple juice every day to replace lost potassium. This drug may also increase the sensitivity of the skin to sunburn in some individuals; therefore, a sunscreen is recommended during periods of prolonged exposure to the sun.

BRAND NAME: Entex, Entex LA, and Entex PSE

GENERIC NAME: Combination products containing various combinations of: phenylephrine, phenylpropanolamine, pseudoephedrine, and guaifenesin

GENERIC FORM AVAILABLE: Yes

THERAPEUTIC CLASS: Decongestant + expectorant

DOSAGE FORMS: Entex capsules: 5 mg phenylephrine/45 mg phenylpropanolamine/200 mg guaifenesin, Entex LA: 75 mg phenylpropanolamine/400 mg guaifenesin long-acting tablets. Entex liquid: 5 mg phenylephrine/20 mg phenylpropanolamine/700 mg guaifenesin per 5 mL. Entex PSE: 120 mg pseudoephedrine/600 mg guaifenesin long-acting tablets.

MAIN USES: Nasal congestion and cough

USUAL DOSE: Entex capsules: one capsule every six hours. Entex LA and Entex PSE: one tablet every 12 hours. Entex liquid: two teaspoons every six hours.

AVERAGE PRICE: $51.68 (B)/$20.88 (G) for Entex; $86.44 (B)/$17.36 (G) for Entex LA; $103.48 (B)/$22.32 (G) for Entex PSE

SIDE EFFECTS: Most common: none. Less common: drowsiness, nausea, giddiness, dry mouth, blurred vision, pounding heartbeat, flushing, and increased irritability or excitability (especially in children).

DRUG INTERACTIONS: Blocadren, Cartrol, Corgard, Inderal, Kerlone, Levatol, Lopressor, Normodyne, Sectral, Tenormin, Toprol-XL,

Trandate, Visken, and Zebeta may increase the effects of the drug. The drug may also reduce the effects of blood-pressure-lowering drugs. Nardil or Parnate may significantly raise blood pressure when taken with this drug.

ALLERGIES: Individuals allergic to phenylpropanolamine, pseudoephedrine, guaifenesin, or any of their derivatives should discuss this with their doctor or pharmacist before using this drug.

PREGNANCY/BREAST-FEEDING: Category C—Risk cannot be ruled out. Human studies are lacking, and animal studies are either positive for fetal risk or lacking as well. However, potential benefits may justify the potential risk in using the drug. The drug is excreted in the breast milk; therefore, extreme caution should be used when breast-feeding.

OTHER BRAND NAMES: Exgest LA

OTHER DRUGS IN THE SAME THERAPEUTIC CLASS: Deconsal II, Duratuss, Exgest LA, Guaifed, Guaifed-PD, and Zephrex LA

IMPORTANT INFORMATION TO REMEMBER: Patients with high blood pressure or heart conditions should consult their doctor before taking this drug. This drug should be taken with plenty of water (eight ounces is preferred). Do not crush or divide tablets—this will destroy the matrix that ensures the delayed release of the drug in the intestine. Swallow the tablets whole. The tablets may, however, be cut in half for easier swallowing. Do not increase the dose without first consulting with your physician.

BRAND NAME: Epivir

GENERIC NAME: lamivudine

GENERIC FORM AVAILABLE: No

THERAPEUTIC CLASS: AIDS antiviral

DOSAGE FORMS: 150-mg tablets and 10 mg/mL solution

MAIN USES: AIDS

USUAL DOSE: 150 mg twice daily

AVERAGE PRICE: $145.22 for 150-mg tablets

SIDE EFFECTS: headache 35%, nausea 33%, tiredness 27%, nasal signs and symptoms (runny nose and stuffy nose) 20%, cough

18%, diarrhea 18%, vomiting 13%, appetite changes 13%, nervous system effects (unusual nerve sensations and damage in the arms, legs, fingers, and toes) 12%, muscle pain 12%, insomnia 11%, dizziness 10%, fever or chills 10%, and blood disorders 7%.

DRUG INTERACTIONS: There are numerous drugs that can cause peripheral neuropathy (unusual nerve sensations and damage in the arms, legs, fingers, and toes) when taken with this drug. Some of these are: alcohol, Aldomet, Apresoline, Bactrim, Biaxin, cisplatin, Clinoril, Cytovene, dapsone, Depakene, Depakote, Dilantin, diuretics (water pills), Doryx, Dynabac, erythromycin, Eskalith, estrogens, Flagyl, isoniazid, Lasix, Lithobid, Macrobid, Macrodantin, pentamidine, Septra, Sumycin, Vibramycin, vincristine, and ZERIT. Bactrim, probenecid, and Septra may increase the blood levels of the drug. Biaxin may decrease the blood levels of the drug. Before taking any prescription drug, discuss it with your doctor.

ALLERGIES: Individuals allergic to lamivudine or any of its derivatives should discuss this with their doctor or pharmacist before using this drug.

PREGNANCY/BREAST-FEEDING: Category C—Risk cannot be ruled out. Human studies are lacking, and animal studies are either positive for fetal risk or lacking as well. However, potential benefits may justify the potential risk in using the drug. It is not known whether the drug is excreted in the breast milk; therefore, caution should be used when breast-feeding.

OTHER BRAND NAMES: None

OTHER DRUGS IN THE SAME THERAPEUTIC CLASS: HIVID, Retrovir, Videx, and ZERIT

IMPORTANT INFORMATION TO REMEMBER: If stomach upset occurs, take the drug with food or milk. Also, take the drug at even intervals around the clock (if two times a day, take every 12 hours). Only take the drug exactly as directed by your physician. Do not stop taking the drug without first consulting with your doctor. It is important to have regular blood and liver function tests while taking this drug. Before taking any prescription or over-the-counter (OTC) drugs, consult your doctor or pharmacist.

BRAND NAME: Epogen

GENERIC NAME: epoetin alfa

GENERIC FORM AVAILABLE: No

THERAPEUTIC CLASS: Blood cell production stimultor

DOSAGE FORMS: 2000 units, 3000 units, 4000 units, and 10000 units per mL

MAIN USES: Anemia in those with chronic renal failure and AIDS

USUAL DOSE: Doses are individualized based on each patient's condition. Usual starting dose is 50 units to 100 units per kg of body weight three times per week. (1 kg = 2.2 pounds)

AVERAGE PRICE: $336.00 for Epogen 2000 (10 vials); $504.00 for Epogen 3000 (10 vials); $672.00 for Epogen 4000 (10 vials)

SIDE EFFECTS: fever 29%–38%, high blood pressure 24%, headache 16%, muscle pains 11%, nausea 11%, tiredness 9%–25%, swelling 9%, diarrhea 9%, vomiting 8%, chest pain 7%, skin reaction at injection site 7%, dizziness 7%, clotted access 7%, and seizures (usually within the first 90 days) 3%.

DRUG INTERACTIONS: None of any clinical significance

ALLERGIES: Individuals allergic to epoetin alfa or any of its derivatives should discuss this with their doctor or pharmacist before using this drug.

PREGNANCY/BREAST-FEEDING: Category C—Risk cannot be ruled out. Human studies are lacking, and animal studies are either positive for fetal risk or lacking as well. However, potential benefits may justify the potential risk in using the drug. It is not known whether the drug is excreted in the breast milk; therefore, caution should be used when breast-feeding.

OTHER BRAND NAMES: Procrit

OTHER DRUGS IN THE SAME THERAPEUTIC CLASS: Procrit

IMPORTANT INFORMATION TO REMEMBER: Patients with high blood pressure should inform their doctor of this before using this drug. Use proper injection technique if you are giving yourself the injections. Only take the drug exactly as directed by your physician and do not increase the dose without first consulting with your physician. This drug should be stored in the refrigerator. Do not shake the bottle before use; this may destroy the active ingredients inside the vial. If the solution is discolored or contains lumps, or particles can be seen, do not use the solution. Consult your doctor or pharmacist before using any over-the-counter medications.

BRAND NAME: Equagesic

GENERIC NAME: Combination product containing: meprobamate and aspirin

GENERIC FORM AVAILABLE: No

THERAPEUTIC CLASS: Muscle relaxant + analgesic

DOSAGE FORMS: 200-mg meprobamate/325-mg aspirin tablets

MAIN USES: Muscle pain, muscle spasms, and tension headaches

USUAL DOSE: one to two tablets three to four times daily

AVERAGE PRICE: $104.91

SIDE EFFECTS: Most common: drowsiness, dizziness, lightheadedness, and unsteadiness. Less common: fast heartbeat, nausea, vomiting, diarrhea, constipation, skin rash, ringing in the ears, headache, and vision problems.

DRUG INTERACTIONS: Alcohol, anxiety medications, and narcotic painkillers may intensify the drowsiness effect of the drug. NSAIDS such as Anaprox, Ansaid, Aleve, aspirin, Cataflam, Clinoril, Daypro, Disalcid, Dolobid, Easprin, Feldene, Indocin, Lodine, Motrin, Nalfon, Naprosyn, Orudis, Oruvail, Relafen, Tolectin, and Voltaren) may decrease the concentration of the drug in the blood. This drug may increase the effects and blood levels of Coumadin, medications for diabetes, Rheumatrex, and Retrovir. The drug may decrease the effects of probenecid and Anturane. The drug may increase the blood levels of Depakene and Depakote, as well as potentially cause other blood disorders.

ALLERGIES: Individuals allergic to meprobamate, aspirin, or any of their derivatives should discuss this with their doctor or pharmacist before using this drug.

PREGNANCY/BREAST-FEEDING: Category D—Positive evidence of risk. Human studies show risk to the fetus. Nevertheless, potential benefits may possibly outweigh the potential risks. This drug should not be taken by nursing mothers.

OTHER BRAND NAMES: None

OTHER DRUGS IN THE SAME THERAPEUTIC CLASS: Norgesic Forte, Robaxisal, and Soma Compound

IMPORTANT INFORMATION TO REMEMBER: This drug does cause drowsiness. Individuals should use caution when driving, operating machinery, or any task where mental alertness is required. Alcohol, anxiety medications, and narcotic painkillers may intensify the drowsiness effect of the drug. Do not increase the dose without first consulting with your physician. This medication is a controlled substance and may be habit-forming.

BRAND NAME: ERYC

GENERIC NAME: erythromycin

GENERIC FORM AVAILABLE: Yes

THERAPEUTIC CLASS: Macrolide antibiotic

DOSAGE FORMS: 250-mg capsules

MAIN USES: Bacterial infections

USUAL DOSE: 250 mg every 6 hours or 500 mg every 12 hours

AVERAGE PRICE: $20.03 (B)/$13.70 (G) for 250 mg (30 capsules)

SIDE EFFECTS: Most common: nausea, vomiting, diarrhea, stomach pain, and loss of appetite. Less common: dizziness, headache, abnormal taste, and confusion.

DRUG INTERACTIONS: *Warning:* This drug should not be used with Seldane, Seldane-D, or Hismanal; the drug may increase the blood levels of these drugs to extremely toxic and possibly life-threatening levels. The drug may also increase the blood levels of Coumadin, Retrovir, rifabutin, Sandimmune, Slo-bid, Theo-Dur, theophylline, Uni-Dur, Uniphyl, and Tegretol. Propulsid and the drug may cause dangerous irregular heartbeats when taken together.

ALLERGIES: Individuals allergic to erythromycin or other macrolide antibiotics (such as those listed in "Other Drugs in the Same Therapeutic Class") should discuss this with their doctor or pharmacist before taking this drug.

PREGNANCY/BREAST-FEEDING: Category B—No evidence of risk in humans. Either animal findings show risk, but human findings do not; or, if no adequate human studies have been done, animal findings show no risk. It is not known whether the drug is excreted in the breast milk; therefore, caution should be used when breast-feeding.

OTHER BRAND NAMES: None

OTHER DRUGS IN THE SAME THERAPEUTIC CLASS: Biaxin, Dynabac, E.E.S., E-Mycin, ERY-TAB, EryPed, Erythrocin, Ilosone, PCE, TAO, and Zithromax

IMPORTANT INFORMATION TO REMEMBER: If stomach upset occurs, take the drug with food or milk. Also, take the drug at even intervals around the clock (if four times a day, take every six hours). Take the drug until all the medication prescribed is gone; otherwise, the infection may return. If severe diarrhea occurs while taking this drug, notify your doctor immediately. Never take the drug with Seldane, Seldane-D, or Hismanal (see "Drug Interactions").

BRAND NAME: Erycette

GENERIC NAME: erythromycin (topical)

See entry for A/T/S

BRAND NAME: Erymax

GENERIC NAME: erythromycin

See entry for A/T/S

BRAND NAME: EryPed

GENERIC NAME: erythromycin ethylsuccinate (oral suspension)

See entry for E.E.S.

BRAND NAME: ERY-TAB

GENERIC NAME: erythromycin base

GENERIC FORM AVAILABLE: Yes

THERAPEUTIC CLASS: Macrolide antibiotic

DOSAGE FORMS: 250-mg, 333-mg, and 500-mg tablets

MAIN USES: Bacterial infections

USUAL DOSE: 250 mg every 6 hours, 333 mg every 8 hours, or 500 mg every 12 hours

AVERAGE PRICE: $14.68 for 333 mg (30 tablets); $16.84 for 500 mg (30 tablets); $12.97 for 250 mg (30 tablets)

SIDE EFFECTS: Most common: nausea, vomiting, stomach pain, diarrhea, and loss of appetite. Less common: dizziness, headache, abnormal taste, and confusion.

DRUG INTERACTIONS: *Warning:* This drug should not be used with Seldane, Seldane-D, or Hismanal; the drug may increase the blood levels of these drugs to extremely toxic and possibly life-threatening levels. The drug may also increase the blood levels of Coumadin, Retrovir, rifabutin, Sandimmune, Slo-bid, Theo-Dur, theophylline, Uni-Dur, Uniphyl, and Tegretol. Propulsid and the drug may cause dangerous irregular heartbeats when taken together.

ALLERGIES: Individuals allergic to erythromycin or other macrolide antibiotics (such as those listed in "Other Drugs in the Same Therapeutic Class") should discuss this with their doctor or pharmacist before taking this drug.

PREGNANCY/BREAST-FEEDING: Category B—No evidence of risk in humans. Either animal findings show risk, but human findings do not; or, if no adequate human studies have been done, animal findings show no risk. The drug is excreted in the breast milk; therefore, extreme caution should be used when breast-feeding.

OTHER BRAND NAMES: E-Mycin

OTHER DRUGS IN THE SAME THERAPEUTIC CLASS: Biaxin, Dynabac, E.E.S., E-Mycin, ERYC, EryPed, Erythrocin, Ilosone, PCE, TAO, and Zithromax

IMPORTANT INFORMATION TO REMEMBER: If stomach upset occurs, take the drug with food or milk. Also, take the drug at even intervals around the clock (if four times a day, take every six hours). Take the drug until all the medication prescribed is gone; otherwise the infection may return. If severe diarrhea occurs while taking this drug, notify your doctor immediately. Never take the drug with Seldane, Seldane-D, or Hismanal (see "Drug Interactions"). The ERY-TAB brand contains an enteric coat that prevents the drug from dissolving until it reaches the intestines. This is supposed to reduce the amount of stomach upset erythromycin usually causes.

BRAND NAME: Erythrocin

GENERIC NAME: erythromycin stearate

GENERIC FORM AVAILABLE: No

THERAPEUTIC CLASS: Macrolide antibiotic

DOSAGE FORMS: 250-mg and 500-mg tablets

MAIN USES: Bacterial infections

USUAL DOSE: 250 mg to 500 mg every 6 or 12 hours

AVERAGE PRICE: $14.25 for 250 mg (30 tablets) and $17.82 for 500 mg (30 tablets)

SIDE EFFECTS: Most common: nausea, vomiting, stomach pain, diarrhea, and loss of appetite. Less common: dizziness, headache, abnormal taste, and confusion.

DRUG INTERACTIONS: *Warning:* This drug should not be used with Seldane, Seldane-D, or Hismanal; the drug may increase the blood levels of these drugs to extremely toxic and possibly life-threatening levels. The drug may also increase the blood levels of Coumadin, Retrovir, rifabutin, Sandimmune, Slo-bid, Theo-Dur, theophylline, Uni-Dur, Uniphyl, and Tegretol. Propulsid and the drug may cause dangerous irregular heartbeats when taken together.

ALLERGIES: Individuals allergic to erythromycin or other macrolide antibiotics (such as those listed in "Other Drugs in the Same Therapeutic Class") should discuss this with their doctor or pharmacist before taking this drug.

PREGNANCY/BREAST-FEEDING: Category B—No evidence of risk in humans. Either animal findings show risk, but human findings do not; or, if no adequate human studies have been done, animal findings show no risk. The drug is excreted in the breast milk; therefore, extreme caution should be used when breast-feeding.

OTHER BRAND NAMES: None

OTHER DRUGS IN THE SAME THERAPEUTIC CLASS: Biaxin, Dynabac, E.E.S., E-Mycin, ERY-TAB, ERYC, EryPed, Ilosone, PCE, TAO, and Zithromax

IMPORTANT INFORMATION TO REMEMBER: If stomach upset occurs, take the drug with food or milk. Also, take the drug at even intervals around the clock (if four times a day, take every six hours). Take the drug until all the medication prescribed is gone; otherwise the infection may return. If severe diarrhea occurs while taking this drug, notify your doctor immediately. Never take the drug with Seldane, Seldane-D, or Hismanal (see "Drug Interactions").

BRAND NAME: Erythromycin (various brand-name manufacturers)

GENERIC NAME: erythromycin

See entry for ERY-TABs

BRAND NAME: Esgic

GENERIC NAME: Combination product containing: butalbital, acetaminophen, and caffeine

See entry for Fioricet

BRAND NAME: Esgic Plus

GENERIC NAME: Combination product containing: butalbital, acetaminophen, and caffeine

Esgic Plus is very similar to Fioricet. Esgic Plus contains an additional 175 mg of acetaminophen. See entry for Fioricet.

BRAND NAME: Esidrix

GENERIC NAME: hydrochlorothiazide

See entry for HydroDIURIL

BRAND NAME: **Esimil**

GENERIC NAME: Combination product containing: guanethidine and hydrochlorothiazide

See individual entries for Ismelin and HydroDIURIL

BRAND NAME: **Eskalith and Eskalith CR**

GENERIC NAME: lithium carbonate

GENERIC FORM AVAILABLE: Yes

THERAPEUTIC CLASS: Anti-manic

DOSAGE FORMS: 300-mg capsules and 450-mg controlled-release (CR) capsules

MAIN USES: Bipolar disorder, manic episodes, and {depression}

USUAL DOSE: 900 mg to 1200 mg per day in divided doses

AVERAGE PRICE: $26.27 (B)/$12.63 (G) for Eskalith; $52.64 for Eskalith CR

SIDE EFFECTS: Most common: slight drowsiness, diarrhea, increased thirst, nausea, increased urination, some limited loss of bladder control, and slight trembling of hands. Less common: irregular heart beat; weight gain; cold arms, legs, feet, and fingers; weakness; skin rash; dry mouth; vision problems; and muscle twitching.

DRUG INTERACTIONS: NSAIDs (such as Anaprox, Ansaid, Aleve, aspirin, Cataflam, Clinoril, Daypro, Disalcid, Dolobid, Easprin, Feldene, Indocin, Lodine, Motrin, Nalfon, Naprosyn, Orudis, Oruvail, Relafen, Tolectin, and Voltaren) may increase the concentration of the drug in the blood. Diuretics (water pills) may increase the blood levels of the drug. The drug may decrease the absorption of Compazine, Mellaril, Prolixin, Serentil, Stelazine, Thorazine, and Trilafon. Haldol and the drug should be used together with extreme caution. Accupril, Altace, Capoten, Lotensin, Monopril, Prinivil, Univasc, Vasotec, and Zestril may increase the toxic effects of the drug.

ALLERGIES: Individuals allergic to lithium carbonate or any of its derivatives should discuss this with their doctor or pharmacist before using this drug.

PREGNANCY/BREAST-FEEDING: Category D—Positive evidence of risk. Human studies show risk to the fetus. Nevertheless, potential benefits may possibly outweigh the potential risk. This drug should not be taken by nursing mothers.

OTHER BRAND NAMES: Lithonate

OTHER DRUGS IN THE SAME THERAPEUTIC CLASS: Lithobid and Lithotabs

IMPORTANT INFORMATION TO REMEMBER: Only take the drug exactly as directed by your physician and do not increase the dose without first consulting with your physician. This drug may cause some drowsiness. Individuals should use caution when driving, operating machinery, or any task where mental alertness is required. Alcohol, anxiety medications, and narcotic painkillers may intensify the drowsiness effect of the drug. Take this drug with plenty of water (eight ounces is preferred), especially during hot weather or while exercising. The drug may require one to three weeks of use before improvement may be noticed. Do not crush or break the controlled-release (CR) tablets. Individuals taking the drug should have regular blood tests to determine if the correct amount of the drug is being taken. Individuals should also have thyroid function tests performed every six months.

BRAND NAME: Estrace

GENERIC NAME: estradiol

GENERIC FORM AVAILABLE: Yes

THERAPEUTIC CLASS: Estrogen replacement

DOSAGE FORMS: 0.5-mg, 1-mg, and 2-mg tablets and 0.01% vaginal cream

MAIN USES: Menopausal disorders, prevention of osteoporosis, and vaginal atrophy (cream only)

USUAL DOSE: Tablets: 0.5 mg to 2 mg every day or daily for three weeks, then off one week. Cream: initially 1 g to 4 g daily, then one to three times weekly.

AVERAGE PRICE: $35.88 (B)/$26.19 (G) for 0.5 mg; $47.81 (B)/$36.19 (G) for 1 mg; $69.80 (B)/$43.49 (G) for 2 mg; $37.38 for 0.01% cream

SIDE EFFECTS: Most common: breast tenderness, breast pain, breast enlargement, swelling of feet and lower legs, stomach cramps, bloating, and nausea. Less common: changes in cervical secretions, yeast infections, headache, diarrhea, vomiting, migraine, depression, weight changes, dizziness, breakthrough bleeding, and changes in sex drive.

DRUG INTERACTIONS: The drug may interfere with the actions of Parlodel. The drug may increase the blood levels of Sandimmune. Liver toxicity may be increased when used with Dantrium.

ALLERGIES: Individuals allergic to estradiol, estrogens, or any of their derivatives should discuss this with their doctor or pharmacist before using this drug.

PREGNANCY/BREAST-FEEDING: Category X—Should not be used during pregnancy. Studies in animals and/or humans have shown fetal abnormalities and birth defects. The risks associated with using this drug clearly outweigh the benefits. This drug should never be used by someone who is pregnant or trying to become pregnant. Also, women should never breast-feed while using this drug.

OTHER BRAND NAMES: None

OTHER DRUGS IN THE SAME THERAPEUTIC CLASS: Climara, Estinyl, Estraderm, ESTRATAB, Ogen, Ortho Dienestrol, Ortho-Est, Premarin, and Tace

IMPORTANT INFORMATION TO REMEMBER: Use the drug exactly as directed by your physician. Do not discontinue the drug without first consulting your physician. Caution should be used by patients with previous or current episodes of cancer, high blood pressure, heart disease, or any other cardiovascular or blood vessel disease. This drug may increase the risk of uterine cancer in women who have been through menopause. Report any abnormal vaginal bleeding to your doctor immediately. If using the vaginal cream, insert the applicator high into the vagina (two-thirds the length of the applicator) and push the plunger to release the cream. Do not use a tampon to hold the cream inside the vagina.

BRAND NAME: Estraderm

GENERIC NAME: estradiol

GENERIC FORM AVAILABLE: No

THERAPEUTIC CLASS: Estrogen replacement

DOSAGE FORMS: estradiol 0.05 mg/day and 0.1 mg/day patches

MAIN USES: Menopausal disorders

USUAL DOSE: One 0.05-mg or 0.1-mg patch applied twice per week every week; or apply one patch twice weekly for three weeks, then off for one week.

AVERAGE PRICE: $24.49 for 0.05 mg (eight patches) and $29.29 for 0.1 mg (eight patches)

SIDE EFFECTS: skin irritation and/or redness at the site of application 17%. Other possible side effects include: Most common: breast tenderness, breast pain, breast enlargement, swelling of feet and lower legs, stomach cramps, bloating, and nausea. Less common: changes in cervical secretions, yeast infections, headache, diarrhea, vomiting, migraine, depression, weight changes, dizziness, breakthrough bleeding, and changes in sex drive.

DRUG INTERACTIONS: The drug may interfere with the actions of Parlodel. The drug may increase the blood levels of Sandimmune. Liver toxicity may be increased when used with Dantrium.

ALLERGIES: Individuals allergic to estradiol, estrogens, other estrogen patches, or any of their derivatives should discuss this with their doctor or pharmacist before using this drug.

PREGNANCY/BREAST-FEEDING: Category X—Should not be used during pregnancy. Studies in animals and/or humans have shown fetal abnormalities and birth defects. The risks associated with using this drug clearly outweigh the benefits. This drug should never be used by someone who is pregnant or trying to become pregnant. Also, women should never breast-feed while using this drug.

OTHER BRAND NAMES: None

OTHER DRUGS IN THE SAME THERAPEUTIC CLASS: Climara and Vivelle

IMPORTANT INFORMATION TO REMEMBER: Use the drug exactly as directed by your physician. Do not discontinue the drug without first consulting your physician. Caution should be used by patients with previous or current episodes of cancer, high blood pressure, heart disease, or any other cardiovascular or blood vessel disease. This drug may increase the risk of uterine cancer in women who have been through menopause. Report any abnormal vaginal bleeding to your doctor immediately.

When using the patches:

1) Do not cut or fold the patch in half. This may cause the medication inside to leak out. Peel off the adhesive liner.
2) Apply the patch to a clean, dry skin area on the stomach. This area should be free of hair, cuts, scars, or irritation. Do not apply the patch to your breasts. Avoid the waistline since tight clothes may rub or remove the patch.
3) Leave the patch on even during swimming, showering, and exercising. If the patch falls off, replace the patch with a new one.
4) When it's time to apply a new patch, use a different site on the skin. Rotate the sites where you apply the patches every time.
5) Make it a habit to apply the patch at the same times each week.
6) Dispose of used patches properly and keep out of reach of children.

BRAND NAME: ESTRATAB, ESTRATEST, and ESTRATEST H.S.

GENERIC NAME: esterified estrogens (ESTRATAB) and esterified estrogens and methyltestosterone (ESTRATEST and ESTRATEST H.S.).

GENERIC FORM AVAILABLE: No

THERAPEUTIC CLASS: Estrogen replacement (ESTRATAB) and estrogen + testosterone (ESTRATEST and ESTRATEST H.S.)

DOSAGE FORMS: 0.3-mg, 0.625-mg, 1.25-mg, and 2.5-mg tablets (ESTRATAB); 1.25-mg estrogen/2.5-mg methyltestosterone tablets (ESTRATEST); and 0.625-mg estrogen/1.25-mg methyltestosterone tablets (ESTRATEST H.S.)

MAIN USES: Menopausal disorders and {prevention of osteoporosis}

USUAL DOSE: For ESTRATAB: 0.3 mg to 2.5 mg every day or daily for three weeks, then off one week. For ESTRATEST and ESTRATEST H.S.: one tablet every day or daily for three weeks, then off one week.

AVERAGE PRICE: $30.28 for 0.3 mg; $42.18 for 0.625 mg; $99.96 for 2.5 mg; $116.50 for ESTRATEST; and $93.57 for ESTRATEST H.S.

SIDE EFFECTS: Most common: breast tenderness, breast pain, breast enlargement, swelling of feet and lower legs, stomach cramps, bloating, and nausea. Less common: changes in cervical secretions, yeast infections, headache, increased hair growth, diarrhea, vomiting, migraine, depression, weight changes, dizziness, breakthrough bleeding, and changes in sex drive.

DRUG INTERACTIONS: The drug may interfere with the actions of Parlodel. The drug may increase the blood levels of Sandimmune. Liver toxicity may be increased when used with Dantrium. In addition for ESTRATEST and ESTRATEST H.S.: the drug may increase the blood levels of Coumadin. The drug may also decrease the amount of insulin needed by diabetics.

ALLERGIES: Individuals allergic to estradiol, estrogens, methyltestosterone, or any of their derivatives should discuss this with their doctor or pharmacist using this drug.

PREGNANCY/BREAST-FEEDING: Category X—Should not be used during pregnancy. Studies in animals and/or humans have shown fetal abnormalities and birth defects. The risks associated with using this drug clearly outweigh the benefits. This drug should never be used by someone who is pregnant or trying to become pregnant. Also, women should never breast-feed while using this drug.

OTHER BRAND NAMES: None

OTHER DRUGS IN THE SAME THERAPEUTIC CLASS: Climara, Estinyl, Estrace, Estraderm, Ogen, Ortho Dienestrol, Ortho-Est, Premarin, and Tace

IMPORTANT INFORMATION TO REMEMBER: Use the drug exactly as directed by your physician. Do not discontinue the drug without first consulting your physician. Caution should be used by patients with previous or current episodes of cancer, high blood pressure, heart disease, or any other cardiovascular or blood vessel disease. This drug may increase the risk of uterine cancer in women who have been through menopause. Report any abnormal vaginal bleeding to your doctor immediately.

BRAND NAME: Estrostep

GENERIC NAME: Combination product containing: norethindrone and ethinyl estradiol

GENERIC FORM AVAILABLE: No

THERAPEUTIC CLASS: Progestin + estrogen contraceptive

DOSAGE FORMS: 1 mg norethindrone/20 micrograms ethinyl estradiol (first five tablets), 1 mg norethindrone/30 micrograms ethinyl estradiol (next seven tablets), and 1 mg norethindrone/35 micrograms ethinyl estradiol (next nine tablets)

MAIN USES: Birth control

USUAL DOSE: Take one tablet daily for 21 or 28 days, beginning on the fifth day of the cycle. Day One of the cycle is the first day of menstrual bleeding.

AVERAGE PRICE: $33.49

SIDE EFFECTS: Most common: stomach cramps, bloating, acne, appetite changes, nausea, swelling of the feet and ankles, weight gain, swelling of the breasts, breast tenderness, and unusual tiredness or weakness. Less common: changes in vaginal bleeding, feeling faint, increased blood pressure, depression, stomach pain, vaginal itching, yeast infections, brown and blotchy spots on the skin, diarrhea, dizziness, headaches, migraines, increased body and facial hair, increased sensitivity of the skin to the sun, irritability, some hair loss from the scalp, vomiting, blood clots, weight loss, and changes in sexual desire.

DRUG INTERACTIONS: Antibiotics may decrease the effectiveness of the drug. The drug may interfere with the effectiveness of Parlodel. The drug may reduce the effects of Coumadin. The drug may increase the blood levels of Anafranil, Asendin, Elavil, Endep, Norpramin, Pamelor, Sinequan, Surmontil, Tofranil, and Vivactil when used for long periods of time. Smoking is not recommended while taking this drug due to the increased risk of heart disease, stroke, and high blood pressure.

ALLERGIES: Individuals allergic to norethindrone and ethinyl estradiol or any of their derivatives should discuss this with their doctor or pharmacist before using this drug.

PREGNANCY/BREAST-FEEDING: Category X—Should not be used during pregnancy. Studies in animals and/or humans have shown fetal abnormalities and birth defects. The risks associated with using this drug clearly outweigh the benefits. This drug should never be used by someone who is pregnant or trying to become pregnant. Also, women should never breast-feed while using this drug.

OTHER BRAND NAMES: None

OTHER DRUGS IN THE SAME THERAPEUTIC CLASS: Ortho-Novum 7/7/7, Ortho Tri-Cylen, Tri-Levlen, Tri-Norinyl, and Triphasil

IMPORTANT INFORMATION TO REMEMBER: Only take the drug exactly as directed by your physician. It is important to take the drug at the same time every day (bedtime). Do not discontinue the drug without first consulting your physician. The drug should not be used by women with a history of heart disease, stroke, high blood pressure, breast cancer, or other blood vessel disease. Breakthrough bleeding may occur during the first few months; if this persists, notify your doctor. This drug does not provide protection against the HIV (AIDS) virus. It is important to use a second method of birth control during the first week when treatment has just begun. It may be necessary to use a second form of birth control when antibiotics are being taken. Also, women who smoke run a higher risk of heart disease, stroke, and high blood pressure when taking this drug. If pregnancy is suspected, stop taking the drug immediately.

BRAND NAME: Etrafon 2-25

GENERIC NAME: Combination product containing: perphenazine and amitriptyline

See entry for Triavil

BRAND NAME: Eulexin

GENERIC NAME: flutamide

GENERIC FORM AVAILABLE: No

THERAPEUTIC CLASS: Anti-androgen and anticancer

DOSAGE FORMS: 125-mg capsules

MAIN USES: Prostate cancer

USUAL DOSE: 250 mg (two capsules) three times daily (every eight hours if possible)

AVERAGE PRICE: $230.35

SIDE EFFECTS: hot flashes 61%, decreased sex drive 36%, impotence 33%, nausea 12%, vomiting 12%, breast enlargement 9%, other stomach disorders (gas, bloating, etc.) 6%, and loss of appetite 4%.

DRUG INTERACTIONS: The drug may increase the effects of Coumadin.

ALLERGIES: Individuals allergic to flutamide or any of its derivatives should discuss this with their doctor or pharmacist before using this drug.

PREGNANCY/BREAST-FEEDING: Category D—Positive evidence of risk. Human studies show risk to the fetus. Nevertheless, potential benefits may possibly outweigh the potential risks. This drug should not be taken by nursing mothers.

OTHER BRAND NAMES: None

OTHER DRUGS IN THE SAME THERAPEUTIC CLASS: Casodex

IMPORTANT INFORMATION TO REMEMBER: Only take the drug exactly as directed by your physician and do not discontinue the drug without first consulting with your physician. Also, take the drug at even intervals around the clock (if three times a day, take every eight hours).

BRAND NAME: Eurax

GENERIC NAME: crotamiton

GENERIC FORM AVAILABLE: No

THERAPEUTIC CLASS: Scabies killer/anti-itch

DOSAGE FORMS: 10% cream and 10% lotion

MAIN USES: Scabies

USUAL DOSE: Apply the drug to the entire body from the chin to the toes and thoroughly rub it in.

AVERAGE PRICE: $14.50 for 10% cream and $15.47 for 10% lotion

SIDE EFFECTS: Most common: none. Less common: allergic skin reactions, itching, and skin irritation.

DRUG INTERACTIONS: None of any clinical significance

ALLERGIES: Individuals allergic to crotamiton or any of its derivatives should discuss this with their doctor or pharmacist before using this drug.

PREGNANCY/BREAST-FEEDING: Category C—Risk cannot be ruled out. Human studies are lacking, and animal studies are either positive for fetal risk or lacking as well. However, potential benefits may justify the potential risk in using the drug. It is not known whether the drug is excreted in the breast milk; therefore, caution should be used when breast-feeding.

OTHER BRAND NAMES: None

OTHER DRUGS IN THE SAME THERAPEUTIC CLASS: Elimite and Kwell Lotion

IMPORTANT INFORMATION TO REMEMBER: This drug is for external use only. Keep the drug away from the face, eyes, nose, mouth, and other mucous membranes. Before applying the drug, take a routine bath or shower and dry off completely. Thoroughly massage the drug into the skin on the entire body from the chin to the toes, including folds and creases in the skin. A second application is recommended 24 hours later, but do not bathe beforehand this time. Clothing and bed linen should be washed in hot, soapy water the next day. A cleansing bath should be taken 48 hours after the last application.

BRAND NAME: Exgest LA

GENERIC NAME: Combination product containing: phenylpropanolamine and guaifenesin

See entry for Entex/Entex LA/Entex PSE

BRAND NAME: Extendryl

GENERIC NAME: Combination product containing: chlorpheniramine, phenylephrine, and methscopolamine

GENERIC FORM AVAILABLE: No

THERAPEUTIC CLASS: Antihistamine + decongestant + anticholingergic

DOSAGE FORMS: For Extendryl chewable tablets: 2-mg chlorpheniramine maleate/10-mg phenylephrine/1.25-mg methscopolamine tablets. For Extendryl syrup: 2 mg chlorpheniramine maleate/10 mg phenylephrine/1.25 mg methscopolamine per 5 mL. For Extendryl SR: 8-mg chlorpheniramine maleate/20-mg phenylephrine/

2.5-mg methscopolamine capsules. For Extendryl JR: 4-mg chlorpheniramine maleate/10-mg phenylephrine/1.25-mg methscopolamine capsules.

MAIN USES: Nasal allergies and congestion

USUAL DOSE: Extendryl JR and Extendyl SR: one capsule every 12 hours. Extendryl chewable tablets: one to two tablets every four hours. Extendryl syrup: one to two teaspoons every four hours.

AVERAGE PRICE: $37.10 Extendyl SR; $33.95 for Extendryl JR

SIDE EFFECTS: Most common: drowsiness. Less common: nausea, giddiness, dry mouth, blurred vision, pounding heartbeat, flushing, and increased irritability or excitability (especially in children).

DRUG INTERACTIONS: Blocadren, Cartrol, Corgard, Inderal, Kerlone, Levatol, Lopressor, Normodyne, Sectral, Tenormin, Toprol-XL, Trandate, Visken, and Zebeta may increase the effects of the drug. The drug may also reduce the effects of blood-pressure-lowering drugs. Nardil or Parnate may significantly raise blood pressure when taken with this drug.

ALLERGIES: Individuals allergic to chlorpheniramine, phenylephrine, methscopolamine, or other antihistamine/decongestant combinations should discuss this with their doctor or pharmacist before taking this drug.

PREGNANCY/BREAST-FEEDING: Category C—Risk cannot be ruled out. Human studies are lacking, and animal studies are either positive for fetal risk or lacking as well. However, potential benefits may justify the potential risk in using the drug. The drug is excreted in the breast milk; therefore, caution should be used when breast-feeding.

OTHER BRAND NAMES: None

OTHER DRUGS IN THE SAME THERAPEUTIC CLASS: Atrohist Plus and Ru-Tuss

IMPORTANT INFORMATION TO REMEMBER: This drug does cause drowsiness. Individuals should use caution when driving, operating machinery, or any task where mental alertness is required. Alcohol, anxiety medications, and narcotic painkillers may intensify the drowsiness effect of the drug. This drug may also cause a dry mouth; sugarless gum or hard candy will help take care of this problem. Patients with glaucoma, high blood pressure, heart conditions, or urinary or prostate problems should consult their doctor before taking this drug.

BRAND NAME: **Famvir**

GENERIC NAME: famciclovir

GENERIC FORM AVAILABLE: No

THERAPEUTIC CLASS: Antiviral

DOSAGE FORMS: 125-mg, 250-mg, and 500-mg tablets

MAIN USES: Shingles, genital herpes, and {viral infections}

USUAL DOSE: 125 mg to 500 mg every 8 hours to 12 hours

AVERAGE PRICE: $175.25 for 125 mg (50 tablets); $167.91 for 250 mg (50 tablets); and $258.30 for 500-mg tablets (50 tablets)

SIDE EFFECTS: headache 23%, nausea 13%, diarrhea 10%, vomiting 5%, tiredness 4%, constipation 4%, itching 4%, dizziness 3%, runny nose 3%, appetite loss 3%, tingling sensations 3%, and muscle pains 2%.

DRUG INTERACTIONS: Tagamet, Slo-bid, Theo-Dur, theophylline, Uni-Dur, and Uniphyl may increase the blood levels of the drug. The drug may increase the blood levels of Lanoxin.

ALLERGIES: Individuals allergic to famciclovir, Cytovene, Valtrex, Zovirax, or any of their derivatives should discuss this with their doctor or pharmacist before using this drug.

PREGNANCY/BREAST-FEEDING: Category B—No evidence of risk in humans. Either animal findings show risk, but human findings do not; or, if no adequate human studies have been done, animal findings show no risk. The drug is excreted in the breast milk; therefore, extreme caution should be used when breast-feeding.

OTHER BRAND NAMES: None

OTHER DRUGS IN THE SAME THERAPEUTIC CLASS: Cytovene, Valtrex, and Zovirax

IMPORTANT INFORMATION TO REMEMBER: Only take the drug exactly as directed by your physician. If stomach upset occurs, take the drug with food or milk. Also, take the drug at even intervals around the clock (if three times a day, take every eight hours). Take the drug for the full course of therapy; otherwise the infection may return. The drug should be started at the first sign of the herpes zoster rash (shingles) for maximum effectiveness. If possible, the drug should be started within the first 72 hours after the appearance of shingles. The effectiveness of the drug has not been studied when used more than 72 hours after the first appearance of shingles.

BRAND NAME: Fansidar

GENERIC NAME: Combination product containing: sulfadoxine and pyrimethamine

GENERIC FORM AVAILABLE: No

THERAPEUTIC CLASS: Sulfonamide + folic acid antagonist

DOSAGE FORMS: 500-mg sulfadoxine/25-mg pyrimethamine tablets

MAIN USES: Prevention and treatment of malaria

USUAL DOSE: For prevention of malaria: one tablet every week starting the week before departure and continuing until four to six weeks after return. For treatment of malaria: two to three tablets in one single dose.

AVERAGE PRICE: $49.56 (10 tablets)

SIDE EFFECTS: Most common: pain or burning sensation in the tongue, loss of taste, blood disorders including anemia, weakness, skin rash, fever, increased sensitivity to the sun, diarrhea, nausea, vomiting, nervousness, and stomach pain. Less common: blood in the urine, lower back pain, hepatitis, aching joints, muscle pain, and Stevens-Johnson syndrome (aching joints and muscles, redness and blistering of the skin, and unusual tiredness or weakness).

DRUG INTERACTIONS: Severe reactions have occurred when used with Aralen. Bactrim or Septra should not be used while taking this drug.

ALLERGIES: Individuals allergic to sulfadoxine, pyrimethamine, other sulfa drugs, or any of their derivatives should discuss this with their doctor or pharmacist before using this drug.

PREGNANCY/BREAST-FEEDING: Category C—Risk cannot be ruled out. Human studies are lacking, and animal studies are either positive for fetal risk or lacking as well. However, potential benefits may justify the potential risk in using the drug. The drug is excreted in the breast milk; therefore, extreme caution should be used when breast-feeding.

OTHER BRAND NAMES: None

OTHER DRUGS IN THE SAME THERAPEUTIC CLASS: None

IMPORTANT INFORMATION TO REMEMBER: Only take the drug exactly as directed by your physician. Take the drug for the full course of therapy, especially if it is being used to prevent malaria. When taking the drug for prevention of malaria, start the medication one week before departure and continue taking it until four to six weeks after returning. Individuals should also use a sunscreen to avoid overexposure to the sun. The drug may increase the skin's sensitivity to sunlight, which may cause one to sunburn more easily. Take the drug with plenty of water (preferably eight ounces) and take with food or milk if stomach upset occurs. At the first sign of a skin rash, contact your doctor immediately and stop taking the drug.

BRAND NAME: Felbatol

GENERIC NAME: felbamate

GENERIC FORM AVAILABLE: No

THERAPEUTIC CLASS: Carbamate anticonvulsant

DOSAGE FORMS: 400-mg and 600-mg tablets; and 600-mg/5 mL suspension

MAIN USES: Epilepsy

USUAL DOSE: 1200 mg to 3600 mg per day in divided doses

AVERAGE PRICE: $97.58 for 400 mg and $111.80 for 600 mg

SIDE EFFECTS: dizziness 18%, insomnia 9%, upset stomach 9%, vomiting 9%, constipation 7%, diarrhea 5%, blurred vision 5%, gait abnormality 5%, runny nose 7%, headache 7%, drowsiness 7%, tiredness 7%, nervousness 5%, acne 3%, rash 3%, weight loss 3%, facial swelling 3%, ear infections 3%, and breakthrough bleeding 3%.

DRUG INTERACTIONS: Dilantin and Tegretol may decrease the blood levels of the drug. The drug itself may decrease blood levels of Tegretol. The drug itself may increase the blood levels of Depakene, Depakote, and Dilantin.

ALLERGIES: Individuals allergic to felbamate or any of its derivatives should discuss this with their doctor or pharmacist before using this drug.

PREGNANCY/BREAST-FEEDING: Category C—Risk cannot be ruled out. Human studies are lacking, and animal studies are either positive for fetal risk or lacking as well. However, potential benefits may justify the potential risk in using the drug. The drug is excreted in the breast milk; therefore, extreme caution should be used when breast-feeding.

OTHER BRAND NAMES: None

OTHER DRUGS IN THE SAME THERAPEUTIC CLASS: None

IMPORTANT INFORMATION TO REMEMBER: This drug has caused serious blood disorders, including aplastic anemia; some individuals taking the drug have died from this condition. This drug should only be used by individuals whose epilepsy is so severe that the risk of aplastic anemia, a serious blood disorder, is deemed acceptable. Only take this drug exactly as directed by your physician and do not increase the dose without first consulting with your physician. Do not stop taking the drug suddenly without consulting with a doctor. Regular visits to a doctor are necessary to monitor progress. This drug may cause some dizziness or drowsiness. Individuals should use caution when driving, operating machinery, or any task where mental alertness is required. Alcohol, anxiety medications, and narcotic painkillers may intensify the dizziness or drowsiness effect of the drug.

BRAND NAME: Feldene

GENERIC NAME: piroxicam

GENERIC FORM AVAILABLE: Yes

THERAPEUTIC CLASS: Nonsteroidal anti-inflammatory drug (NSAID)

DOSAGE FORMS: 10-mg and 20-mg capsules

MAIN USES: Arthritis and pain relief

USUAL DOSE: 20 mg daily in single or divided doses

AVERAGE PRICE: $153.54 (B)/$106.57 (G) for 10 mg and $228.67 (B)/$163.77 (G) for 20 mg

SIDE EFFECTS: nausea 3%–9%, decreases in hemoglobin 3%–9%, decrease in hematocrit 3%–9%, feeling of stomach distress 3%–9%, constipation 1%–3%, stomach discomfort 1%–3%, gas 1%–3%, diarrhea 1%–3%, stomach pain 1%–3%, indigestion 1%–3%, blood disorders 1%–3%, dizziness 1%–3%, tiredness 1%–3%, headache 1%–3%, and ringing in the ear 1%–3%.

DRUG INTERACTIONS: Aspirin will decrease the concentration of this drug in the blood. This drug may also decrease the effects of Lasix, Dyazide, HydroDIURIL, Maxzide, and other water pills. The drug may increase the blood levels of Eskalith, Lithobid, and Sandimmune. The drug may increase the toxic effects of the drug Rheumatrex. Caution should be used when taking the drug with Coumadin.

ALLERGIES: Individuals allergic to piroxicam or other NSAIDs (such as those listed in "Other Drugs in the Same Therapeutic Class") should discuss this with their doctor or pharmacist before taking this drug.

PREGNANCY/BREAST-FEEDING: Category B—No evidence of risk in humans. Either animal findings show risk, but human finding do not; or, if no adequate human studies have been done, animal findings show no risk. The drug should not, however, be used during the late stages (last three months) of pregnancy. The drug is excreted in the breast milk; therefore, extreme caution should be used when breast-feeding.

OTHER BRAND NAMES: None

OTHER DRUGS IN THE SAME THERAPEUTIC CLASS: Anaprox, Ansaid, aspirin, Cataflam, Clinoril, Disalcid, Dolobid, Daypro, Easprin, Indocin, Lodine, Lodine XL, Motrin, Nalfon, Naprosyn, Orudis, Oruvail, Relafen, Tolectin, Toradol, Voltaren, and Voltaren XR

IMPORTANT INFORMATION TO REMEMBER: This drug should be taken with food or milk to reduce the potential for injury to the stomach lining and stomach upset. This drug may take up to two weeks before a noticeable improvement in pain relief associated with arthritis is observed. Drinking alcohol while taking this drug may increase its potential to cause ulcers. This drug should only be used under the direct supervision of a doctor by individuals with a bleeding disorder or ulcer, or those who are currently taking Coumadin. Before taking over-the-counter pain relievers, consult your doctor or pharmacist. No more than one pain reliever should be taken at any one time unless otherwise directed by your doctor.

BRAND NAME: Femstat

GENERIC NAME: butoconazole

GENERIC FORM AVAILABLE: No

THERAPEUTIC CLASS: Antifungal

DOSAGE FORMS: 2% vaginal cream

MAIN USES: Vaginal yeast infections

USUAL DOSE: Apply one applicatorful vaginally at bedtime for three nights.

AVERAGE PRICE: $28.50

SIDE EFFECTS: vaginal burning 2% and itching 1%.

DRUG INTERACTIONS: None of any clinical significance

ALLERGIES: Individuals allergic to butoconazole or other anti-fungals (such as those listed in "Other Drugs in the Same Therapeutic Class") should discuss this with their doctor or pharmacist before taking this drug.

PREGNANCY/BREAST-FEEDING: Category C—Risk cannot be ruled out. Human studies are lacking, and animal studies are either positive for fetal risk or lacking as well. Potential benefits may justify the potential risk in using the drug. However, the drug should not be used during the first trimester (first three months) of pregnancy. It is not known whether the drug is excreted in the breast milk; therefore, caution should be used when breast-feeding.

OTHER BRAND NAMES: The drug is available over-the-counter under the brand name Femstat 3.

OTHER DRUGS IN THE SAME THERAPEUTIC CLASS: Gyne-Lotrimin, Monistat, Mycelex, Terazol, and Vagistat-1

IMPORTANT INFORMATION TO REMEMBER: Use the drug for the full course of therapy even if symptoms disappear; otherwise the infection may return. Continue using the drug even if your menstrual period begins. When using the vaginal cream, insert the applicator high into the vagina (two-thirds the length of the applicator) and push the plunger to release the cream. Do not use a tampon to hold the cream inside the vagina. It is recommended that your sexual partner use a condom until the infection clears up. The drug is now also available over-the-counter without a prescription.

BRAND NAME: **Fioricet and Fioricet with Codeine**

GENERIC NAME: Combination product containing: acetaminophen, butalbital, and caffeine

GENERIC FORM AVAILABLE: Yes

THERAPEUTIC CLASS: Sedative + analgesic

DOSAGE FORMS: 325-mg acetaminophen/50-mg butalbital/40-mg caffeine tablets (Fioricet w/Codeine also has 30 mg of codeine added)

MAIN USES: Tension headache and {pain relief}

USUAL DOSE: one to two tablets or capsules every four hours as needed (not to exceed six tablets per day)

AVERAGE PRICE: $66.75 (B)/$17.56 (G) for Fioricet; $145.82 (B)/$89.87 (G) for Fioricet w/Codeine

SIDE EFFECTS: Most common: drowsiness, lightheadedness, dizziness, sedation, shortness of breath, nausea, vomiting, stomach pain, and drunken feeling. Less common: headache, shaky feeling, dry mouth, gas, constipation, heartburn, muscle fatigue, leg pain, skin rash, nasal congestion, fever, agitation, heavy eyelids, mental confusion, hot flashes, fast heartbeat, and euphoria.

DRUG INTERACTIONS: Nardil and Parnate may enhance the effects of the drug. Alcohol, anxiety medications, and other narcotic painkillers may intensify the drowsiness effect of the drug. The drug may decrease the effects of Aristocort, Coumadin, Blocadren, Cartrol, Corgard, Decadron, Deltasone, estrogens, Fulvicin P/G, Grifulvin V, Gris-PEG, Grisactin, Inderal, Kerlone, Levatol, Lopressor, Medrol, Normodyne, prednisone, Sectral, Slo-bid, Tenormin, Theo-Dur, theophylline, Toprol-XL, Trandate, Uni-Dur, Uniphyl, Vibramycin, Visken, and Zebeta.

ALLERGIES: Individuals allergic to acetaminophen, butalbital, caffeine, codeine, or any of their derivatives should discuss this with their doctor or pharmacist before using this drug.

PREGNANCY/BREAST-FEEDING: Category C—Risk cannot be ruled out. Human studies are lacking, and animal studies are either positive for fetal risk or lacking as well. However, potential benefits may justify the potential risk in using the drug. The drug is excreted in the breast milk; therefore, extreme caution should be used when breast-feeding.

OTHER BRAND NAMES: Esgic

OTHER DRUGS IN THE SAME THERAPEUTIC CLASS: Axocet, Esgic Plus, Fiorinal, and Phrenilin

IMPORTANT INFORMATION TO REMEMBER: This drug does cause drowsiness. Individuals should use caution when driving, operating machinery, or any task where mental alertness is required. Alcohol, anxiety medications, and narcotic painkillers may intensify the drowsiness effect of the drug. If stomach upset occurs, take the drug with food or milk. Do not increase the dose without first consulting with your physician. Before taking over-the-counter pain relievers, consult your doctor or pharmacist. This drug may be habit-forming. Fioricet w/Codeine is a controlled substance.

BRAND NAME: Fiorinal and Fiorinal with Codeine

GENERIC NAME: Combination product containing: aspirin, butalbital, and caffeine

GENERIC FORM AVAILABLE: Yes

THERAPEUTIC CLASS: Sedative + analgesic

DOSAGE FORMS: 325-mg aspirin/50-mg butalbital/40-mg caffeine tablets and capsules (Fiorinal w/Codeine has 30 mg of codeine added)

MAIN USES: Tension headache and {pain relief}

USUAL DOSE: one to two tablets or capsules every four hours (not to exceed six tablets or capsules per day)

AVERAGE PRICE: $68.61 (B)/$12.55 (G) for Fiorinal; $145.82 (B)/$89.27 (G) for Fiorinal w/Codeine

SIDE EFFECTS: Most common: drowsiness, lightheadedness, dizziness, sedation, shortness of breath, nausea, vomiting, stomach pain, and drunken feeling. Less common: headache, shaky feeling, dry mouth, gas, constipation, heartburn, muscle fatigue, leg pain, skin rash, nasal congestion, fever, agitation, heavy eyelids, mental confusion, hot flashes, fast heartbeat, and euphoria.

DRUG INTERACTIONS: Nardil and Parnate may enhance the effects of the drug. Alcohol, anxiety medications, and other narcotic painkillers may intensify the drowsiness effect of the drug. The drug may decrease the effects of Aristocort, Coumadin, Blocadren, Cartrol, Corgard, Decadron, Deltasone, estrogens, Fulvicin P/G, Grifulvin V, Gris-PEG, Grisactin, Inderal, Kerlone, Levatol, Lopressor, Medrol, Normodyne, prednisone, Sectral, Slo-Bid, Tenormin, Theo-Dur, theophylline, Toprol-XL, Trandate, Uni-Dur, Uniphyl, Vibramycin, Visken, and Zebeta. The drug may decrease the effects of probenecid and Anturane. The drug may increase the toxic effects of Depakene, Depakote, and Rheumatrex. The drug should be used cautiously by individuals taking Coumadin.

ALLERGIES: Individuals allergic to aspirin, butalbital, caffeine, or any of their derivatives should discuss this with their doctor or pharmacist before using this drug.

PREGNANCY/BREAST-FEEDING: Category C—Risk cannot be ruled out. Human studies are lacking, and animal studies are either positive for fetal risk or lacking as well. However, potential benefits may justify the potential risk in using the drug. The drug should not, however, be used during the late stages (last three months) of pregnancy. The drug is excreted in the breast milk; therefore, extreme caution should be used when breast-feeding.

OTHER BRAND NAMES: None

OTHER DRUGS IN THE SAME THERAPEUTIC CLASS: Axocet, Esgic Plus, Fioricet, and Phrenilin

IMPORTANT INFORMATION TO REMEMBER: This drug does cause drowsiness. Individuals should use caution when driving, operating machinery, or any task where mental alertness is required. Alcohol, anxiety medications, and narcotic painkillers may intensify the drowsiness effect of the drug. If stomach upset occurs, take the drug with food or milk. Do not increase the dose without first consulting with your physician. This drug may be habit-forming. Fiorinal w/Codeine is a controlled substance. Drinking alcohol while taking this drug may increase its potential to cause ulcers. This drug should only be used under the direct supervision of a doctor by individuals with a bleeding disorder or ulcer, or those who are currently taking Coumadin. Before taking over-the-counter pain relievers, consult your doctor or pharmacist.

BRAND NAME: Flagyl

GENERIC NAME: metronidazole

GENERIC FORM AVAILABLE: Yes

THERAPEUTIC CLASS: Nitroimidazole antibiotic

DOSAGE FORMS: 250-mg and 500-mg tablets

MAIN USES: Protozoal infections, bacterial infections, and trichomoniasis

USUAL DOSE: 250 mg to 750 mg three times a day, or in some instances 2000 mg daily for one day

AVERAGE PRICE: $59.31 (B)/$13.74 (G) for 250 mg (30 tablets) and $83.36 (B)/$22.26 (G) for 500 mg (30 tablets)

SIDE EFFECTS: Most common: lightheadedness, dizziness, nausea, headache, diarrhea, loss of appetite, vomiting, and stomach pain. Less common: change in taste; dry mouth; metallic taste; numbness in hands, feet, toes, and fingers; and rash.

DRUG INTERACTIONS: The drug should never be used with alcohol or with any medication that may contain alcohol. Even small amounts of alcohol will cause intense stomach pain, vomiting, headache, sweating, chest pain, and difficulty breathing. This drug should not be used with Antabuse. In fact, this drug should not be used until at least two weeks after the drug Antabuse has been stopped. The drug may increase the effects of such as Coumadin.

ALLERGIES: Individuals allergic to metronidazole or any of its derivatives should discuss this with their doctor or pharmacist before using this drug.

PREGNANCY/BREAST-FEEDING: Category B—No evidence of risk in humans. Either animal findings show risk, but human findings do not; or, if no adequate human studies have been done, animal findings show no risk. The drug is excreted in the breast milk; therefore, extreme caution should be used when breast-feeding.

OTHER BRAND NAMES: Protostat

OTHER DRUGS IN THE SAME THERAPEUTIC CLASS: Protostat

IMPORTANT INFORMATION TO REMEMBER: This medication should not be taken within 24 hours of using any alcohol. The blood alcohol level of an individual should be zero before therapy is begun. Once treatment has begun, individuals should under no circumstances drink any alcohol. In fact, alcohol should not be used until at least three days after the last dose of the drug. Many cough and cold preparations contain alcohol. Individuals taking this drug should read all over-the-counter medication labels carefully—consult your pharmacist before taking any of these preparations. Also, individuals should check with their physician before taking any narcotic painkillers or anxiety medications. If stomach upset occurs, take the drug with food or milk. Also, take the drug at even intervals around the clock (if three times a day, take every eight hours). Take the drug until all the medication prescribed is gone; otherwise the infection may return. It is recommended that your sexual partner use a condom until the infection clears up.

BRAND NAME: Flarex

GENERIC NAME: fluorometholone acetate

See entry for FML/FML Forte

BRAND NAME: Flexeril

GENERIC NAME: cyclobenzaprine

GENERIC FORM AVAILABLE: Yes

THERAPEUTIC CLASS: Muscle relaxant

DOSAGE FORMS: 10-mg tablets

MAIN USES: Muscle spasms

USUAL DOSE: 10 mg three times daily.

AVERAGE PRICE: $104.15 (B)/$57.62 (G)

SIDE EFFECTS: drowsiness 39%, dry mouth 27%, dizziness 11%, tiredness 1%–3%, weakness 1%–3%, nausea 1%–3%, constipation 1%–3%, blurred vision 1%–3%, headache 1%–3%, fainting 1%–3%, lightheadedness 1%–3%, nervousness 1%–3%, and confusion 1%–3%.

DRUG INTERACTIONS: The drug should not be used with Nardil, Parnate, Matulane, Furoxone, or Eldepryl. In fact, this drug should not be used until at least 14 days after treatment with any of these drugs has stopped. Alcohol, anxiety medications, and narcotic painkillers may intensify the drowsiness effect of the drug.

ALLERGIES: Individuals allergic to cyclobenzaprine or any of its derivatives should discuss this with their doctor or pharmacist before using this drug.

PREGNANCY/BREAST-FEEDING: Category B—No evidence of risk in humans. Either animal findings show risk, but human findings do not; or, if no adequate human studies have been done, animal findings show no risk. It is not known whether the drug is excreted in the breast milk; therefore, caution should be used when breast-feeding.

OTHER BRAND NAMES: None

OTHER DRUGS IN THE SAME THERAPEUTIC CLASS: Lioresal, Parafon Forte DSC, Robaxin, Skelaxin, and Soma

IMPORTANT INFORMATION TO REMEMBER: This drug does cause drowsiness. Individuals should use caution when driving, operating machinery, or any task where mental alertness is required. Alcohol, anxiety medications, and narcotic painkillers may intensify the drowsiness effect of the drug. The drug may cause a dry mouth; sugarless hard candy or gum will help this problem. Do not increase the dose without first consulting with your physician.

BRAND NAME: Flonase

GENERIC NAME: fluticasone

GENERIC FORM AVAILABLE: No

THERAPEUTIC CLASS: Steroid nasal spray

DOSAGE FORMS: 50-micrograms-per-spray nasal spray

MAIN USES: Nasal allergies

USUAL DOSE: one to two sprays in each nostril once daily

AVERAGE PRICE: $56.88

SIDE EFFECTS: bloody nose 3%–6%, nasal burning 3%–6%, blood in nasal mucous 1%–3%, nasal irritation 1%–3%, sore throat 1%–3%, and headache 1%–3%.

DRUG INTERACTIONS: Caution should be used when taking this drug with other oral corticosteroids such as Aristocort, Deltasone, Decadron, Medrol, and prednisone.

ALLERGIES: Individuals allergic to fluticasone or other nasal steroids (such as those listed in "Other Drugs in the Same Therapeutic

Class") should discuss this with their doctor or pharmacist before taking this drug.

PREGNANCY/BREAST-FEEDING: Category C—Risk cannot be ruled out. Human studies are lacking, and animal studies are either positive for fetal risk or lacking as well. However, potential benefits may justify the potential risk in using the drug. It is not known whether the drug is excreted in the breast milk; therefore, caution should be used when breast-feeding.

OTHER BRAND NAMES: None

OTHER DRUGS IN THE SAME THERAPEUTIC CLASS: Beconase, Beconase AQ, Dexacort, Nasacort, Nasalide, Rhinocort, Vancenase, and Vancenase AQ

IMPORTANT INFORMATION TO REMEMBER: The drug is not intended to provide immediate relief of nasal allergies. To receive the full benefits of the drug, use it on a regular basis as a maintenance medication. If some improvements are not seen in seven days, the individual needs to be reassessed by a doctor. The drug may take up to three weeks before the full benefits are seen. Never exceed prescribed dosage unless directed to do so by a doctor—excessive use beyond prescribed dosage is potentially dangerous. This drug should not be used by individuals with fungal, bacterial, systemic viral, or respiratory tract infections; unhealed wounds inside the nose; or tuberculosis.

When using the nasal spray, use the following procedure:

1) Blow your nose gently to clear your nostrils, if necessary.
2) With your other hand, gently place a finger against the side of your nose to close the opposite nostril.
3) Insert the tip of the bottle or aerosol into the open nostril. Point the tip toward the back and outer side of the nostril once inside.
4) After releasing the spray, close your mouth, sniff deeply, hold your breath for a few seconds, then breathe out through your mouth.
5) Tilt your head back slightly for a few seconds to allow the drug to spread to the back of your nose.
6) Repeat the same procedure for the other nostril.
7) If using more than one spray in each nostril, wait five minutes between sprays.

BRAND NAME: **Florone and Florone E**

GENERIC NAME: diflorasone diacetate

GENERIC FORM AVAILABLE: No

THERAPEUTIC CLASS: Topical corticosteroids

DOSAGE FORMS: 0.05% cream, emollient cream, and ointment

MAIN USES: Skin rashes, swelling, and itching

USUAL DOSE: Apply thin film one to four times daily.

AVERAGE PRICE: $47.14 for 0.05% creams and ointment (15 g)

SIDE EFFECTS: Most common: none. Less common: burning, itching, irritation, dry skin, rash, soreness of the skin, and acne.

DRUG INTERACTIONS: None of any clinical significance

ALLERGIES: Individuals allergic to diflorasone diacetate or any of its derivatives should discuss this with their doctor or pharmacist before using this drug.

PREGNANCY/BREAST-FEEDING. Category C—Risk cannot be ruled out. Human studies are lacking, and animal studies are either positive for fetal risk or lacking as well. However, potential benefits may justify the potential risk in using the drug. It is not known whether the drug is excreted in the breast milk; therefore, caution should be used when breast-feeding.

OTHER BRAND NAMES: None

OTHER DRUGS IN THE SAME THERAPEUTIC CLASS: Aclovate, Aristocort, Cordran, Cordran SP, Cutivate, Cyclocort, DesOwen, Diprolene, Diprolene AF, Elocon, Halog, Hytone, Kenalog, Lidex, Synalar, Temovate, Topicort, Tridesilon, Ultravate, Valisone, and Westcort

IMPORTANT INFORMATION TO REMEMBER: This drug is for external use only. Apply only a thin film of drug to skin and rub it in well. Never cover the skin after application with a bandage or wrapping unless directed to do so by a doctor. Never apply to damaged skin or open wounds unless directed to do so by a doctor. Discontinue use if irritation occurs.

BRAND NAME: Flovent

GENERIC NAME: Fluticasone

GENERIC FORM AVAILABLE: No

THERAPEUTIC CLASS: Steroid inhaler

DOSAGE FORMS: 44-micrograms-per-inhalation metered-dose inhaler; 110-micrograms-per-inhalation metered-dose inhaler; and 220-micrograms-per-inhalation metered-dose inhaler

MAIN USES: Asthma and {other diseases causing inflammation in the lungs}

USUAL DOSE: one to four sprays twice daily (88 micrograms to 880 micrograms twice daily)

AVERAGE PRICE: $65.10 for 44-microgram inhaler; $75.30 for 110-microgram inhaler; and $114.01 for 220-microgram inhaler.

SIDE EFFECTS: headache 17%–22%, upper respiratory tract infections 15%–22%, pharyngitis 10%–14%, stuffy nose 8%–16%, runny nose 3%–6%, hoarse throat 3–8%, flu 3%–8%, fungal infection in the mouth 2%–5%, nose pain 1%–3%, muscle and joint pain 1%–3%, irritation in the eyes 1%–3%, diarrhea 1%–3%, nausea 1%–3%, and vomiting 1%–3%.

DRUG INTERACTIONS: Caution should be used when taking this drug with other oral corticosteroids such as Aristocort, Deltasone, Decadron, Medrol, and prednisone.

ALLERGIES: Individuals allergic to fluticasone or other inhaled steroids (such as those listed in "Other Drugs in the Same Therapeutic Class") should discuss this with their doctor or pharmacist before taking this drug.

PREGNANCY/BREAST-FEEDING: Category C—Risk cannot be ruled out. Human studies are lacking, and animal studies are either positive for fetal risk or lacking as well. However, potential benefits may justify the potential risk in using the drug. It is not known whether the drug is excreted in the breast milk; therefore, caution should be used when breast-feeding.

OTHER BRAND NAMES: None

OTHER DRUGS IN THE SAME THERAPEUTIC CLASS: Aerobid, Azmacort, Beclovent, and Vanceril

IMPORTANT INFORMATION TO REMEMBER: The drug is not intended to provide immediate relief of a bronchospasm, shortness of breath, or an asthma attack. To receive the full benefits of the drug, use it on a regular basis as a maintenance medication. The drug may take up to four weeks before noticeable benefits may be seen. Never exceed prescribed dosage unless directed to do so by a doctor—excessive use beyond prescribed dosage is potentially dangerous. If another inhaler is also being used at the same time, use the other one a few minutes prior to using Azmacort.

When using the inhaler, use the following procedure:

1) Shake the canister well.
2) Place the mouthpiece close to the mouth, but not touching the lips.
3) Exhale deeply.
4) Inhale slowly and deeply as you press the top of the canister to release the medication.
5) Hold your breath for a few seconds before exhaling.
6) Wait five minutes between puffs.
7) Rinse your mouth out with water after use; otherwise this drug may cause a fungal infection in the mouth.
8) Be sure to wash the inhaler device (mouthpiece) regularly with warm soapy water to avoid bacterial contamination.

BRAND NAME: Floxin

GENERIC NAME: ofloxacin

GENERIC FORM AVAILABLE: No

THERAPEUTIC CLASS: Quinolone antibiotic

DOSAGE FORMS: 200-mg, 300-mg, and 400-mg tablets

MAIN USES: Bacterial infections

USUAL DOSE: 200 mg to 400 mg twice a day (every 12 hours)

AVERAGE PRICE: $134.32 for 200 mg (30 tablets); $159.72 for 300 mg (30 tablets); $167.41 for 400 mg (30 tablets)

SIDE EFFECTS: nausea 3%, insomnia 3%, headache 1%, dizziness 1%, diarrhea 1%, vomiting 1%, rash 1%, vaginal itching 1%, yeast infections 1% and stomach pain 1%.

DRUG INTERACTIONS: Antacids, Videx, iron supplements, and Carafate may reduce the absorption of the drug. Choledyl, Slo-bid, Theo-Dur, theophylline, Uni-Dur, Uniphyl, and Aminophylline blood levels may be increased when used with this drug. The drug may also increase the effects of Coumadin.

ALLERGIES: Individuals allergic to ofloxacin or other quinolone antibiotics (such as those listed in "Other Drugs in the Same Therapeutic Class") should discuss this with their doctor or pharmacist before taking this drug.

PREGNANCY/BREAST-FEEDING: Category C—Risk cannot be ruled out. Human studies are lacking, and animal studies are either positive for fetal risk or lacking as well. However, potential benefits may justify the potential risk in using the drug. The drug is excreted in the breast milk; therefore, extreme caution should be used when breast-feeding.

OTHER BRAND NAMES: None

OTHER DRUGS IN THE SAME THERAPEUTIC CLASS: Cipro, Maxaquin, Noroxin, Penetrex

IMPORTANT INFORMATION TO REMEMBER: Take the drug at even intervals around the clock (if twice a day, take every 12 hours). Take the drug until all the medication prescribed is gone; otherwise the infection may return. This drug should be taken with plenty of water (eight ounces is preferred). If stomach upset occurs, take the drug with food. Do not take antacids, milk, or iron supplements within four hours of taking this drug. Individuals should also use a sunscreen to avoid overexposure to the sun; the drug may increase the skin's sensitivity to sunlight, which may cause one to sunburn more easily. This drug may also cause a tear in the tendons of the lower leg. Report any soreness or pain of the lower legs to your physician immediately.

BRAND NAME: Flumadine

GENERIC NAME: rimantadine

GENERIC FORM AVAILABLE: No

THERAPEUTIC CLASS: Antiviral

DOSAGE FORMS: 100-mg tablets and 50 mg/5 mL syrup

MAIN USES: Prevention and treatment of influenza Type A infections

USUAL DOSE: 100 mg twice daily

AVERAGE PRICE: $41.89 for 100-mg tablets (20 capsules)

SIDE EFFECTS: nausea 3%, vomiting 2%, loss of appetite 2%, dry mouth 2%, insomnia 2%, dizziness 2%, stomach pain 1%, headache 1%, nervousness 1%, tiredness 1%, confusion 1%, diarrhea 1%, and muscle aches 1%.

DRUG INTERACTIONS: Tagamet may increase the blood levels of the drug.

ALLERGIES: Individuals allergic to rimantadine, Symmetrel, or any of their derivatives should discuss this with their doctor or pharmacist before using this drug.

PREGNANCY/BREAST-FEEDING: Category C—Risk cannot be ruled out. Human studies are lacking, and animals studies are either positive for fetal risk or lacking as well. However, potential benefits may justify the potential risk in using the drug. This drug should not be taken by women who are breast-feeding.

OTHER BRAND NAMES: None

OTHER DRUGS IN THE SAME THERAPEUTIC CLASS: Symmetrel

IMPORTANT INFORMATION TO REMEMBER: Take the drug at even intervals around the clock (if twice a day, take every 12 hours). Take the drug until all the medication prescribed is gone; otherwise the infection may return. If the drug is being used for prevention, it must be taken before exposure to the influenza virus or as soon as possible after exposure. For best effect in treating influenza Type A, the drug should be taken within 48 hours of the first symptoms of flu.

BRAND NAME: FML and FML Forte

GENERIC NAME: fluorometholone

GENERIC FORM AVAILABLE: No

THERAPEUTIC CLASS: Steroid eyedrop

DOSAGE FORMS: fluorometholone 0.1% eyedrop suspension (FML) and fluorometholone 0.25% eyedrop suspension (FML Forte)

MAIN USES: Inflammation of the eye

USUAL DOSE: one drop two to four times daily

AVERAGE PRICE: $22.16 for 0.1% suspension, 5 mL (FML); $25.11 for 0.25% suspension, 5 mL (FML Forte)

SIDE EFFECTS: Most common: temporary, mild blurred vision. Less common: burning, itching, redness, watering of the eyes, and eye pain.

DRUG INTERACTIONS: The drug may decrease the effects of other eyedrops used to treat glaucoma.

ALLERGIES: Individuals allergic to fluorometholone or any of its derivatives should discuss this with their doctor or pharmacist before using this drug.

PREGNANCY/BREAST-FEEDING: Category C—Risk cannot be ruled out. Human studies are lacking, and animal studies are either positive for fetal risk or lacking as well. However, potential benefits may justify the potential risk in using the drug. It is not known whether the drug is excreted in the breast milk; therefore, caution should be used when breast-feeding.

OTHER BRAND NAMES: Flarex

OTHER DRUGS IN THE SAME THERAPEUTIC CLASS: Decadron, Econopred, Flarex, HMS, Inflamase Forte, Inflamase Mild, Maxidex, Pred Mild, and Vexol

IMPORTANT INFORMATION TO REMEMBER: Shake the bottle thoroughly before using the eyedrops. Individuals should not use the drug while wearing contact lenses unless directed otherwise by a doctor. Keep the container tightly closed and avoid touching the applicator tip to the eye—this could contaminate the product over time. Also, only administer one drop at a time. After application, keep the eye open for at least 30 seconds, roll the eyeball around, and avoid squinting. If a second drop is required, wait one to two minutes between drops. If another medication is to be used in the eye, wait at least 10 minutes before administering it.

BRAND NAME: **Fosamax**

GENERIC NAME: alendronate

GENERIC FORM AVAILABLE: No

THERAPEUTIC CLASS: Aminobisphosphonate

DOSAGE FORMS: 10-mg and 40-mg tablets

MAIN USES: Osteoporosis and Paget's disease

USUAL DOSE: For osteoporosis: 10 mg daily immediately after getting up in the morning with a full glass of plain water and at least 30 minutes before any other beverage, food, or medication. For Paget's disease: 40 mg daily immediately after getting up in the morning with a full glass of plain water and at least 30 minutes before any other beverage, food, or medication, for six months.

AVERAGE PRICE: $233.52 for 10 mg and $588.00 for 40 mg

SIDE EFFECTS: stomach pain 6%, muscle pain 4%, nausea 4%, constipation 3%, diarrhea 3%, headache 3%, gas 3%, acid reflux 2%, esophageal ulcer 2%, vomiting 1%, swollen stomach 1%, and taste changes 1%.

DRUG INTERACTIONS: The drug should be taken at least 30 minutes before any other medication is taken. Calcium and antacids may interfere with the absorption of the drug. The drug increases the incidence of stomach problems when taken with Anaprox, Ansaid, Aleve, aspirin, Cataflam, Clinoril, Daypro, Disalcid, Dolobid, Easprin, Feldene, Indocin, Lodine, Motrin, Nalfon, Naprosyn, Orudis, Oruvail, Relafen, Tolectin, or Voltaren.

ALLERGIES: Individuals allergic to alendronate or any of its derivatives should discuss this with their doctor or pharmacist before using this drug.

PREGNANCY/BREAST-FEEDING: Category C—Risk cannot be ruled out. Human studies are lacking, and animal studies are either positive for fetal risk or lacking as well. However, potential benefits may justify the potential risk in using the drug. The drug is excreted in the breast milk; therefore, extreme caution should be used when breast-feeding.

OTHER BRAND NAMES: None

OTHER DRUGS IN THE SAME THERAPEUTIC CLASS: None

IMPORTANT INFORMATION TO REMEMBER: The drug should be taken with a full glass of tap water only (not mineral water) at least 30 minutes before any other food, beverage, or medication is taken. Also, patients should not lie down for at least 30 minutes after taking the drug, to prevent throat irritation. Only take the drug exactly as directed by your physician. Do not stop taking the drug without first consulting with your physician.

BRAND NAME: Fulvicin P/G

GENERIC NAME: griseofulvin

See entry for Gris-PEG

BRAND NAME: Gantanol and Gantrisin

GENERIC NAME: sulfamethoxazole (Gantanol) and sulfisoxazole (Gantrisin)

GENERIC FORM AVAILABLE: Yes

THERAPEUTIC CLASS: Sulfonamide antibiotic

DOSAGE FORMS: 500-mg tablets (Gantanol and Gantrisin) and 500 mg/mL pediatric suspension, (Gantrisin)

MAIN USES: Bacterial infections

USUAL DOSE: For Gantanol: two to four tablets three times daily. For Gantrisin: 2 to 16 tablets daily in four to six divided doses. Doses for children can be less.

AVERAGE PRICE: $69.86 (B)/$23.41 (G) for 500 mg (Gantanol) and $38.81 (B)/$19.78 (G) for 500 mg (Gantrisin)

SIDE EFFECTS: Most common: fever, itching, skin rash, increased sensitivity to sunburn, dizziness, headache, nausea, vomiting, diarrhea, and loss of appetite. Less common: Stevens-Johnson syndrome (aching joints and muscles, redness and blistering of the skin, and unusual tiredness or weakness), weakness, toxic death of skin tissue (Lyell's syndrome), and blood disorders.

DRUG INTERACTIONS: The drug may increase the blood levels of Coumadin, diabetes medications, epilepsy/seizure medications, and Rheumatrex. The drug may cause crystalluria when taken with Hiprex and Urised.

ALLERGIES: Individuals allergic to sulfamethoxazole, sulfisoxazole, other sulfa drugs, or any of their derivatives should discuss this with their doctor or pharmacist before using this drug.

PREGNANCY/BREAST-FEEDING: Category C—Risk cannot be ruled out. Human studies are lacking, and animal studies are either positive for fetal risk or lacking as well. However, potential benefits may justify the potential risk in using the drug. The drug is excreted in the breast milk; therefore, extreme caution should be used when breast-feeding.

OTHER BRAND NAMES: None

OTHER DRUGS IN THE SAME THERAPEUTIC CLASS: None

IMPORTANT INFORMATION TO REMEMBER: Take the drug at even intervals around the clock (if four times a day, take every six hours). Take the drug until all the medication prescribed is gone; otherwise the infection may return. Individuals should also use a sunscreen to avoid overexposure to the sun; the drug may increase the skin's sensitivity to sunlight, which may cause one to sunburn more easily. This drug should be taken with plenty of water (eight ounces is preferred). If stomach upset occurs, take the drug with food or milk. For the pediatric suspension: Shake the bottle well before taking the drug. Also, the suspension tends to taste bad. Placing it in the refrigerator will help hide the bad taste. Otherwise, the drug does not have to be refrigerated.

BRAND NAME: Garamycin

GENERIC NAME: GENTAMICIN

GENERIC FORM AVAILABLE: Yes

THERAPEUTIC CLASS: Aminoglycoside antibiotic

DOSAGE FORMS: 3 mg/mL eyedrops, 3 mg/g eye ointment, and 0.1% topical cream and ointment

MAIN USES: Bacterial infections of the eye and skin

USUAL DOSE: For eyedrops: one to two drops every four hours. For eye ointment: apply a small amount of ointment two to three time daily. For topical cream and ointment: apply gently three to four times daily to skin.

AVERAGE PRICE: $28.36 (B)/$9.33 (G) 5 mL; $25.95 (B)/$9.88 (G) 0.1% cream and ointment (15 mg); and $27.23 (B)/$8.87 (G)

SIDE EFFECTS: For eyedrops: Most common: none. Less common: itching, burning, stinging, and slightly blurred vision after application. For the topical cream and ointment: most common: none. Less common: itching, redness, burning, and irritation.

DRUG INTERACTIONS: None of any clinical significance

ALLERGIES: Individuals allergic to gentamicin or any of its derivatives should discuss this with their doctor or pharmacist before using this drug.

PREGNANCY/BREAST-FEEDING: Category C—Risk cannot be ruled out. Human studies are lacking, and animal studies are either positive for fetal risk or lacking as well. However, potential benefits may justify the potential risk in using the drug. It is not known whether the drug is excreted in the breast milk; therefore, caution should be used when breast-feeding.

OTHER BRAND NAMES: For eyedrops: Genoptic and Gentacidin

OTHER DRUGS IN THE SAME THERAPEUTIC CLASS: For the eyedrops: Tobrex. For the cream and ointment: Bactroban.

IMPORTANT INFORMATION TO REMEMBER: Use the drug for the full course of treatment; otherwise the infection may return. When using the topical cream or ointment, you may cover the affected area with a bandage or dressing. If you are using the eyedrops, you should not use the drug while wearing contact lenses unless directed otherwise by a doctor. Keep the container tightly closed and avoid touching the applicator tip to the eye—this could contaminate the product over time. Also, only administer one drop at a time. After application, keep the eye open for at least 30 seconds, roll the eyeball around, and avoid squinting. If a second drop is required, wait one to two minutes between drops. If another medication is to be used in the eye, wait at least 10 minutes before administering it. If you are using the eye ointment, pull the bottom eyelid down gently. Then apply a small, thin ribbon of ointment along the rim of the lower eyelid between the eyelid and the eyeball. After application, close the eye and roll the eyeball around. Your vision may be slightly blurred after application.

BRAND NAME: Genoptic

GENERIC NAME: gentamicin

See entry for Garamycin

BRAND NAME: **Gentacidin**

GENERIC NAME: gentamicin

See entry for Garamycin

BRAND NAME: **Glucophage**

GENERIC NAME: metformin

GENERIC FORM AVAILABLE: No

THERAPEUTIC CLASS: Anti-diabetic

DOSAGE FORMS: 500-mg and 850-mg tablets

MAIN USES: Diabetes

USUAL DOSE: 500 mg twice daily with meals. Doses of up to 2500 mg per day can be used.

AVERAGE PRICE: $64.77 for 500 mg and $110.12 for 850 mg

SIDE EFFECTS: Most common: diarrhea, nausea, vomiting, stomach bloating, gas, and loss of appetite. Less common: constipation, heartburn, unpleasant taste, metallic taste, and rash.

DRUG INTERACTIONS: The drug may decrease the blood levels of Micronase and DiaβEta. The drug and Lasix, when used together, may increase the blood levels of both. Adalat, Adalat CC, Procardia, Procardia XL, and Tagamet may increase the blood levels of the drug.

ALLERGIES: Individuals allergic to metformin or any of its derivatives should discuss this with their doctor or pharmacist before using this drug.

PREGNANCY/BREAST-FEEDING: Category B—No evidence of risk in humans. Either animal findings show risk, but human findings do not; or, if no adequate human studies have been done, animal findings show no risk. The drug may be excreted in the breast milk; therefore, caution should be used when breast-feeding.

OTHER BRAND NAMES: None

OTHER DRUGS IN THE SAME THERAPEUTIC CLASS: None

IMPORTANT INFORMATION TO REMEMBER: This drug should be taken with food or milk to reduce the potential for injury to the stomach lining and stomach upset. The drug may cause lactic acidosis in some patients; this occurrence is rare. Only take the drug exactly as directed by your physician and do not increase the dose without first consulting with your physician. This drug may be taken alone or with other diabetic medications. Individuals should be aware of the signs and symptoms of blood sugar that is too low: sweating, tremor, blurred vision, weakness hunger, and confusion. If two or more of these symptoms are seen, treat with oral glucose (sugar) and/or contact your doctor. Before taking over-the-counter cold and allergy preparations, consult your doctor or pharmacist—these products may affect your blood sugar.

BRAND NAME: Glucotrol and Glucotrol XL

GENERIC NAME: glipizide

GENERIC FORM AVAILABLE: Yes (Glucotrol only)

THERAPEUTIC CLASS: Second-generation sulfonylurea anti-diabetic

DOSAGE FORMS: 5-mg and 10-mg tablets for both Glucotrol and Glucotrol XL

MAIN USES: Diabetes

USUAL DOSE: 5 mg to 40 mg once or twice daily

AVERAGE PRICE: $42.44 (B)/$28.91 (G) for 5 mg (Glucotrol); $65.87 (B)/$51.46 (G) for 10 mg (Glucotrol); $54.43 for 5 mg (Glucotrol XL); $87.94 for 10 mg (Glucotrol XL)

SIDE EFFECTS: weakness 10%, headache 9%, dizziness 7%, diarrhea 5%, nervousness 4%, tremor 4%, gas 3%, low blood sugar 1%–3%, nausea 1%–3%, constipation 1%–3%, vomiting 1%–3%, changes in appetite 1%–3%, leg cramps 1%–3%, muscle pain 1%–3%, sweating 1%–3%, and increased urination 1%–3%.

DRUG INTERACTIONS: The drug may cause a stomach reaction (nausea, diarrhea, stomach cramps, vomiting, etc.) when taken with alcohol. The drug may initially increase and then decrease the blood levels of itself and Coumadin when taken together. Bactrim, Gantanol, Gantrisin, Ismelin, Nardil, Parnate, Septra, and high doses of aspirin, Easprin, or Disalcid may cause low blood sugar when taken with this drug. Blocadren, Cartrol, Corgard, Inderal, Kerlone, Levatol, Lopressor, Normodyne, Sectral, Tenormin, Toprol-XL, Trandate, Visken, and Zebeta may hide the symptoms of low blood sugar when taken with this drug. Injected insulin may enhance the effects of the drug (low blood sugar).

ALLERGIES: Individuals allergic to glipizide, Diabinese, sulfa drugs, or other sulfonylureas (such as those listed in "Other Drugs in the Same Therapeutic Class") should discuss this with their doctor or pharmacist before taking this drug.

PREGNANCY/BREAST-FEEDING: Category C—Risk cannot be ruled out. Human studies are lacking, and animal studies are either positive for fetal risk or lacking as well. However, potential benefits may justify the potential risk in using the drug. It is not known whether the drug is excreted in the breast milk; therefore, caution should be used when breast-feeding.

OTHER BRAND NAMES: None

OTHER DRUGS IN THE SAME THERAPEUTIC CLASS: DiaβEta, Glynase, and Micronase

IMPORTANT INFORMATION TO REMEMBER: The drug should be taken 30 minutes before meals. To receive optimum effect, regular compliance with therapy is essential; this includes compliance with a prescribed diet. Avoid alcohol while taking this drug; alcohol may cause a severe stomach reaction (vomiting, pain, diarrhea, etc.). This drug lowers blood sugar. Individuals should be aware of the signs and symptoms of blood sugar that is too low: sweating, tremor, blurred vision, weakness, hunger, and confusion. If two or more of these symptoms are seen, treat with oral glucose (sugar) and/or contact your doctor. This drug may increase the risk of cardiovascular disease. Before taking over-the-counter cold and allergy preparations, consult your doctor or pharmacist—these products may affect your blood sugar.

BRAND NAME: Glynase

GENERIC NAME: glyburide (micronized)

GENERIC FORM AVAILABLE: No

THERAPEUTIC CLASS: Second-generation sulfonylurea anti-diabetic

DOSAGE FORMS: 1.5-mg, 3-mg, and 6-mg micronized Pres-Tablets

MAIN USES: Diabetes

USUAL DOSE: 1.5 mg to 12 mg daily in a single or divided dose

AVERAGE PRICE: $45.50 for 1.5 mg; $76.90 for 3 mg; $123.43 for 6 mg

SIDE EFFECTS: nausea 2%, stomach bloating 2%, heartburn 2%, allergic skin reactions 2%, and low blood sugar 1%–2%.

DRUG INTERACTIONS: The drug may cause a stomach reaction (nausea, diarrhea, stomach cramps, vomiting, etc.) when taken with alcohol. The drug may initially increase and then decrease the blood levels of itself and Coumadin when taken together. Bactrim, Gantanol, Gantrisin, Ismelin, Nardil, Parnate, Septra, and high doses of aspirin, Easprin, or Disalcid may cause low blood sugar when taken with this drug. Blocadren, Cartrol, Corgard, Inderal, Kerlone, Levatol, Lopressor, Normodyne, Sectral, Tenormin, Toprol-XL, Trandate, Visken, and Zebeta may hide the symptoms of low blood sugar when taken with this drug. Injected insulin and Cipro may increase the effects of the drug (low blood sugar).

ALLERGIES: Individuals allergic to glyburide, Diabinese, sulfa drugs, or other sulfonylureas (such as those listed in "Other Drugs in the Same Therapeutic Class") should discuss this with their doctor or pharmacist before taking this drug.

PREGNANCY/BREAST-FEEDING: Category B—No evidence of risk in humans. Either animal findings show risk, but human findings do not; or, if no adequate human studies have been done, animal findings show no risk. It is not known whether the drug is excreted in the breast milk; therefore, caution should be used when breast-feeding.

OTHER BRAND NAMES: None

OTHER DRUGS IN THE SAME THERAPEUTIC CLASS: DiaβBeta, Glucotrol, Glucotrol XL, and Micronase

IMPORTANT INFORMATION TO REMEMBER: If taken once daily, the drug should be taken with breakfast or first main meal. To receive optimum effect, regular compliance with therapy is essential; this includes compliance with a prescribed diet. Avoid alcohol while taking this drug; alcohol may cause a severe stomach reaction (vomiting, pain, diarrhea, etc.). This drug lowers blood sugar. Individuals should be aware of the signs and symptoms of blood sugar that is too low: sweating, tremor, blurred vision, weakness, hunger, and confusion. If two or more of these symptoms are seen, treat with oral glucose (sugar) and/or contact your doctor. This drug may increase the risk of cardiovascular disease. Before taking over-the-counter cold and allergy preparations, consult your doctor or pharmacist. These products may affect your blood sugar.

BRAND NAME: GoLYTELY

GENERIC NAME: Combination product containing: polyethylene glycol, sodium chloride, potassium chloride, sodium bicarbonate, and sodium sulfate

Very similar to Colyte. See entry for Colyte.

BRAND NAME: Grifulvin V

GENERIC NAME: griseofulvin

See entry for Gris-PEG

BRAND NAME: Grisactin

GENERIC NAME: griseofulvin

See entry for Gris-PEG

BRAND NAME: Gris-PEG

GENERIC NAME: griseofulvin

GENERIC FORM AVAILABLE: No

THERAPEUTIC CLASS: Antifungal

DOSAGE FORMS: 125-mg and 250-mg tablets

MAIN USES: Fungal infections

USUAL DOSE: 250 mg to 500 mg one to two times daily

AVERAGE PRICE: $61.47 for 125 mg and 107.21 for 250 mg

SIDE EFFECTS: Most common: none. Less common: headache, diarrhea, nausea, vomiting, skin rash, dizziness, insomnia, increased sensitivity to sunburn, and oral thrush.

DRUG INTERACTIONS: The drug may decrease the effects of Coumadin. The drug may increase the toxic effects of alcohol on the liver. The drug may decrease the effectiveness of oral contraceptives (birth control pills).

ALLERGIES: Individuals allergic to griseofulvin or any of its derivatives should discuss this with their doctor or pharmacist before using this drug.

PREGNANCY/BREAST-FEEDING: Category C—Risk cannot be ruled out. Human studies are lacking, and animal studies are either positive for fetal risk or lacking as well. However, potential benefits may justify the potential risk in using the drug. It is not known whether the drug is excreted in the breast milk; therefore, caution should be used when breast-feeding.

OTHER BRAND NAMES: Fulvicin P/G, Fulvicin U/F, Grisactin Ultra, and Grifulvin V

OTHER DRUGS IN THE SAME THERAPEUTIC CLASS: Fulvicin P/G, Fulvicin U/F, Grisactin Ultra, and Grifulvin V

IMPORTANT INFORMATION TO REMEMBER: This drug should be taken with food or milk to reduce the potential for stomach upset. Take the drug at even intervals around the clock (if twice a day, take every 12 hours). Take the drug until all the medication prescribed is gone; otherwise the infection may return. For some infections, the drug may be used for six months or longer. Individuals should also use a sunscreen to avoid overexposure to the sun; the drug may increase the skin's sensitivity to sunlight, which may cause one to sunburn more easily. Women taking birth control pills should use another form of contraception while taking the drug and for the rest of the current menstrual cycle. Avoid alcohol while taking this drug; the drug may increase the toxic effects of alcohol on the liver.

BRAND NAME: Guaifed and Guaifed-PD

GENERIC NAME: Combination product containing: pseudoephedrine and guaifenesin

GENERIC FORM AVAILABLE: No

THERAPEUTIC CLASS: Decongestant + expectorant

DOSAGE FORMS: Guaifed: 120-mg pseudoephedrine/250-mg guaifenesin sustained-release capsules. Guaifed-PD: 60-mg pseudoephedrine/300-mg guaifenesin capsules.

MAIN USES: Nasal congestion and cough

USUAL DOSE: Guaifed capsules: one capsule every 12 hours. Guaifed-PD: one to two capsules every 12 hours.

AVERAGE PRICE: $112.33 for Guaifed; $89.54 for Guaifed-PD

SIDE EFFECTS: Most common: none. Less common: drowsiness, nausea, giddiness, dry mouth, blurred vision, pounding heartbeat, flushing, and increased irritability or excitability (especially in children).

DRUG INTERACTIONS: Blocadren, Cartrol, Corgard, Inderal, Kerlone, Levatol, Lopressor, Normodyne, Sectral, Tenormin, Toprol-XL, Trandate, Visken, and Zebeta may increase the effects of the drug. The drug may also reduce the effects of blood-pressure-lowering drugs. Nardil or Parnate may significantly raise blood pressure when taken with this drug.

ALLERGIES: Individuals allergic to pseudoephedrine, guaifenesin, or any of their derivatives should discuss this with their doctor or pharmacist before using this drug.

PREGNANCY/BREAST-FEEDING: Category C—Risk cannot be ruled out. Human studies are lacking, and animal studies are either positive for fetal risk or lacking as well. However, potential benefits may justify the potential risk in using the drug. The drug is excreted in the breast milk; therefore, extreme caution should be used when breast-feeding.

OTHER BRAND NAMES: None

OTHER DRUGS IN THE SAME THERAPEUTIC CLASS: Deconsal II, Duratuss, Entex, Entex LA, Entex PSE, Exgest LA, and Zephrex LA

IMPORTANT INFORMATION TO REMEMBER: Patients with high blood pressure or heart conditions should consult their doctor before taking this drug. This drug should be taken with plenty of water (eight ounces is preferred). Do not increase the dose without first consulting with your physician.

BRAND NAME: Habitrol

GENERIC NAME: nicotine patch

See entry for Nicoderm

BRAND NAME: Halcion

GENERIC NAME: triazolam

GENERIC FORM AVAILABLE: Yes

THERAPEUTIC CLASS: Benzodiazepine sedative

DOSAGE FORMS: 0.125-mg and 0.25-mg tablets

MAIN USES: Insomnia

USUAL DOSE: 0.125 mg to 0.25 mg at bedtime

AVERAGE PRICE: $99.12 (B)/$72.63 (G) for 0.125 mg and $108.40 (B)/$79.29 (G) for 0.25 mg

SIDE EFFECTS: daytime drowsiness 14%, headache 10%, dizziness 8%, nervousness 5%, lightheadedness 5%, coordination disorders 5%, nausea/vomiting 5%, fast heartbeat 1%, tiredness 1%, confusion 1%, nightmares 1%, memory impairment 1%, depression 1%, and vision problems 1%.

DRUG INTERACTIONS: Central nervous system (CNS) depression may be increased when used with alcohol, narcotic painkillers, or other anxiety medications. Erythromycin and Tagamet may increase the blood levels of the drug.

ALLERGIES: Individuals allergic to triazolam, benzodiazepines, or other sleeping medications (such as those listed in "Other Drugs in the Same Therapeutic Class") should discuss this with their doctor or pharmacist before taking this drug.

PREGNANCY/BREAST-FEEDING: Category X—Should not be used during pregnancy. Studies in animals and/or humans have shown fetal abnormalities and birth defects. The risks associated with using this drug clearly outweigh the benefits. This drug should never be used by someone who is pregnant or trying to become pregnant. Also, women should never breast-feed while using this drug.

OTHER BRAND NAMES: None

OTHER DRUGS IN THE SAME THERAPEUTIC CLASS: Dalmane, Doral, ProSom and Restoril

IMPORTANT INFORMATION TO REMEMBER: This drug will cause drowsiness. Individuals should use caution when driving, operating machinery, or any task where mental alertness is required. The drug may take two to three days before maximum effect is seen. The incidence of drowsiness and unsteadiness increases with age.

Alcohol, anxiety medications, and narcotic painkillers may intensify the drowsiness effect of the drug. This medication is a controlled substance and may be habit-forming. Do not increase the dose of medication without consulting with your doctor; only take the amount prescribed by your doctor. This drug has been associated with some cases of nightmares and amnesia (memory loss).

BRAND NAME: Haldol

GENERIC NAME: haloperidol

GENERIC FORM AVAILABLE: Yes

THERAPEUTIC CLASS: Butyrophenone antipsychotic

DOSAGE FORMS: 0.5-mg, 1-mg, 2-mg, 5-mg, 10-mg, and 20-mg tablets; 2 mg/1 mL oral concentrate

MAIN USES: Psychotic disorders and severe behavioral problems

USUAL DOSE: 0.5 mg to 5 mg two to three times daily

AVERAGE PRICE: $58.27 (B)/$21.97 (G) for 0.5 mg; $78.73 (B)/ $31.87 (G) for 1 mg; $98.97 (B)/$46.17 (G) for 2 mg; $167.17 (B)/ $57.17 (G) for 5 mg; $208.97 (B)/$82.47 (G) for 10 mg

SIDE EFFECTS: Most common: restlessness, muscle spasms of the face, muscle twitching, weakness of the arms and legs, difficulty speaking or swallowing, loss of balance, trembling of hands and fingers, blurred vision, changes in menstrual cycle, constipation, dry mouth, weight gain, sore or swollen breasts in females, milk production from the breasts, and drowsiness. Less common: skin rash, hallucinations, difficulty in urinating, general weakness, dizziness, unusual movements of the tongue and lips, nausea, vomiting, decreased sexual ability, and decreased thirst.

DRUG INTERACTIONS: Alcohol, anxiety medications, and narcotic painkillers may intensify the drowsiness effect of the drug. The drug and either Eskalith or Lithobid, when used together, may cause neurological problems and brain damage. Tegretol may decrease the effectiveness of the drug. Akineton, Artane, Cogentin, and Kemadrin may decrease the increase the severity of side effects caused by the drug.

ALLERGIES: Individuals allergic to haloperidol or any of its derivatives should discuss this with their doctor or pharmacist before using this drug.

PREGNANCY/BREAST-FEEDING: Category C—Risk cannot be ruled out. Human studies are lacking, and animal studies are either positive for fetal risk or lacking as well. However, potential benefits may justify the potential risk in using the drug. The drug is excreted in the breast milk; therefore, extreme caution should be used when breast-feeding.

OTHER BRAND NAMES: None

OTHER DRUGS IN THE SAME THERAPEUTIC CLASS: None

IMPORTANT INFORMATION TO REMEMBER: This drug does cause drowsiness. Individuals should use caution when driving, operating machinery, or any task where mental alertness is required. Alcohol, anxiety medications, and narcotic painkillers may intensify the drowsiness effect of the drug. This drug should not be used by individuals with Parkinson's disease. If stomach upset occurs, take the drug with food or milk. Caution should also be used when exercising and in hot weather while taking this drug; the drug may increase an individual's sensitivity to hot weather. Only take the drug exactly as directed by your physician. Do not stop taking the drug without first consulting your physician. It may take several weeks before an improvement in symptoms is seen.

BRAND NAME: Halog and Halog-E

GENERIC NAME: halcinonide

GENERIC FORM AVAILABLE: No

THERAPEUTIC CLASS: Topical corticosteroids

DOSAGE FORMS: 0.1% ointment, cream, solution, and emollient cream (Halog-E)

MAIN USES: Skin rashes, swelling, and itching

USUAL DOSE: Apply sparingly one to three times daily.

AVERAGE PRICE: $41.93 for 0.1% Halog and Halog-E (30 g)

SIDE EFFECTS: Most common: none. Less common: burning, itching, irritation, dry skin, rash, soreness of the skin, and acne.

DRUG INTERACTIONS: None of any clinical significance

ALLERGIES: Individuals allergic to halcinonide or any of its derivatives should discuss this with their doctor or pharmacist before using this drug.

PREGNANCY/BREAST-FEEDING: Category C—Risk cannot be ruled out. Human studies are lacking, and animal studies are either positive for fetal risk or lacking as well. However, potential benefits may justify the potential risk in using the drug. It is not known whether the drug is excreted in the breast milk; therefore, caution should be used when breast-feeding.

OTHER BRAND NAMES: None

OTHER DRUGS IN THE SAME THERAPEUTIC CLASS: Aclovate, Aristocort, Cordran, Cordran SP, Cutivate, Cyclocort, DesOwen, Diprolene, Diprolene AF, Elocon, Florone, Hytone, Kenalog, Lidex, Synalar, Temovate, Topicort, Tridesilon, Ultravate, Valisone, and Westcort

IMPORTANT INFORMATION TO REMEMBER: This drug is for external use only. Apply only a thin film of drug to skin and rub it in well. Never cover the skin after application with a bandage or wrapping unless directed to do so by a doctor. Never apply to damaged skin or open wounds unless directed to do so by a doctor. Discontinue use if irritation occurs.

BRAND NAME: Helidac

GENERIC NAME: Combination pack of products containing three medications: 1) bismuth subsalicylate, 2) metronidazole, and 3) tetracycline

GENERIC FORM AVAILABLE: No

THERAPEUTIC CLASS: Antibiotic

DOSAGE FORMS: Combination pack of products containing three medication: 1) 262.4-mg bismuth subsalicylate tablets, 2) 250-mg metronidazole tablets, and 3) 500-mg tetracycline capsules

MAIN USES: Active stomach ulcers and active duodenal ulcers (ulcers of the upper part of the small intestine, also called peptic ulcers)

USUAL DOSE: The following regimen should be taken four times daily with meals and at bedtime for 14 days: two bismuth tablets, one metronidazole tablet, and one tetracycline capsule.

AVERAGE PRICE: $85.89 for 14-day pack of medication

SIDE EFFECTS: nausea 10%, diarrhea 5%, stomach pain 3%, anal discomfort 2%, appetite changes 2%, dizziness 2%, numbness 2%, vomiting 2%, weakness 1%, constipation 1%, insomnia 1%, pain 1%, and nasal infection 1%.

DRUG INTERACTIONS: The drug should never be used with alcohol or with any medication that may contain alcohol. Even small amounts of alcohol will cause intense stomach pain, vomiting, headache, sweating, chest pain, and difficulty breathing. This drug should not be used with Antabuse; in fact, this drug should not be used until at least two weeks after the drug Antabuse has been discontinued. The drug may increase the effects of such as Coumadin. Antacids, calcium supplements, iron supplements, magnesium laxatives, and other mineral supplements may bind to the drug in the stomach and intestines and prevent its absorption by the body. The drug may decrease the effectiveness of birth control pills.

ALLERGIES: Individuals allergic to bismuth, aspirin, Sumycin, Flagyl, metronidazole, tetracyclines, or any of their derivatives should discuss this with their doctor or pharmacist before taking this drug.

PREGNANCY/BREAST-FEEDING: Category D—Positive evidence of risk. Human studies show risk to the fetus. Nevertheless, potential benefits may possibly outweigh the potential risks. This drug should not be taken by nursing mothers.

OTHER BRAND NAMES: None

OTHER DRUGS IN THE SAME THERAPEUTIC CLASS: None

IMPORTANT INFORMATION TO REMEMBER: Always complete the full course of therapy, and take the drug only as directed. The drug should be taken with meals and at bedtime with a full glass of water, preferably eight ounces. Individuals may take antacids occasionally for heartburn or temporary flare-ups, but antacids should be taken at least one hour before or two hours after taking the drug. This medication should not be taken within 24 hours of using any alcohol. The blood alcohol level of an individual should be zero before therapy is begun. Once treatment has begun, individuals should under no circumstances drink any alcohol: in fact, alcohol should not be used until at least three days after the last dose of the drug. Many cough and cold preparations contain alcohol. Individuals taking this drug should read all over-the-counter medication labels carefully; consult your pharmacist before taking any of these preparations. Also, individuals should check with their physician before taking any narcotic painkillers or anxiety medications. Avoid taking calcium supplements, iron supplements, magnesium laxatives, and other mineral supplements within two hours of taking the drug. Women taking birth control pills should use another form of contraception while taking the drug and for the rest of the current menstrual cycle. Individuals should also use a sunscreen to avoid overexposure to the sun; the drug may increase the skin's sensitivity to sunlight, which may cause one to sunburn more easily. The drug should not be used for children under eight years of age due to the potential of permanent tooth staining.

BRAND NAME: Hiprex

GENERIC NAME: methenamine hippurate

GENERIC FORM AVAILABLE: No

THERAPEUTIC CLASS: Methenamine derivative antibacterial

DOSAGE FORMS: 1-g tablets

MAIN USES: Bacterial infections (primarily urinary tract infections)

USUAL DOSE: 1 g twice daily

AVERAGE PRICE: $157.92

SIDE EFFECTS: Most common: nausea and vomiting. Less common: skin rash, crystals in the urine, and blood in the urine.

DRUG INTERACTIONS: Drugs that cause the urine to become alkaline (nonacidic), such as antacids, sodium bicarbonate, and diuretics (water pills), may make the drug ineffective.

ALLERGIES: Individuals allergic to methenamine hippurate or any of its derivatives should discuss this with their doctor or pharmacist before using this drug.

PREGNANCY/BREAST-FEEDING: Category C—Risk cannot be ruled out. Human studies are lacking, and animal studies are either positive for fetal risk or lacking as well. However, potential benefits may justify the potential risk in using the drug. It is not known whether the drug is excreted in the breast milk; therefore, caution should be used when breast-feeding.

OTHER BRAND NAMES: Urex

OTHER DRUGS IN THE SAME THERAPEUTIC CLASS: Mandelamine and Urex

IMPORTANT INFORMATION TO REMEMBER: If stomach upset occurs, take the drug with food or milk. Also, take the drug at even intervals around the clock (if two times a day, take every 12 hours). Take the drug until all the medication prescribed is gone; otherwise the infection may return. The drug should be taken with plenty of water (eight ounces is preferred). It also may be necessary to test the urine regularly to assure the pH is acidic (pH = 5.5 or below); discuss this with your physician.

BRAND: **Hismanal**

GENERIC NAME: astemizole

GENERIC FORM AVAILABLE: No

THERAPEUTIC CLASS: Nonsedating antihistamine

DOSAGE FORMS: 10-mg tablets

MAIN USES: Allergies

USUAL DOSE: One tablet daily as directed on an empty stomach.

AVERAGE PRICE: $269.09

SIDE EFFECTS: slight drowsiness 7%, headache 7%, dry mouth 5%, slight tiredness 4%, appetite increase 4%, weight increase 4%, nervousness 2%, dizziness 2%, nausea 2%, diarrhea 2%, and sore throat 2%.

DRUG INTERACTIONS: This drug should not be used with Biaxin, erythromycin, Diflucan, Dynabac, Nizoral, Sporanox, and TAO. This may cause dangerous irregular heartbeats and fast heartbeat. The drug should not be taken with Serzone.

ALLERGIES: Individuals allergic to astemizole or any of their derivatives should discuss this with their doctor or pharmacist before using this drug.

PREGNANCY/BREAST-FEEDING: Category C—Risk cannot be ruled out. Human studies are lacking, and animal studies are either positive for fetal risk or lacking as well. However, potential benefits may justify the potential risk in using the drug. It is not known whether the drug is excreted in the breast milk; therefore, caution should be used when breast-feeding.

OTHER BRAND NAMES: None

OTHER DRUGS IN THE SAME THERAPEUTIC CLASS: Allegra, Claritin, Seldane, and Zyrtec

IMPORTANT INFORMATION TO REMEMBER: It's best to take the drug on an empty stomach—one hour before meals or two hours after meals—if possible. Do not take Hismanal more frequently than every 24 hours. Unless otherwise directed by a physician, take only as needed during allergy seasons. This drug should not be used with Biaxin, erythromycin, Dynabac, Zithromax, Nizoral, Sporanox, TAO, or other macrolide antibiotics. This drug may cause dangerous irregular heartbeats and fast heartbeat. If heart palpitations or fainting occur, report this to your doctor immediately.

BRAND NAME: HIVID

GENERIC NAME: zalcitabine

GENERIC FORM AVAILABLE: No

THERAPEUTIC CLASS: AIDS antiviral

DOSAGE FORMS: 0.375-mg and 0.75-mg tablets

MAIN USES: AIDS

USUAL DOSE: 0.75 mg every eight hours

AVERAGE PRICE: $256.79 for 0.375 mg and $321.88 for 0.75 mg

SIDE EFFECTS: Unusual nerve sensations and nerve damage in the arms, legs, fingers, and toes (tingling, burning, etc.) 28%, abnormal liver function 9%, weakness 4%, stomach pain 4%, blood disorders 3%–13%, rash 3%, nausea 3%, vomiting 3%, diarrhea 3%, mouth sores 3%, vomiting 3%, headache 2%, fever 2%, and convulsions 1%.

DRUG INTERACTIONS: There are numerous drugs that can cause peripheral neuropathy (unusual nerve sensations and nerve damage in the arms, legs, fingers, and toes) when taken with this drug. Some of these are: alcohol, Aldomet, Apresoline, Bactrim, cisplatin, Clinoril, dapsone, Depakene, Depakote, Dilantin, diuretics (water pills), Eskalith, Doryx, estrogens, Flagyl, Gantanol, Gantrisin, isoniazid, Lasix, Lithobid, Macrobid, Macrodantin, Minocin, Monodox, pentamidine, Septra, Sumycin, Vibramycin, vincristine, and ZERIT.

The drug may increase the toxic effects of Biaxin, erythromycin, Dynabac, TAO, and Zithromax. Before taking any prescription drug, discuss it with your doctor.

ALLERGIES: Individuals allergic to zalcitabine or any of its derivatives should discuss this with their doctor or pharmacist before using this drug.

PREGNANCY/BREAST-FEEDING: Category C—Risk cannot be ruled out. Human studies are lacking, and animal studies are either positive for fetal risk or lacking as well. However, potential benefits may justify the potential risk in using the drug. It is not known whether the drug is excreted in the breast milk; therefore, caution should be used when breast-feeding.

OTHER BRAND NAMES: No

OTHER DRUGS IN THE SAME THERAPEUTIC CLASS: Epivir, Retrovir, Videx, and ZERIT

IMPORTANT INFORMATION TO REMEMBER: If stomach upset occurs, take the drug with food or milk; this may, however, decrease the absorption of the drug. Also, take the drug at even intervals around the clock (if threes times a day, take every eight hours). Only take the drug exactly as directed by your physician. Do not stop taking the drug without first consulting with your physician. It is important to have regular blood and liver function tests while taking this drug. Before taking any prescription or over-the-counter (OTC) drugs, consult your physician or pharmacist.

BRAND NAME: Humalog

GENERIC NAME: insulin lispro

GENERIC FORM AVAILABLE: No

THERAPEUTIC CLASS: Insulin replacement

DOSAGE FORMS: 100 units/mL

MAIN USES: Diabetes

USUAL DOSE: varies by patient

AVERAGE PRICE: $28.24 for 10-mL bottle

SIDE EFFECTS: Most common: none. Less common: low blood sugar and allergic reaction (characterized by redness, swelling, and itching at the injection site).

DRUG INTERACTIONS: Alcohol, Aristocort, Blocadren, Cartrol, Corgard, Decadron, Deltasone, Inderal, Kerlone, Levatol, Lopressor, Medrol, Normodyne, prednisone, Sectral, Tenormin, Toprol-XL, Trandate, Visken, Zebeta, smoking, and diuretics (water pills) may cause changes in blood sugar.

ALLERGIES: Individuals allergic to this type or brand of insulin or any of its derivatives should discuss this with their doctor or pharmacist before using this drug.

PREGNANCY/BREAST-FEEDING: Category B—No evidence of risk in humans. Either animal findings show risk, but human findings do not; or, if no adequate human studies have been done, animal findings show no risk. It is not known whether the drug is excreted in the breast milk; therefore, caution should be used when breast-feeding.

OTHER BRAND NAMES: None

OTHER DRUGS IN THE SAME THERAPEUTIC CLASS: Iletin, Novolin, and Velosulin

IMPORTANT INFORMATION TO REMEMBER: When used as a meal-time insulin, it should be taken within 15 minutes before the meal due to its quick onset of action. It's important to follow a prescribed diet carefully even when using insulin. Do not change insulin brands without first discussing this with your doctor or pharmacist. Do not change the order of mixing insulins as prescribed by your doctor. It's important to continue to monitor blood sugar levels at regular intervals as prescribed by your doctor. Bottles of insulin that are not being used should be stored in the refrigerator. Before using a bottle of insulin, roll the bottle gently in your hands. Do not vigorously shake the bottle. If the insulin appears grainy or lumpy or sticks to the bottle, do not use it. Individuals should be aware of the signs and symptoms of both high and low blood sugar and know what action to take. Before taking over-the-counter medications, consult with your doctor or pharmacist; some over-the-counter medications may affect your blood sugar.

BRAND NAME: **Humibid LA, Humibid Sprinkle, Humibid DM, and Humibid DM Sprinkle**

GENERIC NAME: Combination products containing: guaifenesin or dextromethorphan and guaifenesin

GENERIC FORM AVAILABLE: No

THERAPEUTIC CLASS: Expectorant (Humibid LA and Humibid Sprinkle) and expectorant + cough suppressant (Humibid DM)

DOSAGE FORMS: 300-mg guaifenesin capsules (Humibid Sprinkle); 600-mg guaifenesin tablets (Humibid LA); 15-mg dextromethorphan/300-mg guaifenesin capsules (Humibid DM Sprinkle); and 30-mg dextromethorphan/600-mg guaifenesin tablets (Humibid DM)

MAIN USES: Cough and chest congestion

USUAL DOSE: For Humibid LA and Humibd DM: one to two tablets every 12 hours. For the sprinkle capsules: two to four capsules every 12 hours.

AVERAGE PRICE: $99.91 for Humibid DM and $66.78 for Humibid LA

SIDE EFFECTS: Most common: none. Less common: nausea, drowsiness, diarrhea, vomiting, and stomach pain.

DRUG INTERACTIONS: The drug should not be used by individuals currently taking Nardil or Parnate; in fact, the drug should not be used until Nardil or Parnate have been discontinued for 14 days.

ALLERGIES: Individuals allergic to dextromethorphan, guaifenesin, or any of their derivatives should discuss this with their doctor or pharmacist before using this drug.

PREGNANCY/BREAST-FEEDING: Category C—Risk cannot be ruled out. Human studies are lacking, and animal studies are either positive for fetal risk or lacking as well. However, potential benefits may justify the potential risk in using the drug. It is not known whether the drug is excreted in the breast milk; therefore, caution should be used when breast-feeding.

OTHER BRAND NAMES: None

OTHER DRUGS IN THE SAME THERAPEUTIC CLASS: Organidin NR

IMPORTANT INFORMATION TO REMEMBER: Tablets may be split in half, but do not crush them. The sprinkle capsules may be opened, sprinkled on soft food (such as applesauce), and swallowed, making sure not to chew the "sprinkles." The drug should be taken with plenty of water (eight ounces is preferred). Humibid DM may cause some limited drowsiness. Individuals should use caution when driving, operating machinery, or any task where mental alertness is required. Alcohol, anxiety medications, and narcotic painkillers may intensify the drowsiness effect of the drug.

BRAND NAME: Humulin

GENERIC NAME: insulin (human)

GENERIC FORM AVAILABLE: No

THERAPEUTIC CLASS: Insulin replacement

DOSAGE FORMS: Lente, NPH, Regular, Ultralente, 70/30, and 50/50

MAIN USES: Diabetes

USUAL DOSE: varies by patient

AVERAGE PRICE: $28.24 for 10-mL bottle

SIDE EFFECTS: Most common: none. Less common: low blood sugar and allergic reaction (characterized by redness, swelling, and itching at the injection site).

DRUG INTERACTIONS: Alcohol, Aristocort, Blocadren, Cartrol, Corgard, Decadron, Deltasone, Inderal, Kerlone, Levatol, Lopressor, Medrol, Normodyne, prednisone, Sectral, Tenormin, Toprol-XL, Trandate, Visken, Zebeta, smoking, and diuretics (water pills) may cause changes in blood sugar.

ALLERGIES: Individuals allergic to this type or brand of insulin or any of its derivatives should discuss this with their doctor or pharmacist before using this drug.

PREGNANCY/BREAST-FEEDING: Category B—No evidence of risk in humans. Either animal findings show risk, but human findings do not; or, if no adequate human studies have been done, animal findings show no risk. It is not known whether the drug is excreted in the breast milk; therefore, caution should be used when breast-feeding.

OTHER BRAND NAMES: None

OTHER DRUGS IN THE SAME THERAPEUTIC CLASS: Humalog, Iletin, Novolin, and Velosulin

IMPORTANT INFORMATION TO REMEMBER: It's important to follow a prescribed diet carefully even when using insulin. Do not change insulin brands without first discussing this with your doctor or pharmacist. Do not change the order of mixing insulins as prescribed by your doctor. It's important to continue to monitor blood sugar levels at regular intervals as prescribed by your doctor. Bottles of insulin that are not being used should be stored in the refrigerator. Before using a bottle of insulin, roll the bottle gently in your hands. Do not vigorously shake the bottle. If the insulin appears grainy or lumpy or sticks to the bottle, do not use it. Individuals should be aware of the signs and symptoms of both high and low blood sugar and know what action to take. Before taking over-the-counter medications, consult with your doctor or pharmacist; some over-the-counter medications may affect your blood sugar.

BRAND NAME: Hydergine and Hydergine LC

GENERIC NAME: ergoloid mesylates

GENERIC FORM AVAILABLE: Yes

THERAPEUTIC CLASS: Anti-Alzheimer's ergot alkaloid

DOSAGE FORMS: 1.0-mg tablets; 0.5-mg and 1.0-mg sublingual tablets; 1.0-mg capsules; and 1.0 mg/mL liquid

MAIN USES: Mental dementia and Alzheimer's disease

USUAL DOSE: 1 mg three times a day

AVERAGE PRICE: $100.21 (B)/$29.82 (G) for Hydergine and $105.42 (brand only) for Hydergine LC

SIDE EFFECTS: Most common: none. Less common: dizziness, nausea, vomiting, fainting, flushing, stomach pain, headache, slow heartbeat, loss of appetite, drowsiness, slow heart rate, soreness under the tongue (sublingual tablets only), and blurred vision.

DRUG INTERACTIONS: None of any clinical significance

ALLERGIES: Individuals allergic to ergoloid mesylates or any of their derivatives should discuss this with their doctor or pharmacist before using this drug.

PREGNANCY/BREAST-FEEDING: Category D—Positive evidence of risk. Human studies show risk to the fetus. Nevertheless, potential benefits may possibly outweigh the potential risks. This drug should not be taken by nursing mothers.

OTHER BRAND NAMES: None

OTHER DRUGS IN THE SAME THERAPEUTIC CLASS: None

IMPORTANT INFORMATION TO REMEMBER: Only take the drug exactly as directed by your physician and do not increase the dose without first consulting with your physician. Do not stop taking the drug without first consulting with your physician. The drug may take several weeks before any improvement is seen. If you are using the sublingual tablets, allow the tablet to completely dissolve under the tongue.

BRAND NAME: Hydrea

GENERIC NAME: hydroxyurea

GENERIC FORM AVAILABLE: No

THERAPEUTIC CLASS: Anti-metabolite, anticancer

DOSAGE FORMS: 500-mg capsules

MAIN USES: Cancer and (sickle cell anemia)

USUAL DOSE: Various doses for different types of cancer; each is usually individualized based on the patient's weight.

AVERAGE PRICE: $198.70

SIDE EFFECTS: Most common: anemia, blood disorders, diarrhea, drowsiness, loss of appetite, nausea, and vomiting. Less common: constipation, rash, itching, sores in the mouth and lips, decrease in blood platelets, and decrease in white blood cells.

DRUG INTERACTIONS: Probenecid and gout medications may need to be adjusted when taking this drug. Bone marrow depressants (other cancer drugs) and vaccines should be used cautiously when taking this drug.

ALLERGIES: Individuals allergic to hydroxyurea or any of its derivatives should discuss this with their doctor or pharmacist before using this drug.

PREGNANCY/BREAST-FEEDING: Category D—Positive evidence of risk. Human studies show risk to the fetus. Nevertheless, potential benefits may possibly outweigh the potential risks. This drug should not be taken by nursing mothers.

OTHER BRAND NAMES: None

OTHER DRUGS IN THE SAME THERAPEUTIC CLASS: None

IMPORTANT INFORMATION TO REMEMBER: Only take the drug exactly as directed by your physician. Do not stop taking the drug unless directed to do so by your physician. If nausea, vomiting, and/or diarrhea occur, continue taking the drug and contact your physician. If unusual bleeding, bruising, black and tarry stools, a fever, sore throat, blood in the urine, or pinpoint red spots on the skin occur, contact your physician immediately.

BRAND NAME: Hydrocet

GENERIC NAME: Combination product containing: hydrocodone bitartrate and acetaminophen

See entry for Vicodin

BRAND NAME: Hydrocortisone cream, ointment, and lotion (various brand-name manufacturers)

GENERIC NAME: hydrocortisone

See entry for Hytone

BRAND NAME: HydroDIURIL

GENERIC NAME: hydrochlorothiazide

GENERIC FORM AVAILABLE: Yes

THERAPEUTIC CLASS: Thiazide diuretic (water pill)

DOSAGE FORMS: 25-mg, 50-mg, and 100-mg tablets

MAIN USES: High blood pressure and water retention (fluid retention due to congestive heart failure, kidney disease, or cirrhosis of the liver)

USUAL DOSE: 25 mg to 100 mg once or twice a day

AVERAGE PRICE: $28.57 (B)/$9.88 (G) for 25 mg; $30.78 (B)/$13.18 (G) for 50 mg; $46.07 (B)/$14.28 (G) for 100 mg

SIDE EFFECTS: Most common: low potassium, dry mouth, muscle cramps, increased thirst, weakness, nausea, and vomiting. Less common: loss of appetite, constipation, diarrhea, decreased sexual ability, high blood sugar, dizziness, and increased sensitivity to sunburn.

DRUG INTERACTIONS: The drug may require dosage adjustments to diabetic and gout medications. Colestid and Questran may decrease the absorption of the drug. The drug may increase the blood levels of Eskalith and Lithobid.

ALLERGIES: Individuals allergic to hydrochlorothiazide, sulfa drugs, or any of their derivatives should discuss this with their doctor or pharmacist before using this drug.

PREGNANCY/BREAST-FEEDING: Category B—No evidence of risk in humans. Either animal findings show risk, but human findings do not; or, if no adequate human studies have been done, animal findings show no risk. The drug is excreted in the breast milk; therefore, extreme caution should be used when breast-feeding.

OTHER BRAND NAMES: Esidrix and Oretic

OTHER DRUGS IN THE SAME THERAPEUTIC CLASS: Diuril, Enduron, Hydromox, and Hygroton

IMPORTANT INFORMATION TO REMEMBER: If the drug is to be taken once daily, take it in the morning due to increased urine output. Before taking over-the-counter cold and allergy preparations, consult your doctor or pharmacist; these products may raise your blood pressure. The drug may cause the elimination of potassium from the body. It is therefore a good idea to eat a banana or drink orange, grapefruit, or apple juice every day to replace lost potassium. This drug may also increase the sensitivity of the skin to sunburn in some individuals; therefore, a sunscreen is recommended during periods of prolonged exposure to the sun. Individuals with kidney disease should discuss this with their doctor before taking this drug.

BRAND NAME: Hydropres 25 and Hydropres 50

GENERIC NAME: Combination product containing: reserpine and hydrochlorothiazide

GENERIC FORM AVAILABLE: Yes

THERAPEUTIC CLASS: Centrally acting blood vessel dilator + diuretic (water pill)

DOSAGE FORMS: 0.125-mg reserpine/25-mg hydrochlorothiazide tablets (Hydropres 25) and 0.125-mg reserpine/50-mg hydrochlorothiazide tablets (Hydropres 50)

MAIN USES: High blood pressure

USUAL DOSE: one tablet daily

AVERAGE PRICE: $39.41 (B)/$15.97 (G) for Hydropres 25 and $61.74 (B)/$24.94 (G) for Hydropres 50

SIDE EFFECTS: Most common: dizziness and some tiredness. Less common: weakness, depression, low blood pressure, low potassium, drowsiness, headache, restlessness, impotence, decreased sex drive, diarrhea, stomach pain, vomiting, dry mouth, stuffy nose, bloody nose, appetite changes, difficulty sleeping, muscle spasms, muscle aches, irritability, increased sensitivity to sunburn, and slow heartbeat.

DRUG INTERACTIONS: The drug may cause low blood pressure when used with alcohol, Amytal, Butisol, Mebaral, Nembutal, phenobarbital, Seconal, Tuinal, anxiety medications, and narcotic painkillers. The drug may require dosage adjustments to diabetic and gout medications. The drug may increase the effects of muscle relaxers. The drug may increase the blood levels of Eskalith and Lithobid. The drug may cause irregular heartbeat when used with Lanoxin, Quinidex, or Quinaglute. The drug should not be used with Nardil or Parnate.

ALLERGIES: Individuals allergic to reserpine, hydrochlorothiazide, sulfa drugs, or any of their derivatives should discuss this with their doctor or pharmacist before using this drug.

PREGNANCY/BREAST-FEEDING: Category C—Risk cannot be ruled out. Human studies are lacking, and animal studies are either positive for fetal risk or lacking as well. However, potential benefits may justify the potential risk in using the drug. The drug is excreted in the breast milk; therefore, extreme caution should be used when breast-feeding.

OTHER BRAND NAMES: None

OTHER DRUGS IN THE SAME THERAPEUTIC CLASS: Diupres, Enduronyl, and Esimil

IMPORTANT INFORMATION TO REMEMBER: This drug may cause some limited drowsiness. Individuals should use caution when driving, operating machinery, or any task where mental alertness is required. Alcohol, anxiety medications, and narcotic painkillers may intensify the drowsiness effect of the drug. The drug may also cause dizziness when suddenly rising from a sitting or lying-down position. If depression or sleep changes occur, notify your doctor immediately. The drug should be taken with food or milk to reduce the chances of stomach upset. If the drug is to be taken once daily, take it in the morning due to increased urine output. Before taking over-the-counter cold and allergy preparations, consult your doctor or pharmacist; these products may raise your blood pressure. The drug may cause the elimination of potassium from the body. It is therefore a good idea to eat a banana or drink orange, grapefruit, or apple juice every day to replace lost potassium. This drug may also increase the sensitivity of the skin to sunburn in some individuals; therefore, a sunscreen is recommended during periods of prolonged exposure to the sun.

BRAND NAME: Hygroton

GENERIC NAME: chlorthalidone

GENERIC FORM AVAILABLE: Yes

THERAPEUTIC CLASS: Thiazide diuretic (water pill)

DOSAGE FORMS: 25-mg, 50-mg, and 100-mg tablets

MAIN USES: High blood pressure and water retention (fluid retention due to congestive heart failure, kidney disease, or cirrhosis of the liver)

USUAL DOSE: 25 mg to 100 mg daily or 100 mg every other day

AVERAGE PRICE: $86.88 (B)/$10.76 (G) for 25 mg; $107.11 (B)/ $14.27 (G) for 50 mg; 179.06 (B)/$17.56 (G) for 100 mg

SIDE EFFECTS: Most common: low potassium, dry mouth, muscle cramps, increased thirst, weakness, nausea, and vomiting. Less common: loss of appetite, constipation, diarrhea, decreased sexual ability, high blood sugar, dizziness, and increased sensitivity to sunburn.

DRUG INTERACTIONS: The drug may require dosage adjustments to diabetic and gout medications. Colestid and Questran may decrease the absorption of the drug. The drug may increase the blood levels of Eskalith and Lithobid.

ALLERGIES: Individuals allergic to chlorthalidone or any of its derivatives should discuss this with their doctor or pharmacist before using this drug.

PREGNANCY/BREAST-FEEDING: Category B—No evidence of risk in humans. Either animal findings show risk, but human findings do not; or, if no adequate human studies have been done, animal findings show no risk. The drug is excreted in the breast milk; therefore, extreme caution should be used when breast-feeding.

OTHER BRAND NAMES: None

OTHER DRUGS IN THE SAME THERAPEUTIC CLASS: Diuril, Enduron, HydroDIURIL, and Hydromox

IMPORTANT INFORMATION TO REMEMBER: If the drug is to be taken once daily, take it in the morning due to increased urine output. Before taking over-the-counter cold and allergy preparations, consult your doctor or pharmacist; these products may raise your blood pressure. The drug may cause the elimination of potassium from the body. It is therefore a good idea to eat a banana or drink orange, grapefruit, or apple juice every day to replace lost potassium. This drug may also increase the sensitivity of the skin to sunburn in some individuals; therefore, a sunscreen is recommended during periods of prolonged exposure to the sun. Individuals with kidney disease should discuss this with their doctor before taking this drug.

BRAND NAME: **Hytone**

GENERIC NAME: hydrocortisone

GENERIC FORM AVAILABLE: Yes

THERAPEUTIC CLASS: Topical corticosteroid

DOSAGE FORMS: 1% and 2.5% cream, ointment, or lotion

MAIN USES: Skin rashes, swelling, and itching

USUAL DOSE: Apply thin film two to four times daily.

AVERAGE PRICE: $17.58 (B)/$8.78 (G) for 1% cream and ointment (30 g) and $28.58 (B)/$10.98 (G) for 2.5% cream and ointment (30 g)

SIDE EFFECTS: Most common: none. Less common: burning, itching, irritation, dry skin, rash, soreness of the skin, and acne.

DRUG INTERACTIONS: None of any clinical significance

ALLERGIES: Individuals allergic to hydrocortisone or any of its derivatives should discuss this with their doctor or pharmacist before using this drug.

PREGNANCY/BREAST-FEEDING: Category C—Risk cannot be ruled out. Human studies are lacking, and animal studies are either positive for fetal risk or lacking as well. However, potential benefits may justify the potential risk in using the drug. It is not known whether the drug is excreted in the breast milk; therefore, caution should be used when breast-feeding.

OTHER BRAND NAMES: Nutracort

OTHER DRUGS IN THE SAME THERAPEUTIC CLASS: Aclovate, Aristocort, Cordran, Cordran SP, Cutivate, Cyclocort, DesOwen, Diprolene, Diprolene AF, Elocon, Florone, Halog, Kenalog, Lidex, Synalar, Temovate, Topicort, Tridesilon, Ultravate, Valisone, and Westcort

IMPORTANT INFORMATION TO REMEMBER: This drug is for external use only. Apply only a thin film of drug to skin and rub it in well. Never cover the skin after application with a bandage or wrapping unless directed to do so by a doctor. Never apply to damaged skin or open wounds unless directed to do so by a doctor. Discontinue use if irritation occurs. If using the lotion, be sure to shake it well. Hydrocortisone cream 1% is available over-the-counter without a prescription.

<u>BRAND NAME:</u> **Hytrin**

GENERIC NAME: terazosin

GENERIC FORM AVAILABLE: Yes

THERAPEUTIC CLASS: Selective alpha-1-blood-vessel dilator

DOSAGE FORMS: 1-mg, 2-mg, 5-mg, and 10-mg capsules

MAIN USES: High blood pressure and benign prostatic hyperplasia (BPH)

USUAL DOSE: 1 mg to 10 mg once daily, usually at bedtime

AVERAGE PRICE: $167.78 for 1 mg; $178.41 for 2 mg; $184.54 for 5 mg; and $189.72 for 10 mg

SIDE EFFECTS: dizziness 9%–19%, weakness 7%–11%, headache 5%–16%, drowsiness 4%–5%, stuffy nose 2%–6%, nausea 2%–4%, trouble breathing 2%–3%, nervousness 2%, blurred vision 2%, swelling in legs 1%–6%, low blood pressure after lying down or sitting 1%–4%, pounding heartbeat 1%–4%, impotence 1%, and low blood pressure 1%.

DRUG INTERACTIONS: Caution should be used when taken with other drugs for high blood pressure; the combination may cause blood pressure to go too low.

ALLERGIES: Individuals allergic to terazosin or any of its derivatives should discuss this with their doctor or pharmacist before using this drug.

PREGNANCY/BREAST-FEEDING: Category C—Risk cannot be ruled out. Human studies are lacking, and animal studies are either positive for fetal risk or lacking as well. However, potential benefits may justify the potential risk in using the drug. It is not known whether the drug is excreted in the breast milk; therefore, caution should be used when breast-feeding.

OTHER BRAND NAMES: None

OTHER DRUGS IN THE SAME THERAPEUTIC CLASS: Cardura and Minipress

IMPORTANT INFORMATION TO REMEMBER: The first dose should be taken at bedtime to avoid dizziness and fainting. Only take the drug exactly as directed by your physician. Do not discontinue the drug without first consulting your physician. Before taking over-the-counter cold and allergy preparations, consult your doctor or pharmacist; these products may raise your blood pressure. This drug may cause some drowsiness at first. Individuals should use caution when driving, operating machinery, or any task where mental alertness is required. Individuals should get up slowly from the sitting or lying-down position; otherwise dizziness may occur.

BRAND NAME: Hyzaar

GENERIC NAME: Combination product containing: losartan and hydrochlorothiazide

See individuals entries for Cozaar and HydroDIURIL

BRAND NAME: Iletin Insulin

GENERIC NAME: insulin (beef/pork mixture)

GENERIC FORM AVAILABLE: No

THERAPEUTIC CLASS: Insulin replacement

DOSAGE FORMS: Regular, Semilente, Lente, Ultralente, NPH, and Protamine Zinc

MAIN USES: Diabetes

USUAL DOSE: varies by patient

AVERAGE PRICE: $23.53 for 10-mL bottle

SIDE EFFECTS: Most common: none. Less common: low blood sugar and allergic reaction (characterized by redness, swelling, and itching at the injection site).

DRUG INTERACTIONS: Alcohol, Aristocort, Blocadren, Cartrol, Corgard, Decadron, Deltasone, Inderal, Kerlone, Levatol, Lopressor, Medrol, Normodyne, prednisone, Sectral, Tenormin, Toprol-XL, Trandate, Visken, Zebeta, smoking, and diuretics (water pills) may cause changes in blood sugar.

ALLERGIES: Individuals allergic to beef/pork mixture insulins or any of its derivatives should discuss this with their doctor or pharmacist before using this drug.

PREGNANCY/BREAST-FEEDING: Category B—No evidence of risk in humans. Either animal findings show risk, but human findings do not; or, if no adequate human studies have been done, animal findings show no risk. It is not known whether the drug is excreted in the breast milk; therefore, caution should be used when breast-feeding.

OTHER BRAND NAMES: None

OTHER DRUGS IN THE SAME THERAPEUTIC CLASS: Humalog, Humulin, Novolin, Velosulin

IMPORTANT INFORMATION TO REMEMBER: It's important to follow a prescribed diet carefully even when using insulin. Do not change insulin brands without first discussing this with your doctor or pharmacist. Do not change the order of mixing insulins as prescribed by your doctor. It's important to continue to monitor blood sugar levels at regular intervals as prescribed by your doctor. Bottles of insulin that are not being used should be stored in the refrigerator. Before using a bottle of insulin, roll the bottle gently in your hands. Do not vigorously shake the bottle. If the insulin appears grainy or lumpy or sticks to the bottle, do not use it. Individuals should be aware of the signs and symptoms of both high and low blood sugar and know what action to take. Before taking over-the-counter medications, consult with your doctor or pharmacist; some over-the-counter medications may affect your blood sugar.

BRAND NAME: Ilosone

GENERIC NAME: erythromycin estolate

GENERIC FORM AVAILABLE: Yes

THERAPEUTIC CLASS: Macrolide antibiotic

DOSAGE FORMS: 250-mg capsules, 500-mg tablets, and 125 mg/5 mL and 250 mg/5 mL suspension

MAIN USES: Bacterial infections

USUAL DOSE: 250 mg to 500 mg every six hours. Doses for children may be less.

AVERAGE PRICE: $24.21 (B)/$15.67 (G) for 250 mg (30 capsules) and $41.31 (brand only) for 500 mg (30 tablets)

SIDE EFFECTS: Most common: nausea, vomiting, itching, stomach pain, diarrhea, rash, allergic reactions, and appetite changes. Less common: dizziness, headache, abnormal taste, and confusion.

DRUG INTERACTIONS: *Warning:* This drug should not be used with Seldane, Seldane-D, or Hismanal—the drug may increase the blood levels of these drugs to extremely toxic and possibly life-threatening levels. The drug may also increase the blood levels of Coumadin, Retrovir, rifabution, Sandimmune, Slo-bid, Theo-Dur, theophylline, Uni-Dur, Uniphyl, and Tegretol. Propulsid and the drug may cause dangerous irregular heartbeats when taken together.

ALLERGIES: Individuals allergic to erythromycin or other macrolide antibiotics (such as those listed in "Other Drugs in the Same Therapeutic Class") should discuss this with their doctor or pharmacist before taking this drug.

PREGNANCY/BREAST-FEEDING: Category B—No evidence of risk in humans. Either animal findings show risk, but human findings do not; or, if no adequate human studies have been done, animal findings show no risk. The drug is excreted in the breast milk; therefore, extreme caution should be used when breast-feeding.

OTHER BRAND NAMES: None

OTHER DRUGS IN THE SAME THERAPEUTIC CLASS: Biaxin, Dynabac, E.E.S., E-Mycin, ERY-TAB, ERYC, EryPed, Erythrocin, PCE, Pediazole, TAO, and Zithromax

IMPORTANT INFORMATION TO REMEMBER: *Warning:* This drug has caused liver problems in some individuals, mostly in adults. This has made the drug somewhat unpopular. Caution should be used when taking this drug. Individuals with liver disorders should never use this drug. If stomach upset occurs, take the drug with food or milk. Also, take the drug at even intervals around the clock (if four times a day, take very six hours). Take the drug until all the medication prescribed is gone; otherwise the infection may return. Individuals taking the liquid form should shake it thoroughly before use and store the medication in the refrigerator. If severe diarrhea occurs while taking the drug, notify your doctor immediately. Never take the drug with Seldane, Seldane-D, or Hismanal (see "Drug Interactions").

BRAND NAME: Imdur

GENERIC NAME: isosorbide mononitrate

GENERIC FORM AVAILABLE: No

THERAPEUTIC CLASS: Nitrate anti-anginal

DOSAGE FORMS: 30-mg, 60-mg, and 120-mg extended-release tablets

MAIN USES: Prevention of angina

USUAL DOSE: 60 mg to 120 mg once daily

AVERAGE PRICE: $123.47 for 30 mg; $144.90 for 60 mg; and $202.86 for 120 mg

SIDE EFFECTS: headache 38%–57% and dizziness 8%–11% are the most common. Less common: flushing, restlessness, weakness, nausea, vomiting, and sweating.

DRUG INTERACTIONS: Alcohol and the drug may produce low blood pressure. Apresoline, Loniten, or Vasodilan and the drug may also produce low blood pressure.

ALLERGIES: Individuals allergic to isosorbide mononitrate or other nitrates (such as those listed in "Other Drugs in the Same Therapeutic Class") should discuss this with their doctor or pharmacist before taking this drug.

PREGNANCY/BREAST-FEEDING: Category B—No evidence of risk in humans. Either animal findings show risk, but human findings do not; or, if no adequate human studies have been done, animal findings show no risk. It is not known whether the drug is excreted in the breast milk; therefore, caution should be used when breast-feeding.

OTHER BRAND NAMES: None

OTHER DRUGS IN THE SAME THERAPEUTIC CLASS: Dilatrate-SR, Ismo, Isordil, Monoket, and Sorbitrate

IMPORTANT INFORMATION TO REMEMBER: This drug does not relieve angina attacks—it only prevents them. Only take the drug exactly as directly by your physician. Do not discontinue the drug or increase the dose without first consulting your physician. Do not crush tablets—this will destroy the mechanism that delays the release of the medication. Tablets may, however, be cut in half for easier swallowing. Do not drink alcohol while taking this drug. The headache that is common with this drug usually goes away with continued use. If it does not, contact your doctor. Before taking over-the-counter cold and allergy preparations, consult your doctor or pharmacist.

BRAND NAME: Imitrex

GENERIC NAME: sumatriptan

GENERIC FORM AVAILABLE: No

THERAPEUTIC CLASS: Anti-migraine

DOSAGE FORMS: 6 mg/0.5 mL subcutaneous injection, and 25-mg and 50-mg tablets

MAIN USES: Migraines

USUAL DOSE: For the injection: one 6 mg/0.5 mL subcutaneous injection. Another injection may be used in one hour if the first one provides some, but not complete, relief. For the tablets: 25 mg at the onset of migraine, with an additional dose of up to 100 mg two hours later if the headache is not relieved.

AVERAGE PRICE: $98.03 for injection kit; $135.32 for 25 mg (nine tablets); and $153.46 for 50 mg (nine tablets)

SIDE EFFECTS: injection site reaction (redness, swelling, itching, etc.) 59%, abnormal sensations 42%, tingling 14%, dizziness 12%, warm sensations 11%, burning sensations 8%, pressure sensations 7%, flushing 7%, discomfort of the mouth/tongue 5%, weakness 5%, neck pain 5%, numbness 5%, chest discomfort 5%, throat discomfort 3%, drowsiness 3%, feeling of tightness in the chest 3%, nasal discomfort 2%, pressure in chest 2%, feeling strange 2%, jaw discomfort 2%, muscle pain 2%, cold sensation 1%, blurred vision 1%, and stomach discomfort 1%.

DRUG INTERACTIONS: Bellergal-S, Cafergot, ergotamine, Hydergine, and Wigraine should not be used within 24 hours after using this drug. Nardil or Parnate should not be taken with this drug.

ALLERGIES: Individuals allergic to sumatriptan or any of its derivatives should discuss this with their doctor or pharmacist before using this drug.

PREGNANCY/BREAST-FEEDING: Category C—Risk cannot be ruled out. Human studies are lacking, and animal studies are either positive for fetal risk or lacking as well. However, potential benefits may justify the potential risk in using the drug. The drug is excreted in the breast milk; therefore, extreme caution should be used when breast-feeding.

OTHER BRAND NAMES: None

OTHER DRUGS IN THE SAME THERAPEUTIC CLASS: None

IMPORTANT INFORMATION TO REMEMBER: Patients with high blood pressure, heart disease, or other cardiovascular problems should discuss this with their physician before using this drug. This drug may cause some drowsiness. Individuals should use caution when driving, operating machinery, or any task where mental alertness is required. Alcohol, anxiety medications, and narcotic painkillers may intensify the drowsiness effect of the drug. It is important to take the drug at the first sign of a migraine. Only take the drug exactly as directed by your physician and do not increase the dose without first consulting with your physician—using more than the prescribed amount can be very dangerous. The tablets must be swallowed whole. If the first dose does not provide substantial relief, additional doses are not likely to be effective for that attack. Additional doses should only be used for the return of a migraine after initial relief was obtained, and only if directed to do so by your physician.

BRAND NAME: Imodium

GENERIC NAME: loperamide

GENERIC FORM AVAILABLE: Yes

THERAPEUTIC CLASS: Antidiarrheal

DOSAGE FORMS: 2-mg capsules

MAIN USES: Diarrhea

USUAL DOSE: For acute (short-term) diarrhea: 4 mg initially, then 2 mg after each unformed stool, with a maximum daily dose of 16 mg. For chronic (long-term) diarrhea: 4 mg to 8 mg daily in divided doses.

AVERAGE PRICE: $85.76 (B)/$45.91 (G)

SIDE EFFECTS: Most common: none. Less common: drowsiness, dizziness, constipation, stomach pain, nausea, vomiting, allergic reactions, and dry mouth.

DRUG INTERACTIONS: Narcotic painkillers may increase the risk of constipation.

ALLERGIES: Individuals allergic to loperamide or any of its derivatives should discuss this with their doctor or pharmacist before using this drug.

PREGNANCY/BREAST-FEEDING: Category B—No evidence of risk in humans. Either animal findings show risk, but human findings do not; or, if no adequate human studies have been done, animal findings show no risk. It is not known whether the drug is excreted in the breast milk; therefore, caution should be used when breast-feeding.

OTHER BRAND NAMES: None

OTHER DRUGS IN THE SAME THERAPEUTIC CLASS: Lomotil

IMPORTANT INFORMATION TO REMEMBER: This drug may cause some limited drowsiness. Individuals should use caution when driving, operating machinery, or any task where mental alertness is required. Alcohol, anxiety medications, and narcotic painkillers may intensify the drowsiness effect of the drug. Contact your physician if the diarrhea is not controlled within 48 hours of the start of treatment. Drink plenty of liquids to avoid the dehydration that may occur due to the diarrhea. Do not increase the dose without first consulting with your physician. This drug is also available over-the-counter in the same 2mg strength.

BRAND NAME: Imuran

GENERIC NAME: azathioprine

GENERIC FORM AVAILABLE: Yes

THERAPEUTIC CLASS: Immune suppressant

DOSAGE FORMS: 50-mg tablets

MAIN USES: Arthritis and prevention of organ transplant rejection

USUAL DOSE: 50 mg to 100 mg per day in one or two doses

AVERAGE PRICE: $165.04 (B)/$131.95 (G)

SIDE EFFECTS: Most common: blood disorders, infections, anemia, loss of appetite, nausea, and vomiting. Less common: hepatitis, thrombocytopenia, black and tarry stools, blood in the urine, skin rash, and pinpoint red spots on the skin.

DRUG INTERACTIONS: Zyloprim (allopurinol) may increase the blood levels of the drug to three to four times the normal amount. Accupril, Altace, Capoten, Lotensin, Monopril, Prinivil, Univasc,

Vasotec, or Zestril and the drug, when taken together, may cause severe blood disorders. The drug may inhibit the effects of Coumadin.

ALLERGIES: Individuals allergic to azathioprine or any of its derivatives should discuss this with their doctor or pharmacist before using this drug.

PREGNANCY/BREAST-FEEDING: Category D—Positive evidence of risk. Human studies show risk to the fetus. Nevertheless, potential benefits may possibly outweigh the potential risks. This drug should not be taken by nursing mothers.

OTHER BRAND NAMES: None

OTHER DRUGS IN THE SAME THERAPEUTIC CLASS: None

IMPORTANT INFORMATION TO REMEMBER: Only take the drug exactly as directed by your physician. If stomach upset occurs, take the drug with food or milk. When used long-term, the drug may increase the risk of cancer. Individuals taking this drug need to be monitored very closely by their doctor for blood disorders. Patients should avoid immunizations, such as flu and pneumonia vaccines, while taking this drug. If any of the following symptoms occur during therapy—aches; flu-like symptoms; soreness of the mouth, gums, or throat; black, tarry stools; blood in the urine; sore joints; pinpoint red spots on the skin; or any unusual bleeding or bruising—contact your doctor immediately. The drug may take up to three months before benefits are seen in arthritis.

BRAND NAME: Inderal and Inderal LA

GENERIC NAME: propranolol

GENERIC FORM AVAILABLE: Yes

THERAPEUTIC CLASS: Noncardioselective beta-blocker

DOSAGE FORMS: 10-mg, 20-mg, 40-mg, 60-mg, and 80-mg tablets; and 60-mg, 80-mg, 120-mg, and 160-mg sustained-release capsules

MAIN USES: High blood pressure, irregular heartbeat, angina, after heart attacks, and migraines

USUAL DOSE: 30 mg to 240 mg daily in single or divided doses

AVERAGE PRICE: $36.39 (B)/$12.41 (G) for 10 mg; $45.98 (B)/$14.72 (G) for 20 mg; $69.94 (B)/$15.71 (G) for 40 mg; $91.17 (B)/$16.48 (G) for 60 mg; $102.17 (B)/$18.46 (G) for 80 mg; $93.99 (B)/$52.89 (G) for 60 mg (Inderal LA); $109.87 (B)/$57.29 (G) for 80 mg (Inderal LA); $142.28 (B)/$68.07 (G) for 120 mg (Inderal LA); $173.89 (B)/$96.78 (G) for 160 mg (Inderal LA)

SIDE EFFECTS: Most common: decreased sexual ability, drowsiness, trouble sleeping, and unusual tiredness or weakness. Less common: slow heart rate, dizziness, difficulty breathing, congestive heart failure, cold hands and feet, nervousness, diarrhea, constipation, nausea, vomiting, stomach discomfort, and depression.

DRUG INTERACTIONS: The drug may cause additive effects when used with reserpine. The drug may increase the effects of Calan, Cardene, Cardizem, Catapres, Dilacor XR, DynaCirc, Isoptin, Lanoxin, Norvasc, Plendil, Procardia, Sular, Tiazac, Verelan, and Wytensin. Diabetic medications, insulin, Slo-bid, Theo-Dur, theophylline, Uni-Dur, and Uniphyl dosages may need to be adjusted when taking this drug. The drug may also interfere with glaucoma screening tests. Tagamet and Thorazine may increase the blood levels of the drug Antacids and alcohol may decrease the absorption of the drug. Dilantin may decrease the blood levels of the drug.

ALLERGIES: Individuals allergic to propranolol or other beta-blockers (such as those listed in "Other Drugs in the Same Therapeutic Class") should discuss this with their doctor or pharmacist before taking this drug.

PREGNANCY/BREAST-FEEDING: Category C—Risk cannot be ruled out. Human studies are lacking, and animal studies are either positive for fetal risk or lacking as well. However, potential benefits may justify the potential risk in using the drug. The drug is excreted in the breast milk; therefore, extreme caution should be used when breast-feeding.

OTHER BRAND NAMES: None

OTHER DRUGS IN THE SAME THERAPEUTIC CLASS: Blocadren, Cartrol, Corgard, Levatol, Normodyne, Trandate, and Visken

IMPORTANT INFORMATION TO REMEMBER: Only take the drug exactly as directed by your physician. Do not discontinue the drug without first consulting your physician. This drug may cause some tiredness, especially at first. Individuals should use caution when driving, operating machinery, or any task where mental alertness is required. Alcohol, anxiety medications, or narcotic painkillers may intensify the tiredness effect of the drug. Before taking over-the-counter cold and allergy preparations, consult your doctor or pharmacist—these products may raise your blood pressure. This drug may mask the symptoms of low blood sugar in diabetics.

BRAND NAME: Inderide and Inderide LA

GENERIC NAME: Combination product containing: propranolol and hydrochlorothiazide

See individual entries for Inderal/Inderal LA and HydroDIURIL

BRAND NAME: Indocin

GENERIC NAME: indomethacin

GENERIC FORM AVAILABLE: Yes

THERAPEUTIC CLASS: Nonsteroidal anti-inflammatory drug (NSAID)

DOSAGE FORMS: 25-mg and 50-mg capsules; 75-mg sustained-release capsules; 50-mg suppositories; and 25 mg/5 mL suspension

MAIN USES: Arthritis and {general pain relief}

USUAL DOSE: 25 mg to 50 mg three times daily or 75 mg twice daily

AVERAGE PRICE: $63.12 (B)/$19.23 (G) for 25 mg; $111.07 (B)/$36.27 (G) for 50 mg; $177.07 (B)/$97.87 (G) for 75 mg (Indocin SR)

SIDE EFFECTS: headache 12%, nausea 3%–9%, dizziness 3%–9%, indigestion 3%–9%, heartburn 3%–9%, vomiting 1%–3%, diarrhea 1%–3%, stomach pain 1%–3%, drowsiness 1%–3%, dizziness 1%–3%, tiredness 1%–3%, constipation 1%–3%, and ringing in the ears 1%–3%.

DRUG INTERACTIONS: Aspirin will decrease the concentration of this drug in the blood. This drug may also decrease the effects of Lasix, Dyazide, HydroDIURIL, Maxzide, and other water pills. The drug may increase the blood levels of Eskalith, Lithobid, and Sandimmune. The drug may increase the toxic effects of the drug Rheumatrex. Caution should be used when taking the drug with

Coumadin. Dolobid and the drug should not be used at the same time. The drug increases the blood levels of Retrovir.

ALLERGIES: Individuals allergic to indomethacin or other NSAIDs (such as those listed in "Other Drugs in the Same Therapeutic Class") should discuss this with their doctor or pharmacist before taking this drug.

PREGNANCY/BREAST-FEEDING: Category B—No evidence of risk in humans. Either animal findings show risk, but human findings do not; or, if no adequate human studies have been done, animal findings show no risk. The drug should not, however, be used during the late stages (last three months) of pregnancy. The drug is excreted in the breast milk; therefore, extreme caution should be used when breast-feeding.

OTHER BRAND NAMES: None

OTHER DRUGS IN THE SAME THERAPEUTIC CLASS: Anaprox, Ansaid, aspirin, Cataflam, Clinoril, Daypro, Disalcid, Dolobid, Easprin, Feldene, Lodine, Lodine XL, Motrin, Nalfon, Naprosyn, Orudis, Oruvail, Relafen, Tolectin, Toradol, Voltaren, and Voltaren XR

IMPORTANT INFORMATION TO REMEMBER: This drug should be taken with food or milk to reduce the potential for injury to the stomach lining and stomach upset. This drug may take up to two weeks before a noticeable improvement in pain relief associated with arthritis is observed. Drinking alcohol while taking this drug may increase its potential to cause ulcers. This drug should only be used under the direct supervision of a doctor by individuals with a bleeding disorder or ulcer, or those who are currently taking Coumadin. Before taking over-the-counter pain relievers, consult your doctor or pharmacist. No more than one pain reliever should be taken at any one time unless directed by your doctor.

BRAND NAME: Inflamase Mild and Inflamase Forte

GENERIC NAME: prednisolone sodium phosphate

GENERIC FORM AVAILABLE: Yes

THERAPEUTIC CLASS: Steroid eyedrop

DOSAGE FORMS: 1% eyedrop solution (Forte) and 1/8% eyedrop solution (Mild)

MAIN USES: Inflammation of the eye

USUAL DOSE: one or two drops three to six times daily

AVERAGE PRICE: $19.16 (B)/$11.24 (G) for Inflamase Mild (5 mL) and $31.31 (B)/$16.32 (G) for Inflamase Forte (10 mL)

SIDE EFFECTS: Most common: temporary, mild blurred vision. Less common: burning, itching, redness, watering of the eyes, and eye pain.

DRUG INTERACTIONS: The drug may decrease the effects of other eyedrops used to treat glaucoma.

ALLERGIES: Individuals allergic to prednisolone sodium phosphate or any of its derivatives should discuss this with their doctor or pharmacist before using this drug.

PREGNANCY/BREAST-FEEDING: Category C—Risk cannot be ruled out. Human studies are lacking, and animal studies are either positive for fetal risk or lacking as well. However, potential benefits may justify the potential risk in using the drug. It is not known whether the drug is excreted in the breast milk; therefore, caution should be used when breast-feeding.

OTHER BRAND NAMES: None

OTHER DRUGS IN THE SAME THERAPEUTIC CLASS: Decadron, Econopred, Flarex, FML, FML Forte, HMS, Maxidex, Pred Mild, Pred Forte, and Vexol

IMPORTANT INFORMATION TO REMEMBER: Individuals should not use the drug while wearing contact lenses unless directed otherwise by a physician. Keep the container tightly closed and avoid touching the applicator tip to the eye—this could contaminate the product over time. Also, only administer one drop at a time. After application, keep the eye open for at least 30 seconds, roll the eyeball around, and avoid squinting. If a second drop is required, wait one to two minutes between drops. If another medication is to be used in the eye, wait at least 10 minutes before administering it.

BRAND NAME: Insulin

GENERIC NAME: insulin

See entries for Humulin Insulin and Iletin Insulin

BRAND NAME: Intal

GENERIC NAME: cromolyn sodium

GENERIC FORM AVAILABLE: Yes (ampule solution only)

THERAPEUTIC CLASS: Asthma preventative

DOSAGE FORMS: 20 mg/2 mL ampule solution for a nebulizer; and 800-micrograms-per-spray metered-dose inhaler

MAIN USES: Asthma and prevention of bronchospasms

USUAL DOSE: Inhaler: two sprays inhaled four times a day. Nebulizer solution: one ampule administered via a nebulizer four times a day. Capsules: contents of one capsule inhaled via a Spinhaler four times a day.

AVERAGE PRICE: $67.55 (B)/$61.91 (G) for 60 ampules of solution and $55.30 for 100-spray inhaler.

SIDE EFFECTS: Most common: cough, dry mouth, dry throat, nausea, stuffy nose, unpleasant taste, and throat irritation. Less common: hoarseness, watering of the eyes, muscle pain, and weakness.

DRUG INTERACTIONS: This drug and Isuprel should not be used together during pregnancy.

ALLERGIES: Individuals allergic to cromolyn sodium or any of its derivatives should discuss this with their doctor or pharmacist before using this drug.

PREGNANCY/BREAST-FEEDING: Category B—No evidence of risk in humans. Either animal findings show risk, but human findings do not; or, if no adequate human studies have been done, animal findings show no risk. It is not known whether the drug is excreted in the breast milk; therefore, caution should be used when breast-feeding.

OTHER BRAND NAMES: None

OTHER DRUGS IN THE SAME THERAPEUTIC CLASS: None

IMPORTANT INFORMATION TO REMEMBER: The drug is not intended to provide immediate relief of a bronchospasm, shortness of breath, or an asthma attack; it is used only for prevention of attacks. To receive the full benefits of the drug, use it on a regular basis as a maintenance medication. The drug may take up to four weeks before noticeable benefits may be seen. Never exceed the prescribed dosage unless directed to do so by a physician; excessive use beyond prescribed dosage is potentially dangerous. If another inhaler is also being used at the same time, use the other one a few minutes prior to using Intal. Do not swallow the Intal capsules for use in the Spinhaler.

When using the inhaler, use the following procedure:

1) Shake the canister well.
2) Place the mouthpiece close to the mouth, but not touching the lips.
3) Exhale deeply.
4) Inhale slowly and deeply as you press the top of the canister to release the medication.
5) Hold your breath for a few seconds before exhaling.
6) Wait five minutes between puffs.
7) Rinse your mouth out with water after use.
8) Be sure to wash the inhaler device (mouthpiece) regularly with warm soapy water to avoid bacterial contamination.

BRAND NAME: Invirase

GENERIC NAME: saquinavir

GENERIC FORM AVAILABLE: No

THERAPEUTIC CLASS: Protease inhibitor

DOSAGE FORMS: 200-mg capsules

MAIN USES: AIDS

USUAL DOSE: 600 mg three times daily

AVERAGE PRICE: $296.62

SIDE EFFECTS: diarrhea 4%, mouth sores 3%, stomach pain 2%, nausea 2%, headache 1%, numbness 1%, weakness 1%, rash 1%, muscle pain 1%, and stomach discomfort 1%.

DRUG INTERACTIONS: Dilantin, Mycobutin, phenobarbital, Rifadin, Rimactine, and Tegretol may decrease the blood levels of the drug. The drug may increase the blood levels of Calan, Cardene, Cardizem, Catapres, Dilacor XR, DynaCirc, Halcion, Isoptin, Norvasc, Plendil, Procardia, Quinidex, Quinaglute, Sular, Tiazac, and Verelan. Nizoral may increase the blood levels of the drug. The drug should never be used with Hismanal, Seldane, or Seldane-D.

ALLERGIES: Individuals allergic to saquinavir or any of its derivatives should discuss this with their doctor or pharmacist before using this drug.

PREGNANCY/BREAST-FEEDING: Category B—No evidence of risk in humans. Either animal findings show risk, but human findings do not; or, if no adequate human studies have been done, animal findings show no risk. It is not known whether the drug is excreted in the breast milk; therefore, caution should be used when breast-feeding.

OTHER BRAND NAMES: None

OTHER DRUGS IN THE SAME THERAPEUTIC CLASS: Crixivan and Norvir

IMPORTANT INFORMATION TO REMEMBER: The drug should always be taken within two hours of a full meal. Never take the drug on an empty stomach; food increases the absorption of the drug. Also, take the drug at even intervals around the clock (if three times a day, take every eight hours). Only take the drug exactly as directed by your physician. Do not stop taking the drug without first consulting with your physician. It is important to have regular blood and liver function tests while taking this drug. Before taking any prescription or over-the-counter drugs, consult your physician or pharmacist.

BRAND NAME: Iopidine

GENERIC NAME: apraclonidine

GENERIC FORM AVAILABLE: No

THERAPEUTIC CLASS: Anti-glaucoma

DOSAGE FORMS: 0.5% eyedrop solution

MAIN USES: Glaucoma

USUAL DOSE: one to two drops three times daily

AVERAGE PRICE: $49.43 for 5 mL

SIDE EFFECTS: Most common: dryness of mouth, eye discomfort, allergic reactions, redness, itching, and tearing of the eye. Less common: paleness of the eyelid, crusting of the eyelid, nausea, nervousness, increased sensitivity of the eye to sunlight, runny nose, drowsiness, feeling of a foreign body in the eye, headache, and insomnia.

DRUG INTERACTIONS: The drug should not be used with Nardil or Parnate.

ALLERGIES: Individuals allergic to apraclonidine, Catapres, clonidine, or any of their derivatives should discuss this with their doctor or pharmacist before using this drug.

PREGNANCY/BREAST-FEEDING: Category C—Risk cannot be ruled out. Human studies are lacking, and animal studies are either positive for fetal risk or lacking as well. However, potential benefits may justify the potential risk in using the drug. It is not known whether the drug is excreted in the breast milk; therefore, caution should be used when breast-feeding.

OTHER BRAND NAMES: None

OTHER DRUGS IN THE SAME THERAPEUTIC CLASS: Alphagan

IMPORTANT INFORMATION TO REMEMBER: This drug may cause some limited drowsiness. Individuals should use caution when driving, operating machinery, or any task where mental alertness is required. Alcohol, anxiety medications, and narcotic painkillers may intensify the drowsiness effect of the drug. Keep the container tightly closed and avoid touching the applicator tip to the eye—this could contaminate the product over time. Also, only administer one drop at a time. After application, keep the eye open for at least 30 seconds, roll the eyeball around, and avoid squinting. If a second drop is required, wait one to two minutes between drops. If another medication is to be used in the eye, wait at least 10 minutes before administering it. Only use the drug exactly as directly by your physician. Do not discontinue the drug without first consulting your physician. Keep the bottle out of the light.

BRAND NAME: Ismelin

GENERIC NAME: guanethidine

GENERIC FORM AVAILABLE: No

THERAPEUTIC CLASS: Centrally acting blood vessel dilator

DOSAGE FORMS: 10-mg and 25-mg tablets

MAIN USES: High blood pressure

USUAL DOSE: 10 mg to 50 mg daily

AVERAGE PRICE: $72.32 for 10 mg and $118.18 for 25 mg

SIDE EFFECTS: Most common: swelling of the feet and legs, slow heartbeat, diarrhea, increased bowel movements, difficulty in ejaculating, stuffy nose, low blood pressure, dizziness, lightheadedness, and weakness. Less common: blurred vision, drooping eyelids, dry mouth, headaches, loss of hair, drowsiness, confusion, constipation, muscle pain, tremors, nausea, vomiting, nighttime urination, chest pain, and shortness of breath.

DRUG INTERACTIONS: Drugs used to treat depression, Loxitane, Navane, and Temaril may decrease the effects of the drug. Minoxidil and the drug may cause low blood pressure. Nardil or Parnate and the drug may cause severe high blood pressure. Medications used to treat diabetes, including insulin, and the drug may cause low blood sugar.

ALLERGIES: Individuals allergic to guanethidine or any of its derivatives should discuss this with their doctor or pharmacist before using this drug.

PREGNANCY/BREAST-FEEDING: Category C—Risk cannot be ruled out. Human studies are lacking, and animal studies are either positive for fetal risk or lacking as well. However, potential benefits may justify the potential risk in using the drug. The drug is excreted in the breast milk; therefore, extreme caution should be used when breast-feeding.

OTHER BRAND NAMES: None

OTHER DRUGS IN THE SAME THERAPEUTIC CLASS: reserpine

IMPORTANT INFORMATION TO REMEMBER: Only take the drug exactly as directed by your physician. Do not discontinue the drug without first consulting your physician. Before taking over-the-counter cold and allergy preparations, consult your doctor or pharmacist—these products may raise your blood pressure. This drug may cause some drowsiness at first. Individuals should use caution when driving, operating machinery, or any task where mental alertness is required. Individuals should get up slowly from the sitting or lying-down position; otherwise dizziness may occur.

BRAND NAME: Ismo

GENERIC NAME: isosorbide mononitrate

GENERIC FORM AVAILABLE: No

THERAPEUTIC CLASS: Nitrate anti-anginal

DOSAGE FORMS: 20-mg tablets

MAIN USES: Prevention of angina

USUAL DOSE: 20 mg upon awakening, then 20 mg seven hours later

AVERAGE PRICE: $95.65

SIDE EFFECTS: headache 19%–38%, dizziness 3%–5%, and nausea 2%–4% are the most common. Less common: flushing, restlessness, dizziness, weakness, vomiting, and sweating.

DRUG INTERACTIONS: Alcohol and the drug may produce low blood pressure. Apresoline, Loniten, or Vasodilan and the drug may also produce low blood pressure.

ALLERGIES: Individuals allergic to isosorbide mononitrate or other nitrates (such as those listed in "Other Drugs in the Same Therapeutic Class") should discuss this with their doctor or pharmacist before taking this drug.

PREGNANCY/BREAST-FEEDING: Category C—Risk cannot be ruled out. Human studies are lacking, and animal studies are either positive for fetal risk or lacking as well. However, potential benefits may justify the potential risk in using the drug. It is not known whether the drug is excreted in the breast milk; therefore, caution should be used when breast-feeding.

OTHER BRAND NAMES: None

OTHER DRUGS IN THE SAME THERAPEUTIC CLASS: Dilatrat-SR, Imdur, Isordil, Monoket, and Sorbitrate

IMPORTANT INFORMATION TO REMEMBER: This drug does not relieve angina attacks—it only prevents them. Only take the drug exactly as directed by your physician. Do not discontinue the drug or increase the dose without first consulting your physician. Do not drink alcohol while taking this drug. The headache that is common with this drug usually goes away with continued use; if it does not, contact your doctor. Before taking over-the-counter cold and allergy preparations, consult your doctor or pharmacist.

BRAND NAME: Isoptin and Isoptin SR

GENERIC NAME: verapamil

See entry for Calan

BRAND NAME: Isopto Atropine

GENERIC NAME: atropine

GENERIC FORM AVAILABLE: Yes

THERAPEUTIC CLASS: Mydriatic anti-glaucoma

DOSAGE FORMS: 0.5% and 1% eyedrop solution

MAIN USES: Glaucoma

USUAL DOSE: one to two drops one to four times daily

AVERAGE PRICE: $17.97 (B)/$9.91 (G) for 5 mL of both strengths

SIDE EFFECTS: Most common: none. Less common: blurred vision, eye irritation, increased sensitivity of the eyes to light, and swelling of the eyelids.

DRUG INTERACTIONS: None of any clinical significance

ALLERGIES: Individuals allergic to atropine or any of its derivatives should discuss this with their doctor or pharmacist before using this drug.

PREGNANCY/BREAST-FEEDING: Category C—Risk cannot be ruled out. Human studies are lacking, and animal studies are either positive for fetal risk or lacking as well. However, potential benefits may justify the potential risk in using the drug. The drug may be excreted in the breast milk; therefore, caution should be used when breast-feeding.

OTHER BRAND NAMES: None

OTHER DRUGS IN THE SAME THERAPEUTIC CLASS: Cyclogyl and Mydriacyl

IMPORTANT INFORMATION TO REMEMBER: This medication may cause blurred vision and increased sensitivity of the eyes to sunlight. If these effects last more than 14 days after discontinuing use, contact your doctor. Keep the container tightly closed and avoid touching the applicator tip to the eye—this could contaminate the product over time. Also, only administer one drop at a time. After application, keep the eye open for at least 30 seconds, roll the eyeball around, and avoid squinting. If a second drop is required, wait one to two minutes between drops. If another medication is to be used in the eye, wait at least 10 minutes before administering it. Do not discontinue the drug without first consulting your physician, and use exactly as directed.

BRAND NAME: Isopto Carbachol

GENERIC NAME: carbachol

GENERIC FORM AVAILABLE: No

THERAPEUTIC CLASS: Miotic anti-glaucoma

DOSAGE FORMS: 0.75%, 1.5%, 2.25%, and 3% eyedrop solution

MAIN USES: Glaucoma

USUAL DOSE: one to two drops one to three times daily

AVERAGE PRICE: $24.50 for 0.75% (15 mL); $25.81 for 1.5% (15 mL); $27.13 for 2.25% (15 mL); and $29.47 for 3% (15 mL)

SIDE EFFECTS: Most common: blurred vision, changes in near or distance vision, eye pain, and stinging or burning of the eye. Less common: headache, irritation or redness of the eye, and twitching of the eyelids.

DRUG INTERACTIONS: None of any clinical significance

ALLERGIES: Individuals allergic to carbachol, hydroxypropyl methylcellulose, or any of their derivatives should discuss this with their doctor or pharmacist before using this drug.

PREGNANCY/BREAST-FEEDING: Category C—Risk cannot be ruled out. Human studies are lacking, and animal studies are either positive for fetal risk or lacking as well. However, potential benefits may justify the potential risk in using the drug. It is not known whether the drug is excreted in the breast milk; therefore, caution should be used when breast-feeding.

OTHER BRAND NAMES: None

OTHER DRUGS IN THE SAME THERAPEUTIC CLASS: Isopto Carpine, Ocusert Pilo, Pilocar, and Pilopine HS

IMPORTANT INFORMATION TO REMEMBER: Caution should be used when driving or doing other activities at night or in dim light.

Changes in near or distance vision can occur with this drug. Keep the container tightly closed and avoid touching the applicator tip to the eye—this could contaminate the product over time. Also, only administer one drop at a time. After application, keep the eye open for at least 30 seconds, roll the eyeball around, and avoid squinting. If a second drop is required, wait one to two minutes between drops. If another medication is to be used in the eye, wait at least 10 minutes before administering it. Do not discontinue the drug without first consulting your physician, and use exactly as directed.

BRAND NAME: Isopto Carpine

GENERIC NAME: pilocarpine

GENERIC FORM AVAILABLE: Yes

THERAPEUTIC CLASS: Miotic anti-glaucoma

DOSAGE FORMS: 0.25%, 0.5%, 1%, 2%, 3%, 4%, 5%, 6%, 8%, and 10% eyedrop solution

MAIN USES: Glaucoma

USUAL DOSE: one to two drops three to six times daily

AVERAGE PRICE: $23.07 (B)/$10.98 (G) for 0.5%, 1%, and 2% (15 mL); $24.17 (B)/$12.08 (G) for 4% (15 mL)

SIDE EFFECTS: Most common: blurred vision, changes in near or far vision, and decrease in night vision. Less common: eye irritation, headache, eyebrow ache, and eye pain.

DRUG INTERACTIONS: None of any clinical significance

ALLERGIES: Individuals allergic to pilocarpine or any of its derivatives should discuss this with their doctor or pharmacist before using this drug.

PREGNANCY/BREAST-FEEDING: Category C—Risk cannot be ruled out. Human studies are lacking, and animal studies are either positive for fetal risk or lacking as well. However, potential benefits may justify the potential risk in using the drug. It is not known whether the drug is excreted in the breast milk; therefore, caution should be used when breast-feeding.

OTHER BRAND NAMES: Pilocar

OTHER DRUGS IN THE SAME THERAPEUTIC CLASS: Isopto Carbachol, Ocusert Pilo, Pilocar, and Pilopine HS

IMPORTANT INFORMATION TO REMEMBER: Caution should be used when driving or doing other activities at night or in dim light. Changes in near or distance vision can occur with this drug. Keep the container tightly closed and avoid touching the applicator tip to the eye—this could contaminate the product over time. Also, only administer one drop at a time. After application, keep the eye open for at least 30 seconds, roll the eyeball around, and avoid squinting. If a second drop is required, wait one to two minutes between drops. If another medication is to be used in the eye, wait at least 10 minutes before administering it. Do not discontinue the drug without first consulting your physician, and use exactly as directed.

BRAND NAME: Isordil

GENERIC NAME: isosorbide dinitrate

GENERIC FORM AVAILABLE: Yes

THERAPEUTIC CLASS: Nitrate anti-anginal

DOSAGE FORMS: 5-mg, 10-mg, 20-mg, 30-mg, and 40-mg tablets; 2.5-mg, 5-mg, and 10-mg sublingual tablets; 40-mg sustained-release tablets; and 40-mg sustained-release capsules

MAIN USES: Treatment and prevention of angina

USUAL DOSE: For prevention of angina attacks: 5 mg to 40 mg four times a day, or 40 mg sustained-release tablets or capsules every 6 to 12 hours. For treatment of angina attacks: 2.5 mg to 10 mg of the sublingual tablets dissolved under the tongue every two to three hours as needed.

AVERAGE PRICE: $35.17 (B)/$12.40 (G) for 5 mg; $39.57 (B)/$13.17 (G) for 10 mg; $70.15 (B)/$17.57 (G) for 20 mg; $79.01 (B)/$19.78 (G) for 30 mg; $85.57 (B)/$29.67 (G) for 40 mg sustained-release tablets and capsules

SIDE EFFECTS: Most common: headache, nausea, and dizziness. Less common: flushing, restlessness, weakness, vomiting, and sweating.

DRUG INTERACTIONS: Alcohol and the drug may produce low blood pressure. Apresoline, Loniten, or Vasodilan and the drug may also produce low blood pressure.

ALLERGIES: Individuals allergic to isosorbide dinitrate or other nitrates (such as those listed in "Other Drugs in the Same Therapeutic Class") should discuss this with their doctor or pharmacist before taking this drug.

PREGNANCY/BREAST-FEEDING: Category C—Risk cannot be ruled out. Human studies are lacking, and animal studies are either positive for fetal risk or lacking as well. However, potential benefits may justify the potential risk in using the drug. It is not known whether the drug is excreted in the breast milk; therefore, caution should be used when breast-feeding.

OTHER BRAND NAMES: Sorbitrate and Sorbitrate SL

OTHER DRUGS IN THE SAME THERAPEUTIC CLASS: Dilatrate-SR, Imdur, Ismo, Monoket, and Sorbitrate

IMPORTANT INFORMATION TO REMEMBER. The tablet and sustained-release forms of the drug do not relieve angina attacks—they only prevent them. The sublingual tablets can be used to relieve an angina attack. Only take the drug exactly as directed by your physician. Do not discontinue the drug or increase the dose without first consulting your physician. Do not crush or chew the sustained-release tablets (Tembids) or capsules—this will destroy the mechanism that delays the release of the medication. Tablets may, however, be cut in half for easier swallowing. Do not drink alcohol while taking this drug. The headache that is common with this drug usually goes away with continued use; if it does not, contact your doctor. Before taking over-the-counter cold and allergy preparations, consult your physician or pharmacist.

When using the sublingual tablets for acute angina attacks:

1) Dissolve the tablet under the tongue (do not swallow) at the first sign of an angina attack; do not wait until the attack is severe.
2) If the angina is not relieved in five minutes after placing the first tablet under the tongue, dissolve a second tablet and then a third if necessary.
3) If the pain continues or increases, notify your physician or go to the nearest emergency room immediately.

BRAND NAME: **Isuprel**

GENERIC NAME: isoproterenol

GENERIC FORM AVAILABLE: Yes

THERAPEUTIC CLASS: Nonselective beta-agonist bronchodilator

DOSAGE FORMS: 0.131mg-per-inhalation metered-dose inhaler (Mistometer); 10-mg and 15-mg sublingual tablets; and 1:100 and 1:200 solution for inhalation

MAIN USES: Asthma, emphysema, chronic bronchitis, (and other breathing disorders)

USUAL DOSE: For the metered-dose inhaler (Mistometer): one to two inhalations every three to four hours as needed. For the tablets: 10 mg under the tongue every three to four hours (maximum three times per day). For the solution: doses vary with the individual.

AVERAGE PRICE: $44.12 for 15 mL (Mistometer); $34.73 (B)/ $21.75 (G) for solution (10 mL)

SIDE EFFECTS: Most common: dryness, irritation of the mouth, irritation of the throat, nervousness, restlessness, trouble sleeping, and pinkish or red color of saliva. Less common: coughing, dizziness, lightheadedness, fast heartbeat, headache, flushing, redness of the face or skin, increased sweating, nausea, increase in blood pressure, pounding heartbeat, trembling, vomiting, and weakness.

DRUG INTERACTIONS: Decongestants contained in cold, cough, and allergy products may increase the toxicity of this drug. The drug and Intal should never be used by a woman who is pregnant. Blocadren, Cartrol, Corgard, Inderal, Kerlone, Levatol, Lopressor, Normodyne, Sectral, Tenormin, Toprol-XL, Trandate, Visken, and Zebeta may decrease the effect of the drug. This drug should be used with caution by patients taking Lanoxin and Ludiomil.

ALLERGIES: Individuals allergic to isoproterenol or any of its derivatives should discuss this with their doctor or pharmacist before using this drug.

PREGNANCY/BREAST-FEEDING: Category C—Risk cannot be ruled out. Human studies are lacking, and animal studies are either positive for fetal risk or lacking as well. However, potential benefits may justify the potential risk in using the drug. It is not known

whether the drug is excreted in the breast milk; therefore, caution should be used when breast-feeding.

OTHER BRAND NAMES: None

OTHER DRUGS IN THE SAME THERAPEUTIC CLASS: None

IMPORTANT INFORMATION TO REMEMBER: Only take the drug exactly as directed by your physician. Never take more of the drug than what is prescribed without first consulting with your physician. Due to its potential to cause insomnia, take the drug a few hours before bedtime if possible.

When using the inhaler, follow the following procedure:

1) Shake the canister well.
2) Place the mouthpiece close to the mouth, but not touching the lips.
3) Exhale deeply.
4) Inhale slowly and deeply as you press the top of the canister to release the medication.
5) Hold your breath for a few seconds before exhaling.
6) Wait five minutes between puffs.
7) Be sure to wash the inhaler device (mouthpiece) regularly with warm soapy water to avoid bacterial contamination.

BRAND NAME: **KAON-CL 10**

GENERIC NAME: potassium chloride

See entry for K-Tab

BRAND NAME: K-Dur

GENERIC NAME: potassium chloride

GENERIC FORM AVAILABLE: No

THERAPEUTIC CLASS: Potassium supplement

DOSAGE FORMS: 10 mEq (750 mg) and 20 mEq (1500 mg) tablets

MAIN USES: Low potassium

USUAL DOSE: 10 mEq to 40 mEq per day in divided doses

AVERAGE PRICE: $30.18 for 10 mEq and $54.89 for 20 mEq

SIDE EFFECTS: Most common: none. Less common: diarrhea, vomiting, gas, nausea, and stomach discomfort.

DRUG INTERACTIONS: Aldactazide, Aldactone, Dyazide, Dyrenium, Hygroton, Maxzide, Midamor, and Moduretic may cause potassium levels to become too high when taken with this drug. Accupril, Altace, Capoten, Lotensin, Monopril, Prinivil, Univasc, Vasotec, Zestril, and salt substitutes may cause potassium levels to become too high when taken with this drug. Caution should be used with patients taking Lanoxin and this drug.

ALLERGIES: Individuals allergic to potassium, potassium chloride, or any of their derivatives should discuss this with their doctor or pharmacist before using this drug.

PREGNANCY/BREAST-FEEDING: Category C—Risk cannot be ruled out. Human studies are lacking, and animal studies are either positive for fetal risk or lacking as well. However, potential benefits may justify the potential risk in using the drug. It is not known whether the drug is excreted in the breast milk; therefore, caution should be used when breast-feeding.

OTHER BRAND NAMES: None

OTHER DRUGS IN THE SAME THERAPEUTIC CLASS: KAON-CL, Kay Ciel, K-Lor, Klor-Con, Klorvess, Klotrix, K-Lyte, K-Lyte/Cl, K-Norm, K-Tab, Micro-K, and Slow-K

IMPORTANT INFORMATION TO REMEMBER: This drug should be taken with food or milk to reduce the potential for injury to the stomach lining and stomach upset. The drug should also be taken with a full glass of water (eight ounces is preferred). Only take the drug exactly as directed by your doctor; do not increase the dose or discontinue taking the drug without first consulting with your doctor. Do not crush or crew the tablets. The tablets can, however, be cut in half at the scored line on the tablet. Individuals should avoid salt substitutes that contain potassium. The tablets may be dissolved in four ounces of water, and the liquid drank. When doing this, allow two to three minutes for the tablet to disintegrate, and stir for one minute after disintegration.

BRAND NAME: Keflex, Keflet, and Keftab

GENERIC NAME: cephalexin

GENERIC FORM AVAILABLE: Yes

THERAPEUTIC CLASS: Cephalosporin antibiotic

DOSAGE FORMS: For Keflex: 250-mg and 500-mg capsules, and 125 mg/5 mL and 250 mg/5 mL oral suspensions. For Keflet: 250-mg and 500-mg tablets. For Keftab: 500-mg tablets.

MAIN USES: Bacterial infections

USUAL DOSE: 250 mg to 500 mg every 6 hours or 500 mg every 12 hours

AVERAGE PRICE: $61.59 (B)/$17.59 (G) for 250 mg (30 capsules of Keflex); $119.67 (B)/$32.97 (G) for 500 mg (30 capsules of Keflex); $106.74 for 500 mg (30 tablets of 500-mg Keftab and Keflet)

SIDE EFFECTS: Most common: diarrhea. Less common: nausea, vomiting, hives, itching, rash, and vaginal yeast infections.

DRUG INTERACTIONS: These drugs may decrease the effectiveness of oral contraceptives used for birth control. Women may become pregnant while taking these drugs and oral contraceptives. The drug probenecid will decrease elimination of these drugs by the kidneys.

ALLERGIES: Individuals allergic to cephalexin, penicillins (including amoxicillin and ampicillin), or other cephalosporins (such as those listed in "Other Drugs in the Same Therapeutic Class") should discuss this with their doctor or pharmacist before taking this drug.

PREGNANCY/BREAST-FEEDING: Category B—No evidence of risk in humans. Either animal findings show risk, but human findings do not; or, if no adequate human studies have been done, animal findings show no risk. The drug is excreted in the breast milk; therefore, caution should be used when breast-feeding.

OTHER BRAND NAMES: None

OTHER DRUGS IN THE SAME THERAPEUTIC CLASS: Ceclor, Cedax, Ceftin, Cefzil, Duricef, Suprax, Ultracef, Vantin, and Velosef

IMPORTANT INFORMATION TO REMEMBER: If stomach upset occurs, the drug can be taken with food or milk. Also, take the drug at even intervals around the clock (if four times a day, take every six hours). Take the drug until all the medication prescribed is gone; otherwise the infection may return. Women taking birth control pills should use another form of contraception while taking the drug and for the rest of the current menstrual cycle. Individuals taking the liquid form should shake it thoroughly before use, store the medication in the refrigerator, and discard any remaining medication after 14 days. The drug may produce a false positive for some glucose and protein urine tests.

BRAND NAME: Kenalog

GENERIC NAME: triamcinolone acetonide

GENERIC FORM AVAILABLE: Yes

THERAPEUTIC CLASS: Topical corticosteroid

DOSAGE FORMS: 0.025%, 0.1%, and 0.5% cream and ointment; 0.025% and 0.1% lotion; 0.2% aerosol spray; and 0.1% paste form (Kenalog in Orabase)

MAIN USES: Skin rashes, swelling, itching, and canker sores (Kenalog in Orabase)

USUAL DOSE: Apply to the affected area as a thin film two to four times daily.

AVERAGE PRICE: $19.78 (B)/$7.68 (G) for 0.025% and 0.1% cream and ointment (15 g); $45.59 (B)/$14.48 (G) for 0.5% cream (15 g); $38.96 for the 0.2% aerosol spray; and $23.37 (B)/$13.21 (G) for the Kenalog in Orabase

SIDE EFFECTS: Most common: none. Less common: burning, itching, irritation, dry skin, rash, soreness of the skin, and acne.

DRUG INTERACTIONS: None of any clinical significance

ALLERGIES: Individuals allergic to triamcinolone acetonide or any of its derivatives should discuss this with their doctor or pharmacist before using this drug.

PREGNANCY/BREAST-FEEDING: Category C—Risk cannot be ruled out. Human studies are lacking, and animal studies are either positive for fetal risk or lacking as well. However, potential benefits may justify the potential risk in using the drug. It is not known whether the drug is excreted in the breast milk; therefore, caution should be used when breast-feeding.

OTHER BRAND NAMES: None

OTHER DRUGS IN THE SAME THERAPEUTIC CLASS: Aclovate, Aristocort, Cordran, Cordran SP, Cutivate, Cyclocort, DesOwen, Diprolene, Diprolene AF, Elocon, Florone, Florone E, Halog, Hytone,

Lidex, Synalar, Temovate, Topicort, Tridesilon, Ultravate, Valisone, and Westcort

IMPORTANT INFORMATION TO REMEMBER: This drug is for external use only. Apply only a thin film of drug to skin and rub it in well. Never cover the skin after application with a bandage or wrapping unless directed to do so by a doctor. Never apply to damaged skin or open wounds unless directed to do so by a doctor. Discontinue use if irritation occurs.

BRAND NAME: Kerlone

GENERIC NAME: betaxolol

GENERIC FORM AVAILABLE: No

THERAPEUTIC CLASS: Cardioselective beta-blocker

DOSAGE FORMS: 10-mg and 20-mg tablets

MAIN USES: High blood pressure

USUAL DOSE: 10 mg to 20 mg once daily

AVERAGE PRICE: $105.91 for 10 mg and $158.81 for 20 mg

SIDE EFFECTS: slow heart rate 8%, headache 7%, upset stomach 5%, dizziness 5%, tiredness 3%, muscle pain 3%, swelling 2%, difficulty breathing 2%, diarrhea 2%, chest pain 2%–7%, nausea 2%, drowsiness 1%, insomnia 1%–5%, pounding heartbeat 1%, and impotence 1%.

DRUG INTERACTIONS: The drug may cause additive effects when used with reserpine. The drug may increase the effects of Calan, Cardene, Cardizem, Catapres, Dilacor XR, DynaCirc, Isoptin, Lanoxin, Norvasc, Plendil, Procardia, Sular, Tiazac, Verelan, and Wytensin. Diabetic medications, insulin, Slo-bid, Theo-Dur, theophylline, Uni-Dur, and Uniphyl dosages may need to be adjusted when taking this drug. The drug may also interfere with glaucoma screening tests.

ALLERGIES: Individuals allergic to betaxolol or any of its derivatives should discuss this with their doctor or pharmacist before taking this drug.

PREGNANCY/BREAST-FEEDING: Category C—Risk cannot be ruled out. Human studies are lacking, and animal studies are either positive for fetal risk or lacking as well. However, potential benefits

may justify the potential risk in using the drug. The drug is excreted in the breast milk; therefore, extreme caution should be used when breast-feeding.

OTHER BRAND NAMES: None

OTHER DRUGS IN THE SAME THERAPEUTIC CLASS: Lopressor, Sectral, Tenormin, Torpol-XL, and Zebeta

IMPORTANT INFORMATION TO REMEMBER: Only take the drug exactly as directed by your physician. Do not discontinue the drug without first consulting your physician. This drug may cause some limited drowsiness, especially at first. Individuals should use caution when driving, operating machinery, or any task where mental alertness is required. Alcohol, anxiety medications, and narcotic painkillers may intensify the drowsiness effect of the drug. Before taking over-the-counter cold and allergy preparations, consult your doctor or pharmacist—these products may raise your blood pressure. This drug may mask the symptoms of low blood sugar in diabetics.

BRAND NAME: Klonopin

GENERIC NAME: clonazepam

GENERIC FORM AVAILABLE: Yes

THERAPEUTIC CLASS: Benzodiazepine anticonvulsant

DOSAGE FORMS: 0.5-mg, 1-mg, and 2-mg tablets

MAIN USES: Epilepsy and seizures

USUAL DOSE: 0.5 mg to 2 mg three times daily

AVERAGE PRICE: $128.84 (B)/$94.09 (G) for 0.5 mg; $129.88 (B)/$97.79 (G) for 1 mg; and $175.99 (B)/$134.99 (G) for 2 mg

SIDE EFFECTS: Most common: drowsiness, shaky movements, behavioral problems, dizziness, lightheadedness, clumsiness, and slurred speech. Less common: abnormal eye movements, stomach pain, blurred vision, headache, tremor, dizziness, confusion, depression, increased sex drive, insomnia, pounding heartbeat, muscle weakness, appetite changes, dry mouth, constipation, sore gums, diarrhea, and nausea.

DRUG INTERACTIONS: Central nervous system (CNS) depression may be increased when used with alcohol, antidepressants, narcotic painkillers, or other anxiety medications.

ALLERGIES: Individuals allergic to clonazepam or other benzodiazepines (such as those listed in "Other Drugs in the Same Therapeutic Class") should discuss this with their doctor or pharmacist before taking this drug.

PREGNANCY/BREAST-FEEDING: Category D—Positive evidence of risk. Human studies show risk to the fetus. Nevertheless, potential benefits may possibly outweigh the potential risks. This drug should not be taken by nursing mothers.

OTHER BRAND NAMES: None

OTHER DRUGS IN THE SAME THERAPEUTIC CLASS: Valium

IMPORTANT INFORMATION TO REMEMBER: This drug may cause drowsiness. Individuals should use caution when driving, operating machinery, or any task where mental alertness is required. The incidence of drowsiness and unsteadiness increases with age. Alcohol, anxiety medications, or narcotic painkillers may intensify the drowsiness effect of the drug. This medication is a controlled substance and may be habit-forming. Do not increase the dose of medication without consulting with your doctor; only take the amount prescribed by your doctor.

BRAND NAME: K-Lor

GENERIC NAME: potassium chloride

GENERIC FORM AVAILABLE: Yes

THERAPEUTIC CLASS: Potassium supplement

DOSAGE FORMS: 20-mEq powder for solution

MAIN USES: Low potassium

USUAL DOSE: 10 mEq to 40 mEq per day in divided doses

AVERAGE PRICE: $43.37 (B)/$15.49 (G) for 30 packets

SIDE EFFECTS: Most common: none. Less common: diarrhea, vomiting, gas, nausea, and stomach discomfort.

DRUG INTERACTIONS: Aldactazide, Aldactone, Dyazide, Dyrenium, Hygroton, Maxzide, Midamor, and Moduretic may cause potassium levels to become too high when taken with this drug. Accupril, Altace, Capoten, Lotensin, Monopril, Prinivil, Univasc, Vasotec, Zestril, and salt substitutes may cause potassium levels to become too high when taken with this drug. Patients taking Lanoxin and this drug should do so with caution.

ALLERGIES: Individuals allergic to potassium, potassium chloride, or any of their derivatives should discuss this with their doctor or pharmacist before using this drug.

PREGNANCY/BREAST-FEEDING: Category C—Risk cannot be ruled out. Human studies are lacking, and animal studies are either positive for fetal risk or lacking as well. However, potential benefits may justify the potential risk in using the drug. It is not known whether the drug is excreted in the breast milk; therefore, caution should be used when breast-feeding.

OTHER BRAND NAMES: None

OTHER DRUGS IN THE SAME THERAPEUTIC CLASS: KAON-CL, Kay Ciel, K-Dur, Klor-Con, Klorvess, Klotrix, K-Lyte, K-Lyte/Cl, K-Norm, K-Tab, Micro-K, and Slow-K

IMPORTANT INFORMATION TO REMEMBER: This drug should be taken with food or milk to reduce the potential for injury to the stomach lining and stomach upset. The drug should also be taken with a full glass of water (eight ounces is preferred). Only take the drug exactly as directed by your doctor; do not increase the dose or discontinue taking the drug without first consulting with your doctor. Individuals should avoid salt substitutes that contain potassium. The packet of powder should be mixed in four ounces of cold water or fruit juice and drank slowly over a 5- to 10-minute period.

BRAND NAME: Klor-Con

GENERIC NAME: potassium chloride

GENERIC FORM AVAILABLE: Yes

THERAPEUTIC CLASS: Potassium supplement

DOSAGE FORMS: 20-mEq and 25-mEq powder; 8-mEq (600-mg) and 10-mEq (750-mg) tablets

MAIN USES: Low potassium

USUAL DOSE: 8 mEq to 40 mEq per day in divided doses

AVERAGE PRICE: $15.89 (B)/$12.91 (G) for 80mEq tablets and $19.97 (B)/$16.71 (G) for 10-mEq tablets

SIDE EFFECTS: Most common: none. Less common: diarrhea, vomiting, gas, nausea, stomach discomfort, and wax matrix of the tablet may be seen in the stool.

DRUG INTERACTIONS: Aldactazide, Aldactone, Dyazide, Dyrenium, Hygroton, Maxzide, Midamor, and Moduretic may cause potassium levels to become too high when taken with this drug. Accupril, Altace, Capoten, Lotensin, Monopril, Prinivil, Univasc, Vasotec, Zestril, and salt substitutes may cause potassium levels to become too high when taken with this drug. Patients taking Lanoxin and this drug should do so with caution.

ALLERGIES: Individuals allergic to potassium, potassium chloride, or any of their derivatives should discuss this with their doctor or pharmacist before using this drug.

PREGNANCY/BREAST-FEEDING: Category C—Risk cannot be ruled out. Human studies are lacking, and animal studies are either positive for fetal risk or lacking as well. However, potential benefits may justify the potential risk in using the drug. It is not known whether the drug is excreted in the breast milk; therefore, caution should be used when breast-feeding.

OTHER BRAND NAMES: None

OTHER DRUGS IN THE SAME THERAPEUTIC CLASS: KAON-CL, Kay Ciel, K-Dur, K-Lor, Klorvess, Klotrix, K-Lyte, L-Lyte/Cl, K-Norm, K-Tab, Micro-K, and Slow-K

IMPORTANT INFORMATION TO REMEMBER: This drug should be taken with food or milk to reduce the potential for injury to the stomach lining and stomach upset. The drug should also be taken with a full glass of water (eight ounces is preferred). Only take the drug exactly as directed by your doctor; do not increase the dose or discontinue taking the drug without first consulting with your doctor. Swallow the tablets whole. Do not crush or chew the tablets—this will destroy the wax matrix that delays the release of the drug. Individuals should avoid salt substitutes that contain potassium.

BRAND NAME: Klotrix

GENERIC NAME: potassium chloride

See entry for Klor-Con

BRAND NAME: K-Lyte, K-Lyte DS, and K-Lyte/Cl

GENERIC NAME: potassium bicarbonate (K-Lyte and K-Lyte DS) and potassium chloride (K-Lyte/Cl)

GENERIC FORM AVAILABLE: Yes

THERAPEUTIC CLASS: Potassium supplement

DOSAGE FORMS: 25-mEq and 50-mEq effervescent tablets

MAIN USES: Low potassium

USUAL DOSE: 25 mEq to 100 mEq per day in divided doses

AVERAGE PRICE: $132.38 (B)/$45.99 (G) for K-Lyte; and $211.13 (B)/$74.77 (G) for K-Lyte DS

SIDE EFFECTS: Most common: none. Less common: diarrhea, vomiting, gas, nausea, and stomach discomfort.

DRUG INTERACTIONS: Aldactazide, Aldactone, Dyazide, Dyrenium, Hygroton, Maxzide, Midamor, and Moduretic may cause potassium levels to become too high when taken with this drug. Accupril, Altace, Capoten, Lotensin, Monopril, Prinivil, Univasc, Vasotec, Zestril, and salt substitutes may cause potassium levels to become too high when taken with this drug. Patients taking Lanoxin and this drug should do so with caution.

ALLERGIES: Individuals allergic to potassium bicarbonate, potassium chloride, or any of their derivatives should discuss this with their doctor or pharmacist before using this drug.

PREGNANCY/BREAST-FEEDING: Category C—Risk cannot be ruled out. Human studies are lacking, and animal studies are either positive for fetal risk or lacking as well. However, potential benefits may justify the potential risk in using the drug. It is not known whether the drug is excreted in the breast milk; therefore, caution should be used when breast-feeding.

OTHER BRAND NAMES: None

OTHER DRUGS IN THE SAME THERAPEUTIC CLASS: KAON-CL, Kay Ciel, K-Dur, K-Lor, Klor-Con, Klorvess, Klotrix, K-Norm, K-Tab, Micro-K, and Slow-K

IMPORTANT INFORMATION TO REMEMBER: This drug should be taken with food or milk to reduce the potential for injury to the stomach lining and stomach upset. Only take the drug exactly as directed by your doctor; do not increase the dose or discontinue taking the drug without first consulting with your doctor. Individuals should avoid salt substitutes that contain potassium. Do not swallow the tablet. The tablet should be mixed in four ounces of cold water or fruit juice and drank slowly over a 5- to 10-minute period. The DS tablets should be mixed with eight ounces of water.

BRAND NAME: K-Norm

GENERIC NAME: potassium chloride

See entry for Micro-K

BRAND NAME: K-Tab

GENERIC NAME: potassium chloride

GENERIC FORM AVAILABLE: Yes

THERAPEUTIC CLASS: Potassium supplement

DOSAGE FORMS: 10-mEq (750-mg) extended-release tablets

MAIN USES: Low potassium

USUAL DOSE: 20 mEq to 80 mEq daily in one or two divided doses

AVERAGE PRICE: $47.25 (B)/$18.25 (G)

SIDE EFFECTS: Most common: none. Less common: diarrhea, vomiting, gas, nausea, and stomach discomfort.

DRUG INTERACTIONS: Aldactazide, Aldactone, Dyazide, Dyrenium, Hygroton, Maxzide, Midamor, and Moduretic may cause potassium levels to become too high when taken with this drug. Accupril, Altace, Capoten, Lotensin, Monopril, Prinivil, Univasc, Vasotec, Zestril, and salt substitutes may cause potassium levels to become too high when taken with this drug. Patients taking Lanoxin and this drug should do so with caution.

ALLERGIES: Individuals allergic to potassium, potassium chloride, or any of their derivatives should discuss this with their doctor or pharmacist before using this drug.

PREGNANCY/BREAST-FEEDING: Category C—Risk cannot be ruled out. Human studies are lacking, and animal studies are either positive for fetal risk or lacking as well. However, potential benefits may justify the potential risk in using the drug. It is not known whether the drug is excreted in the breast milk; therefore, caution should be used when breast-feeding.

OTHER BRAND NAMES: None

OTHER DRUGS IN THE SAME THERAPEUTIC CLASS: KAON-CL, Kay Ciel, K-Dur, K-Lor, Klor-Con, Klorvess, Klotrix, K-Lyte, K-Lyte/Cl, K-Norm, Micro-K, and Slow-K

IMPORTANT INFORMATION TO REMEMBER: This drug should be taken with food or milk to reduce the potential for injury to the stomach lining and stomach upset. The drug should also be taken with a full glass of water (eight ounces is preferred). Only take the drug exactly as directed by your doctor; do not increase the dose or discontinue taking the drug without first consulting with your doctor. Swallow the tablets whole. Do not crush or chew the tablets—this will destroy the mechanism that delays the release of the drug. Individuals should avoid salt substitutes that contain potassium.

BRAND NAME: Kwell

GENERIC NAME: lindane

GENERIC FORM AVAILABLE: Yes

THERAPEUTIC CLASS: Anti-lice and anti-scabies

DOSAGE FORMS: 1% cream, lotion, and shampoo

MAIN USES: Head lice, crab lice, and scabies

USUAL DOSE: Cream and lotion: apply and leave in place for 8 to 12 hours. Shampoo: Work in and allow to remain in place for four minutes; lather, rinse thoroughly, and gently dry.

AVERAGE PRICE: $16.47 (B)/$9.33 (G) for shampoo (60 mL); $16.15 (B)/$9.87 (G) for lotion (6 mL)

SIDE EFFECTS: Most common: itching of the skin. Less common: skin or scalp irritation and skin rash.

DRUG INTERACTIONS: None of any clinical significance

ALLERGIES: Individuals allergic to lindane or any of its derivatives should discuss this with their doctor or pharmacist before using this drug.

PREGNANCY/BREAST-FEEDING: Category B—No evidence of risk in humans. Either animal findings show risk, but human findings do not; or, if no adequate human studies have been done, animal findings show no risk. The drug is excreted in the breast milk; therefore, caution should be used when breast-feeding.

OTHER BRAND NAMES: None

OTHER DRUGS IN THE SAME THERAPEUTIC CLASS: None

IMPORTANT INFORMATION TO REMEMBER: Avoid contact with the eyes. For the cream and lotion: take a warm bath and dry off thoroughly before applying drug. Apply enough drug to cover the entire area from the chin to the toes and rub it in. Leave the medication on for 8 to 12 hours only and follow with a bath or shower. For the shampoo: work it in well with small amounts of water; allow shampoo to stay on the hair for four minutes, and then rinse thoroughly. It is then necessary to remove the nits and nit shells with a pair of tweezers or a fine-toothed comb, (a metal lice comb is preferred). All clothing and bedding should be washed in hot water immediately to prevent contracting the problem again after treatment. It is important not to exceed the recommended dose prescribed by your physician.

BRAND NAME: Kytril

GENERIC FORM: granisetron

GENERIC FORM AVAILABLE: No

THERAPEUTIC CLASS: Antinausea

DOSAGE FORMS: 1-mg tablets

MAIN USES: Prevention of chemotherapy-induced nausea

USUAL DOSE: 1 mg up to 1 hour before chemotherapy and 1 mg 12 hours after the first dose

AVERAGE PRICE: $110.25 for two tablets

SIDE EFFECTS: headache 14%–21%, weakness 5%–14%, drowsiness 4%, dizziness 4%, diarrhea 4%–8%, and constipation 3%–18%.

DRUG INTERACTIONS: None of any clinical significance

ALLERGIES: Individuals allergic to granisetron or any of its derivatives should discuss this with their doctor or pharmacist before using this drug.

PREGNANCY/BREAST-FEEDING: Category B—No evidence of risk in humans. Either animal findings show risk, but human findings do not; or, if no adequate human studies have been done, animal findings show no risk. It is not known whether the drug is excreted in the breast milk; therefore, caution should be used when breast-feeding.

OTHER BRAND NAMES: None

OTHER DRUGS IN THE SAME THERAPEUTIC CLASS: Zofran

IMPORTANT INFORMATION TO REMEMBER: This drug may cause some drowsiness. Individuals should use caution when driving, operating machinery, or any task where mental alertness is required. Alcohol, anxiety medications, and narcotic painkillers intensify the drowsiness effect of the drug. Only take the drug exactly as directed by your physician; do not increase the dose without first consulting your physician.

BRAND NAME: Lac-Hydrin

GENERIC NAME: ammonium lactate (12% lactic acid)

GENERIC FORM AVAILABLE: No

THERAPEUTIC CLASS: Emollient

DOSAGE FORMS: ammonium lactate (12% lactic acid) lotion and cream

MAIN USES: Dry skin and scaly skin

USUAL DOSE: Apply to affected area and rub it in twice daily.

AVERAGE PRICE: $34.04 for 225-g bottle of lotion and $18.36 for cream (140 g)

SIDE EFFECTS: stinging 3%, burning 3%, redness 2%, and peeling 2%. In severe skin conditions, these side effects may occur as often as 10%.

DRUG INTERACTIONS: None of any clinical significance

ALLERGIES: Individuals allergic to ammonium lactate, lactic acid, mineral oil, or any of their derivatives should discuss this with their doctor or pharmacist before using this drug.

PREGNANCY/BREAST-FEEDING: Category C—Risk cannot be ruled out. Human studies are lacking, and animal studies are either positive for fetal risk or lacking as well. However, potential benefits may justify the potential risk in using the drug. It is not known whether the drug is excreted in the breast milk; therefore, caution should be used when breast-feeding.

OTHER BRAND NAMES: None

OTHER DRUGS IN THE SAME THERAPEUTIC CLASS: None

IMPORTANT INFORMATION TO REMEMBER: This drug is for external use only. Rub it in thoroughly to affected areas. Discontinue use if irritation occurs. Do not cover the area with a bandage unless instructed to do so by your physician.

BRAND NAME: Lamictal

GENERIC NAME: lamotrigine

GENERIC FORM AVAILABLE: No

THERAPEUTIC CLASS: Phenyltriazine antiepileptic

DOSAGE FORMS: 25-mg, 100-mg, 150-mg, and 200-mg tablets

MAIN USES: Epilepsy and seizures

USUAL DOSE: 100 mg to 500 mg daily in two divided doses

AVERAGE PRICE: $214.18 for 25 mg; $231.84 for 100 mg; $243.60 for 150 mg; and $255.36 for 200 mg

SIDE EFFECTS: dizziness 38%, headache 29%, double vision 28%, abnormal body movements 22%, nausea 19%, blurred vision 16%, runny nose 14%, rash 10%, vomiting 9%, flu-like symptoms 7%, fever 6%, insomnia 6%, clumsiness 6%, diarrhea 6%, stomach pain 5%, tremor 4%, depression 4%, constipation 4%, convulsions 3%, tooth disorder 3%, neck pain 3%, joint and muscle pain

2%, loss of appetite 2%, tiredness 2%, worse seizures 2%, chills 1%, hot flashes 1%, and dry mouth 1%.

DRUG INTERACTIONS: The drug may decrease the blood levels of Depakene and Depakote. Depakene and Depakote may significantly increase the blood levels of Lamictal. Dilantin, Mysoline, phenobarbital, and Tegretol may decrease the blood levels of the drug.

ALLERGIES: Individuals allergic to lamotrigine or any of its derivatives should discuss this with their doctor or pharmacist before using this drug.

PREGNANCY/BREAST-FEEDING: Category C—Risk cannot be ruled out. Human studies are lacking, and animal studies are either positive for fetal risk or lacking as well. However, potential benefits may justify the potential risk in using the drug. The drug is excreted in the breast milk; therefore, extreme caution should be used when breast-feeding.

OTHER BRAND NAMES: None

OTHER DRUGS IN THE SAME THERAPEUTIC CLASS: None

IMPORTANT INFORMATION TO REMEMBER: This drug does cause some dizziness. Individuals should use caution when driving, operating machinery, or any task where mental alertness is required. Alcohol, anxiety medications, and narcotic painkillers may intensify the dizziness effect of the drug. Avoid drinking alcohol while taking his drug. Only take the drug exactly as directed by your physician. Do not discontinue the drug or increase the dose without first consulting your physician. Before taking over-the-counter medications, consult your physician or pharmacist.

BRAND NAME: Lamisil

GENERIC NAME: terbinafine

GENERIC FORM AVAILABLE: No

THERAPEUTIC CLASS: Allylamine antifungal

DOSAGE FORMS: 1% cream and 250-mg tablets

MAIN USES: Fungal infections (mainly ringworm, jock itch, athlete's foot, toenail fungus, and fingernail fungus)

USUAL DOSE: For the cream: apply one to two times daily. For the tablets: one tablet daily.

AVERAGE PRICE: $35.11 for 1% cream (15 g) and $187.64 for 250-mg tablets (30 tablets)

SIDE EFFECTS: For the cream: irritation 1% and burning 1%. For the tablets: headache 13%, diarrhea 6%, rash 6%, stomach pain 4%, nausea 3%, itching 3%, taste changes 3%, gas 2%, hives 1%, and vision problems 1%.

DRUG INTERACTIONS: Rifampin may decrease the blood levels of the drug.

ALLERGIES: Individuals allergic to terbinafine or any of its derivatives should discuss this with their doctor or pharmacist before using this drug.

PREGNANCY/BREAST-FEEDING: Category B—No evidence of risk in humans. Either animal findings show risk, but human findings do not; or, if no adequate human studies have been done, animal findings show no risk. It is not known whether the drug is excreted in the breast milk; therefore, caution should be used when breast-feeding.

OTHER BRAND NAMES: None

OTHER DRUGS IN THE SAME THERAPEUTIC CLASS: Naftin

IMPORTANT INFORMATION TO REMEMBER: For the cream: this drug is for external use only. Apply and gently rub in enough of the cream to cover the affected area and surrounding areas. Use the drug for the full course of treatment or the fungal infection may return. Never cover the skin after application with a bandage or wrapping unless directed to do so by a doctor. Discontinue use if irritation occurs. If taking the tablets, continue taking the medication for the full course of treatment; otherwise the infection may return.

BRAND NAME: Lanoxin and Lanoxicaps

GENERIC NAME: digoxin

GENERIC FORM AVAILABLE: No

THERAPEUTIC CLASS: Cardiac glycoside

DOSAGE FORMS: 0.125-mg, 0.25-mg, and 0.5-mg tablets; 0.05-mg, 0.1-mg, and 0.2-mg capsules; and 0.05-mg-per-1-ml pediatric elixir

MAIN USES: Congestive heart failure, irregular heartbeat, and fast heartbeat

USUAL DOSE: 0.125 mg to 0.5 mg daily in a single dose

AVERAGE PRICE: $16.53 for 0.125 mg and 0.25 mg

SIDE EFFECTS: Most of the drug's side effects are related to a patient taking too high of a dose. These side effects may include: nausea, vomiting, diarrhea, lower stomach pain, loss of appetite, slow heartbeat, blurred vision, seeing colored halos around objects, drowsiness, dizziness, irregular heartbeat, headache, fainting, and tiredness.

DRUG INTERACTIONS: Cordarone, erythromycin, Quinidex, Quinaglute, quinine, Rythmol, Sandimmune, and Sumycin may increase the blood levels of the drug. Some cancer drugs may decrease the blood levels of the drug. Some drugs used to treat irregular heartbeats; calcium supplements; and decongestants found in cough, cold, and allergy products may cause irregular heartbeats when used with the drug. Diuretics (water pills) may cause toxicity when used together with this drug. Patients taking potassium supplements should use this drug with caution. Calan or Isoptin taken with Lanoxin may have additive effects. Colestid and Questran may prevent the drug from being absorbed.

ALLERGIES: Individuals allergic to digoxin or any of its derivatives should discuss this with their doctor or pharmacist before using this drug.

PREGNANCY/BREAST-FEEDING: Category C—Risk cannot be ruled out. Human studies are lacking, and animal studies are either positive for fetal risk or lacking as well. However, potential benefits may justify the potential risk in using the drug. The drug is excreted in the breast milk; therefore, extreme caution should be used when breast-feeding.

OTHER BRAND NAMES: None

OTHER DRUGS IN THE SAME THERAPEUTIC CLASS: Crystodigin

IMPORTANT INFORMATION TO REMEMBER: Only take the drug exactly as directed by your physician. Do not discontinue the drug or increase the dose without first consulting your physician. Before taking over-the-counter medications, consult your physician or pharmacist. Report to your physician any nausea, diarrhea, vomiting, loss of appetite, or extremely slow pulse—these may be possible signs of overdose.

BRAND NAME: Lariam

GENERIC NAME: mefloquine

GENERIC FORM AVAILABLE: No

THERAPEUTIC CLASS: Antimalarial

DOSAGE FORMS: 250-mg tablets

MAIN USES: Prevention and treatment of malaria

USUAL DOSE: Treatment: 1250 mg (five tablets) in a single dose. Prevention: 250 mg weekly, starting one week before departure and continuing during the entire stay and for four weeks after returning home.

AVERAGE PRICE: $59.18 for six tablets

SIDE EFFECTS: Most common: nausea, dizziness, vomiting, muscle pain, fever, headache, insomnia, lightheadedness, chills, diarrhea, stomach pain, rash, loss of appetite, vision disturbances, and ringing in the ears. Less common: slow heartbeat, nervousness, confusion, seizures, depression, mental illness, and restlessness.

DRUG INTERACTIONS: The drug should not be used with Aralen, quinine, Quinidex, or Quinaglute. The drug may lower the blood levels of Depakene and Depakote. Blocadren, Cartrol, Corgard, Inderal, Kerlone, Levatol, Lopressor, Normodyne, Sectral, Tenormin, Toprol-XL, Trandate, Visken, or Zebeta and the drug may cause irregular heartbeats. Calan, Cardene, Cardizem, Dilacor XR, DynaCirc, Isoptin, Norvasc, Plendil, Procardia, Sular, Tiazac, or Verelan and the drug may cause irregular heartbeats.

ALLERGIES: Individuals allergic to mefloquine or any of its derivatives should discuss this with their doctor or pharmacist before using this drug.

PREGNANCY/BREAST-FEEDING: Category C—Risk cannot be ruled out. Human studies are lacking, and animal studies are either positive for fetal risk or lacking as well. However, potential benefits may justify the potential risk in using the drug. The drug is excreted in the breast milk; therefore, extreme caution should be used when breast-feeding.

OTHER BRAND NAMES: None

OTHER DRUGS IN THE SAME THERAPEUTIC CLASS: Aralen and Plaquenil

IMPORTANT INFORMATION TO REMEMBER: This drug should be taken with food or milk to reduce the potential for stomach upset. The drug should also be taken with plenty of water (eight ounces in preferred). Use exactly as directed by your physician. Always complete the full course of therapy for both prevention and treatment uses. Patients with epilepsy or seizures should discuss this with their doctor before taking the drug.

BRAND NAME: Larodopa

GENERIC NAME: levodopa

GENERIC FORM AVAILABLE: No

THERAPEUTIC CLASS: Dopamine precursor, anti-Parkinson's

DOSAGE FORMS: 100-mg, 250-mg, and 500-mg tablets

MAIN USES: Parkinson's disease

USUAL DOSE: 500 mg to 100 mg daily in divided doses

AVERAGE PRICE: $31.96 for 100 mg; $51.03 for 250 mg; and $87.65 for 500 mg

SIDE EFFECTS: Most common: dizziness, difficulty in urinating, dizziness when getting up suddenly, irregular heartbeat, nausea, diarrhea, aggressive behavior, unusual or uncontrolled body movements, nervousness, and confusion. Less common: loss of appetite, diarrhea, dry mouth, headache, diarrhea, muscle twitching, flushing, and muscle weakness.

DRUG INTERACTIONS: Compazine, Dilantin, Haldol, Mellaril, Prolixin, Serentil, Stelazine, Thorazine, and Trilafon may decrease the effects of the drug. The drug should not be used with Nardil or Parnate. Eldepryl and the drug should be used together with caution. Vitamin B_6 supplements may reduce the effectiveness of the drug.

ALLERGIES: Individuals allergic to levodopa or any of its derivatives should discuss this with their doctor or pharmacist before using this drug.

PREGNANCY/BREAST-FEEDING: Category C—Risk cannot be ruled out. Human studies are lacking, and animal studies are either positive for fetal risk or lacking as well. However, potential benefits may justify the potential risk in using the drug. It is not known whether the drug is excreted in the breast milk; therefore, caution should be used when breast-feeding.

OTHER BRAND NAMES: Dopar

OTHER DRUGS IN THE SAME THERAPEUTIC CLASS: Dopar

IMPORTANT INFORMATION TO REMEMBER: Only take the drug exactly as directed by your physician; do not stop taking the drug without first consulting with your physician. This drug should be taken with food or milk to reduce the potential for stomach upset. Individuals should avoid vitamins supplements containing large amounts of vitamin B_6. Individuals with glaucoma or urinary problems should discuss this with their physician before taking this drug. Individuals should get up slowly from the sitting or lying-down position; otherwise dizziness may occur. The drug may take several weeks before noticeable improvements are seen.

BRAND NAME: Larotid

GENERIC NAME: amoxicillin

See entry for Amoxil

BRAND NAME: Lasix

GENERIC NAME: furosemide

GENERIC FORM AVAILABLE: Yes

THERAPEUTIC CLASS: Loop diuretic (water pill)

DOSAGE FORMS: 20-mg, 40-mg, and 80-mg tablets and 10 mg/mL oral solution

MAIN USES: Water retention (fluid retention due to congestive heart failure, kidney disease, or cirrhosis of the liver) and high blood pressure

USUAL DOSE: 20 mg to 80 mg daily in a single or divided doses

AVERAGE PRICE: $21.87 (B)/$6.47 (G) for 20 mg; $30.56 (B)/$8.78 (G) for 40 mg; $42.00 (B)/$11.64 (G) for 80 mg

SIDE EFFECTS: Most common: dizziness when getting up from a sitting or lying-down position, muscle cramps, and some weakness. Less common: low potassium, blurred vision, diarrhea, headache, increased sensitivity to sunburn, loss of appetite, anemia, and stomach pain.

DRUG INTERACTIONS: The drug may increase the levels of Coumadin, Eskalith, and Lithobid in the blood. The drug may increase the chance of ototoxicity (hearing loss) when used with amphotericin B and cisplatin.

ALLERGIES: Individuals allergic to furosemide or any of its derivatives should discuss this with their doctor or pharmacist before using this drug.

PREGNANCY/BREAST-FEEDING: Category C—Risk cannot be ruled out. Human studies are lacking, and animal studies are either positive for fetal risk or lacking as well. However, potential benefits may justify the potential risk in using the drug. The drug is excreted in the breast milk; therefore, extreme caution should be used when breast-feeding.

OTHER BRAND NAMES: None

OTHER DRUGS IN THE SAME THERAPEUTIC CLASS: Bumex, Demadex, and Edecrin

IMPORTANT INFORMATION TO REMEMBER: If stomach upset occurs, the drug may be taken with food or milk. If the drug is to be taken once daily, take it in the morning due to increased urine output. Individuals with kidney disease should discuss this with their doctor before taking this drug. Before taking over-the-counter cold and allergy preparations, consult your doctor or pharmacist—these products may raise your blood pressure. The drug may cause the elimination of potassium from the body. It is therefore a good idea to eat a banana or drink orange, grapefruit, or apple juice every day to replace lost potassium. Individuals should get up slowly from the sitting or lying-down position; otherwise dizziness may occur.

BRAND NAME: Lescol

GENERIC NAME: fluvastatin

GENERIC FORM AVAILABLE: No

THERAPEUTIC CLASS: Cholesterol-lowering agent

DOSAGE FORMS: 20-mg and 40-mg capsules

MAIN USES: High cholesterol

USUAL DOSE: 20 mg to 80 mg daily

AVERAGE PRICE: $160.86 for 20 mg and $179.84 for 40 mg

SIDE EFFECTS: headache 9%, diarrhea 6%, stomach pain 6%, back pain 6%, hoarse throat 4%, runny nose 4%, tiredness 4%, muscle pain 3%, rash 3%, nausea 3%, gas 3%, constipation 3%, dizziness 3%, insomnia 3%, and bronchitis 2%.

DRUG INTERACTIONS: Sandimmune, Lopid, and niacin may cause kidney problems when taken with the drug. Tagamet, Prilosec, and Zantac may increase the blood levels of the drug. The drug may increase the effects of Coumadin. Lopid and the drug, when taken together, may increase the risk of developing rhabdomyolysis (destruction and death of muscle tissue); symptoms are muscle pain and dark, red-brown colored urine.

ALLERGIES: Individuals allergic to fluvastatin, Mevacor, Pravachol, Zocor, or any of their derivatives should discuss this with their doctor or pharmacist before using this drug.

PREGNANCY/BREAST-FEEDING: Category X—Should not be used during pregnancy. Studies in animals and/or humans have shown fetal abnormalities and birth defects. The risks associated with using this drug clearly outweigh the benefits. This drug should never be used by someone who is pregnant or trying to become pregnant. Also, women should never breast-feed while using this drug.

OTHER BRAND NAMES: None

OTHER DRUGS IN THE SAME THERAPEUTIC CLASS: Lipitor, Mevacor, Pravachol, and Zocor

IMPORTANT INFORMATION TO REMEMBER: If stomach upset occurs, the drug may be taken with food or milk. Only take the drug exactly as directed by your physician. It is also important to follow the prescribed low cholesterol diet. Report any sign of unexplained muscle pain or tenderness to your doctor, especially if it is accompanied by tiredness or fever.

BRAND NAME: Leukeran

GENERIC NAME: chlorambucil

GENERIC FORM AVAILABLE: No

THERAPEUTIC CLASS: Alkylating agent, anticancer

DOSAGE FORMS: 2-mg tablets

MAIN USES: Cancer

USUAL DOSE: 4 mg to 10 mg daily based on body weight

AVERAGE PRICE: $82.76 for 50 tablets

SIDE EFFECTS: Most common: blood disorders and bone marrow suppression. Less common: changes in menstrual periods, nausea, vomiting, itching, sores in the mouth, and allergic reaction.

DRUG INTERACTIONS: The drug may increase the blood levels of probenecid and Anturane. The drug may increase bone marrow suppression when used with radiation or other bone marrow suppressants.

ALLERGIES: Individuals allergic to chlorambucil or any of its derivatives should discuss this with their doctor or pharmacist before using this drug.

PREGNANCY/BREAST-FEEDING: Category D—Positive evidence of risk. Human studies show risk to the fetus. Nevertheless, potential benefits may possibly outweigh the potential risks. This drug should not be taken by nursing mothers.

OTHER BRAND NAMES: None

OTHER DRUGS IN THE SAME THERAPEUTIC CLASS: Alkeran and Cytoxan

IMPORTANT INFORMATION TO REMEMBER: It is extremely important to follow the dosing schedule set by your physician; do not deviate from this schedule. If unusual bleeding, bruising, black and tarry stools, blood in the urine, blood in the stool, or pinpoint red spots on the skin occur, contact your physician immediately. Nausea and vomiting may occur while taking this drug. Do not discontinue use unless directed by your physician. The drug may also lower the body's resistance to infection. At the first sign of infection—sore throat, fever, or chills—contact your physician immediately.

BRAND NAME: Levatol

GENERIC NAME: penbutolol

GENERIC FORM AVAILABLE: No

THERAPEUTIC CLASS: Noncardioselective beta-blocker

DOSAGE FORMS: 20-mg tablets

MAIN USES: High blood pressure

USUAL DOSE: 20 mg to 40 mg daily

AVERAGE PRICE: $156.32

SIDE EFFECTS: headache 8%, dizziness 5%, tiredness 4%, nausea 4%, diarrhea 3%, muscle pain 2%, chest pain 2%, cough 2%, trouble breathing 2%, excessive sweating 2%, insomnia 2%, impotence 1%.

DRUG INTERACTIONS: The drug may increase the effects of reserpine. The drug may increase the effects of Calan, Cardene, Cardizem, Catapres, Dilacor XR, DynaCirc, Isoptin, Lanoxin, Norvasc, Plendil, Procardia, Sular, Tiazac, Verelan, and Wytensin. Diabetic medications, insulin, Slo-bid, Theo-Dur, theophylline, Uni-Dur, and Uniphyl dosages may need to be adjusted when taking this drug.

ALLERGIES: Individuals allergic to penbutolol or other beta-blockers (such as those listed in "Other Drugs in the Same Therapeutic Class") should discuss this with their doctor or pharmacist before taking this drug.

PREGNANCY/BREAST-FEEDING: Category C—Risk cannot be ruled out. Human studies are lacking, and animal studies are either positive for fetal risk or lacking as well. However, potential benefits may justify the potential risk in using the drug. It is not known whether the drug is excreted in the breast milk; therefore, caution should be used when breast-feeding.

OTHER BRAND NAMES: None

OTHER DRUGS IN THE SAME THERAPEUTIC CLASS: Blocadren, Cartrol, Corgard, Inderal, Normodyne, Trandate, and Visken

IMPORTANT INFORMATION TO REMEMBER: Only take the drug exactly as directed by your physician. Do not discontinue the drug without first consulting your physician. This drug may cause some tiredness, especially at first. Individuals should use caution when driving, operating machinery, or any task where mental alertness is required. Alcohol, anxiety medications, and narcotic painkillers may intensify the drowsiness effect of the drug. Before taking over-the-counter cold and allergy preparations, consult your doctor or pharmacist; these products may raise your blood pressure. This drug may mask the symptoms of low blood sugar in diabetics.

BRAND NAME: Levlen

GENERIC NAME: Combination product containing: ethinyl estradiol and levonorgestrel

See entry for Nordette

BRAND NAME: Levothroid

GENERIC NAME: levothyroxine

See entry for Synthroid

BRAND NAME: Levoxyl

GENERIC NAME: levothyroxine

See entry for Synthroid

BRAND NAME: Levsin and Levsinex

GENERIC NAME: hyoscyamine

GENERIC FORM AVAILABLE: Yes

THERAPEUTIC CLASS: Anticholinergic

DOSAGE FORMS: 0.125-mg tablets, 0.125-mg sublingual tablets, 0.375-mg capsules (Levsinex), 0.125-mg/5 mL elixir, and 0.125-mg/mL drops

MAIN USES: Peptic ulcers, stomach spasms, and irritable bowel syndrome

USUAL DOSE: For the tablets: 0.125 mg to 0.25 mg every four hours as needed. For the Levsinex capsules: one capsule every 8 to 12 hours.

AVERAGE PRICE: $44.63 (B)/$17.92 (G) for 0.125-mg and $88.88 (B)/$64.33 (G) for 0.375-mg capsules (Levsinex)

SIDE EFFECTS: Most common: decreased sweating, dry mouth, and dry throat. Less common: constipation, difficulty in swallowing, blurred vision, decreased flow of breast milk, and increased sensitivity of the eyes to light.

DRUG INTERACTIONS: The drug may cause additive adverse effects when used with Compazine, Haldol, Mellaril, Nardil, Parnate, Prolixin, Serentil, Stelazine, Thorazine, and Trilafon. Antacids may decrease the absorption of the drug.

ALLERGIES: Individuals allergic to hyoscyamine or any of its derivatives should discuss this with their doctor or pharmacist before using this drug.

PREGNANCY/BREAST-FEEDING: Category C—Risk cannot be ruled out. Human studies are lacking, and animal studies are either positive for fetal risk or lacking as well. However, potential benefits may justify the potential risk in using the drug. The drug is excreted in the breast milk; therefore, extreme caution should be used when breast-feeding.

OTHER BRAND NAMES: Anaspaz

OTHER DRUGS IN THE SAME THERAPEUTIC CLASS: Bentyl, Cantil, Pro-Banthīne, Robinul, and Spacol

IMPORTANT INFORMATION TO REMEMBER: It's best to take the drug on an empty stomach, 30 minutes before meals. This drug does cause drowsiness. Individuals should use caution when driving, operating machinery, or any task where mental alertness is required. Alcohol, anxiety medications, and narcotic painkillers may intensify the drowsiness effect of the drug. This drug may also cause a dry mouth; sugarless gum or hard candy will help take care of this problem. Patients with glaucoma, urinary or prostate problems, GI obstruction, or severe ulcerative colitis should consult their doctor before taking this drug.

BRAND NAME: Librax

GENERIC NAME: Combination product containing: chlordiazepoxide and clidinium bromide

GENERIC FORM AVAILABLE: Yes

THERAPEUTIC CLASS: Benzodiazepine antianxiety + antispasmatic

DOSAGE FORMS: 5-mg chlordiazepoxide/2.5-mg clidinium bromide capsules

MAIN USES: Peptic ulcer and irritable bowel syndrome

USUAL DOSE: one to two capsules three to four times daily before meals and at bedtime

AVERAGE PRICE: $79.51 (B)/$9.77 (G)

SIDE EFFECTS: Most common: drowsiness, and dry mouth and throat. Less common: decreased sweating, confusion, dizziness, blurred vision, decreased flow of breast milk, constipation, and difficulty in urinating.

DRUG INTERACTIONS: Central nervous system (CNS) depression may be increased when used with alcohol, narcotic painkillers, or anxiety medications. The drug may cause additive adverse effects when used with Compazine, Haldol, Mellaril, Nardil, Parnate, Prolixin, Serentil, Stelazine, Thorazine, and Trilafon.

ALLERGIES: Individuals allergic to chlordiazepoxide, Librium, clidinium bromide, or any of their derivatives should discuss this with their doctor or pharmacist before using this drug.

PREGNANCY/BREAST-FEEDING: Category C—Risk cannot be ruled out. Human studies are lacking, and animal studies are either positive for fetal risk or lacking as well. However, potential benefits may justify the potential risk in using the drug. It is not known whether the drug is excreted in the breast milk; therefore, caution should be used when breast-feeding.

OTHER BRAND NAMES: Clindex

OTHER DRUGS IN THE SAME THERAPEUTIC CLASS: None

IMPORTANT INFORMATION TO REMEMBER: The drug should be taken 30–60 minutes before meals. This drug may cause drowsiness. Individuals should use caution when driving, operating machinery, or any task where mental alertness is required. The incidence of drowsiness and unsteadiness increases with age. Alcohol, anxiety medications, and narcotic painkillers may intensify the drowsiness effect of the drug. This medication may be habit-forming. Do not increase the dose of medication without consulting with your doctor—take only the amount prescribed by your doctor. Patients with glaucoma, urinary or prostate problems, GI obstruction, or severe ulcerative colitis should consult their doctors before taking this drug.

BRAND NAME: Librium

GENERIC NAME: chlordiazepoxide

GENERIC FORM AVAILABLE: Yes

THERAPEUTIC CLASS: Benzodiazepine antianxiety

DOSAGE FORMS: 5-mg, 10-mg, and 25-mg tablets and capsules

MAIN USES: Anxiety

USUAL DOSE: 5 mg to 25 mg two to four times daily

AVERAGE PRICE: $41.89 (B)/$8.78 (G) for 5 mg; $60.92 (B)/$9.88 (G) for 10 mg; 104.26 (B)/$13.51 (G) for 25 mg

SIDE EFFECTS: Most common: drowsiness, clumsiness, and dizziness. Less common: confusion, depression, stomach cramps, nausea, vomiting, dry mouth, changes in sex drive, sleep disturbances, and fast heartbeat.

DRUG INTERACTIONS: Central nervous system (CNS) depression may be increased when used with alcohol, narcotic painkillers, or other anxiety medications.

ALLERGIES: Individuals allergic to chlordiazepoxide or other benzodiazepines (such as those listed in "Other Drugs in the Same Therapeutic Class") should discuss this with their doctor or pharmacist before taking this drug.

PREGNANCY/BREAST-FEEDING: Category D—Positive evidence of risk. Human studies show risk to the fetus. Nevertheless, potential benefits may possibly outweigh the potential risks. This drug should not be taken by nursing mothers.

OTHER BRAND NAMES: None

OTHER DRUGS IN THE SAME THERAPEUTIC CLASS: Ativan, Serax, Tranxene, Valium, and Xanax

IMPORTANT INFORMATION TO REMEMBER: This drug may cause drowsiness. Individuals should use caution when driving, operating machinery, or any task where mental alertness is required. The incidence of drowsiness and unsteadiness increases with age. Alcohol or central nervous system depressants may intensify the drowsiness effect of the drug. This medication is a controlled substance and may be habit-forming. Do not increase the dose of medication without consulting with your doctor—take only the amount prescribed by your doctor.

BRAND NAME: Lidex and Lidex-E

GENERIC NAME: fluocinonide

GENERIC FORM AVAILABLE: Yes

THERAPEUTIC CLASS: Topical corticosteroid

DOSAGE FORMS: 0.05% ointment, gel, cream, and solution

MAIN USES: Skin rashes, swelling, and itching

USUAL DOSE: Apply to the affected area as a thin film two to four times daily.

AVERAGE PRICE: $24.96 (B)/$14.24 (G) for Lidex 0.05% cream and ointment (15 g); and $26.89 (B)/$14.94 (G) for Lidex-E cream (15 g)

SIDE EFFECTS: Most common: none. Less common: burning, itching, irritation, dry skin, rash, and soreness of the skin.

DRUG INTERACTIONS: None of any clinical significance

ALLERGIES: Individuals allergic to fluocinonide or any of its derivatives should discuss this with their doctor or pharmacist before using this drug.

PREGNANCY/BREAST-FEEDING: Category C—Risk cannot be ruled out. Human studies are lacking, and animal studies are either positive for fetal risk or lacking as well. However, potential benefits may justify the potential risk in using the drug. It is not known whether the drug is excreted in the breast milk; therefore, caution should be used when breast-feeding.

OTHER BRAND NAMES: None

OTHER DRUGS IN THE SAME THERAPEUTIC CLASS: Aclovate, Aristocort, Cordran, Cordran SP, Cutivate, Cyclocort, DesOwen, Diprolene, Diprolene AF, Elocon, Florone, Florone E, Halog, Hytone, Kenalog, Synalar, Temovate, Topicort, Tridesilon, Ultravate, Valisone, and Westcort

IMPORTANT INFORMATION TO REMEMBER: This drug is for external use only. Apply only a thin film of drug to skin and rub it in well. Never cover the skin after application with a bandage or wrapping unless directed to do so by a doctor. Never apply to damaged skin or open wounds unless directed to do so by a doctor. Discontinue use if irritation occurs.

BRAND NAME: Limbitrol and Limbitrol DS

GENERIC NAME: Combination product containing: chlordiazepoxide and amitriptyline

GENERIC FORM AVAILABLE: Yes

THERAPEUTIC CLASS: Benzodiazepine antianxiety + tricyclic antidepressant

DOSAGE FORMS: 5-mg chlordiazepoxide/12.5-mg amitriptyline tablets (Limbitrol) and 10-mg chlordiazepoxide/25-mg amitriptyline tablets (Limbitrol DS)

MAIN USES: Depression with anxiety

USUAL DOSE: three to four tablets daily in divided doses

AVERAGE PRICE: $76.98 (B)/$25.72 (G) for Limbitrol and $108.55 (B)/$32.54 (G) for Limbitrol DS

SIDE EFFECTS: Most common: drowsiness, clumsiness, and dizziness. Less common: confusion, depression, stomach cramps, nausea, vomiting, dry mouth, changes in sex drive, sleep disturbances, restlessness, changes in appetite, headache, and fast heartbeat.

DRUG INTERACTIONS: Central nervous system (CNS) depression may be increased when used with alcohol, narcotic painkillers, or other anxiety medications. The drug may block the action of Ismelin. Tagamet may increase the blood levels of the drug. The drug should not be taken within 14 days of taking Nardil or Parnate.

ALLERGIES: Individuals allergic to chlordiazepoxide, Librium, amitriptyline, or any of their derivatives should discuss this with their doctor or pharmacist before using this drug.

PREGNANCY/BREAST-FEEDING: Category D—Positive evidence of risk. Human studies show risk to the fetus. Nevertheless, potential benefits may possibly outweigh the potential risk. This drug should not be taken by nursing mothers.

OTHER BRAND NAMES: None

OTHER DRUGS IN THE SAME THERAPEUTIC CLASS: None

IMPORTANT INFORMATION TO REMEMBER: This drug may cause drowsiness. Individuals should use caution when driving, operating machinery, or any task where mental alertness is required. The incidence of drowsiness and unsteadiness increases with age. Alcohol, anxiety medications, and narcotic painkillers may intensify the drowsiness effect of the drug. This medication may be habit-forming. Do not increase the dose of medication without consulting with your doctor—take only the amount prescribed by your doctor. This drug should be discontinued if any kind of surgery is required. The drug may take several weeks before a significant improvement is seen.

BRAND NAME: Lioresal

GENERIC NAME: baclofen

GENERIC FORM AVAILABLE: Yes

THERAPEUTIC CLASS: Muscle relaxant

DOSAGE FORMS: 10-mg and 20-mg tablets

MAIN USES: Muscle spasms

USUAL DOSE: 40 mg to 80 mg daily in divided doses

AVERAGE PRICE: $57.29 (B)/$24.07 (G) for 10 mg

SIDE EFFECTS: drowsiness (usually goes away after a few days), 10%–63%, dizziness 5%–15%, weakness 5%–15%, nausea 4%–12%, headache 4%–8%, insomnia 2%–7%, constipation 2%–6%, increased urination 2%–6%, tiredness 2%–4%, confusion 1%–11%, and low blood pressure 1%–9%.

DRUG INTERACTIONS: Central nervous system (CNS) depression may be increased when used with alcohol, narcotic painkillers, or other anxiety medications.

ALLERGIES: Individuals allergic to baclofen or any of its derivatives should discuss this with their doctor or pharmacist before using this drug.

PREGNANCY/BREAST-FEEDING: Category C—Risk cannot be ruled out. Human studies are lacking, and animal studies are either positive for fetal risk or lacking as well. However, potential benefits may justify the potential risk in using the drug. The drug is excreted in the breast milk; therefore, extreme caution should be used when breast-feeding.

OTHER BRAND NAMES: Atrofen

OTHER DRUGS IN THE SAME THERAPEUTIC CLASS: Flexeril, Parafon Forte DSC, Robaxin, Skelaxin, and Soma

IMPORTANT INFORMATION TO REMEMBER: This drug does cause drowsiness. Individuals should use caution when driving, operating machinery, or any task where mental alertness is required. Alcohol, anxiety medications, and narcotic painkillers may intensify the drowsiness effect of the drug. Do not increase the dose without first consulting with your physician and do not suddenly stop taking the drug.

BRAND NAME: Lipitor

GENERIC NAME: atorvastatin

GENERIC FORM AVAILABLE: No

THERAPEUTIC CLASS: Cholesterol-lowering agent

DOSAGE FORMS: 10-mg, 20-mg, and 40-mg tablets

MAIN USES: High cholesterol

USUAL DOSE: 10 mg to 80 mg once daily

AVERAGE PRICE: $187.47 for 10 mg; $274.91 for 20 mg; and $395.15 for 40 mg

SIDE EFFECTS: headache 3%–17%, muscle pain 3%–6%, stomach pain 3%–4%, diarrhea 3%–4%, skin rash 3%–4%, back pain 3%–4%, joint pain 2%–5%, weakness 2%–4%, nausea 2%–3%, nasal congestion 2%–3%, constipation 2%, flu-like symptoms 2%, allergic reaction 1%–3%, and gas 1%–3%.

DRUG INTERACTIONS: Antacids may decrease the absorption of the drug. Colestid and Questran may decrease the blood levels of the drug. Erythromycin may increase the blood levels of the drug. Lopid and the drug, when taken together, may increase the risk of developing rhabdomyolysis (destruction and death of muscle tissue); symptoms are muscle pain and dark, red-brown colored urine.

ALLERGIES: Individuals allergic to atorvastatin, Lescol, Mevacor, Pravachol, Zocor, or any of their derivatives should discuss this with their doctor or pharmacist before using this drug.

PREGNANCY/BREAST-FEEDING: Category X—Should not be used during pregnancy. Studies in animals and/or humans have shown fetal abnormalities and birth defects. The risks associated with using this drug clearly outweigh the benefits. This drug should never be used by someone who is pregnant or trying to become pregnant. Also, women should never breast-feed while using this drug.

OTHER BRAND NAMES: None

OTHER DRUGS IN THE SAME THERAPEUTIC CLASS: Lescol, Mevacor, and Pravachol

IMPORTANT INFORMATION TO REMEMBER: The drug may be taken with food or milk if stomach upset occurs. Only take the drug exactly as directed by your physician. It is also important to follow the prescribed low cholesterol diet. Report any sign of unexplained muscle pain or tenderness to your doctor, especially if it is accompanied by tiredness or fever.

BRAND NAME: Lithobid

GENERIC NAME: lithium carbonate

GENERIC FORM AVAILABLE: No

THERAPEUTIC CLASS: Anti-manic

DOSAGE FORMS: 300-mg slow-release tablets

MAIN USES: Bipolar disorder and manic episodes

USUAL DOSE: 900 mg to 1200 mg per day in two or three divided doses

AVERAGE PRICE: $34.16

SIDE EFFECTS: Most common: drowsiness, diarrhea, increased thirst, nausea, increased urination, some limited loss of bladder control, and slight trembling of hands. Less common: irregular heartbeat; weight gain; cold arms, legs, feet, and fingers; weakness; and muscle twitching.

DRUG INTERACTIONS: NSAIDs (such as Anaprox, Ansaid, Aleve, aspirin, Cataflam, Clinoril, Daypro, Disalcid, Dolobid, Easprin,

Feldene, Indocin, Lodine, Motrin, Nalfon, Naprosyn, Orudis, Oruvail, Relafen, Tolectin, and Voltaren) and Tegretol may increase the concentration of the drug in the blood. Diuretics (water pills) may increase the blood levels of the drug. The drug may decrease the absorption of Compazine, Mellaril, Prolixin, Serentil, Stelazine, Thorazine, and Trilafon. Haldol and the drug, when used together, may cause brain damage. Accupril, Altace, Capoten, Lotensin, Monopril, Prinivil, Univasc, Vasotec, and Zestril may increase the toxic effects of the drug.

ALLERGIES: Individuals allergic to lithium carbonate, Eskalith, or any of their derivatives should discuss this with their doctor or pharmacist before using this drug.

PREGNANCY/BREAST-FEEDING: Category D—Positive evidence of risk. Human studies show risk to the fetus. Nevertheless, potential benefits may possibly outweigh the potential risks. This drug should not be taken by nursing mothers.

OTHER BRAND NAMES: None

OTHER DRUGS IN THE SAME THERAPEUTIC CLASS: Eskalith, Eskalith CR, and Lithotabs

IMPORTANT INFORMATION TO REMEMBER: Only take the drug exactly as directed by your physician and do not increase the dose without first consulting with your physician. This drug may cause some drowsiness. Individuals should use caution when driving, operating machinery, or any task where mental alertness is required. Alcohol, anxiety medications, and narcotic painkillers may intensify the drowsiness effect of the drug. Take this drug with plenty of water (eight ounces is preferred), especially during hot weather or while exercising. The drug may require one to three weeks of use before improvement may be noticed. Do not crush or break the tablets—this will destroy the mechanism that delays the release of the drug. Individuals taking the drug should have regular blood tests to determine if the correct amount of the drug is being taken. Individuals should also have thyroid function tests performed every six months.

BRAND NAME: Lithonate and Lithotabs

GENERIC NAME: lithium carbonate

See entry for Eskalith/Eskalith CR

BRAND NAME: Livostin

GENERIC NAME: levocabastine

GENERIC FORM AVAILABLE: No

THERAPEUTIC CLASS: Antihistamine eyedrop

DOSAGE FORMS: 0.05% eyedrop suspension

MAIN USES: Eye allergies

USUAL DOSE: one drop four times daily

AVERAGE PRICE: $36.31 for 5 mL

SIDE EFFECTS: Most common: burning and stinging upon use. Less common: headache, blurred vision, and dry eyes.

DRUG INTERACTIONS: None of any clinical significance

ALLERGIES: Individuals allergic to levocabastine or any of its derivatives should discuss this with their doctor or pharmacist before using this drug.

PREGNANCY/BREAST-FEEDING: Category C—Risk cannot be ruled out. Human studies are lacking, and animal studies are either positive for fetal risk or lacking as well. However, potential benefits may justify the potential risk in using the drug. The drug is excreted in the breast milk; therefore, caution should be used when breast-feeding.

OTHER BRAND NAMES: None

OTHER DRUGS IN THE SAME THERAPEUTIC CLASS: None

IMPORTANT INFORMATION TO REMEMBER: Individuals should not use the drug while wearing contact lenses unless otherwise directed by a physician. Keep the container tightly closed and avoid touching the applicator tip to the eye—this could contaminate the product over time. Also, only administer one drop at a time. After application, keep the eye open for at least 30 seconds, roll the eyeball around, and avoid squinting. If a second drop is required, wait one to two minutes between drops. If another medication is to be used in the eye, wait at least 10 minutes before administering it.

BRAND NAME: Lodine and Lodine XL

GENERIC NAME: etodolac

GENERIC FORM AVAILABLE: No

THERAPEUTIC CLASS: Nonsteroidal anti-inflammatory drug (NSAID)

DOSAGE FORMS: 200-mg and 300-mg capsules, and 400-mg and 500-mg tablets (Lodine); and 400-mg and 600-mg extended-release tablets (Lodine XL)

MAIN USES: Arthritis and pain relief

USUAL DOSE: 600 mg to 1200 mg per day in divided doses (Lodine) and 400 mg to 1000 mg once daily (Lodine XL)

AVERAGE PRICE: For Lodine: $141.90 for 200 mg; $149.04 for 300 mg; $156.97 for 400 mg; and $198.39 for 500 mg. For Lodine XL: $164.09 for 400 mg and $245.30 for 600 mg.

SIDE EFFECTS: upset stomach 10%, stomach pain 3%–9%, gas 3%–9%, diarrhea 3%–9%, dizziness 3%–9%, constipation 1%–3%, vomiting 1%–3%, depression 1%–3%, nervousness 1%–3%, itching 1%–3%, rash 1%–3%, urinary problems 1%–3%, ringing in the ears 1%–3%, and blurred vision 1%–3%.

DRUG INTERACTIONS: Aspirin will decrease the concentration of this drug in the blood. This drug may also decrease the effects of Lasix, Dyazide, HydroDIURIL, Maxzide, and other water pills. The drug may increase the blood levels of Eskalith, Lithobid, and Sandimmune. The drug may increase the toxic effects of the drug Rheumatrex. Caution should be used when taking the drug with Coumadin.

ALLERGIES: Individuals allergic to etodolac or other NSAIDs (such as those listed in "Other Drugs in the Same Therapeutic Class") should discuss this with their doctor or pharmacist before taking this drug.

PREGNANCY/BREAST-FEEDING: Category C—Risk cannot be ruled out. Human studies are lacking, and animal studies are either positive for fetal risk or lacking as well. However, potential benefits may justify the potential risk in using the drug. The drug should not, however, be used during the late stages (last three months) of pregnancy. It is not known whether the drug is excreted in the breast milk; therefore, caution should be used when breast-feeding.

OTHER BRAND NAMES: None

OTHER DRUGS IN THE SAME THERAPEUTIC CLASS: Anaprox, Ansaid, aspirin, Cataflam, Clinoril, Daypro, Disalcid, Dolobid, Easprin, Feldene, Indocin, Motrin, Nalfon, Naprosyn, Orudis, Oruvail, Relafen, Tolectin, Toradol, Voltaren, and Voltaren XR

IMPORTANT INFORMATION TO REMEMBER: This drug should be taken with food or milk to reduce the potential for injury to the stomach lining and stomach upset. This drug may take up to two weeks before a noticeable improvement in pain relief associated with arthritis is observed. Drinking alcohol while taking this drug may increase its potential to cause ulcers. This drug should only be used under the direct supervision of a doctor by individuals with a bleeding disorder or ulcer, or those who are currently taking Coumadin. Before taking over-the-counter pain relievers, consult your doctor or pharmacist. No more than one pain reliever should be taken at any one time unless otherwise directed by your doctor.

BRAND NAME: Loestrin and Loestrin FE

GENERIC NAME: Combination product containing: norethindrone and ethinyl estradiol

GENERIC FORM AVAILABLE: No

THERAPEUTIC CLASS: Progestin + estrogen contraceptive

DOSAGE FORMS: 7-mg norethindrone/20-micrograms/ethinyl estradiol (Loestrin 1/20) and 1.5-mg norethindrone/30-micrograms/ethinyl estradiol (Loestrin 1.5/30). The Loestrin FE is same as the Loestrin, except the last seven tablets (the inactive ones) contain iron as a supplement.

MAIN USES: Birth control

USUAL DOSE: Take one tablet daily for 21 or 28 days, beginning on the fifth day of the cycle. Day One of the cycle is the first day of menstrual bleeding.

AVERAGE PRICE: $29.94

SIDE EFFECTS: Most common: stomach cramps, bloating, acne, appetite changes, nausea, swelling of the feet and ankles, weight gain, swelling of the breasts, breast tenderness, and unusual tiredness or weakness. Less common: changes in vaginal bleeding, feeling faint, increased blood pressure, depression, stomach pain, vaginal itching, yeast infections, brown and blotchy spots on the skin, diarrhea, dizziness, headaches, migraines, increased body and facial hair, increased sensitivity of the skin to the sun, irritability, some hair loss from the scalp, vomiting, blood clots, weight loss, and changes in sexual desire.

DRUG INTERACTIONS: Antibiotics may decrease the effectiveness of the drug. The drug may interfere with the effectiveness of Parlodel. The drug may reduce the effects of Coumadin. The drug may increase the blood levels of Anafranil, Asendin, Elavil, Endep, Norpramin, Pamelor, Sinequan, Surmontil, Tofranil, and Vivactil when used for long periods of time. Smoking is not recommended while taking this drug due to the increased risk of heart disease, stroke, and high blood pressure.

ALLERGIES: Individuals allergic to norethindrone, ethinyl estradiol, ferrous fumarate (if taking Loestrin FE), or any of their derivatives should discuss this with their doctor or pharmacist before using this drug.

PREGNANCY/BREAST-FEEDING: Category X—Should not be used during pregnancy. Studies in animals and/or humans have shown fetal abnormalities and birth defects. The risks associated with using this drug clearly outweigh the benefits. This drug should never be used by someone who is pregnant or trying to become pregnant. Also, women should never breast-feed while using this drug.

OTHER BRAND NAMES: None

OTHER DRUGS IN THE SAME THERAPEUTIC CLASS: Brevicon, Demulen, Desogen, Levlen, Lo/Ovral, Modicon, Nordette, Norinyl, Ortho-Cept, Ortho-Cyclen, Ortho-Novum, Ovcon, and Orval

IMPORTANT INFORMATION TO REMEMBER: Only take the drug exactly as directed by your physician. It is important to take the drug at the same time every day (bedtime). Do not discontinue the drug without first consulting your physician. The drug should not be used by women with a history of heart disease, stroke, high blood pressure, breast cancer, or other blood vessel disease. Breakthrough bleeding may occur during the first few months; if this persists, notify your doctor. This drug will not provide protection against the HIV (AIDS) virus. It is important to use a second method of birth control during the first week when treatment has just begun. It may be necessary to use a second form of birth control when antibiotics are being taken. Also, women who smoke run a higher risk of heart disease, stroke, and high blood pressure when taking this drug. If pregnancy is suspected, stop taking the drug immediately.

BRAND NAME: Lomotil

GENERIC NAME: Combinaton product containing: diphenoxylate and atropine

GENERIC FORM AVAILABLE: Yes

THERAPEUTIC CLASS: Narcotic antidiarrheal + antispasmatic

DOSAGE FORMS: 2.5-mg diphenoxylate/0.025-mg atropine tablets; 2.5 mg diphenoxylate/0.025 mg atropine per 5 mL liquid

MAIN USES: Diarrhea

USAL DOSE: Short-term use: two tablets or two teaspoons four times a day until diarrhea is under control. Long-term use: one tablet or one teaspoon once or twice daily.

AVERAGE PRICE: $31.96 (B)/$9.61 (G) for 30 tablets; liquid price $25.99 (B)/$13.81 (G) for 120 ml

SIDE EFFECTS: Most common: drowsiness and constipation. Less common: appetite changes, stomach pain, dry mouth, nausea, vomiting, confusion, headaches, and dizziness.

DRUG INTERACTIONS: Central nervous system (CNS) depression may be increased when used with alcohol, narcotic painkillers, or other anxiety medications. Eldepryl, Furoxone, Matulane, Nardil, and Parnate may cause severe high blood pressure when taken with this drug.

ALLERGIES: Individuals allergic to diphenoxylate, atropine, or any of their derivatives should discuss this with their doctor or pharmacist before using this drug.

PREGNANCY/BREAST-FEEDING: Category C—Risk cannot be ruled out. Human studies are lacking, and animal studies are either positive for fetal risk or lacking as well. However, potential benefits may justify the potential risk in using the drug. The drug is excreted in the breast milk; therefore, caution should be used when breast-feeding.

OTHER BRAND NAMES: None

OTHER DRUGS IN THE SAME THERAPEUTIC CLASS: None

IMPORTANT INFORMATION TO REMEMBER: This drug may cause some limited drowsiness. Individuals should use caution when driving, operating machinery, or any task where mental alertness is required. Alcohol, anxiety medications, and narcotic painkillers may intensify the drowsiness effect of the drug. Contact your physician if the diarrhea is not controlled within 48 hours of the start of treatment. Drink plenty of liquids to avoid the dehydration that may occur due to the diarrhea. Do not increase the dose without first consulting with your physician. This drug is a controlled substance and may be habit-forming.

BRAND NAME: Loniten

GENERIC NAME: minoxidil

GENERIC FORM AVAILABLE: Yes

THERAPEUTIC CLASS: Blood vessel dilator

DOSAGE FORMS: 2.5-mg and 10-mg tablets

MAIN USES: High blood pressure

USUAL DOSE: 5 mg to 40 mg per day in single or divided doses

AVERAGE PRICE: $65.66 (B)/$46.55 (G) for 2.5 mg and $144.24 (B)/$75.53 (G) for 10 mg

SIDE EFFECTS: Most common: increased body hair growth, temporary swelling, fast heartbeat, pounding heartbeat, and bloating. Less common: headache, drowsiness, tiredness, breast tenderness in males and females, and chest pain.

DRUG INTERACTIONS: Dilatrate, Imdur, Ismelin, Isordil, Monoket, nitroglycerin patches, or Sorbitrate may produce low blood pressure when used with this drug.

ALLERGIES: Individuals allergic to minoxidil, Rogaine, or any of their derivatives should discuss this with their doctor or pharmacist before using this drug.

PREGNANCY/BREAST-FEEDING: Category C—Risk cannot be ruled out. Human studies are lacking, and animal studies are either positive for fetal risk or lacking as well. However, potential benefits may justify the potential risk in using the drug. Nursing mothers should not take this drug.

OTHER BRAND NAMES: None

OTHER DRUGS IN THE SAME THERAPEUTIC CLASS: Apresoline

IMPORTANT INFORMATION TO REMEMBER: Loniten should be used only by those individuals who did not respond to other high-blood-pressure medications. Do not stop taking the drug without first consulting with a doctor. The drug may cause drowsiness, headache, or heart palpitations during the first few days of therapy. Drowsiness may occur, but usually goes away once the body adjusts to the medication. Before taking over-the-counter cold and allergy preparations, consult your doctor or pharmacist—these products may raise your blood pressure. Weight gain (two to three pounds) during the beginning of treatment is normal and is usually lost with continued treatment. If a lot of weight is gained or swelling is seen, contact your doctor.

BRAND NAME: Lo/Ovral

GENERIC NAME: Combination product containing: norgestrel and ethinyl estradiol

See entry for Ovral

BRAND NAME: Lopid

GENERIC NAME: gemfibrozil

GENERIC FORM AVAILABLE: Yes

THERAPEUTIC CLASS: Anti-cholesterol

DOSAGE FORMS: 600-mg tablets

MAIN USES: High cholesterol and high triglycerides

USUAL DOSE: 600 mg twice daily 30 minutes prior to morning and evening meals

AVERAGE PRICE: $177.07 (B)/$94.57 (G)

SIDE EFFECTS: upset stomach 20%, stomach pain 10%, diarrhea 7%, tiredness 4%, vomiting 2%, eczema 2%, rash 2%, dizziness 2%, constipation 1%, headache 1%, and appendicitis 1%.

DRUG INTERACTIONS: The drug may increase the effects of Coumadin. Lescol, Mevacor, Pravachol, or Zocor and the drug, when used together, may increase the risk of developing rhabdomyolysis (destruction and death of muscle tissue); symptoms are muscle pain and dark, red-brown colored urine.

ALLERGIES: Individuals allergic to gemfibrozil or any of its derivatives should discuss this with their doctor or pharmacist before using this drug.

PREGNANCY/BREAST-FEEDING: Category C—Risk cannot be ruled out. Human studies are lacking, and animal studies are either positive for fetal risk or lacking as well. However, potential benefits may justify the potential risk in using the drug. It is not known whether the drug is excreted in the breast milk; therefore, caution should be used when breast-feeding.

OTHER BRAND NAMES: None

OTHER DRUGS IN THE SAME THERAPEUTIC CLASS: Atromid-S

IMPORTANT INFORMATION TO REMEMBER: The drug should be taken 30 minutes before breakfast and dinner for best results. Only take the drug exactly as directed by your physician. If the following symptoms occur—muscle pain, muscle tenderness, or muscle weakness—contact your physician. These symptoms may be from a dangerous condition, called myositis, which affects the muscles of the body.

BRAND NAME: Lopressor

GENERIC NAME: metoprolol tartrate

GENERIC FORM AVAILABLE: Yes

THERAPEUTIC CLASS: Cardioselective beta-blocker

DOSAGE FORMS: 50-mg and 100-mg tablets

MAIN USES: High blood pressure, angina, and after a heart attack

USUAL DOSE: 100 mg to 450 mg per day in single or divided doses

AVERAGE PRICE: $57.17 (B)/$39.57 (G) for 50 mg and $101.17 (B)/ $71.47 (G) for 100 mg

SIDE EFFECTS: low blood pressure 27%, tiredness 10%, dizziness 10%, depression 5%, rash 5%, diarrhea 5%, shortness of breath 3%, slow heartbeat 3%, cold feet and hands 1%, swelling 1%, wheezing 1%, nausea 1%, dry mouth 1%, constipation 1%, stomach pain 1%, gas 1%, and heartburn 1%.

DRUG INTERACTIONS: The drug may cause additive effects when used with reserpine. The drug may increase the effects of Calan, Cardene, Cardizem, Catapres, Covera-HS, Dilacor XR, DynaCirc, Isoptin, Lanoxin, Norvasc, Plendil, Procardia, Sular, Tiazac, Verelan, and Wytensin. Diabetic medications, insulin, Slo-bid, Theo-Dur, theophylline, Uni-Dur, and Uniphyl dosages may need to be adjusted when taking this drug. The drug may also interfere with glaucoma screening tests.

ALLERGIES: Individuals allergic to metoprolol or other beta-blockers (such as those listed in "Other Drugs in the Same Therapeutic Class") should discuss this with their doctor or pharmacist before taking this drug.

PREGNANCY/BREAST-FEEDING: Category C—Risk cannot be ruled out. Human studies are lacking, and animal studies are either positive for fetal risk or lacking as well. However, potential benefits may justify the potential risk in using the drug. The drug is excreted in the breast milk; therefore, extreme caution should be used when breast-feeding.

OTHER BRAND NAMES: None

OTHER DRUGS IN THE SAME THERAPEUTIC CLASS: Kerlone, Sectral, Tenormin, Toprol-XL, and Zebeta

IMPORTANT INFORMATION TO REMEMBER: Only take the drug exactly as directed by your physician. Do not discontinue the drug without first consulting your physician. This drug may cause some tiredness, especially at first. Individuals should use caution when driving, operating machinery, or any task where mental alertness is required. Alcohol, anxiety medications, and narcotic painkillers may intensify the tiredness effect of the drug. Before taking over-the-counter cold and allergy preparations, consult your doctor or pharmacist—these products may raise your blood pressure. This drug may mask the symptoms of low blood sugar in diabetics.

BRAND NAME: Lopressor HCT

GENERIC NAME: Combination product containing: metoprolol tartrate and hydrochlorothiazide

See individual entries for Lopressor and HydroDIURIL

BRAND NAME: **Loprox**

GENERIC NAME: ciclopiroxolamine

GENERIC FORM AVAILABLE: No

THERAPEUTIC CLASS: Antifungal

DOSAGE FORMS: 1% cream and lotion

MAIN USES: fungal infections (mainly ringworm, jock itch, and athlete's foot)

USUAL DOSE: Apply and massage into affected area twice daily.

AVERAGE PRICE: $15.21 for 15 g of cream and $29.89 for 30 mL of lotion

SIDE EFFECTS: Most common: None. Less common: irritation and burning.

DRUG INTERACTIONS: None of any clinical significance

ALLERGIES: Individuals allergic to ciclopiroxolamine or any of its derivatives should discuss this with their doctor or pharmacist before using this drug.

PREGNANCY/BREAST-FEEDING: Category B—No evidence of risk in humans. Either animal findings show risk, but human findings do not; or, if no adequate human studies have been done, animal findings show no risk. It is not known whether the drug is excreted in the breast milk; therefore, caution should be used when breast-feeding.

OTHER BRAND NAMES: None

OTHER DRUGS IN THE SAME THERAPEUTIC CLASS: None

IMPORTANT INFORMATION TO REMEMBER: This drug is for external use only. Apply and gently rub in enough of the cream to cover the affected area and surrounding areas. Use the drug for the full course of treatment or the fungal infection may return. Do not cover the skin after application with a bandage or wrapping unless directed to do so by a doctor. Discontinue use if irritation occurs.

BRAND NAME: **Lopurin**

GENERIC NAME: allopurinol

See entry for Zyloprim

BRAND NAME: **Lorabid**

GENERIC NAME: loracarbef

GENERIC FORM AVAILABLE: No

THERAPEUTIC CLASS: Carbacephem antibiotic

DOSAGE FORMS: 200-mg and 400-mg capsules, 100 mg/5 mL suspension, and 200 mg/5 mL suspension

MAIN USES: Bacterial infections

USUAL DOSE: 200 mg to 400 mg every 12 hours

AVERAGE PRICE: $88.06 for 200 mg (20 capsules) and $110.60 for 400 mg (20 capsules)

SIDE EFFECTS: diarrhea 4%, headache 3%, runny nose 2%, nausea 2%, vomiting 1%, stomach pain 1%, and skin rash 1%.

DRUG INTERACTIONS: The drug may decrease the effectiveness of oral contraceptives used for birth control. Probenecid will decrease elimination of the drug by the kidneys.

ALLERGIES: Individuals allergic to loracarbef, penicillins, cephalosporins, or any of its derivatives should discuss this with their doctor or pharmacist before using this drug.

PREGNANCY/BREAST-FEEDING: Category B—No evidence of risk in humans. Either animal findings show risk, but human findings do not; or, if no adequate human studies have been done, animal findings show no risk. It is not known whether the drug is excreted in the breast milk; therefore, caution should be used when breast-feeding.

OTHER BRAND NAMES: None

OTHER DRUGS IN THE SAME THERAPEUTIC CLASS: None

IMPORTANT INFORMATION TO REMEMBER: If possible, take the drug on an empty stomach—one hour before meals or two hours after meals. Also, take the drug at even intervals around the clock (if two times a day, take every 12 hours). Take the drug until all the medication prescribed is gone; otherwise the infection may return. Women taking birth control pills should use another form of contraception while taking the drug and for the rest of the current menstrual cycle. Individuals taking the liquid form should shake it thoroughly before use, store the medication in the refrigerator, and discard any remaining medication after 14 days.

BRAND NAME: Lorcet-HD

GENERIC NAME: Combination product containing: acetaminophen and hydrocodone

See entry for Vicodin/Vicodin ES/Vicodin HP

BRAND NAME: Lorcet Plus and Lorcet 10/650

GENERIC NAME: Combination product containing: acetaminophen and hydrocodone

GENERIC FORM AVAILABLE: No

THERAPEUTIC CLASS: Narcotic analgesic + pain reliever

DOSAGE FORMS: 7.5-mg hydrocodone/650-mg acetaminophen tablets (Lorcet Plus) and 10-mg hydrocodone/650-mg acetaminophen tablet (Lorcet 10/650)

MAIN USES: Moderate to severe pain

USUAL DOSE: one tablet every four to six hours as needed for pain

AVERAGE PRICE: $69.56 for Lorcet Plus and $90.32 for Lorcet 10/650

SIDE EFFECTS: Most common: drowsiness, dizziness, tiredness, nausea, vomiting, and histamine release (symptoms include decreased blood pressure, sweating, fast heartbeat, flushing, and wheezing). Less common: confusion, decreased urination, dry mouth, constipation, stomach pain, skin rash, anxiety, headache, weakness, minor vision disturbances, and hallucinations.

DRUG INTERACTIONS: Alcohol, anxiety medications, and other narcotic painkillers may intensify the drowsiness effect of the drug. Liver toxicity may occur when used long-term with Anturane, Dilantin, or Mesantoin. This drug, when taken with Nardil or Parnate, may cause severe and sometimes fatal reactions.

ALLERGIES: Individuals allergic to acetaminophen, hydrocodone, or any of their derivatives should discuss this with their doctor or pharmacist before using this drug.

PREGNANCY/BREAST-FEEDING: Category C—Risk cannot be ruled out. Human studies are lacking, and animal studies are either positive for fetal risk or lacking as well. However, potential benefits

may justify the potential risk in using the drug. It is not known whether the drug is excreted in the breast milk; therefore, caution should be used when breast-feeding.

OTHER BRAND NAMES: None

OTHER DRUGS IN THE SAME THERAPEUTIC CLASS: Bancap-HC, Darvocet-N 50, Darvocet-N 100, Darvon, Darvon Compound, DHCplus, Empirin #3, Empirin #4, Hydrocet, Lortab, Percocet, Percodan, Phenaphen w/Codeine, Synalgos DC, Talacen, Tylenol #2, Tylenol #3, Tylenol #4, Tylox, Vicodin, and Zydone

IMPORTANT INFORMATION TO REMEMBER: This drug does cause drowsiness. Individuals should use caution when driving, operating machinery, or any task where mental alertness is required. Alcohol, anxiety medications, and other narcotic painkillers may intensify the drowsiness effect of the drug. If stomach upset occurs, take the drug with food or milk. Do not increase the dose without first consulting with your physician. This medication is a controlled substance and may be habit-forming.

BRAND NAME: Lortab

GENERIC NAME: Combination product containing: acetaminophen and hydrocodone

GENERIC FORM AVAILABLE: Yes (Lortab 5/500 only)

THERAPEUTIC CLASS: Narcotic analgesic + pain reliever

DOSAGE FORMS: 2.5-mg hydrocodone/500-mg acetaminophen tablets (Lortab 2.5/500), 5-mg hydrocodone/500-mg acetaminophen tablets (Lortab 5/500), 7.5-mg hydrocodone/500-mg acetaminophen tablets (Lortab 7.5/500), 70-mg hydrocodone/500-mg acetaminophen tablets (Lortab 10/500), and 7.5 mg hydrocodone/500 mg acetaminophen tablets per 15 mL (Lortab Elixir)

MAIN USES: Moderate to severe pain

USUAL DOSE: one to two tablets every four to six hours as needed for pain (maximum of eight tablets per day)

AVERAGE PRICE: $58.51 (B) for 2.5/500; $63.42 (B)/$26.99 (G) for 5/500; and $70.91 for 7.5/500; and $91.23 for 10/500

SIDE EFFECTS: Most common: drowsiness, dizziness, tiredness, nausea, vomiting, and histamine release (symptoms include decreased blood pressure, sweating, fast heartbeat, flushing, and wheezing). Less common: confusion, decreased urination, dry mouth, constipation, stomach pain, skin rash, headache, weakness, minor vision disturbances, and hallucinations.

DRUG INTERACTIONS: Alcohol, anxiety medications, and other narcotic painkillers may intensify the drowsiness effect of the drug. Liver toxicity may occur with long-term use of Anturane, Dilantin, or Mesantoin. This drug, when taken with Nardil or Parnate, may cause severe and sometimes fatal reactions.

ALLERGIES: Individuals allergic to acetaminophen, hydrocodone, or any of their derivatives should discuss this with their doctor or pharmacist before using this drug.

PREGNANCY/BREAST-FEEDING: Category C—Risk cannot be ruled out. Human studies are lacking, and animal studies are either positive for fetal risk or lacking as well. However, potential benefits may justify the potential risk in using the drug. It is not known whether the drug is excreted in the breast milk; therefore, caution should be used when breast-feeding.

OTHER BRAND NAMES: None

OTHER DRUGS IN THE SAME THERAPEUTIC CLASS: Bancap-HC, Darvocet-N 50, Darvocet-N 100, Darvon, Darvon Compound, DHCplus, Empirin #3, Empirin #4, Hydrocet, Lorcet Plus, Lorcet 10/650, Perocet, Percodan, Phenaphen w/Codeine, Synalgos DC, Talacen, Tylenol #2, Tylenol #3, Tylenol #4, Tylox, Vicodin, and Zydone

IMPORTANT INFORMATION TO REMEMBER: This drug does cause drowsiness. Individuals should use caution when driving, operating machinery, or any task where mental alertness is required. Alcohol, anxiety medications, and other narcotic painkillers may intensify the drowsiness effect of the drug. If stomach upset occurs, take the drug with food or milk. Do not increase the dose without first consulting with your physician. This medication is a controlled substance and may be habit-forming.

BRAND NAME: Lotensin

GENERIC NAME: benazepril

GENERIC FORM AVAILABLE: No

THERAPEUTIC CLASS: ACE inhibitor

DOSAGE FORMS: 5-mg, 10-mg, 20-mg, and 40-mg tablets

MAIN USES: High blood pressure

USUAL DOSE: 10 mg and 40 mg daily in one or two doses

AVERAGE PRICE: $85.55 for 5 mg; $93.53 for 10 mg; $99.63 for 20 mg; and $109.42 for 40 mg

SIDE EFFECTS: headache 6%, dizziness 4%, tiredness 2%, weakness 2%, dizziness upon arising from a sitting or lying-down position 2%, nausea 1%, and cough 1%.

DRUG INTERACTIONS: The drug may decrease the absorption of the antibiotic Sumycin and other tetracyclines. High potassium levels may occur when used together with Dyrenium, Aldactone, and potassium supplements such as Micro-K, K-Dur, Klor-Con, K-Lyte, and Slow-K. Patients on water pills, especially those recently started on a water pill, may experience low blood pressure. The drug may also increase the toxic effects of Eskalith and Lithobid, especially when taken with a water pill.

ALLERGIES: Individuals allergic to benazepril or other ACE inhibitors (such as those listed in "Other Drugs in the Same Therapeutic Class") should discuss this with their doctor or pharmacist before using this drug.

PREGNANCY/BREAST-FEEDING: Category C (first trimester)—Risk cannot be ruled out. Human studies are lacking, and animal studies are either positive for fetal risk or lacking as well. However, potential benefits may justify the potential risk in using the drug. Category D (second and third trimesters)—Positive evidence of risk. Human studies show risk to the fetus. Nevertheless, potential benefits may possibly outweigh the potential risk. This drug should not be taken by nursing mothers.

OTHER BRAND NAMES: None

OTHER DRUGS IN THE SAME THERAPEUTIC CLASS: Accupril, Altace, Capoten, Mavik, Monopril, Prinivil, Univasc, Vasotec, and Zestril

IMPORTANT INFORMATION TO REMEMBER: Take this drug regularly and exactly as directed by your physician. Do not stop taking drug unless otherwise directed by your doctor. Avoid salt substitutes containing potassium. Before taking over-the-counter cold and allergy preparations, consult your doctor or pharmacist—these products may raise your blood pressure. If you experience swelling of the face, lips, or tongue or difficulty in breathing, contact your doctor immediately.

BRAND NAME: Lotrel

GENERIC NAME: Combination product containing: amlodipine and benazepril

See individual entries for Norvasc and Lotensin

BRAND NAME: Lotrimin

GENERIC NAME: clotrimazole

See entry for Lotrisone (Lotrimin is now also available without a prescription as Lotrimin AF).

BRAND NAME: Lotrisone

GENERIC NAME: Combination product containing: clotrimazole and betamethasone dipropionate

GENERIC FORM AVAILABLE: No

THERAPEUTIC CLASS: Topical corticosteroid + antifungal

DOSAGE FORMS: 1.0% clotrimazole/0.05% betamethasone dipropionate cream

MAIN USES: Fungal infections (mainly ringworm, jock itch, and athlete's foot)

USUAL DOSE: Apply to the affected area twice daily in the morning and evening.

AVERAGE PRICE: $25.58 for 15 g

SIDE EFFECTS: Most common: None. Less common: stinging, redness, irritation, rash, itching, skin dryness, and tingling or prickling sensation on the skin.

DRUG INTERACTIONS: None of any clinical significance

ALLERGIES: Individuals allergic to clotrimazole, betamethasone dipropionate, Lotrimin, Valisone, or any of their derivatives should discuss this with their doctor or pharmacist before using this drug.

PREGNANCY/BREAST-FEEDING: Category C—Risk cannot be ruled out. Human studies are lacking, and animal studies are either positive for fetal risk or lacking as well. However, potential benefits may justify the potential risk in using the drug. It is not known whether the drug is excreted in the breast milk; therefore, caution should be used when breast-feeding.

OTHER BRAND NAMES: None

OTHER DRUGS IN THE SAME THERAPEUTIC CLASS: Mycolog-II

IMPORTANT INFORMATION TO REMEMBER: This drug is for external use only. The drug may stain clothing. Apply and gently rub in enough of the cream to cover the affected area and surrounding areas. Use the drug for the full course of treatment or the fungal infection may return. Never cover the skin after application with a bandage or wrapping unless directed to do so by a doctor. Discontinue use if irritation occurs.

BRAND NAME: Lozol

GENERIC NAME: indapamide

GENERIC FORM AVAILABLE: Yes

THERAPEUTIC CLASS: Indoline diuretic (water pill)

DOSAGE FORMS: 1.25-mg and 2.5-mg tablets

MAIN USES: Water retention (fluid retention due to congestive heart failure, kidney disease, or cirrhosis of the liver) and high blood pressure

USUAL DOSE: 1.25 mg to 5 mg once daily in the morning

AVERAGE PRICE: $123.16 (B)/$102.27 (G) for 2.5 mg

SIDE EFFECTS: Most common: muscle cramps. Less common: loss of appetite, diarrhea, headache, dry mouth, increased sensitivity to sunlight, dizziness upon arising from a sitting or lying-down position, insomnia, and upset stomach.

DRUG INTERACTIONS: The drug may increase the toxic effects of Eskalith and Lithobid. Individuals taking Lanoxin should inform their doctor of this before taking this drug. Anti-diabetic medications may need to be adjusted when taking this drug.

ALLERGIES: Individuals allergic to indapamide or any of its derivatives should discuss this with their doctor or pharmacist before using this drug.

PREGNANCY/BREAST-FEEDING: Category B—No evidence of risk in humans. Either animal findings show risk, but human findings do not; or, if no adequate human studies have been done, animal findings show no risk. It is not known whether the drug is excreted in the breast milk; therefore, caution should be used when breast-feeding.

OTHER BRAND NAMES: None

OTHER DRUGS IN THE SAME THERAPEUTIC CLASS: None

IMPORTANT INFORMATION TO REMEMBER: If the drug is to be taken once daily, take it in the morning due to increased urine output. If stomach upset occurs, take the drug with food or milk. Before taking over-the-counter cold and allergy preparations, consult your doctor or pharmacist—these products may raise your blood pressure. The drug may cause the elimination of potassium from the body. It is therefore a good idea to eat a banana or drink orange, grapefruit, or apple juice every day to replace lost potassium. Individuals with kidney disease should discuss this with their doctor before taking this drug.

BRAND NAME: Ludiomil

GENERIC NAME: maprotiline

GENERIC FORM AVAILABLE: Yes

THERAPEUTIC CLASS: Tetracyclic antidepressant

DOSAGE FORMS: 25-mg, 50-mg, and 75-mg tablets

MAIN USES: Depression

USUAL DOSE: 75 mg to 150 mg daily in a single or divided doses

AVERAGE PRICE: $63.15 (B)/$32.89 (G) for 25 mg; $90.16 (B)/$55.90 (G) for 50 mg; $123.84 (B)/$76.45 (G) for 75 mg

SIDE EFFECTS: dry mouth 22%, drowsiness 16%, dizziness 8%, constipation 6%, nervousness 6%, blurred vision 4%, headache 4%, weakness 4%, anxiety 3%, tremors 3%, insomnia 2%, agitation 2%, and nausea 2%.

DRUG INTERACTIONS: Central nervous system (CNS) depression may be increased when used with alcohol, narcotic painkillers, or other anxiety medications. The drug should not be taken within 14 days of taking Nardil or Parnate. Decongestants found in cough, cold, and allergy products may cause fast heartbeat, irregular heartbeat, and/or high blood pressure when taken with this drug. Tagamet may increase the blood levels of the drug. Dilantin may decrease the blood levels of the drug.

ALLERGIES: Individuals allergic to maprotiline or any of its derivatives should discuss this with their doctor or pharmacist before using this drug.

PREGNANCY/BREAST-FEEDING: Category B—No evidence of risk in humans. Either animal findings show risk, but human findings do not; or, if no adequate human studies have been done, animal findings show no risk. The drug is excreted in the breast milk; therefore, extreme caution should be used when breast-feeding.

OTHER BRAND NAMES: None

OTHER DRUGS IN THE SAME THERAPEUTIC CLASS: None

IMPORTANT INFORMATION TO REMEMBER: Only take the drug exactly as directed by your physician. Do not discontinue the drug without first consulting your physician. The drug may require three weeks of use before improvement may be noticed. This drug does cause drowsiness. Individuals should use caution when driving, operating machinery, or any task where mental alertness is required. Alcohol, anxiety medications, and narcotic painkillers may intensify the drowsiness effect of the drug. The drug may cause a slight amount of dizziness or lightheadedness when rising from a sitting or lying-down position.

BRAND NAME: Luvox

GENERIC NAME: fluvoxamine

GENERIC FORM AVAILABLE: No

THERAPEUTIC CLASS: Serotonin reuptake inhibitor antidepressant

DOSAGE FORMS: 50-mg and 100-mg tablets

MAIN USES: Obsessive-compulsive disorder

USUAL DOSE: 100 mg to 300 mg per day

AVERAGE PRICE: $267.44 for 50 mg and $285.11 for 100 mg

SIDE EFFECTS: nausea 40%, drowsiness 22%, insomnia 21%, dry mouth 14%, weakness 14%, nervousness 12%, diarrhea 11%, dizziness 11%, constipation 10%, abnormal ejaculation 8%, sweating 7%, appetite changes 6%, vomiting 5%, anxiety 5%, and tremor 5%.

DRUG INTERACTIONS: The drug should not be used with Hismanal, Seldane, or Seldane-D. The drug may increase the blood levels of Coumadin, Inderal, Lopressor, Slo-bid, Theo-Dur, theophylline, Uni-Dur, Uniphyl, Toprol-XL, and Valium. Eskalith and Lithobid may increase the effects of the drug. The drug should not be taken within 14 days of taking Nardil or Parnate.

ALLERGIES: Individuals allergic to fluvoxamine or any of its derivatives should discuss this with their doctor or pharmacist before using this drug.

PREGNANCY/BREAST-FEEDING: Category C—Risk cannot be ruled out. Human studies are lacking, and animal studies are either positive for fetal risk or lacking as well. However, potential benefits may justify the potential risk in using the drug. The drug is excreted in the breast milk; therefore, extreme caution should be used when breast-feeding.

OTHER BRAND NAMES: None

OTHER DRUGS IN THE SAME THERAPEUTIC CLASS: Paxil, Prozac, and Zoloft

IMPORTANT INFORMATION TO REMEMBER: Only take the drug exactly as directed by your physician. Do not discontinue the drug without first consulting your physician. The drug may require four weeks or longer of use before improvement may be noticed. This drug does cause drowsiness. Individuals should use caution when driving, operating machinery, or any task where mental alertness is required. Alcohol, anxiety medications, and narcotic painkillers may intensify the drowsiness effect of the drug. The drug may cause a slight amount of dizziness or lightheadedness when rising from a sitting or lying-down position.

BRAND NAME: **Macrodantin and Macrobid**

GENERIC NAME: nitrofurantoin

GENERIC FORM AVAILABLE: Yes (Macrodantin only)

THERAPEUTIC CLASS: Urinary antibiotic

DOSAGE FORMS: 25-mg, 50-mg, and 100-mg capsules (Macrodantin); and 100-mg capsules (Macrobid)

MAIN USES: Urinary tract infections and {prevention of urinary tract infections}

USUAL DOSE: For Macrodantin: 50 mg to 100 mg four times daily with food. For Macrobid: 100 mg every 12 hours. For the prevention of urinary tract infections; 50 mg to 100 mg at bedtime.

AVERAGE PRICE: $47.46 (B)/$37.57 (G) for 50-mg Macrodantin (40 capsules) and $76.07 (B)/$55.27 (G) for 100-mg Macrodantin (40 capsules); $50.97 for 100-mg Macrobid (20 capsules)

SIDE EFFECTS: Most common: pneumonitis (symptoms are chest pains, chills, cough, fever, and trouble breathing), stomach pain, nausea, vomiting, diarrhea, and loss of appetite. Less common: low white blood cell count, anemia, numbness, tingling or burning sensation of the face and mouth, and weakness.

DRUG INTERACTIONS: Antacids may decrease the absorption of the drug. Probenecid and Anturane may increase the blood levels of the drug.

ALLERGIES: Individuals allergic to nitrofurantoin or any of its derivatives should discuss this with their doctor or pharmacist before using this drug.

PREGNANCY/BREAST-FEEDING: Category B—No evidence of risk in humans. Either animal findings show risk, but human findings do not; or, if no adequate human studies have been done, animal findings show no risk. The drug is excreted from the breast in small amounts of milk; therefore, caution should be used when breast-feeding.

OTHER BRAND NAMES: None

OTHER DRUGS IN THE SAME THERAPEUTIC CLASS: None

IMPORTANT INFORMATION TO REMEMBER: The drug should be taken with food or milk. This helps the body absorb the drug better, which increases its effectiveness. Also, take the drug at even intervals around the clock (if four times a day, take every six hours). Take the drug until all the medication prescribed is gone; otherwise the infection may return. The drug may cause a slight discoloration of the urine, but this is rare. If symptoms of pneumonitis occur (chest pains, chills, cough, fever, and trouble breathing), contact your physician immediately.

BRAND NAME: Marinol

GENERIC NAME: dronabinol

GENERIC FORM AVAILABLE: No

THERAPEUTIC CLASS: Antinausea

DOSAGE FORMS: 2.5-mg, 5-mg, and 10-mg capsules

MAIN USES: Weight loss in persons with AIDS (increases appetite) and nausea and vomiting associated with cancer chemotherapy

USUAL DOSE: To increase appetite: 2.5 mg to 10 mg twice daily before lunch and supper. For nausea and vomiting: 5 mg four to six times daily.

AVERAGE PRICE: $418.15 for 2.5 mg; $822.29 for 5 mg; $1,856.00 for 10 mg

SIDE EFFECTS: Most common: drowsiness, unsteadiness, dizziness, and trouble concentrating and thinking. Less common: vision changes, low blood pressure, dry mouth, restlessness, fast heartbeat, changes in mood, hallucinations, and depression.

DRUG INTERACTIONS: Alcohol, anxiety medications, and narcotic painkillers may intensify the drowsiness effect of the drug.

ALLERGIES: Individuals allergic to dronabinol or any of its derivatives should discuss this with their doctor or pharmacist before using this drug.

PREGNANCY/BREAST-FEEDING: Category C—Risk cannot be ruled out. Human studies are lacking, and animal studies are either positive for fetal risk or lacking as well. However, potential benefits may justify the potential risk in using the drug. The drug should not be used by women who are breast-feeding.

OTHER BRAND NAMES: None

OTHER DRUGS IN THE SAME THERAPEUTIC CLASS: None

IMPORTANT INFORMATION TO REMEMBER: This drug does cause drowsiness. Individuals should use caution when driving, operating machinery, or performing any task where mental alertness is required. Alcohol, anxiety medications, and narcotic painkillers may intensify the drowsiness effect of the drug. Do not increase the dose without first consulting with your physician. This medication is a controlled substance and may be habit-forming. Caution should be used when getting up suddenly from a sitting or lying-down position—this may cause dizziness or unsteadiness.

BRAND NAME: Materna

GENERIC NAME: Prenatal multivitamin

Very similar to Natalins Rx. See entry for Natalins Rx.

BRAND NAME: Mavik

GENERIC NAME: trandolapril

GENERIC FORM AVAILABLE: No

THERAPEUTIC CLASS: ACE inhibitor

DOSAGE FORM: 1-mg, 2-mg, and 4-mg tablets

MAIN USES: High blood pressure

USUAL DOSE: 1 mg to 4 mg once daily

AVERAGE PRICE: $89.73 for the 1-mg, 2-mg, and 4-mg tablets

SIDE EFFECTS: cough 2%, headache 1%–2%, tiredness 1%–2%, dizziness 1%, and diarrhea 1%.

DRUG INTERACTIONS: May decrease the absorption of the antibiotic Sumycin and other tetracyclines. High potassium levels may occur when used together with Dyrenium and Aldactone, and potassium supplements such as Micro-K, K-Dur, Klor-Con, K-Lyte, and Slow-K. Patients on water pills, especially those recently started on a water pill, may experience low blood pressure. The drug may also increase the toxic effects of Eskalith and Lithobid, especially when taken with a water pill.

ALLERGIES: Individuals allergic to trandolapril or other ACE inhibitors (such as those listed under "Other Drugs in the Same

Therapeutic Class") should discuss this with their doctor or pharmacist before using this drug.

PREGNANCY/BREAST-FEEDING: Category C (first trimester)—Risk cannot be ruled out. Human studies are lacking, and animal studies are either positive for fetal risk or lacking as well. However, potential benefits may justify the potential risk in using the drug. Category D (second and third trimesters)—Positive evidence of risk. Human studies show risk to the fetus. Nevertheless, potential benefits may possibly outweigh the potential risk. This drug should not be taken by nursing mothers.

OTHER BRAND NAMES: None

OTHER DRUGS IN THE SAME THERAPEUTIC CLASS: Accupril, Altace, Capoten, Lotensin, Monopril, Prinivil, Univasc, Vasotec, and Zestril

IMPORTANT INFORMATION TO REMEMBER: Take this drug regularly and exactly as directed by your physician. Do not stop taking this drug unless otherwise directed by your doctor. Avoid salt substitutes containing potassium. Before taking over-the-counter cold and allergy preparations, consult your doctor or pharmacist—these products may raise your blood pressure. If you experience swelling of the face, lips, or tongue or difficulty in breathing, contact your doctor immediately.

BRAND NAME: Maxair

GENERIC NAME: pirbuterol

GENERIC FORM AVAILABLE: No

THERAPEUTIC CLASS: Beta-2-agonist bronchodilator

DOSAGE FORMS: 0.2 mg of pirbuterol per inhalation

MAIN USES: Asthma, {chronic bronchitis, emphysema, and other breathing disorders}

USUAL DOSE: one to two inhalations every four to six hours as needed

AVERAGE PRICE: $13.44 for 0.2 mg, 2.8 g (80 inhalations)

SIDE EFFECTS: nervousness 7%, tremors 6%, nausea 2%, headache 2%, pounding heartbeat 2%, fast heartbeat 1%, cough 1%, dizziness 1%, chest tightness 1%, diarrhea 1%, and dry mouth 1%.

DRUG INTERACTIONS: Anafranil, Asendin, Elavil, Endep, Ludiomil, Nardil, Norpramin, Pamelor, Parnate, Sinequan, Surmontil, Tofranil, and Vivactil may increase the toxicity of this drug. Decongestants in cough, cold, and allergy products may increase the toxicity of this drug. Blocadren, Cartrol, Corgard, Inderal, Levatol, Normodyne, Sectral, and Visken may decrease the effect of the drug.

ALLERGIES: Individuals allergic to pirbuterol or any of its derivatives should discuss this with their doctor or pharmacist before using this drug.

PREGNANCY/BREAST-FEEDING: Category C—Risk cannot be ruled out. Human studies are lacking, and animal studies are either positive for fetal risk or lacking as well. However, potential benefits may justify the potential risk in using the drug. It is not known whether the drug is excreted in the breast milk; therefore, caution should be used when breast-feeding.

OTHER DRUGS IN THE SAME THERAPEUTIC CLASS: Alupent, Brethaire, Bronkometer, Metaprel, Proventil, Serevent, Tornalate, and Ventolin

IMPORTANT INFORMATION TO REMEMBER: Only take the drug exactly as directed by your physician. Never increase the dose of the drug without consulting with your physician. Prolonged use of the drug may cause tolerance to its effects to develop.

When using the inhaler, use the following procedure (instructions for the autoinhaler are different and are enclosed with the drug):

1) Shake the canister well.
2) Place the mouthpiece close to the mouth, but not touching the lips.
3) Exhale deeply.
4) Inhale slowly and deeply as you press the top of the canister to release the medication.
5) Hold your breath for a few seconds before exhaling.
6) Wait five minutes between puffs.
7) Be sure to wash the inhaler device (mouthpiece) regularly with warm soapy water to avoid bacterial contamination.

BRAND NAME: Maxaquin

GENERIC NAME: lomefloxacin

GENERIC FORM AVAILABLE: No

THERAPEUTIC CLASS: Quinolone antibiotic

DOSAGE FORMS: 400-mg tablets

MAIN USES: Bacterial infections

USUAL DOSE: 400 mg once daily

AVERAGE PRICE: $98.04 (10 tablets)

SIDE EFFECTS: nausea 4%, headache 3%, increased sensitivity of the skin to sunburn 3%, dizziness 2%, and diarrhea 1%.

DRUG INTERACTIONS: Antacids, Videx, iron supplements, and Carafate may reduce the absorption of the drug. Choledyl, Slo-bid, Theo-Dur, theophylline, Uni-Dur, Uniphyl, and aminophylline blood levels may be increased when used with this drug. The drug may also increase the effects of Coumadin. The drug may increase the blood levels of Sandimmune.

ALLERGIES: Individuals allergic to lomefloxacin or other quinolone antibiotics (such as those listed under "Other Drugs in the Same Therapeutic Class") should discuss this with their doctor or pharmacist before taking this drug.

PREGNANCY/BREAST-FEEDING: Category C—Risk cannot be ruled out. Human studies are lacking, and animal studies are either positive for fetal risk or lacking as well. However, potential benefits may justify the potential risk in using the drug. It is not known whether the drug is excreted in the breast milk; therefore, caution should be used when breast-feeding.

OTHER BRAND NAMES: None

OTHER DRUGS IN THE SAME THERAPEUTIC CLASS: Cipro, Floxin, Noroxin, Penetrex

IMPORTANT INFORMATION TO REMEMBER: Take the drug at even intervals around the clock (if twice a day, take every 12 hours). Take the drug until all the medication prescribed is gone; otherwise the infection may return. This drug should be taken with plenty of water (eight ounces is preferred). If stomach upset occurs, take with food. Do not take antacids, milk, or iron supplements within four hours of taking this drug. Individuals should also use a sunscreen to avoid overexposure to the sun; the drug may increase the skin's sensitivity to sunlight, which may cause one to sunburn more easily. This drug may also cause a tear in the tendons of the lower leg. Report any soreness or pain of the lower legs to your physician immediately.

BRAND NAME: Maxitrol and Maxidex

GENERIC NAME: Combination product containing: dexamethasone, neomycin, and polymyxin B (Maxitrol); and dexamethasone only (Maxidex)

GENERIC FORM AVAILABLE: Yes

THERAPEUTIC CLASS: Antibiotic + steroid eyedrops (Maxitrol) and steroid eyedrops (Maxidex)

DOSAGE FORMS: 0.1% dexamethasone, 3.5 mg/mL neomycin, and 10,000 units/mL polymyxin B eyedrops and eye ointment (Maxitrol); and 0.1% dexamethasone eyedrops and eye ointment (Maxidex)

MAIN USES: Bacterial eye infections (Maxitrol) and inflammation of the eye (Maxidex)

USUAL DOSE: For the eyedrops: one to two drops every three to six hours. For the ointment: apply 1/2 ribbon three to four times daily.

AVERAGE PRICE: $28.86 (B)/$14.89 (G) for Maxitrol ointment and suspension drops; $25.81 (B)/$12.63 (G) for Maxidex ointment and suspension drops

SIDE EFFECTS: Most common: temporary, mild blurred vision. Less common: burning, itching, redness, watering of the eyes, and eye pain.

DRUG INTERACTIONS: The drug may decrease the effectiveness of other eyedrops used to treat glaucoma.

ALLERGIES: Individuals allergic to dexamethasone, neomycin, polymyxin B, or any of their derivatives should discuss this with their doctor or pharmacist before using this drug.

PREGNANCY/BREAST-FEEDING: Category C—Risk cannot be ruled out. Human studies are lacking, and animal studies are either positive for fetal risk or lacking as well. However, potential benefits may justify the potential risk in using the drug. It is not known

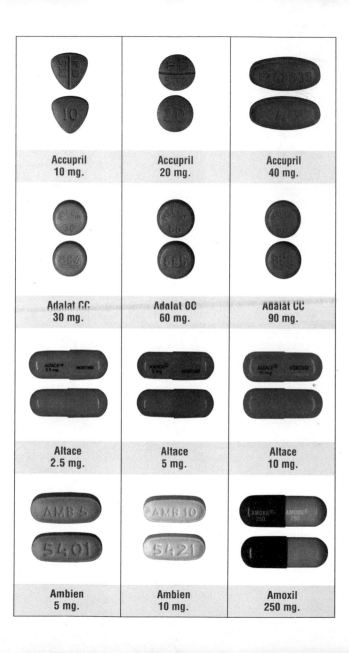

Accupril 10 mg.	Accupril 20 mg.	Accupril 40 mg.
Adalat CC 30 mg.	Adalat CC 60 mg.	Adalat CC 90 mg.
Altace 2.5 mg.	Altace 5 mg.	Altace 10 mg.
Ambien 5 mg.	Ambien 10 mg.	Amoxil 250 mg.

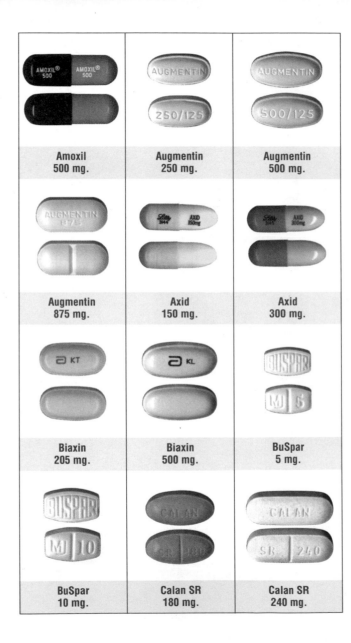

Amoxil 500 mg.	Augmentin 250 mg.	Augmentin 500 mg.
Augmentin 875 mg.	Axid 150 mg.	Axid 300 mg.
Biaxin 205 mg.	Biaxin 500 mg.	BuSpar 5 mg.
BuSpar 10 mg.	Calan SR 180 mg.	Calan SR 240 mg.

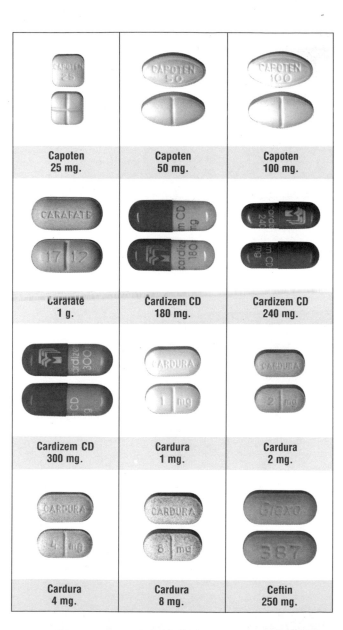

Capoten
25 mg.

Capoten
50 mg.

Capoten
100 mg.

Carafate
1 g.

Cardizem CD
180 mg.

Cardizem CD
240 mg.

Cardizem CD
300 mg.

Cardura
1 mg.

Cardura
2 mg.

Cardura
4 mg.

Cardura
8 mg.

Ceftin
250 mg.

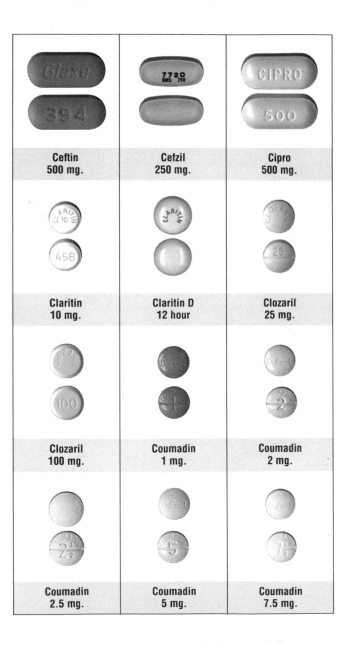

Ceftin 500 mg.	**Cefzil** 250 mg.	**Cipro** 500 mg.
Claritin 10 mg.	**Claritin D** 12 hour	**Clozaril** 25 mg.
Clozaril 100 mg.	**Coumadin** 1 mg.	**Coumadin** 2 mg.
Coumadin 2.5 mg.	**Coumadin** 5 mg.	**Coumadin** 7.5 mg.

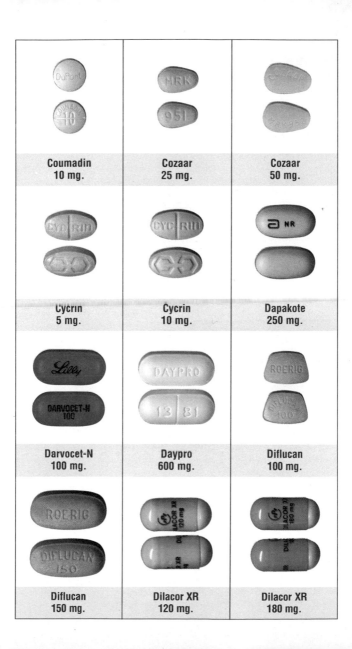

Coumadin 10 mg.	**Cozaar** 25 mg.	**Cozaar** 50 mg.
Cycrin 5 mg.	**Cycrin** 10 mg.	**Dapakote** 250 mg.
Darvocet-N 100 mg.	**Daypro** 600 mg.	**Diflucan** 100 mg.
Diflucan 150 mg.	**Dilacor XR** 120 mg.	**Dilacor XR** 180 mg.

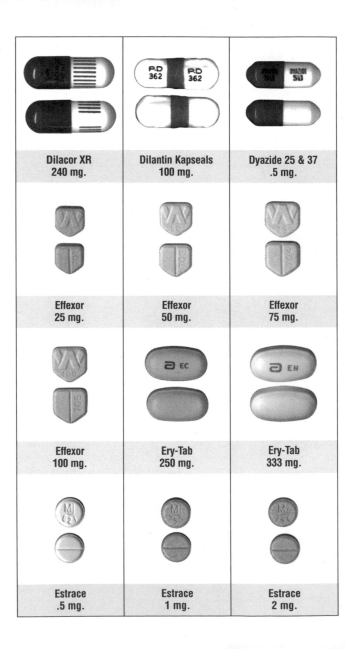

Dilacor XR 240 mg.	Dilantin Kapseals 100 mg.	Dyazide 25 & 37 .5 mg.
Effexor 25 mg.	Effexor 50 mg.	Effexor 75 mg.
Effexor 100 mg.	Ery-Tab 250 mg.	Ery-Tab 333 mg.
Estrace .5 mg.	Estrace 1 mg.	Estrace 2 mg.

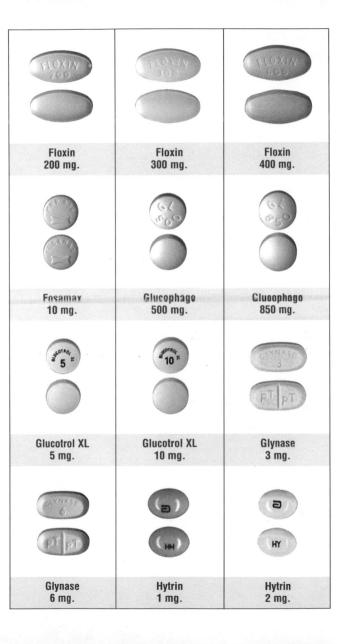

Floxin 200 mg.	Floxin 300 mg.	Floxin 400 mg.
Fosamax 10 mg.	Glucophage 500 mg.	Glucophage 850 mg.
Glucotrol XL 5 mg.	Glucotrol XL 10 mg.	Glynase 3 mg.
Glynase 6 mg.	Hytrin 1 mg.	Hytrin 2 mg.

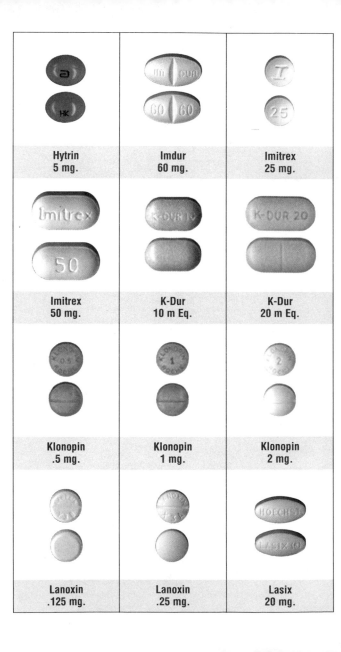

Hytrin 5 mg.	**Imdur** 60 mg.	**Imitrex** 25 mg.
Imitrex 50 mg.	**K-Dur** 10 m Eq.	**K-Dur** 20 m Eq.
Klonopin .5 mg.	**Klonopin** 1 mg.	**Klonopin** 2 mg.
Lanoxin .125 mg.	**Lanoxin** .25 mg.	**Lasix** 20 mg.

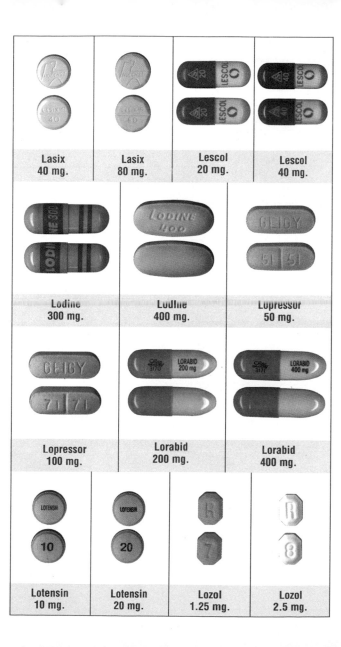

| Lasix 40 mg. | Lasix 80 mg. | Lescol 20 mg. | Lescol 40 mg. |

| Lodine 300 mg. | Lodine 400 mg. | Lopressor 50 mg. |

| Lopressor 100 mg. | Lorabid 200 mg. | Lorabid 400 mg. |

| Lotensin 10 mg. | Lotensin 20 mg. | Lozol 1.25 mg. | Lozol 2.5 mg. |

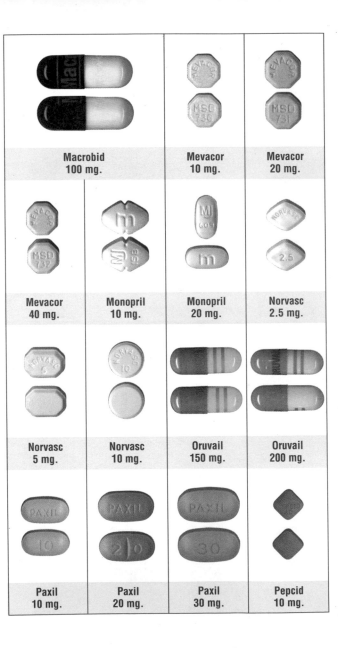

Macrobid 100 mg.	**Mevacor** 10 mg.	**Mevacor** 20 mg.
Mevacor 40 mg.	**Monopril** 10 mg.	**Monopril** 20 mg.
	Norvasc 2.5 mg.	
Norvasc 5 mg.	**Norvasc** 10 mg.	**Oruvail** 150 mg.
Oruvail 200 mg.		
Paxil 10 mg.	**Paxil** 20 mg.	**Paxil** 30 mg.
Pepcid 10 mg.		

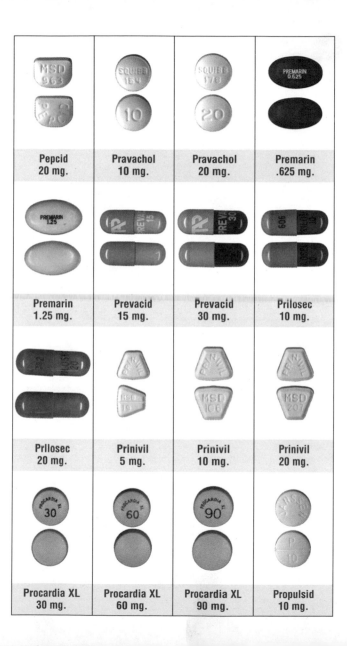

Pepcid 20 mg.	Pravachol 10 mg.	Pravachol 20 mg.	Premarin .625 mg.
Premarin 1.25 mg.	Prevacid 15 mg.	Prevacid 30 mg.	Prilosec 10 mg.
Prilosec 20 mg.	Prinivil 5 mg.	Prinivil 10 mg.	Prinivil 20 mg.
Procardia XL 30 mg.	Procardia XL 60 mg.	Procardia XL 90 mg.	Propulsid 10 mg.

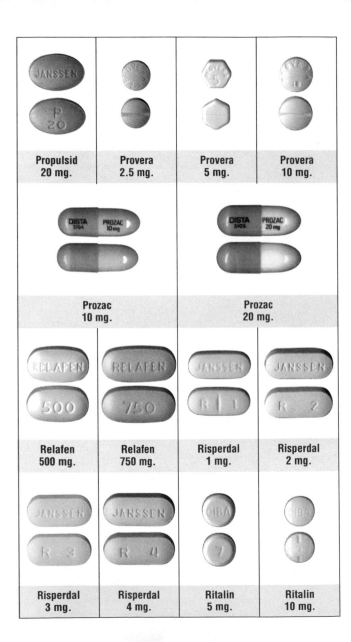

Propulsid 20 mg.	**Provera** 2.5 mg.	**Provera** 5 mg.	**Provera** 10 mg.
Prozac 10 mg.		**Prozac** 20 mg.	
Relafen 500 mg.	**Relafen** 750 mg.	**Risperdal** 1 mg.	**Risperdal** 2 mg.
Risperdal 3 mg.	**Risperdal** 4 mg.	**Ritalin** 5 mg.	**Ritalin** 10 mg.

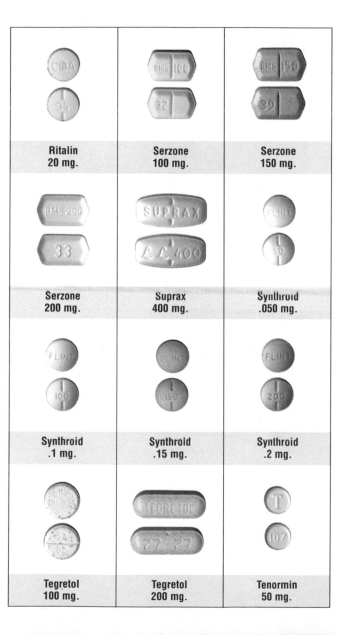

Ritalin 20 mg.	**Serzone** 100 mg.	**Serzone** 150 mg.
Serzone 200 mg.	**Suprax** 400 mg.	**Synthroid** .050 mg.
Synthroid .1 mg.	**Synthroid** .15 mg.	**Synthroid** .2 mg.
Tegretol 100 mg.	**Tegretol** 200 mg.	**Tenormin** 50 mg.

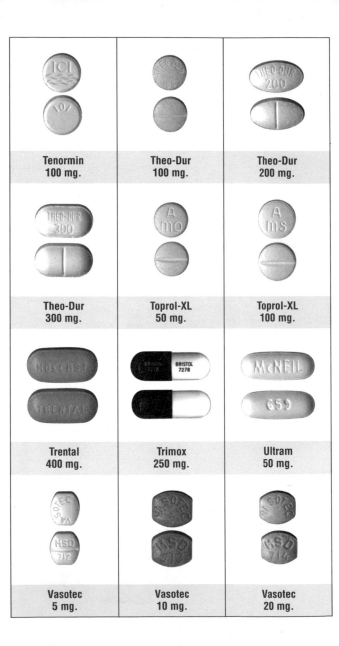

Tenormin 100 mg.	**Theo-Dur** 100 mg.	**Theo-Dur** 200 mg.
Theo-Dur 300 mg.	**Toprol-XL** 50 mg.	**Toprol-XL** 100 mg.
Trental 400 mg.	**Trimox** 250 mg.	**Ultram** 50 mg.
Vasotec 5 mg.	**Vasotec** 10 mg.	**Vasotec** 20 mg.

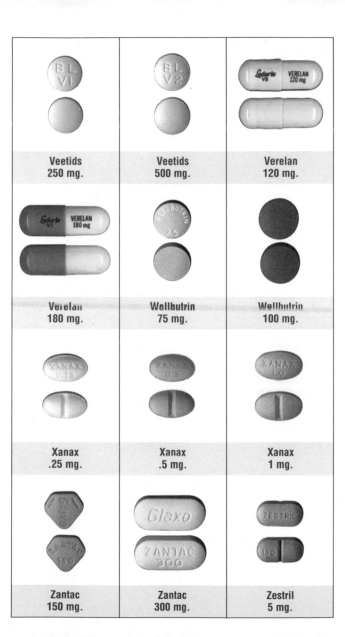

Veetids 250 mg.	Veetids 500 mg.	Verelan 120 mg.
Verelan 180 mg.	Wellbutrin 75 mg.	Wellbutrin 100 mg.
Xanax .25 mg.	Xanax .5 mg.	Xanax 1 mg.
Zantac 150 mg.	Zantac 300 mg.	Zestril 5 mg.

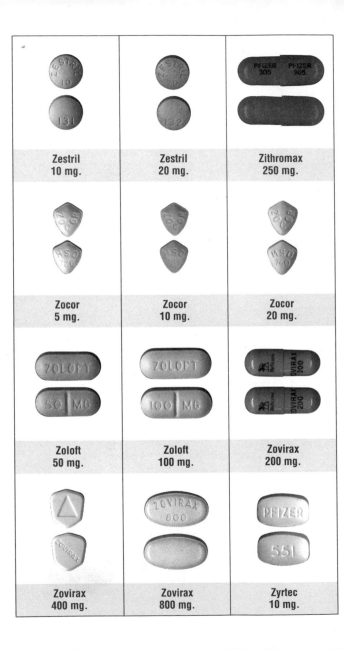

Zestril 10 mg.	Zestril 20 mg.	Zithromax 250 mg.
Zocor 5 mg.	Zocor 10 mg.	Zocor 20 mg.
Zoloft 50 mg.	Zoloft 100 mg.	Zovirax 200 mg.
Zovirax 400 mg.	Zovirax 800 mg.	Zyrtec 10 mg.

whether the drug is excreted in the breast milk; therefore, caution should be used when breast-feeding.

OTHER BRAND NAMES: None

OTHER DRUGS IN THE SAME THERAPEUTIC CLASS: For Maxidex: Decadron, Econopred, Flarex, HMS, Inflamase Forte, Inflamase Mild, Pred Mild, and Vexol. For Maxitrol: Cortisporin, FML-S, Isopto Cetapred, Metimyd, Neodecadron, Poly-Pred, TobraDex, and Vasocidin

IMPORTANT INFORMATION TO REMEMBER: Shake the bottle thoroughly before using the eyedrops. Individuals should not use the drug while wearing contact lenses unless directed otherwise by a doctor. Keep the container tightly closed and avoid touching the applicator tip to the eye—this could contaminate the product over time. Also, only administer one drop at a time. After application, keep the eye open for at least 30 seconds, roll the eyeball around, and avoid squinting. If a second drop is required, wait one to two minutes between drops. If another medication is to be used in the eye, wait at least 10 minutes before administering it. For Maxitrol, use the drug for the full duration of treatment; otherwise the infection may return. If using the eye ointment, insert a small ribbon of the ointment inside the lower eyelid, then close the eye and roll the eyeball around in all directions. Do not touch the tip of the ointment tube to the eye if possible. When using the eye ointment, your vision may become temporarily blurred after use.

BRAND NAME: Maxzide and Maxzide-25

GENERIC NAME: Combination product containing: triamterene and hydrochlorothiazide

GENERIC FORM AVAILABLE: Yes

THERAPEUTIC CLASS: Potassium-sparing diuretic + thiazide diuretic (water pill)

DOSAGE FORMS: 37.5-mg triamterene/25-mg hydrochlorothiazide tablets (Maxzide-25) and 75-mg triamterene/50-mg hydrochlorothiazide tablets (Maxzide)

USUAL DOSE: one or two tablets daily

AVERAGE PRICE: $93.04 (B)/$25.83 (G) for Maxzide and $57.76 (B)/$24.16 (G) for Maxzide-25

SIDE EFFECTS: Most common: none. Less common: dizziness, nausea, vomiting, stomach pain, diarrhea, high potassium, muscle cramps, headache, increased sensitivity to sunlight (sunburn), dry mouth, and skin rash.

DRUG INTERACTIONS: The drug may increase the toxic effects of Eskalith or Lithobid. The drug may also cause high blood sugar when used with Indocin. High potassium levels may occur when used together with Accupril, Altace, Capoten, Lotensin, Monopril, Prinivil, Univasc, Vasotec, and potassium supplements such as Micro-K, K-Dur, Klor-Con, K-Lyte, K-Tab, and Slow-K. The drug may decrease the effects of Coumadin. Individuals taking Lanoxin should inform their doctor of this before taking this drug.

ALLERGIES: Individuals allergic to triamterene, hydrochlorothiazide, Dyrenium, HydroDIURIL, Maxzide, Moduretic, sulfa drugs, or any of their derivatives should discuss this with their doctor or pharmacist before using this drug.

PREGNANCY/BREAST-FEEDING: Category C—Risk cannot be ruled out. Human studies are lacking, and animal studies are either positive for fetal risk or lacking as well. However, potential benefits may justify the potential risk in using the drug. It is not known whether the drug is excreted in the breast milk; therefore, caution should be used when breast-feeding.

OTHER BRAND NAMES: None

OTHER DRUGS IN THE SAME THERAPEUTIC CLASS: Aldactazide, Dyazide, and Moduretic

IMPORTANT INFORMATION TO REMEMBER: If the drug is to be taken once daily, take it in the morning due to increased urine output. If stomach upset occurs, take the drug with food or milk. This drug may also increase the sensitivity of the skin to sunburn in some individuals; therefore, a sunscreen is recommended during periods of prolonged exposure to the sun. Individuals with kidney disease should discuss this with their doctor before taking this drug. Before taking over-the-counter cold and allergy preparations, consult your doctor or pharmacist—these products may raise your blood pressure.

BRAND NAME: Mebaral

GENERIC NAME: mephobarbital

GENERIC FORM AVAILABLE: No

THERAPEUTIC CLASS: Barbiturate sedative

DOSAGE FORMS: 32-mg, 50-mg, and 100-mg tablets

MAIN USES: Seizures and sedative

USUAL DOSE: For seizures: 400 mg to 600 mg daily in divided doses. For sedation: 32 mg to 100 mg three to four times daily.

AVERAGE PRICE: $23.97 for 32 mg; $34.32 for 50 mg; $46.00 for 100 mg

SIDE EFFECTS: Most common: drowsiness, dizziness, unsteadiness, and "hangover effect." Less common: nervousness, constipation, feeling faint, headache, nausea, vomiting, slow heartbeat, insomnia, nightmares, and depression.

DRUG INTERACTIONS. Alcohol, anxiety medications, and narcotic painkillers will intensify the drowsiness effect of the drug. The drug may decrease the blood levels of Aristocort, Coumadin, Decadron, Deltasone, Medrol, prednisone, and Tegretol. The drug may also decrease the effectiveness of birth control pills. Depakene and Depakote may increase the blood levels of the drug.

ALLERGIES: Individuals allergic to mephobarbital or other barbiturates (such as those listed under "Other Drugs in the Same Therapeutic Class") should discuss this with their doctor or pharmacist before taking this drug.

PREGNANCY/BREAST-FEEDING: Category D—Positive evidence of risk. Human studies show risk to the fetus. Nevertheless, potential benefits may possibly outweigh the potential risks. This drug should not be taken by nursing mothers.

OTHER BRAND NAMES: None

OTHER DRUGS IN THE SAME THERAPEUTIC CLASS: Amytal, Butisol, Nembutal, phenobarbital, Seconal, and Tuinal

IMPORTANT INFORMATION TO REMEMBER: This drug does cause drowsiness. Individuals should use caution when driving, operating machinery, or performing any task where mental alertness is required. Alcohol, anxiety medications, or narcotic painkillers may intensify the drowsiness effect of the drug. This medication is a controlled substance and may be habit-forming. Only take the drug exactly as directed by your physician. Do not increase the dose without first consulting with your physician. Women taking birth control pills should use another form of contraception while taking the drug and for the rest of the current menstrual cycle.

BRAND NAME: Meclomen

GENERIC NAME: meclofenamate

GENERIC FORM AVAILABLE: Yes

THERAPEUTIC CLASS: Nonsteroidal anti-inflammatory drug (NSAID)

DOSAGE FORMS: 50-mg and 100-mg capsules

MAIN USES: Arthritis and pain relief

USUAL DOSE: 50 mg to 100 mg three or four times daily

AVERAGE PRICE: $96.75 (B)/$52.70 (G) for 50 mg and $128.66 (B)/$67.67 (G) for 100 mg

SIDE EFFECTS: nausea 3%–9%, upset stomach 3%–9%, diarrhea 3%–9%, stomach pain 3%–9%, heartburn 3%–9%, rash 3%–9%, gas 3%–9%, constipation 1%–3%, vomiting 1%–3%, tiredness 1%–3%, insomnia 1%–3%, ringing in the ears 1%–3%, itching 1%–2%, and dizziness 1%–3%.

DRUG INTERACTIONS: Aspirin will decrease the concentration of this drug in the blood. This drug may also decrease the effects of Lasix, Dyazide, HydroDIURIL, Maxzide, and other water pills. The drug may increase the blood levels of Eskalith, Lithobid, and Sandimmune. The drug may increase the toxic effects of the drug Rheumatrex. Caution should be used when taking the drug with Coumadin.

ALLERGIES: Individuals allergic to meclofenamate or other NSAIDs (such as those listed under "Other Drugs in the Same Therapeutic Class") should discuss this with their doctor or pharmacist before taking this drug.

PREGNANCY/BREAST-FEEDING: Category C—Risk cannot be ruled out. Human studies are lacking, and animal studies are either positive for fetal risk or lacking as well. However, potential benefits may justify the potential risk in using the drug. The drug should not, however, be used during the late stages (last three months) of pregnancy. The drug is excreted in the breast milk; therefore, extreme caution should be used when breast-feeding.

OTHER BRAND NAMES: None

OTHER DRUGS IN THE SAME THERAPEUTIC CLASS: Anaprox, Ansaid, aspirin, Cataflam, Clinoril, Daypro, Disalcid, Dolobid, Easprin, Feldene, Indocin, Lodine, Motrin, Nalfon, Naprosyn, Orudis, Oruvail, Relafen, Tolectin, and Voltaren

IMPORTANT INFORMATION TO REMEMBER: This drug should be taken with food or milk to reduce the potential for injury to the stomach lining and stomach upset. This drug may take up to two weeks before a noticeable improvement in pain relief associated with arthritis is observed. Drinking alcohol while taking this drug may increase its potential to cause ulcers. This drug should only be used under the direct supervision of a doctor by individuals with a bleeding disorder or ulcer, or those who are currently taking Coumadin. Before taking over-the-counter pain relievers, consult your doctor or pharmacist.

BRAND NAME: Medrol

GENERIC NAME: methylprednisolone

GENERIC FORM AVAILABLE: Yes (4 mg only)

THERAPEUTIC CLASS: Glucocorticoid steroid

DOSAGE FORMS: 2-mg, 4-mg, 8-mg, 16-mg, 24-mg, and 32-mg tablets, and 4-mg Dosepak

MAIN USES: Endocrine disorders, and {multiple uses for its ability to reduce inflammation in various part of the body, including asthma}

USUAL DOSE: normal doses range from 4 mg to 48 mg daily

AVERAGE PRICE: $49.62 (B)/for 2 mg; $78.02 (B)/$49.11 (G) for 4 mg; $131.70 (B) for 8 mg; and $23.07 (B)/$18.68 (G) for Dosepak

SIDE EFFECTS: Short-term use of the tablets: Most common: none. Less common: diarrhea, nausea, dizziness, insomnia, nervousness, headache, and stomach pain. Long-term use of the tablets: high blood pressure, muscle weakness, peptic ulcer, hemorrhage, thin fragile skin, facial swelling, weight gain, menstrual irregularities, glaucoma, and many others. Long-term use of the tablets should be avoided if possible.

DRUG INTERACTIONS: Antacids may decrease the absorption of the drug. Amytal, Butisol, Dilantin, Mebaral, Mesantoin, Nembutal, Rifadin, Rifamate, Rifater, Seconal, and Tuinal may decrease the effects of the drug. The drug may increase blood glucose levels. Patients taking drugs for diabetes, including insulin, may need to adjust their dose. The drug may decrease the effects of water pills used to treat high blood pressure and potassium supplements such as K-Dur, Klor-Con, K-Lyte, K-Tab, Micro-K, and Slow-K.

ALLERGIES: Individuals allergic to methylprednisolone or other steroids (such as those listed under "Other Drugs in the Same Therapeutic Class") should discuss this with their doctor or pharmacist before taking this drug.

PREGNANCY/BREAST-FEEDING: Category C—Risk cannot be ruled out. Human studies are lacking, and animal studies are either positive for fetal risk or lacking as well. However, potential benefits may justify the potential risk in using the drug. The drug is excreted in the breast milk; therefore, extreme caution should be used when breast-feeding.

OTHER BRAND NAMES: None

OTHER DRUGS IN THE SAME THERAPEUTIC CLASS: Aristocort, Celestone, Decadron, Deltasone, Pediapred, and Prelone

IMPORTANT INFORMATION TO REMEMBER: This drug should be taken with food or milk to reduce the potential for injury to the stomach lining and stomach upset. Drinking alcohol while taking this drug may increase its potential to cause ulcers. Use exactly as directed by your physician. Never suddenly stop taking the drug without first consulting with your physician—this can be very dangerous. The drug may also cause some weight gain when used for long periods of time.

BRAND NAME: Megace

GENERIC NAME: megestrol

GENERIC FORM AVAILABLE: Yes

THERAPEUTIC CLASS: Progestin anticancer

DOSAGE FORMS: 20-mg and 40-mg tablets; and 40 mg/mL suspension

MAIN USES: Cancer, increase appetite, and {increase in weight gain}

USUAL DOSE: For cancer: 20 mg to 40 mg four times a day. Doses for endometrial cancer may be higher. To increase appetite: 400 mg to 800 mg daily.

AVERAGE PRICE: $96.04 (B)/$72.91 (G) for 20 mg; $171.30 (B)/$102.87 (G) for 40 mg

SIDE EFFECTS: Most common: changes in vaginal bleeding, irregular menstrual cycle time, spotting, breakthrough bleeding, complete lack of bleeding, changes in appetite, changes in weight, swelling of the ankles and feet, tiredness, and weakness. Less common: acne, fever, increased body and facial hair, nausea, vomiting, insomnia, breast tenderness, blood clots, headaches, depression, and some loss of scalp hair.

DRUG INTERACTIONS: The drug may interfere with the effects of Parlodel.

ALLERGIES: Individuals allergic to megestrol or any of its derivatives should discuss this with their doctor or pharmacist before using this drug.

PREGNANCY/BREAST-FEEDING: Category D—Positive evidence of risk. Human studies show risk to the fetus. Nevertheless, potential benefits may possibly outweigh the potential risks. This drug should not be taken by nursing mothers.

OTHER BRAND NAMES: None

OTHER DRUGS IN THE SAME THERAPEUTIC CLASS: None

IMPORTANT INFORMATION TO REMEMBER: It is extremely important to follow the dosing schedule set by your physician—do not deviate from this schedule. Nausea and vomiting may be occur while taking this drug. Do not discontinue use unless directed by your physician; however, stop taking the drug if you suspect you are pregnant. Notify your physician if one of the following occurs: sudden loss of vision, double vision, migraine headache, or pain in the calves of the legs with warmth and tenderness.

BRAND NAME: Mellaril

GENERIC NAME: thioridazine

GENERIC FORM AVAILABLE: Yes

THERAPEUTIC CLASS: Piperidine phenothiazine antipsychotic

DOSAGE FORMS: 10-mg, 15-mg, 25-mg, 50-mg, 100-mg, 150-mg, and 200-mg tablets; 25 mg/5 mL and 100 mg/5 mL suspensions

MAIN USES: Psychotic disorders

USUAL DOSE: 10 mg to 200 mg two to four times daily

AVERAGE PRICE: $33.42 (B)/$13.29 (G) for 10 mg; $46.95 (B)/ $17.36 (G) for 25 mg; $56.96 (B)/$17.47 (G) for 50 mg; $66.75 (B)/$20.00 (G) for 100 mg; $103.36 (B)/$35.93 (G) for 150 mg; $122.60 (B)/$49.81 (G) for 200 mg

SIDE EFFECTS: Most common: drowsiness; restlessness; blurred vision; Parkinson's-like symptoms; low blood pressure; stuffy nose; involuntary movements of the tongue, arms, or legs; muscle spasms; dry mouth; constipation; and dizziness. Less common: increased sensitivity to sunburn, difficulty in urinating, nausea, vomiting, stomach pain, trembling of fingers and hands, stomach pain, changes in menstrual period, decreased sexual ability, swelling and/or pain in the breasts, weight gain, and secretion of milk from the breasts.

DRUG INTERACTIONS: Drugs used to treat depression and Mellaril may increase the severity and frequency of side effects. Alcohol, anxiety medications, and narcotic painkillers may intensify the drowsiness effect of the drug. Eskalith and Lithobid may decrease the absorption of the drug. Eskalith or Lithobid and the drug may cause disorientation and for one to black out. The drug may decrease the effects of Larodopa. Inderal may increase the blood levels of the drug.

ALLERGIES: Individuals allergic to thioridazine or any of their derivatives should discuss this with their doctor or pharmacist before using this drug.

PREGNANCY/BREAST-FEEDING: Category C—Risk cannot be ruled out. Human studies are lacking, and animal studies are either positive for fetal risk or lacking as well. However, potential benefits may justify the potential risk in using the drug. The drug is excreted in the breast milk; therefore, extreme caution should be used when breast-feeding.

OTHER BRAND NAMES: None

OTHER DRUGS IN THE SAME THERAPEUTIC CLASS: Compazine, Prolixin, Serentil, Stelazine, Thorazine, and Trilafon

IMPORTANT INFORMATION TO REMEMBER: This drug does cause drowsiness. Individuals should use caution when driving, operating machinery, or performing any task where mental alertness is required. Alcohol, anxiety medications, and narcotic painkillers may intensify the drowsiness effect of the drug. Do not increase the dose or stop taking the drug without first consulting with your physician. Individuals should report any involuntary movements of the tongue, arms, or legs to their physician. This drug may also increase the sensitivity of the skin to sunburn in some individuals; therefore, a sunscreen is recommended during periods of prolonged exposure to the sun. Caution should be used during hot weather, due to decreased tolerance to the heat.

BRAND NAME: Mesantoin

GENERIC NAME: mephenytoin

GENERIC FORM AVAILABLE: No

THERAPEUTIC CLASS: Hydantoin antiepileptic

DOSAGE FORMS: 100-mg tablets

MAIN USES: Epilepsy and seizures

USUAL DOSE: 200 mg to 600 mg daily in single or divided doses

AVERAGE PRICE: $39.31

SIDE EFFECTS: Most common: central nervous system toxicity (mood changes, rolling eye movements, unsteadiness, nervousness, etc.), increase in gum tissue, bleeding or tender gums, constipation, mild dizziness, mild drowsiness, nausea, and vomiting. Less common: diarrhea, widening of nasal tip, thickening of the lips, swelling of the breasts, headache, unusual hair growth, insomnia, and muscle twitching.

DRUG INTERACTIONS: There are several drugs that interact with Mesantoin. Before taking any medication, consult with your doctor or pharmacist. Some of these drug are listed below: Antabuse, Bactrim, chloramphenicol, Cordarone, Diflucan, isoniazid, Coumadin, Septra, Gantanol, Gantrisin, Pediazole, Tagamet, and trimethoprim may increase the blood levels of the drug. Cancer drugs may decrease the effects of the drug. The drug may decrease the blood levels of Tegretol. Carafate, folic acid, rifampin, Slo-bid, Theo-Dur, theophylline, Uni-Dur, Uniphyl, and may decrease blood levels of the drug. Depakene and Depakote may increase the effects of the drug. The drug may decrease the blood levels of steroids (such as Aristocort, Deltasone, Decadron, Medrol, and prednisone), doxycycline, Mexitil, Norpace, Quinidex, Quinaglute, Slo-bid, Theo-Dur, theophylline, Uni-Dur, Uniphyl, and Vibramycin. The drug may decrease the effects of birth control pills, Larodopa, and some muscle relaxers. The drug may increase the blood levels of Mysoline.

ALLERGIES: Individuals allergic to mephenytoin or any of its derivatives should discuss this with their doctor or pharmacist before using this drug.

PREGNANCY/BREAST-FEEDING: Category D—Positive evidence of risk. Human studies show risk to the fetus. Nevertheless, potential benefits may possibly outweigh the potential risks. This drug should not be taken by nursing mothers.

OTHER BRAND NAMES: None

OTHER DRUGS IN THE SAME THERAPEUTIC CLASS: Dilantin

IMPORTANT INFORMATION TO REMEMBER: This drug does cause some drowsiness. Individuals should use caution when driving, operating machinery, or performing any task where mental alertness is required. Alcohol, anxiety medications, and narcotic painkillers may intensify the drowsiness effect of the drug. Avoid drinking alcohol while taking his drug. Only take the drug exactly as directed by your physician. Do not discontinue the drug or increase the dose without first consulting your physician. Before taking over-the-counter medications, consult your doctor or pharmacist. Birth control pills may be ineffective while taking this drug; another method of birth control is recommended. Practice good oral hygiene to help prevent gum disease associated with taking this drug. Diabetics should monitor their blood sugar carefully while taking this drug.

BRAND NAME: Mestinon

GENERIC NAME: pyridostigmine

GENERIC FORM AVAILABLE: No

THERAPEUTIC CLASS: Cholinesterase inhibitor

DOSAGE FORMS: 180-mg sustained-release tablets (Timespan); 60 mg/5 mL syrup; and 60-mg tablets

MAIN USES: Myasthenia gravis

USUAL DOSE: 600 mg daily in divided doses of the tablets or syrup; or one to three sustained-release tablets once or twice daily

AVERAGE PRICE: $127.31 for 180-mg sustained-release and $58.18 for 60-mg tablets

SIDE EFFECTS: Most common: diarrhea, increased sweating, watering of the mouth, nausea, vomiting, and stomach pain. Less common: frequent urge to urinate, muscle cramps, weakness, increase bronchial secretions, unusually small pupils, and watering of the eyes.

DRUG INTERACTIONS: Hylorel, Ismelin, and Procan may decrease the effects of the drug.

ALLERGIES: Individuals allergic to pyridostigmine or any of its derivatives should discuss this with their doctor or pharmacist before using this drug.

PREGNANCY/BREAST-FEEDING: Category C—Risk cannot be ruled out. Human studies are lacking, and animal studies are either positive for fetal risk or lacking as well. However, potential benefits may justify the potential risk in using the drug. The drug is excreted in the breast milk; therefore, extreme caution should be used when breast-feeding.

OTHER BRAND NAMES: None

OTHER DRUGS IN THE SAME THERAPEUTIC CLASS: Prostigmin

IMPORTANT INFORMATION TO REMEMBER: Only take the drug exactly as directed by your physician. Do not discontinue the drug without first consulting your physician. Also, do not increase the dose without first consulting with your physician. Swallow the tablets whole—do not crush or chew the tablets (sustained-release tablets only, Timespan); this will destroy the sustained-release mechanism of the tablet. Before taking over-the-counter medications, consult your doctor or pharmacist.

BRAND NAME: Metaprel

GENERIC NAME: metaproterenol

See entry for Alupent

BRAND NAME: Methergine

GENERIC NAME: methylergonovine

GENERIC FORM AVAILABLE: No

THERAPEUTIC CLASS: Uterine constrictor

DOSAGE FORMS: 0.2-mg tablets

MAIN USES: Bleeding after delivery, lack of muscle tone in the uterus, and failure of the uterus to return to normal size after delivery

USUAL DOSE: 0.2 mg three to four times daily after delivery for a maximum of one week

AVERAGE PRICE: $28.66 (30 tablets)

SIDE EFFECTS: Most common: nausea, high blood pressure, uterine cramping, and vomiting. Less common: stomach pain, chest pain, slow heartbeat, diarrhea, headache, low blood pressure, heart attack, leg cramps, difficulty breathing, dizziness, sweating, and ringing in the ears.

DRUG INTERACTIONS: The drug should be used cautiously with cough, cold, and allergy products that contain decongestants, as well as Cafergot, Midrin, Sansert, and Wigraine.

ALLERGIES: Individuals allergic to methylergonovine or any of its derivatives should discuss this with their doctor or pharmacist before using this drug.

PREGNANCY/BREAST-FEEDING: Category C—Risk cannot be ruled out. Human studies are lacking, and animal studies are either positive for fetal risk or lacking as well. However, potential benefits may justify the potential risk in using the drug. The drug is excreted in the breast milk; therefore, caution should be used when breast-feeding.

OTHER BRAND NAMES: None

OTHER DRUGS IN THE SAME THERAPEUTIC CLASS: None

IMPORTANT INFORMATION TO REMEMBER: Only take the drug exactly as directed by your physician. Do not discontinue the drug or increase the dose without first consulting your physician. If you have high blood pressure, discuss this with your physician before taking the drug.

BRAND NAME: Methotrexate

GENERIC NAME: methotrexate

See entry for Rheumatrex

BRAND NAME: MetroGel and MetroGel Vaginal

GENERIC NAME: metronidazole

GENERIC FORM AVAILABLE: No

THERAPEUTIC CLASS: Topical antibiotic

DOSAGE FORMS: 0.75% aqueous gel and 0.75% vaginal gel

MAIN USES: Skin infections (MetroGel) and bacterial vaginal infections (MetroGel Vaginal)

USUAL DOSE: Apply in a thin film twice daily (MetroGel). Insert one applicatorful into the vagina twice daily for five days (MetroGel Vaginal).

AVERAGE PRICE: $33.25 for 0.75% gel (28 g of MetroGel), and $36.96 for 0.75% gel (70 g of MetroGel Vaginal)

SIDE EFFECTS: Most common: None. Less common: vaginal cramps, dry skin, redness, skin irritation, vaginal rash, stinging, vaginal yeast infection, itching, and burning.

DRUG INTERACTIONS: Individuals should not drink alcohol or take cough or cold medications that may contain alcohol while using MetroGel Vaginal, and for at least 24 hours after the last dose. The drug may increase the effects of Coumadin.

ALLERGIES: Individuals allergic to metronidazole, Flagyl, or any of their derivatives should discuss this with their doctor or pharmacist before using this drug.

PREGNANCY/BREAST-FEEDING: Category B—No evidence of risk in humans. Either animal findings show risk, but human findings do not; or, if no adequate human studies have been done, animal findings show no risk. It is not known whether the drug is excreted in the breast milk; therefore, caution should be used when breast-feeding.

OTHER BRAND NAMES: None

OTHER DRUGS IN THE SAME THERAPEUTIC CLASS: AVC Vaginal Cream, Cleocin Vaginal, and Sultrin Vaginal Cream

IMPORTANT INFORMATION TO REMEMBER: This drug is for external and vaginal use only. Apply and gently rub in enough of the gel to cover the affected area and surrounding areas. Use the drug for the full course of treatment or the infection may return. Never cover the skin after application with a bandage or wrapping unless directed to do so by a doctor. Discontinue use if irritation occurs. For the vaginal gel: insert the applicator high into the vagina (two-thirds the length of the applicator) and push the plunger to release the cream. Also, when using the vaginal gel, do not use a tampon to hold the gel inside the vagina. If the drug is to be used twice daily, apply it in the morning and in the evening. The vaginal gel may stain clothing. Avoid sexual intercourse until therapy is complete.

BRAND NAME: Mevacor

GENERIC NAME: lovastatin

GENERIC FORM AVAILABLE: No

THERAPEUTIC CLASS: Cholesterol-lowering agent

DOSAGE FORMS: 10-mg, 20-mg and 40-mg tablets

MAIN USES: High cholesterol

USUAL DOSE: 10 mg to 80 mg per day in single or divided doses

AVERAGE PRICE: $171.94 for 10 mg; $308.60 for 20 mg; $545.67 for 40 mg

SIDE EFFECTS: gas 4%–6%, diarrhea 3%–6%, headache 3%–9%, stomach pain 2%–6%, constipation 3%–5%, nausea 2%, muscle cramps 1%, dizziness 1%–2%, skin rash 1%–5%, and blurred vision 1%–2%.

DRUG INTERACTIONS: Sandimmune, Lopid, and niacin may cause kidney problems when taken with the drug. Tagamet, Prilosec, and Zantac may increase the blood levels of the drug. The drug may increase the effects of Coumadin. Lopid and the drug, when taken together, may increase the risk of developing rhabdomyolysis (destruction and death of muscle tissue). Symptoms are muscle pain and dark, red-brown colored urine.

ALLERGIES: Individuals allergic to lovastatin, Lescol, Pravachol, Zocor, or any of their derivatives should discuss this with their doctor or pharmacist before using this drug.

PREGNANCY/BREAST-FEEDING: Category X—Should not be used during pregnancy. Studies in animals and/or humans have shown fetal abnormalities and birth defects. The risks associated with using this drug clearly outweigh the benefits. This drug should never be used by someone who is pregnant or trying to become pregnant. Also, women should never breast-feed while using this drug.

OTHER BRAND NAMES: None

OTHER DRUGS IN THE SAME THERAPEUTIC CLASS: Lescol, Lipitor, Pravachol, and Zocor

IMPORTANT INFORMATION TO REMEMBER: The drug should be taken with food or milk (preferably an evening meal). Only take the drug exactly as directed by your physician. It is also important to follow the prescribed low cholesterol diet. Report any sign of unexplained muscle pain or tenderness to your doctor, especially if it is accompanied by tiredness or fever.

BRAND NAME: Mexitil

GENERIC NAME: mexiletine

GENERIC FORM AVAILABLE: Yes

THERAPEUTIC CLASS: Class 1B antiarrhythmic

DOSAGE FORMS: 150-mg, 200-mg, and 250-mg capsules

MAIN USES: Irregular heartbeats and {diabetic neuropathy}

USUAL DOSE: 150 mg to 300 mg every eight hours

AVERAGE PRICE: $105.00 (B)/$72.14 (G) for 150 mg; $126.81 (B)/$91.58 (G) for 200 mg; and $147.27 (B)/$105.17 (G) for 250 mg

SIDE EFFECTS: nausea 39%, dizziness 19%–26%, tremor 13%, clumsiness 10%, changes in sleep habits 7%, blurred vision 6%–8%, headache 6%–8%, nervousness 5%–11%, diarrhea 5%, constipation 4%, rash 4%, pounding heartbeat 4%, changes in appetite 3%, speech difficulties 3%, trouble breathing 3%, dry mouth 3%, chest pain 3%, tiredness 2%–4%, anginalike pain 2%, weakness 2%–5%, depression 2%, numbness 2%–4%, joint pain 2%, increased irregular heartbeats 1%, and stomach pain 1%.

DRUG INTERACTIONS: Dilantin, Mesantoin, phenobarbital, and rifampin may lower blood levels of the drug. The drug may increase the blood levels of Slo-bid, Theo-Dur, theophylline, Uni-Dur, and Uniphyl. Tagamet may alter the blood levels of the drug.

ALLERGIES: Individuals allergic to mexiletine or any of its derivatives should discuss this with their doctor or pharmacist before using this drug.

PREGNANCY/BREAST-FEEDING: Category C—Risk cannot be ruled out. Human studies are lacking, and animal studies are either positive for fetal risk or lacking as well. However, potential benefits may justify the potential risk in using the drug. The drug is excreted in the breast milk; therefore, extreme caution should be used when breast-feeding.

OTHER BRAND NAMES: None

OTHER DRUGS IN THE SAME THERAPEUTIC CLASS: None

IMPORTANT INFORMATION TO REMEMBER: The drug should be taken with food or milk to reduce the potential for stomach upset. The drug may cause some limited amount of dizziness. Only take the drug exactly as directed by your physician. Do not discontinue the drug or increase the dose without first consulting your physician.

BRAND NAME: Miacalcin

GENERIC NAME: calcitonin–salmon

GENERIC FORM AVAILABLE: No

THERAPEUTIC CLASS: Hormone for bone disorders

DOSAGE FORMS: 200-units-per-spray nasal spray

MAIN USES: Osteoporosis and Paget's disease

USUAL DOSE: one spray daily in one nostril

AVERAGE PRICE: $37.04

SIDE EFFECTS: runny nose 12%, other nasal symptoms 11%, back pain 5%, muscle pain 4%, bloody nose 4%, headache 3%, tiredness 1%–3%, upper respiratory infection 1%–3%, constipation 1%–3%, diarrhea 1%–3%, nausea 1%–3%, stomach pain 1%–3%, dizziness 1%–3%, muscle soreness 1%–3%, rash 1%–3%, numbness 1%–3%, and depression 1%–3%.

DRUG INTERACTIONS: None of any clinical significance

ALLERGIES: Individuals allergic to calcitonin, salmon, or any of their derivatives should discuss this with their doctor or pharmacist before using this drug.

PREGNANCY/BREAST-FEEDING: Category C—Risk cannot be ruled out. Human studies are lacking, and animal studies are either positive for fetal risk or lacking as well. However, potential benefits may justify the potential risk in using the drug. It is not known whether the drug is excreted in the breast milk; therefore, caution should be used when breast-feeding.

OTHER BRAND NAMES: None

OTHER DRUGS IN THE SAME THERAPEUTIC CLASS: Calcimar

IMPORTANT INFORMATION TO REMEMBER: Only use the drug exactly as directed by your physician. Do not discontinue the drug or increase the dose without first consulting with your physician. Use the drug at the same time every day. Also, alternate the nostril you spray every other day. Unopened bottles of the drug should be stored in the refrigerator.

BRAND NAME: Micro-K

GENERIC NAME: potassium chloride

GENERIC FORM AVAILABLE: Yes

THERAPEUTIC CLASS: Potassium supplement

DOSAGE FORMS: 8-mEq (600-mg) and 10-mEq (750-mg) sustained-release capsules; and 20-mEq powder

MAIN USES: Low potassium

USUAL DOSE: 10 mEq to 40 mEq per day in divided doses

AVERAGE PRICE: $19.35 (B)/$13.79 (G) for 8 mEq; and $22.15 (B)/ $15.66 (G) for 10 mEq

SIDE EFFECTS: Most common: none. Less common: diarrhea, vomiting, gas, nausea, and stomach discomfort.

DRUG INTERACTIONS: Aldactazide, Aldactone, Dyazide, Dyrenium, Hygroton, Maxzide, Midamor, and Moduretic may cause potassium levels to become too high when taken with this drug. Accupril, Altace, Capoten, Lotensin, Monopril, Prinivil, Univasc, Vasotec, Zestril, and salt substitutes may cause potassium levels to become too high when taken with this drug. Caution should be used by patients taking Lanoxin and this drug.

ALLERGIES: Individuals allergic to potassium, potassium chloride, or any of their derivatives should discuss this with their doctor or pharmacist before using this drug.

PREGNANCY/BREAST-FEEDING: Category C—Risk cannot be ruled out. Human studies are lacking, and animal studies are either positive for fetal risk or lacking as well. However, potential benefits may justify the potential risk in using the drug. It is not known whether the drug is excreted in the breast milk; therefore, caution should be used when breast-feeding.

OTHER BRAND NAMES: K-Norm

OTHER DRUGS IN THE SAME THERAPEUTIC CLASS: KAON-CL, Kay Ciel, K-Dur, K-Lor, Klor-Con, Klorvess, Klotrix, K-Lyte, K-Lyte/Cl, K-Norm, K-Tab, and Slow-K

IMPORTANT INFORMATION TO REMEMBER: This drug should be taken with food or milk to reduce the potential for injury to the stomach lining and stomach upset. The drug should also be taken with a full glass of water (eight ounces is preferred). Only take the drug exactly as directed by your doctor; do not increase the dose or discontinue taking the drug without first consulting with your doctor. Individuals should avoid salt substitutes that contain potassium. Individuals unable to swallow the capsules may sprinkle the contents on some soft food (such as applesauce) and swallow it without chewing.

BRAND NAME: Micronase

GENERIC NAME: glyburide

GENERIC FORM AVAILABLE: Yes

THERAPEUTIC CLASS: Second-generation sulfonylurea anti-diabetic

DOSAGE FORMS: 1.25-mg, 2.5-mg, and 5.0-mg tablets

MAIN USES: Diabetes

USUAL DOSE: 1.25 mg to 20 mg daily in divided doses

AVERAGE PRICE: $55.96 (B)/$33.42 (G) for 2.5 mg and $94.73 (B)/ $40.13 (G) for 5 mg

SIDE EFFECTS: nausea 2%, stomach bloating 2%, heartburn 2%, allergic skin reactions 2%, and low blood sugar 1%–2%.

DRUG INTERACTIONS: The drug may cause a stomach reaction (nausea, diarrhea, stomach cramps, vomiting, etc.) when taken with alcohol. The blood levels of the drug and Coumadin may initially increase and then decrease when these are taken together. Bactrim, Gantanol, Gantrisin, Ismelin, Nardil, Parnate, and Septra, and high doses of aspirin, Easprin, or Disalcid may cause low blood sugar when taken with this drug. Blocadren, Cartrol, Corgard, Inderal, Kerlone, Levatol, Lopressor, Normodyne, Sectral, Tenormin, Toprol-XL, Trandate, Visken, and Zebeta may hide the symptoms of low blood sugar when taken with this drug. Injected insulin and Cipro may increase the effects of the drug (low blood sugar).

ALLERGIES: Individuals allergic to glyburide, Glynase, sulfa drugs, or other sulfonylureas (such as those listed under "Other Drugs in the Same Therapeutic Class") should discuss this with their doctor or pharmacist before taking this drug.

PREGNANCY/BREAST-FEEDING: Category B—No evidence of risk in humans. Either animal findings show risk, but human findings do not; or, if no adequate human studies have been done, animal findings show no risk. It is not known whether the drug is excreted in the breast milk; therefore, caution should be used when breast-feeding.

OTHER BRAND NAMES: Diaβeta

OTHER DRUGS IN THE SAME THERAPEUTIC CLASS: Diaβeta, Glucotrol, Glucotrol XL, and Glynase

IMPORTANT INFORMATION TO REMEMBER: If taken once daily, the drug should be taken with breakfast or the first main meal. To receive optimum effect, regular compliance with therapy is essential. This includes compliance with a prescribed diet. Avoid alcohol while taking this drug; alcohol may cause a severe stomach reaction (vomiting, pain, diarrhea, etc.). This drug lowers blood sugar. Individuals should be aware of the signs and symptoms of blood sugar that is too low: sweating, tremor, blurred vision, weakness, hunger, and confusion. If two or more of these symptoms are seen, treat with oral glucose (sugar) and/or contact your doctor. This drug may increase the risk of cardiovascular disease. Before taking over-the-counter cold and allergy preparations, consult your doctor or pharmacist—these products may affect your blood sugar.

BRAND NAME: Midamor

GENERIC NAME: amiloride

GENERIC FORM AVAILABLE: Yes

THERAPEUTIC CLASS: Potassium-sparing diuretic (water pill)

DOSAGE FORMS: 5-mg tablets

MAIN USES: Swelling and water retention due to congestive heart failure, kidney or liver disease, and high blood pressure

USUAL DOSE: 5 mg to 10 mg daily

AVERAGE PRICE: $64.51 (B)/$59.71 (G)

SIDE EFFECTS: headache 3%–8%, nausea 3%–8%, diarrhea 3%–8%, vomiting 3%–8%, weakness 1%–3%, stomach pain 1%–3%, gas 1%–3%, appetite changes 1%–3%, dizziness 1%–3%, tiredness 1%–3%, constipation 1%–3%, muscle cramps 1%–3%, cough 1%–3%, and impotence 1%–3%.

DRUG INTERACTIONS: The drug may increase the toxic effects of Eskalith or Lithobid. May also cause high potassium when used with Indocin. High potassium levels may occur when used together with Accupril, Altace, Capoten, Lotensin, Monopril, Prinivil, Univasc, and Vasotec, and potassium supplements such as Micro-K, K-Dur, Klor-Con, K-Lyte, and Slow-K. The drug may decrease the effects of Coumadin. Individuals taking Lanoxin should inform their doctor of this before taking this drug.

ALLERGIES: Individuals allergic to amiloride or any of its derivatives should discuss this with their doctor or pharmacist before using this drug.

PREGNANCY/BREAST-FEEDING: Category B—No evidence of risk in humans. Either animal findings show risk, but human findings do not; or, if no adequate human studies have been done, animal findings show no risk. It is not known whether the drug is excreted in the breast milk; therefore, caution should be used when breast-feeding.

OTHER BRAND NAMES: None

OTHER DRUGS IN THE SAME THERAPEUTIC CLASS: Aldactone and Dyrenium

IMPORTANT INFORMATION TO REMEMBER: If the drug is to be taken once daily, take it in the morning due to increased urine output. If stomach upset occurs, take with food or milk. Individuals with kidney disease should discuss this with their doctor before taking this drug. Before taking over-the-counter cold and allergy preparations, consult your doctor or pharmacist—these products may raise your blood pressure.

BRAND NAME: Midrin

GENERIC NAME: Combination product containing: isometheptene, dichloralphenazone, and acetaminophen

GENERIC FORM AVAILABLE: Yes

THERAPEUTIC CLASS: Blood vessel constrictor + sedative + analgesic

DOSAGE FORMS: 65-mg isometheptene/100-mg dichloralphenazone/325-mg acetaminophen capsules

MAIN USES: Tension headaches and migraine headaches

USUAL DOSE: For a tension headache: one to two capsules every four hours as needed (maximum of eight capsules per day). For a migraine headache: two capsules at the onset of the headache, followed by one capsule every hour until relieved (maximum of five capsules within 12 hours).

AVERAGE PRICE: $61.57 (B)/$36.27 (G)

SIDE EFFECTS: Most common: drowsiness. Less common: dizziness, rash, fast heartbeat, irregular heartbeat, anemia, and unusual tiredness or weakness.

DRUG INTERACTIONS: The drug may increase the severity and occurrence of side effects when used with Nardil or Parnate.

ALLERGIES: Individuals allergic to isometheptene, dichloralphenazone, acetaminophen, or any of their derivatives should discuss this with their doctor or pharmacist before using this drug.

PREGNANCY/BREAST-FEEDING: This drug has not been rated; therefore, extreme caution should be used when breast-feeding.

OTHER BRAND NAMES: None

OTHER DRUGS IN THE SAME THERAPEUTIC CLASS: None

IMPORTANT INFORMATION TO REMEMBER: Patients with high blood pressure or heart disease should discuss this with their physician before taking this drug. The drug is most effective if it is taken at the first sign of a migraine attack. If the usual dose of the drug does not provide relief, contact your physician. Only take the drug exactly as directed by your physician. Do not increase the dose without first consulting with your physician. The drug may cause some drowsiness. Individuals should use caution when driving, operating machinery, or performing any task where mental alertness is required. Alcohol, anxiety medications, and narcotic painkillers may intensify the drowsiness effect of the drug. Avoid drinking alcohol while taking this drug.

BRAND NAME: Minipress

GENERIC NAME: prazosin

GENERIC FORM AVAILABLE: Yes

THERAPEUTIC CLASS: Selective alpha-1-blood-vessel dilator

DOSAGE FORMS: 1-mg, 2-mg, and 5-mg capsules

MAIN USES: High blood pressure and {benign prostatic hyperplasia (BPH)}

USUAL DOSE: 3 mg to 20 mg per day in divided doses

AVERAGE PRICE: $60.44 (B)/$29.65 (G) for 1 mg; $83.54 (B)/$40.66 (G) for 2 mg; $140.78 (B)/$69.27 (G) for 5 mg

SIDE EFFECTS: dizziness 10%, headache 8%, drowsiness 8%, lack of energy 7%, weakness 7%, pounding heartbeat 5%, nausea 5%, diarrhea 1%–4%, vomiting 1%–4%, low blood pressure when getting up from a sitting or lying down position 1%–4%, depression 1%–4%, nervousness 1%–4%, dry mouth 1%–4%, nasal congestion 1%–4%, blurred vision 1%–4%, swelling 1%–4%, and increased frequency in urination 1%–4%.

DRUG INTERACTIONS: Calan and Isoptin may increase the blood levels of the drug. Caution should be used when this drug is taken with other drugs for high blood pressure; the combination may cause blood pressure to go too low.

ALLERGIES: Individuals allergic to prazosin or any of its derivatives should discuss this with their doctor or pharmacist before using this drug.

PREGNANCY/BREAST-FEEDING: Category C—Risk cannot be ruled out. Human studies are lacking, and animal studies are either positive for fetal risk or lacking as well. However, potential benefits may justify the potential risk in using the drug. The drug is excreted in the breast milk; therefore, extreme caution should be used when breast-feeding.

OTHER BRAND NAMES: None

OTHER DRUGS IN THE SAME THERAPEUTIC CLASS: Cardura and Hytrin

IMPORTANT INFORMATION TO REMEMBER: The first dose should be taken at bedtime to avoid dizziness and fainting. Only take the drug exactly as directed by your physician. Do not discontinue the drug without first consulting your physician. Before taking over-the-counter cold and allergy preparations, consult your doctor or pharmacist—these products may raise your blood pressure. This drug may cause some drowsiness at first. Individuals should use caution when driving, operating machinery, or performing any task where mental alertness is required. Individuals should get up slowly from the sitting or lying-down position; otherwise dizziness may occur.

BRAND NAME: Minitran

GENERIC NAME: nitroglycerin patch

See entry for Nitro-Dur

BRAND NAME: **Minocin**

GENERIC NAME: minocycline

GENERIC FORM AVAILABLE: Yes

THERAPEUTIC CLASS: Tetracycline antibiotic

DOSAGE FORMS: 50-mg and 100-mg capsules; and 50 mg/5 mL powder for oral suspension

MAIN USES: Bacterial infections and acne

USUAL DOSE: 50 mg to 100 mg every 12 hours

AVERAGE PRICE: $125.33 (B)/$84.86 (G) for 50 mg (50 capsules) and $161.17 (B)/$114.17 (G) for 100 mg (50 capsules)

SIDE EFFECTS: Most common: discoloration of infants and children's teeth, dizziness, diarrhea, nausea, vomiting, stomach pain, and burning stomach. Less common: sore or darkened tongue, headache, discoloration of the skin and mucous membranes, increased sensitivity to sunburn, and fungal overgrowth.

DRUG INTERACTIONS: Antacids, milk, dairy products, calcium supplements, iron supplements, magnesium laxatives, and other mineral supplements may bind to the drug in the stomach and intestines and prevent its absorption by the body. The drug may decrease the effectiveness of birth control pills.

ALLERGIES: Individuals allergic to minocycline or other tetracyclines (such as those listed under "Other Drugs in the Same Therapeutic Class") should discuss this with their doctor or pharmacist before taking this drug.

PREGNANCY/BREAST-FEEDING: Category D—Positive evidence of risk. Human studies show risk to the fetus. Nevertheless, potential benefits may possibly outweigh the potential risk. This drug should not be taken by nursing mothers.

OTHER BRAND NAMES: None

OTHER DRUGS IN THE SAME THERAPEUTIC CLASS: Achromycin V, Doryx, Monodox, Sumycin, Vibramycin, and Vibra-Tabs

IMPORTANT INFORMATION TO REMEMBER: If stomach upset occurs, take the drug with food. Take the drug at the same time every day. Also, take the drug until all the medication prescribed is gone; otherwise the infection may return. This drug should be taken with plenty of water (eight ounces is preferred) and the capsules should be swallowed whole. Avoid taking antacids, calcium supplements, iron supplements, magnesium laxatives, and other mineral supplements within two hours of taking the drug. Women taking birth control pills should use another form of contraception while taking the drug and for the rest of the current menstrual cycle. Individuals should also use a sunscreen to avoid overexposure to the sun. The drug may increase the skin's sensitivity to sunlight, which may cause one to sunburn more easily. The drug should not be used by children under eight years of age due to the potential of permanent tooth staining.

BRAND NAME: Moban

GENERIC NAME: molindone

GENERIC FORM AVAILABLE: No

THERAPEUTIC CLASS: Dihydroindolone antipsychotic

DOSAGE FORMS: 5-mg, 10-mg, 25-mg, 50 mg, and 100-mg tablets

MAIN USES: Psychotic disorders

USUAL DOSE: 5 mg to 25 mg three or four times a day. Severe cases may require higher doses.

AVERAGE PRICE: $82.26 for 5 mg; $176.26 for 25 mg; $235.38 for 50 mg; $314.45 for 100 mg

SIDE EFFECTS: Most common: drowsiness; severe restlessness; need to keep moving; muscle spasms of the face, neck, and back; twitching; weakness of the arms and legs; inability to move the eyes; trembling and shaking of the hands; Parkinson's-like symptoms; lip smacking or puckering; uncontrollable movements of the tongue; blurred vision; constipation; decreased sweating; dry mouth; increased heart rate; headache; low blood pressure; nausea; and difficulty in urinating. Less common: changes in menstrual periods, decreased sexual ability, false sense of well-being, swelling of the breasts, unusual secretion of milk, and depression.

DRUG INTERACTIONS: Eskalith or Lithobid and the drug may produce toxic effects. Alcohol, anxiety medications, and narcotic painkillers may intensify the drowsiness effect of the drug. The drug may decrease the blood levels of tetracycline antibiotics and Dilantin.

ALLERGIES: Individuals allergic to molindone or any of its derivatives should discuss this with their doctor or pharmacist before using this drug.

PREGNANCY/BREAST-FEEDING: Category C—Risk cannot be ruled out. Human studies are lacking, and animal studies are either positive for fetal risk or lacking as well. However, potential benefits may justify the potential risk in using the drug. It is not known whether the drug is excreted in the breast milk; therefore, caution should be used when breast-feeding.

OTHER BRAND NAMES: None

OTHER DRUGS IN THE SAME THERAPEUTIC CLASS: None

IMPORTANT INFORMATION TO REMEMBER: This drug does cause drowsiness. Individuals should use caution when driving, operating machinery, or performing any task where mental alertness is required. Alcohol, anxiety medications, and narcotic painkillers may intensify the drowsiness effect of the drug. Do not increase the dose or stop taking the drug without first consulting with your physician. The drug may require several weeks before optimal effects are seen. Individuals should report any involuntary movements of the tongue, arms, or legs to their physician. This drug may also increase the sensitivity of the individual to heat and sun; caution should be used in hot weather. Individuals should not take antacids or antidiarrheal medications within two hours of taking this drug. Individuals should get up slowly from a sitting or lying-down position; otherwise dizziness may occur.

BRAND NAME: Modicon

GENERIC NAME: Combination product containing: norethindrone and ethinyl estradiol

Very similar to Ortho-Novum. See entry for Ortho-Novum.

BRAND NAME: Moduretic

GENERIC NAME: Combination product containing: amiloride and hydrochlorothiazide

GENERIC FORM AVAILABLE: Yes

THERAPEUTIC CLASS: Potassium-sparing diuretic (water pill) + thiazide diuretic (water pill)

DOSAGE FORMS: 5-mg amiloride/50-mg hydrochlorothiazide tablets

MAIN USES: Swelling and water retention due to congestive heart failure, kidney or liver disease, and high blood pressure

USUAL DOSE: one tablet daily with food

AVERAGE PRICE: $67.07 (B)/$31.87 (G)

SIDE EFFECTS: headache 3%–8%, weakness 3%–8%, nausea 3%–8%, dizziness 3%–8%, rash 3%–8%, tiredness 1%–3%, diarrhea 1%–3%, irregular heartbeat 1%–3%, stomach pain 1%–3%, difficulty breathing 1%–3%, and leg aches 1%–3%.

DRUG INTERACTIONS: The drug may increase the toxic effects of Eskalith or Lithobid. The drug may also cause high potassium levels when used with Indocin. High potassium levels may also occur when the drug is used together with Accupril, Altace, Capoten, Lotensin, Monopril, Prinivil, Univasc, and Vasotec, and potassium supplements such as Micro-K, K-Dur, Klor-Con, K-Lyte, K-Tab, and Slow-K. The drug may decrease the effects of Coumadin. Individuals taking Lanoxin should inform their doctor of this before taking this drug.

ALLERGIES: Individuals allergic to amiloride, hydrochlorothiazide, Dyazide, HydroDIURIL, Maxzide, or sulfa drugs or any of their derivatives should discuss this with their doctor or pharmacist before using this drug.

PREGNANCY/BREAST-FEEDING: Category B—No evidence of risk in humans. Either animal findings show risk, but human findings do not; or, if no adequate human studies have been done, animal findings show no risk. The drug is excreted in the breast milk; therefore, extreme caution should be used when breast-feeding.

OTHER BRAND NAMES: None

OTHER DRUGS IN THE SAME THERAPEUTIC CLASS: Aldactazide, Dyazide, and Maxzide

IMPORTANT INFORMATION TO REMEMBER: If the drug is to be taken once daily, take it in the morning due to increased urine output. If stomach upset occurs, take the drug with food or milk. This drug may also increase the sensitivity of the skin to sunburn in some individuals; therefore, a sunscreen is recommended during periods of prolonged exposure to the sun. Individuals with kidney disease should discuss this with their doctor before taking this drug. Before taking over-the-counter cold and allergy preparations, consult your doctor or pharmacist—these products may raise your blood pressure.

BRAND NAME: Monistat and Monistat-Derm

GENERIC NAME: miconazole

GENERIC FORM AVAILABLE: Yes

THERAPEUTIC CLASS: Imidazole antifungal

DOSAGE FORMS: 100-mg and 200-mg vaginal suppositories, 2% vaginal cream, and 2% skin cream

MAIN USES: Vaginal yeast infections and fungal skin infections

USUAL DOSE: one suppository (vaginally) at bedtime for three days (Monistat 3) or seven days (Monistat 7); one applicatorful (vaginally) of cream at bedtime for seven days (Monistat 7); and application twice daily (Monistat-Derm)

AVERAGE PRICE: $27.98 (B)/$14.82 (G) for 2% vaginal cream; $35.28 (B)/$29.24 (G) for 200-mg suppositories; and $36.28 for cream (30 g) (Monistat-Derm)

SIDE EFFECTS: burning 2%, itching 2%, irritation 2%, cramping (Monistat vaginal products only) 2%, rash 1%, and headaches 1%.

DRUG INTERACTIONS: None of any clinical significance

ALLERGIES: Individuals allergic to miconazole or any of its derivatives should discuss this with their doctor or pharmacist before using this drug.

PREGNANCY/BREAST-FEEDING: Category C—Risk cannot be ruled out. Human studies are lacking, and animal studies are either positive for fetal risk or lacking as well. Potential benefits may justify the potential risk in using the drug. However, the drug should not be used during the first trimester (first three months) of pregnancy. It is not known whether the drug is excreted in the breast milk; therefore, caution should be used when breast-feeding.

OTHER BRAND NAMES: None

OTHER DRUGS IN THE SAME THERAPEUTIC CLASS: For Monistat vaginal products: Femstat, Gyne-Lotrimin, Mycelex, Mycelex-G, Terazol, and Vagistat-1. For Monistat-Derm: Lotrimin, Nizoral, Oxistat, and Spectazole.

IMPORTANT INFORMATION TO REMEMBER: For Monistat-Derm: this drug is for external use only. Apply and gently rub in enough of the cream to cover the affected area and surrounding areas. Use the drug for the full course of treatment or the infection may return. Never cover the skin after application with a bandage or wrapping unless directed to do so by a doctor. Discontinue use if irritation occurs. For the vaginal cream and suppositories: insert the applicator high into the vagina (two-thirds the length of the applicator) and push the plunger to release the cream. Also, when using the vaginal cream or suppositories, do not use a tampon to hold them inside the vagina. These products may stain clothing. It is important to continue using the products even during your menstrual period unless otherwise directed by your doctor. The vaginal cream and suppositories are available over-the-counter (OTC) without a prescription.

BRAND NAME: Monodox

GENERIC NAME: doxycycline monohydrate

GENERIC FORM AVAILABLE: No

THERAPEUTIC CLASS: Tetracycline antibiotic

DOSAGE FORMS: 50-mg and 100-mg capsules

MAIN USES: Bactcrial infections and severe acne

USUAL DOSE: 50 mg to 100 mg once daily or every 12 hours

AVERAGE PRICE: $132.72 for 50 mg and $216.72 for 100 mg

SIDE EFFECTS: Most common: discoloration of infants and children's teeth, increased sensitivity to sunburn, dizziness, diarrhea, nausea, vomiting, stomach pain, and burning stomach. Less common: sore or darkened tongue, discoloration of the skin and mucous membranes, and fungal overgrowth.

DRUG INTERACTIONS: Antacids, calcium supplements, iron supplements, magnesium laxatives, and other mineral supplements may bind to the drug in the stomach and intestines and prevent its absorption by the body. The drug may decrease the effectiveness of birth control pills.

ALLERGIES: Individuals allergic to doxycycline or other tetracyclines (such as those listed under "Other Drugs in the Same Therapeutic Class") should discuss this with their doctor or pharmacist before taking this drug.

PREGNANCY/BREAST-FEEDING: Category D—Positive evidence of risk. Human studies show risk to the fetus. Nevertheless, potential benefits may possibly outweigh the potential risks. This drug should not be taken by nursing mothers.

OTHER BRAND NAMES: None

OTHER DRUGS IN THE SAME THERAPEUTIC CLASS: Achromycin V, Doryx, Minocin, Sumycin, Vibramycin, and Vibra-Tabs

IMPORTANT INFORMATION TO REMEMBER: If stomach upset occurs, take the drug with food. Take the drug at the same time every day. Also, take the drug until all the medication prescribed is gone; otherwise the infection may return. This drug should be taken with plenty of water (eight ounces is preferred) and the capsules should be swallowed whole. Avoid taking antacids, calcium supplements, iron supplements, magnesium laxatives, and other mineral supplements within two hours of taking the drug. Women taking birth control pills should use another form of contraception while taking the drug and for the rest of the current menstrual cycle. Individuals should also use a sunscreen to avoid overexposure to the sun; the drug may increase the skin's sensitivity to sunlight, which may cause one to sunburn more easily. The drug should not be used by children under eight years of age due to the potential of permanent tooth staining.

BRAND NAME: Monoket

GENERIC NAME: isosorbide mononitrate

GENERIC FORM AVAILABLE: No

THERAPEUTIC CLASS: Nitrate anti-anginal

DOSAGE FORMS: 10-mg and 20-mg tablets

MAIN USES: Prevention of angina

USUAL DOSE: 10 mg to 20 mg upon awakening, and 10 mg to 20 mg seven hours later

AVERAGE PRICE: $77.47 for 10 mg and $81.59 for 20 mg

SIDE EFFECTS: Most common: headache 13%–35%, dizziness 3%–4%, and nausea 2%–3%. Less common: flushing, restlessness, dizziness, weakness, vomiting, and sweating.

DRUG INTERACTIONS: Alcohol and the drug may produce low blood pressure. Apresoline, Loniten, or Vasodilan and the drug may also produce low blood pressure.

ALLERGIES: Individuals allergic to isosorbide mononitrate or other nitrates (such as those listed under "Other Drugs in the Same Therapeutic Class") should discuss this with their doctor or pharmacist before taking this drug.

PREGNANCY/BREAST-FEEDING: Category B—No evidence of risk in humans. Either animal findings show risk, but human findings do not; or, if no adequate human studies have been done, animal findings show no risk. It is not known whether the drug is excreted in the breast milk; therefore, caution should be used when breast-feeding.

OTHER BRAND NAMES: None

OTHER DRUGS IN THE SAME THERAPEUTIC CLASS: Dilatrate-SR, Imdur, Isordil, Ismo, and Sorbitrate

IMPORTANT INFORMATION TO REMEMBER: This drug does not relieve angina attacks—it only prevents them. Take the drug only exactly as directed by your physician. Do not discontinue the drug without first consulting your physician. Also, do not increase the dose without first consulting with your physician. Do not drink alcohol while taking this drug. The headache that is common with this drug usually goes away with continued use; if it does not, contact your doctor. Before taking over-the-counter cold and allergy preparations, consult your doctor or pharmacist.

BRAND NAME: Monopril

GENERIC NAME: fosinopril

GENERIC FORM AVAILABLE: No

THERAPEUTIC CLASS: ACE inhibitor

DOSAGE FORMS: 10-mg, 20-mg, and 40-mg tablets

MAIN USES: High blood pressure and congestive heart failure

USUAL DOSE: 20 mg to 40 mg daily in one or two doses

AVERAGE PRICE: $102.17 for 10 mg and $109.35 for 20 mg

SIDE EFFECTS: headache 3%, cough 2%, dizziness 2%, diarrhea 2%, tiredness 2%, nausea 1%, vomiting 1%, and sexual dysfunction 1%.

DRUG INTERACTIONS: May decrease the absorption of the antibiotic Sumycin. High potassium levels may occur when used together with Dyrenium and Aldactone, and potassium supplements such as Micro-K, K-Dur, Klor-Con, K-Lyte, and Slow-K. Patients using water pills, especially those recently started on a water pill, may experience low blood pressure. The drug may also increase the toxic effects of Eskalith and Lithobid, especially when taken with a water pill.

ALLERGIES: Individuals allergic to fosinopril or other ACE inhibitors (such as those listed under "Other Drugs in the Same Therapeutic Class") should discuss this with their doctor or pharmacist before using this drug.

PREGNANCY/BREAST-FEEDING: Category C (first trimester)—Risk cannot be ruled out. Human studies are lacking, and animal studies are either positive for fetal risk or lacking as well. However, potential benefits may justify the potential risk in using the drug. Category D (second and third trimesters)—Positive evidence of risk. Human studies show risk to the fetus. Nevertheless, potential benefits may possibly outweigh the potential risk. This drug should not be taken by nursing mothers.

OTHER BRAND NAMES: None

OTHER DRUGS IN THE SAME THERAPEUTIC CLASS: Accupril, Altace, Capoten, Mavik, Lotensin, Prinivil, Univasc, Vasotec, and Zestril

IMPORTANT INFORMATION TO REMEMBER: Take this drug regularly and exactly as directed by your physician. Do not stop taking the drug unless otherwise directed by your doctor. Avoid salt substitutes containing potassium. Before taking over-the-counter cold and allergy preparations, consult your doctor or pharmacist—these products may raise your blood pressure. If you experience swelling of the face, lips, or tongue or difficulty in breathing, contact your doctor immediately.

BRAND NAME: Motrin

GENERIC NAME: ibuprofen

GENERIC FORM AVAILABLE: Yes

THERAPEUTIC CLASS: Nonsteroidal anti-inflammatory drug (NSAID)

DOSAGE FORMS: 300-mg, 400-mg, 600-mg, and 800-mg tablets

MAIN USES: Arthritis, pain relief, fever, and menstrual pain

USUAL DOSE: 300 mg to 800 mg three to four times daily

AVERAGE PRICE: $26.25 (B)/$14.28 (G) for 400 mg; $32.65 (B)/$16.04 (G) for 600 mg; $42.85 (B)/$20.88 (G) for 800 mg

SIDE EFFECTS: nausea 3%–9%, stomach pain 3%–9%, heartburn 3%–9%, dizziness 3%–9%, rash 3%–9%, diarrhea 1%–3%, vomiting 1%–3%, indigestion 1%–3%, constipation 1%–3%, bloating 1%–3%, gas 1%–3%, headache 1%–3%, nervousness 1%–3%, decreased appetite 1%–3%, ringing in the ears 1%–3%, and stomach cramps 1%–3%.

DRUG INTERACTIONS: Aspirin may decrease the concentration of this drug in the blood. This drug may also decrease the effects of Lasix, Dyazide, HydroDIURIL, Maxzide, and other water pills. The drug may increase the blood levels of Eskalith, Lithobid, and Sandimmune. The drug may increase the toxic effects of the drug Rheumatrex. Caution should be used when taking the drug with Coumadin.

ALLERGIES: Individuals allergic to ibuprofen or other NSAIDs (such as those listed under "Other Drugs in the Same Therapeutic Class") should discuss this with their doctor or pharmacist before taking this drug.

PREGNANCY/BREAST-FEEDING: Category B—No evidence of risk in humans. Either animal findings show risk, but human findings do not; or, if no adequate human studies have been done, animal findings show no risk. The drug should not, however, be used during the late stages (last three months) of pregnancy. It is not known whether the drug is excreted in the breast milk; therefore, caution should be used when breast-feeding.

OTHER BRAND NAMES: Advil, Nuprin, Excedrin IB, and Motrin IB (all of which are available over-the-counter without a prescription in 200-mg strength)

OTHER DRUGS IN THE SAME THERAPEUTIC CLASS: Anaprox, Ansaid, aspirin, Cataflam, Clinoril, Daypro, Disalcid, Dolobid, Easprin, Feldene, Indocin, Lodine, Lodine XL, Nalfon, Naprosyn, Orudis, Oruvail, Relafen, Tolectin, Toradol, Voltaren, and Voltaren XR

IMPORTANT INFORMATION TO REMEMBER: This drug should be taken with food or milk to reduce the potential for injury to the stomach lining and stomach upset. This drug may take up to two weeks before a noticeable improvement in pain relief associated with arthritis is observed. Drinking alcohol while taking this drug may increase its potential to cause ulcers. This drug should only be used under the direct supervision of a doctor by individuals with a bleeding disorder or ulcer, or those who are currently taking Coumadin. Before taking over-the-counter pain relievers, consult your doctor or pharmacist. No more than one pain reliever should be taken at any one time unless otherwise directed by your doctor. This drug is available over-the-counter (OTC) as 200-mg tablets for adults, a 100 mg/5 mL suspension, and 40 mg/mL drops for children.

BRAND NAME: MS Contin

GENERIC NAME: morphine

GENERIC FORM AVAILABLE: No

THERAPEUTIC CLASS: Narcotic analgesic

DOSAGE FORMS: 15-mg, 30-mg, 60-mg, 100-mg, and 200-mg sustained-release tablets

MAIN USES: Moderate to severe pain

USUAL DOSE: 15 mg to 60 mg every 8 to 12 hours

AVERAGE PRICE: $130.98 for 15 mg; $228.98 for 30 mg; $446.79 for 60 mg; $661.50 for 100 mg; and $1211.46 for 200 mg (sustained-release tablets)

SIDE EFFECTS: Most common: lightheadedness, dizziness, drowsiness, tiredness, constipation, nausea, vomiting, and sweating. Less common: weakness, agitation, tremor, depressed breathing, hallucinations, dry mouth, loss of appetite, low blood pressure, disorientation, vision problems, muscle spasms, and slow heartbeat.

DRUG INTERACTIONS: The effects of the drug may be increased when used with Compazine, Mellaril, Prolixin, Serentil, Stelazine,

Thorazine, or Trilafon. Alcohol, anxiety medications, or other narcotic painkillers may intensify the drowsiness and depressive respiratory effects of the drug. This drug and Nardil or Parnate may cause severe and sometimes fatal reactions. The drug may increase the blood levels of Retrovir.

ALLERGIES: Individuals allergic to morphine or any of its derivatives should discuss this with their doctor or pharmacist before using this drug.

PREGNANCY/BREAST-FEEDING: Category C—Risk cannot be ruled out. Human studies are lacking, and animal studies are either positive for fetal risk or lacking as well. However, potential benefits may justify the potential risk in using the drug. The drug is excreted in the breast milk; therefore, extreme caution should be used when breast-feeding.

OTHER BRAND NAMES: None

OTHER DRUGS IN THE SAME THERAPEUTIC CLASS: Demerol, Dolophine, Dilaudid, Durogesic, Levo Dromoran, MSIR, Oramorph SR, Roxanol, and Stadol

IMPORTANT INFORMATION TO REMEMBER: This is a very potent drug and may cause a lot of drowsiness. Individuals should use extreme caution when driving, operating machinery, or performing any task where mental alertness is required. Alcohol, anxiety medications, and other narcotic painkillers may intensify the drowsiness effect of the drug. Do not increase the dose without first consulting with your physician—this could be very dangerous and possibly life-threatening. If stomach upset occurs, take the drug with food or milk. This medication is a controlled substance, may be habit-forming, and should only be used as needed for pain relief. This prescription cannot be refilled; a new written prescription must be obtained each time. The potential for abuse with this medication is high. Do not crush or chew the tablets—this will destroy the mechanism that ensures the delayed release of the medication.

BRAND NAME: MSIR

GENERIC NAME: morphine

GENERIC FORM AVAILABLE: No

THERAPEUTIC CLASS: Narcotic analgesic

DOSAGE FORMS: 15-mg and 30-mg tablets and capsules; and 10 mg/5 mL and 20 mg/5 mL solution

MAIN USES: Moderate to severe pain

USUAL DOSE: 5 mg to 30 mg every four hours as needed

AVERAGE PRICE: $31.02 for 15-mg tablets; $48.72 for 30-mg tablets; $49.01 for 15-mg capsules; $84.01 for 30-mg capsules; and $19.43 for the solutions (120 mL)

SIDE EFFECTS: Most common: lightheadedness, dizziness, drowsiness, tiredness, constipation, nausea, vomiting, and sweating. Less common: weakness, agitation, tremor, depressed breathing, hallucinations, dry mouth, loss of appetite, low blood pressure, disorientation, vision problems, muscle spasms, and slow heartbeat.

DRUG INTERACTIONS: The effects of the drug may be increased when used with Compazine, Mellaril, Prolixin, Serentil, Stelazine, Thorazine, or Trilafon. Alcohol, anxiety medications, or other narcotic painkillers may intensify the drowsiness and depressive respiratory effects of the drug. This drug and Nardil or Parnate may cause severe and sometimes fatal reactions. The drug may increase the blood levels of Retrovir.

ALLERGIES: Individuals allergic to morphine or any of its derivatives should discuss this with their doctor or pharmacist before using this drug.

PREGNANCY/BREAST-FEEDING: Category C—Risk cannot be ruled out. Human studies are lacking, and animal studies are either positive for fetal risk or lacking as well. However, potential benefits may justify the potential risk in using the drug. The drug is excreted in the breast milk; therefore, extreme caution should be used when breast-feeding.

OTHER BRAND NAMES: None

OTHER DRUGS IN THE SAME THERAPEUTIC CLASS: Demerol, Dolophine, Dilaudid, Duragesic, Levo-Dromoran, MS Contin, Oramorph SR, Roxanol, and Stadol

IMPORTANT INFORMATION TO REMEMBER: This is a very potent drug and may cause a lot of drowsiness. Individuals should use extreme caution when driving, operating machinery, or performing any task where mental alertness is required. Alcohol, anxiety medications, and other narcotic painkillers may intensify the drowsiness effect of the drug. Do not increase the dose without first consulting with your physician—this could be very dangerous and possibly life-threatening. If stomach upset occurs, take the drug with food or milk. This medication is a controlled substance, may be habit-forming, and should only be used as needed for pain relief. This prescription cannot be refilled; a new written prescription must be obtained each time. The potential for abuse with this medication is high.

BRAND NAME: Mycelex Cream

GENERIC NAME: clotrimazole

See entry for Lotrisone

BRAND NAME: Mycelex Troches

GENERIC NAME: clotrimazole

GENERIC FORM AVAILABLE: No

THERAPEUTIC CLASS: Imidazole antifungal

DOSAGE FORMS: 10-mg troches

MAIN USES: Prevention and treatment of oral fungal infections

USUAL DOSE: Dissolve the tablet slowly in mouth like a lozenge. Treatment: one troche five times daily. Prevention: one troche three times daily.

AVERAGE PRICE: $110.43

SIDE EFFECTS: Most common: stomach pain, stomach cramps, nausea, diarrhea, and vomiting. Less common: unpleasant taste and abnormal liver function tests.

DRUG INTERACTIONS: Propulsid and the drug may cause dangerous irregular heartbeats when taken together.

ALLERGIES: Individuals allergic to clotrimazole or any of its derivatives should discuss this with their doctor or pharmacist before using this drug.

PREGNANCY/BREAST-FEEDING: Category C—Risk cannot be ruled out. Human studies are lacking, and animal studies are either

positive for fetal risk or lacking as well. However, potential benefits may justify the potential risk in using the drug. It is not known
whether the drug is excreted in the breast milk; therefore, caution
should be used when breast-feeding.

OTHER BRAND NAMES: None

OTHER DRUGS IN THE SAME THERAPEUTIC CLASS: Nizoral

IMPORTANT INFORMATION TO REMEMBER: Dissolve the tablet
slowly in mouth like a lozenge, swallowing the saliva as it dissolves. Do not swallow or chew the tablet. Food or liquid should
not be put into the mouth during or immediately after dissolving
the tablet. Also, take the drug for the full course of treatment;
otherwise the infection may return.

BRAND NAME: Mycobutin

GENERIC NAME: rifabutin

GENERIC FORM AVAILABLE: No

THERAPEUTIC CLASS: Rifamycin antibiotic

DOSAGE FORMS: 150-mg capsules

MAIN USES: Prevention of disseminated *Mycobacterium avium-
intracellulare complex* (MAC) disease in advanced AIDS

USUAL DOSE: 300 mg once daily

AVERAGE PRICE: $63.28 (10 capsules)

SIDE EFFECTS: discoloration of the urine 30%, rash 11%, nausea
6%, stomach pain 4%, headache 3%, diarrhea 3%, taste changes
3%, fever 2%, loss of appetite 2%, gas 2%, muscle pain 2%, and
vomiting 1%.

DRUG INTERACTIONS: The drug may decrease the blood levels of
Retrovir. The drug may increase the blood levels of Amytal, Aristo-
cort, Butisol, Calan, Coumadin, Decadron, Deltasone, Isoptin,
Lanoxin, Mebaral, Medrol, methadone, Nembutal, Nizoral, pheno-
barbital, prednisone, Quinidex, Quinaglute, Seconal, Slo-bid, Theo-
Dur, theophylline, Tuinal, Uni-Dur, Uniphyl, and birth control pills.

ALLERGIES: Individuals allergic to rifabutin or any of its derivatives should discuss this with their doctor or pharmacist before
using this drug.

PREGNANCY/BREAST-FEEDING: Category B—No evidence of risk in humans. Either animal findings show risk, but human findings do not; or, if no adequate human studies have been done, animal findings show no risk. It is not known whether the drug is excreted in the breast milk; therefore, caution should be used when breast-feeding.

OTHER BRAND NAMES: None

OTHER DRUGS IN THE SAME THERAPEUTIC CLASS: Rifadin

IMPORTANT INFORMATION TO REMEMBER: It's best to take the drug on an empty stomach—one hour before or two hours after meals. If stomach upset occurs, however, the drug can be taken with food or milk. Do not stop taking the drug without first consulting with your physician. The drug may cause the tears, urine, or any body fluid to turn reddish-orange to reddish-brown in color; this is normal. However, the drug may permanently discolor contact lenses; therefore, contact lenses should not be used during treatment.

BRAND NAME. Mycolog-II

GENERIC NAME: Combination product containing: triamcinolone acetonide and nystatin

GENERIC FORM AVAILABLE: Yes

THERAPEUTIC CLASS: Topical corticosteroid + antifungal

DOSAGE FORMS: 0.1% triamcinolone acetonide/100,000-units nystatin per-gram cream and ointment

MAIN USES: Fungal infections (mainly ringworm, jock itch, and athlete's foot)

USUAL DOSE: Apply a thin layer two to four times daily.

AVERAGE PRICE: $19.11 (B)/$8.56 (G) for 15 g of cream and ointment

SIDE EFFECTS: Most common: none. Less common: stinging, redness, dry skin, irritation, and tingling or prickling sensation on the skin.

DRUG INTERACTIONS: None of any clinical significance

ALLERGIES: Individuals allergic to triamcinolone acetonide, nystatin, Aristocort, Kenalog, or any of their derivatives should discuss this with their doctor or pharmacist before using this drug.

PREGNANCY/BREAST-FEEDING: Category C—Risk cannot be ruled out. Human studies are lacking, and animal studies are either positive for fetal risk or lacking as well. However, potential benefits may justify the potential risk in using the drug. It is not known whether the drug is excreted in the breast milk; therefore, caution should be used when breast-feeding.

OTHER BRAND NAMES: None

OTHER DRUGS IN THE SAME THERAPEUTIC CLASS: Lotrisone

IMPORTANT INFORMATION TO REMEMBER: The drug may stain clothing. This drug is for external use only. Apply and gently rub in enough of the cream to cover the affected area and surrounding areas. Use the drug for the full course of treatment or the fungal infection may return. Never cover the skin after application with a bandage or wrapping unless directed to do so by a doctor. Discontinue use if irritation occurs.

BRAND NAME: Mycostatin

GENERIC NAME: nystatin

GENERIC FORM AVAILABLE: Yes

THERAPEUTIC CLASS: Antifungal

DOSAGE FORMS: 100,000 units/g cream, ointment, powder, and vaginal tablets; 100,00 units/mL suspension; 200,000-unit pastilles; and 500,000-unit tablets

MAIN USES: Fungal infections

USUAL DOSE: Cream, ointment, or powder: apply twice daily. Vaginal tablets: insert one vaginal tablet one or two times daily for 14 days. Suspension: 1 mL to 2 mL of the suspension four times daily. Pastilles: dissolve one to two 200,000-unit pastilles in the mouth four or five times daily. Tablets: one or two 500,000-unit tablets three times daily.

AVERAGE PRICE: $22.02 (B)/$8.78 (G) for 60-mL suspension; $32.02 (B)/$13.43 (G) for the cream and ointment (30 g); $28.97 (B)/$14.47 (G) for the vaginal tablets (15 tablets); and $47.61 for 200,000-unit pastilles (30 tablets)

SIDE EFFECTS: For the cream, ointment, powder, and vaginal tablets: Most common: none. Less common: stinging, redness, irritation, and tingling or prickling sensation on the skin. For the suspension, pastilles, and tablets: Most common: none. Less common: diarrhea, nausea, vomiting, and stomach pain.

DRUG INTERACTIONS: None of any clinical significance

ALLERGIES: Individuals allergic to nystatin or any of its derivatives should discuss this with their doctor or pharmacist before using this drug.

PREGNANCY/BREAST-FEEDING: Category C—Risk cannot be ruled out. Human studies are lacking, and animal studies are either positive for fetal risk or lacking as well. However, potential benefits may justify the potential risk in using the drug. It is not known whether the drug is excreted in the breast milk; therefore, caution should be used when breast-feeding.

OTHER BRAND NAMES: None

OTHER DRUGS IN THE SAME THERAPEUTIC CLASS: None

IMPORTANT INFORMATION TO REMEMBER: For the cream, ointment, powder: this drug is for external use only. The drug may stain clothing. Apply and gently rub in enough of the cream to cover the affected area and surrounding areas. Use the drug for the full course of treatment or the fungal infection may return. Never cover the skin after application with a bandage or wrapping unless directed to do so by a doctor. Discontinue use if irritation occurs. For the vaginal tablets: use the drug for the full course of treatment or the fungal infection may return. Insert the vaginal tablet high into the vagina. Never use a tampon with the vaginal tablets, and continue using the products even during a menstrual period unless otherwise directed by your doctor. The drug may stain clothing. For the pastilles: dissolve the tablet slowly in mouth like a lozenge, swallowing the saliva as it dissolves. Do not swallow or chew the pastilles. Food or liquid should not be put into the mouth during or immediately after dissolving the tablet. Also, take the drug for the full course of treatment; otherwise the infection may return.

BRAND NAME: Mykrox

GENERIC NAME: metolazone

See entry for Zaroxolyn

BRAND NAME: Mysoline

GENERIC NAME: primidone

GENERIC FORM AVAILABLE: Yes

THERAPEUTIC CLASS: Anticonvulsant

DOSAGE FORMS: 50-mg and 250-mg tablets; and 250 mg/5 mL suspension

MAIN USES: Epilepsy and seizures

USUAL DOSE: 125 mg to 250 mg three to four times daily

AVERAGE PRICE: $61.34 (B)/$40.24 (G) for 250 mg

SIDE EFFECTS: Most common: drowsiness, unsteadiness, clumsiness, and dizziness. Less common: loss of appetite, impotence, mood or mental changes, double vision, nausea, and vomiting.

DRUG INTERACTIONS: Alcohol, anxiety medications, and narcotic painkillers may intensify the drowsiness effect of the drug. The drug may decrease the effects of Aristocort, Coumadin, Decadron, Deltasone, estrogens, Medrol, prednisone, and birth control pills. Tegretol may decrease the effects of the drug. Depakene may increase the blood levels of the drug. The drug may also decrease the blood levels of Depakene. Nardil and Parnate may prolong the effects of the drug.

ALLERGIES: Individuals allergic to primidone or any of its derivatives should discuss this with their doctor or pharmacist before using this drug.

PREGNANCY/BREAST-FEEDING: Category D—Positive evidence of risk. Human studies show risk to the fetus. Nevertheless, potential benefits may possibly outweigh the potential risks. This drug should not be taken by nursing mothers.

OTHER BRAND NAMES: None

OTHER DRUGS IN THE SAME THERAPEUTIC CLASS: None

IMPORTANT INFORMATION TO REMEMBER: This drug may cause some drowsiness or dizziness. Individuals should use caution when driving, operating machinery, or performing any task where mental alertness is required. Alcohol, anxiety medications, and narcotic painkillers may intensify the drowsiness effect of the drug. If stomach upset occurs, take the drug with food or milk. Avoid drinking alcohol while taking this drug. Only take the drug exactly as directed by your physician. Do not discontinue the drug or increase the dose without first consulting your physician. Before taking over-the-counter medications, consult your doctor or pharmacist. Birth control pills may be ineffective while taking this drug; another method of birth control is recommended. Individuals should get up slowly from the sitting or lying-down position; otherwise dizziness may occur.

BRAND NAME: Naftin

GENERIC NAME: naftifine

GENERIC FORM AVAILABLE: No

THERAPEUTIC CLASS: Allylamine antifungal

DOSAGE FORMS: 1% cream and 1% gel

MAIN USES: Fungal infections (mainly ringworm, jock itch, and athlete's foot)

USUAL DOSE: Apply one to two times daily.

AVERAGE PRICE: $33.32 for 1% cream (30 g) and $42.37 for 1% gel (30 g)

SIDE EFFECTS: burning and stinging 5%–6%, dryness 3%, redness 2%, itching 2%, and irritation 2%.

DRUG INTERACTIONS: None of any clinical significance

ALLERGIES: Individuals allergic to naftifine or any of its derivatives should discuss this with their doctor or pharmacist before using this drug.

PREGNANCY/BREAST-FEEDING: Category B—No evidence of risk in humans. Either animal findings show risk, but human findings do not; or, if no adequate human studies have been done, animal findings show no risk. It is not known whether the drug is excreted in the breast milk; therefore, caution should be used when breast-feeding.

OTHER BRAND NAMES: None

OTHER DRUGS IN THE SAME THERAPEUTIC CLASS: Lamisil

IMPORTANT INFORMATION TO REMEMBER: This drug is for external use only. Apply and gently rub in enough of the cream to cover the affected area and surrounding areas. Use the drug for the full course of treatment or the fungal infection may return. Never cover the skin after application with a bandage or wrapping unless directed to do so by a doctor. Discontinue use if irritation occurs.

BRAND NAME: Naldecon, Naldecon Syrup, and Naldecon Pediatric Syrup

GENERIC NAME: Combination product containing: chlorpheniramine, phenylephrine, phenylpropanolamine, and phenyltoloxamine

GENERIC FORM AVAILABLE: Yes

THERAPEUTIC CLASS: Antihistamine + decongestant

DOSAGE FORMS: 5-mg chlorpheniramine/10-mg phenylephrine/40-mg phenylpropanolamine/15-mg phenyltoloxamine sustained-release tablets; 2.5-mg chlorpheniramine/5-mg phenylephrine/20-mg phenylpropanolamine/7.5-mg phenyltoloxamine per 5 mL syrup; and 0.5-mg chlorpheniramine/1.25-mg phenylephrine/5-mg phenylpropanolamine/2-mg phenyltoloxamine per 5 mL pediatric syrup

MAIN USES: Nasal allergies and congestion

USUAL DOSE: One tablet three times daily or one teaspoon every three to four hours for the syrup. For the pediatric syrup: 1/2 to 2 teaspoons every three to four hours.

AVERAGE PRICE: $94.58 (B)/$14.83 (G) for Naldecon

SIDE EFFECTS: Most common: drowsiness. Less common: nausea, giddiness, dry mouth, blurred vision, pounding heartbeat, flushing, and increased irritability or excitability (especially in children).

DRUG INTERACTIONS: Blocadren, Cartrol, Corgard, Inderal, Kerlone, Levatol, Lopressor, Normodyne, Sectral, Tenormin, Toprol-XL, Trandate, Visken, and Zebeta may increase the effects of the drug. The drug may also reduce the effects of blood-pressure-lowering drugs. Nardil or Parnate may significantly raise blood pressure when taken with this drug.

ALLERGIES: Individuals allergic to chlorpheniramine, phenylephrine, phenylpropanolamine, phenyltoloxamine, or other antihistamine/decongestant combinations (such as those listed under

"Other Drugs in the Same Therapeutic Class") should discuss this with their doctor or pharmacist before taking this drug.

PREGNANCY/BREAST-FEEDING: Category C—Risk cannot be ruled out. Human studies are lacking, and animal studies are either positive for fetal risk or lacking as well. However, potential benefits may justify the potential risk in using the drug. It is not known whether the drug is excreted in the breast milk; therefore, caution should be used when breast-feeding.

OTHER BRAND NAMES: None

OTHER DRUGS IN THE SAME THERAPEUTIC CLASS: Bromfed, Bromfed PD, Claritin-D, Comhist LA, Deconamine SR, Fedahist, Nolamine, Novafed-A, Ornade, Poly-Histine-D, Rondec, Rynatan, Seldane-D, Semprex-D, Tavist-D, and Trinalin

IMPORTANT INFORMATION TO REMEMBER: This drug does cause drowsiness. Individuals should use caution when driving, operating machinery, or performing any task where mental alertness is required. Alcohol, anxiety medications, and narcotic painkillers may intensify the drowsiness effect of the drug. This drug may also cause a dry mouth; sugarless gum or hard candy will help take care of this problem. Patients with glaucoma, high blood pressure, heart conditions, or urinary or prostate problems should consult their doctor before taking this drug.

BRAND NAME: **Nalfon**

GENERIC NAME: fenoprofen

GENERIC FORM AVAILABLE: Yes

THERAPEUTIC CLASS: Nonsteroidal anti-inflammatory drug (NSAID)

DOSAGE FORMS: 200-mg and 300-mg capsules; and 600-mg tablets

MAIN USES: Arthritis and pain relief

USUAL DOSE: 200 mg to 600 mg three to four times daily

AVERAGE PRICE: $67.98 (B)/$62.98 (G) for 200 mg; $69.98 (B)/$57.98 (G) for 300 mg; $90.62 (B)/$39.58 (G) for 600 mg

SIDE EFFECTS: nausea 8%–10%, headache 8%, tiredness 8%, constipation 7%, dizziness 6%, nervousness 6%, increased sweating 5%, ringing in the ears 5%, itching 4%, rash 4%, vomiting 3%, pounding heartbeat 3%, stomach pain 2%, diarrhea 2%, decreased hearing 2%, and blurred vision 2%.

DRUG INTERACTIONS: Aspirin will decrease the concentration of this drug in the blood. This drug may also decrease the effects of Lasix, Dyazide, HydroDIURIL, Maxzide, and other water pills. The drug may increase the blood levels of Eskalith, Lithobid, and Sandimmune. The drug may increase the toxic effects of the drug Rheumatrex. Caution should be used when taking the drug with Coumadin.

ALLERGIES: Individuals allergic to fenoprofen or other NSAIDs (such as those listed under "Other Drugs in the Same Therapeutic Class") should discuss this with their doctor or pharmacist before taking this drug.

PREGNANCY/BREAST-FEEDING: Category C—Risk cannot be ruled out. Human studies are lacking, and animal studies are either positive for fetal risk or lacking as well. However, potential benefits may justify the potential risk in using the drug. The drug should not, however, be used during the late stages (last three months) of pregnancy. The drug is excreted in the breast milk; therefore, extreme caution should be used when breast-feeding.

OTHER BRAND NAMES: None

OTHER DRUGS IN THE SAME THERAPEUTIC CLASS: Anaprox, Ansaid, aspirin, Cataflam, Clinoril, Daypro, Disalcid, Dolobid, Easprin, Feldene, Indocin, Lodine, Lodine XL, Motrin, Naprosyn, Orudis, Oruvail, Relafen, Tolectin, Toradol, Voltaren, and Voltaren XR

IMPORTANT INFORMATION TO REMEMBER: This drug should be taken with food or milk to reduce the potential for injury to the stomach lining and stomach upset. This drug may take up to two weeks before a noticeable improvement in pain relief associated with arthritis is observed. Drinking alcohol while taking this drug may increase its potential to cause ulcers. This drug should only be used under the direct supervision of a doctor by individuals with a bleeding disorder or ulcer, or those who are currently taking Coumadin. Before taking over-the-counter pain relievers, consult your doctor or pharmacist. No more than one pain reliever should be taken at any one time unless otherwise directed by your doctor.

BRAND NAME: Naprosyn and Naprosyn-EC

GENERIC NAME: naproxen

GENERIC FORM AVAILABLE: Yes

THERAPEUTIC CLASS: Nonsteroidal anti-inflammatory drug (NSAID)

DOSAGE FORMS: Naprosyn: 250-mg, 375-mg, and 500-mg tablets; and 125 mg/5 mL suspension. Naprosyn-EC: 375-mg and 500-mg enteric coated tablets

MAIN USES: Arthritis, pain relief, and (menstrual pain)

USUAL DOSE: 250 mg to 500 mg twice daily

AVERAGE PRICE: For Naprosyn: $94.08 (B)/$26.98 (G) for 250 mg; $103.00 (B)/$32.28 (G) for 375 mg; $118.50 (B)/$41.27 (G) for 500 mg. For Naprosyn-EC: $84.71 for 375 mg; and $126.56 for 500 mg

SIDE EFFECTS: constipation 3%–9%, nausea 3%–9%, heartburn 3%–9%, stomach pain 3%–9%, headache 3%–9%, dizziness 3%–9%, swelling 3%–9%, drowsiness 3%–9%, itching 3%–9%, rash 3%–9%, ringing in the ears 3%–9%, trouble breathing 3%–9%, hearing disturbances 1%–3%, vision disturbances 1%–3%, light-headedness 1%–3%, diarrhea 1%–3%, sweating 1%–3%, pounding heartbeat 1%–3%, and thirst 1%–3%.

DRUG INTERACTIONS: Aspirin will decrease the concentration of this drug in the blood. This drug may also decrease the effects of Lasix, Dyazide, HydroDIURIL, Maxzide, and other water pills. The drug may increase the blood levels of Eskalith, Lithobid, and Sandimmune. The drug may increase the toxic effects of the drug Rheumatrex. Caution should be used when taking the drug with Coumadin.

ALLERGIES: Individuals allergic to naproxen, Aleve, or other NSAIDs (such as those listed under "Other Drugs in the Same Therapeutic Class") should discuss this with their doctor or pharmacist before taking this drug.

PREGNANCY/BREAST-FEEDING: Category B—No evidence of risk in humans. Either animal findings show risk, but human findings do not; or, if no adequate human studies have been done, animal findings show no risk. The drug should not, however, be used during the late stages (last three months) of pregnancy. The drug is excreted in the breast milk; therefore, extreme caution should be used when breast-feeding.

OTHER BRAND NAMES: None

OTHER DRUGS IN THE SAME THERAPEUTIC CLASS: Anaprox, Ansaid, aspirin, Cataflam, Clinoril, Daypro, Disalcid, Dolobid, Easprin, Feldene, Indocin, Lodine, Lodine XL, Motrin, Nalfon, Orudis, Oruvail, Relafen, Tolectin, Toradol, Voltaren, and Voltaren XR

IMPORTANT INFORMATION TO REMEMBER: This drug should be taken with food or milk to reduce the potential for injury to the stomach lining and stomach upset. This drug may take up to two weeks before a noticeable improvement in pain relief associated with arthritis is observed. Drinking alcohol while taking this drug may increase its potential to cause ulcers. This drug should only be used under the direct supervision of a doctor by individuals with a bleeding disorder or ulcer, or those who are currently taking Coumadin. Before taking over-the-counter pain relievers, consult your doctor or pharmacist. No more than one pain reliever should be taken at any one time unless otherwise directed by your doctor.

BRAND NAME: Nardil

GENERIC NAME: phenelzine

GENERIC FORM AVAILABLE: No

THERAPEUTIC CLASS: Monoamine oxidase (MAO) inhibitor antidepressant

DOSAGE FORMS: 15-mg tablets

MAIN USES: Depression and {psychotic disorders}

USUAL DOSE: 15 mg three times daily

AVERAGE PRICE: $56.33

SIDE EFFECTS: Most common: low blood pressure; constipation; dry mouth; severe dizziness or lightheadedness, especially when getting up from a sitting or lying-down position; decreased urine output; insomnia; muscle twitching; restlessness; drowsiness; decreased sexual ability; headache; increased appetite; weight gain; increased sweating; shakiness; and weakness. Less common: chills, diarrhea, blurred vision, swelling of the feet and legs, nervousness, fast heartbeat, and pounding heartbeat.

DRUG INTERACTIONS: This drug interacts with many prescription and over-the-counter (OTC) medications. Before taking this drug, discuss the medications you are currently taking with your doctor and pharmacist; many of these interactions can be severe.

ALLERGIES: Individuals allergic to phenelzine or any of its derivatives should discuss this with their doctor or pharmacist before using this drug.

PREGNANCY/BREAST-FEEDING: Category C—Risk cannot be ruled out. Human studies are lacking, and animal studies are either positive for fetal risk or lacking as well. However, potential benefits may justify the potential risk in using the drug. It is not known whether the drug is excreted in the breast milk; therefore, caution should be used when breast-feeding.

OTHER BRAND NAMES: None

OTHER DRUGS IN THE SAME THERAPEUTIC CLASS: Parnate

IMPORTANT INFORMATION TO REMEMBER: This drug does cause drowsiness. Individuals should use caution when driving, operating machinery, or performing any task where mental alertness is required. Alcohol, anxiety medications, and narcotic painkillers may intensify the drowsiness effect of the drug. Take the drug exactly as directed by your physician. Never suddenly stop taking the drug without first consulting with your physician. Before taking any prescription or over-the-counter (OTC) medications, consult with your doctor or pharmacist. The drug may take three to four weeks before a noticeable improvement is seen. While taking the drug and for at least 14 days after stopping, observe the precautions for 14 days as given by your physician. Individuals should avoid tyramine-containing foods (red wines, sherry, liquors, aged cheese, smoked or pickled meats, sauerkraut, beer, and overripe fruits, including avocados, raisins, and overripe bananas), alcoholic beverages, vitamin supplements containing yeast, and large quantities of caffeine-containing beverages.

BRAND NAME: Nasacort

GENERIC NAME: triamcinolone acetonide

GENERIC FORM AVAILABLE: No

THERAPEUTIC CLASS: Steroid nasal spray

DOSAGE FORMS: 55-micrograms-per-spray nasal inhaler and water-based spray

MAIN USES: Nasal allergies

USUAL DOSE: one to two sprays in each nostril once a day

AVERAGE PRICE: $54.85 for 10-g nasal inhaler and water-based spray

SIDE EFFECTS: nasal irritation 3%, dry mucous membranes 1%–5%, stuffy nose 1%–5%, throat discomfort 1%–5%, bloody nose 1%–5%, and sneezing 1%–5%.

DRUG INTERACTIONS: Caution should be used when taking this drug with other oral corticosteroids such as Aristocort, Deltasone, Decadron, Medrol, and prednisone.

ALLERGIES: Individuals allergic to triamcinolone or other nasal steroids (such as those listed under "Other Drugs in the Same Therapeutic Class") should discuss this with their doctor or pharmacist before taking this drug.

PREGNANCY/BREAST-FEEDING: Category C—Risk cannot be ruled out. Human studies are lacking, and animal studies are either positive for fetal risk or lacking as well. However, potential benefits may justify the potential risk in using the drug. It is not known whether the drug is excreted in the breast milk; therefore, caution should be used when breast-feeding.

OTHER BRAND NAMES: None

OTHER DRUGS IN THE SAME THERAPEUTIC CLASS: Beconase, Beconase AQ, Dexacort, Flonase, Nasalide, Rhinocort, Vancenase, and Vancenase AQ

IMPORTANT INFORMATION TO REMEMBER: The drug is not intended to provide immediate relief of nasal allergies. To receive the full benefits of the drug, use it on a regular basis as a maintenance medication. If some improvements are not seen in seven days, the individual needs to be reassessed by a doctor. The drug may take up to three weeks before the full benefits are seen. Never exceed the prescribed dosage unless directed to do so by a doctor—excessive use beyond the prescribed dosage is potentially dangerous. This drug should not be used by individuals with fungal, bacterial, systemic viral, or respiratory tract infections; unhealed wounds inside the nose; or tuberculosis.

When using the nasal spray, use the following procedure:

1) Blow your nose gently to clear your nostrils, if necessary.
2) With your other hand, gently place a finger against the side of your nose to close the opposite nostril.
3) Insert the tip of the bottle or aerosol into the open nostril. Point the tip toward the back and outer side of the nostril once inside.
4) After releasing the spray, close your mouth, sniff deeply, hold your breath for a few seconds, then breathe out through your mouth.
5) Tilt your head back slightly for a few seconds to allow the drug to spread to the back of your nose.
6) Repeat the same procedure for the other nostril.
7) If using more than one spray in each nostril, wait five minutes between sprays.

BRAND NAME: Nasalcrom

GENERIC NAME: cromolyn sodium

GENERIC FORM AVAILABLE: No

THERAPEUTIC CLASS: Nasal allergy controller

DOSAGE FORMS: 5.2-mg-per-spray nasal spray

MAIN USES: Nasal allergies

USUAL DOSE: one spray in each nostril three to four times daily

AVERAGE PRICE: $31.19 for 13 mL

SIDE EFFECTS: sneezing 10%, stinging 5%, nasal burning 4%, irritation 2%, bad taste 2%, and headaches 2%.

DRUG INTERACTIONS: The drug, when used with Isuprel, may increase the chance of birth defects in pregnant women.

ALLERGIES: Individuals allergic to cromolyn sodium or any of its derivatives should discuss this with their doctor or pharmacist before using this drug.

PREGNANCY/BREAST-FEEDING: Category B—No evidence of risk in humans. Either animal findings show risk, but human findings do not; or, if no adequate human studies have been done, animal findings show no risk. It is not known whether the drug is excreted in the breast milk; therefore, caution should be used when breast-feeding.

OTHER BRAND NAMES: None

OTHER DRUGS IN THE SAME THERAPEUTIC CLASS: None

IMPORTANT INFORMATION TO REMEMBER: The drug is not intended to provide immediately relief of nasal allergies. To receive the full benefits of the drug, use it on a regular basis as a maintenance medication. The drug may take up to four weeks before the full benefits are seen. Never exceed the prescribed dosage unless directed to do so by a doctor—excessive use beyond the prescribed dosage is potentially dangerous. Do not clean the spraying device; just replace it every six months. The drug is also now available over-the-counter without a prescription.

When using the nasal spray, use the following procedure:

1) Blow your nose gently to clear your nostrils, if necessary.
2) Hold the spray bottle with your thumb at the bottom and your index and middle finger on the shoulder attached to the neck of the bottle (top of the canister for the aerosol).
3) With your other hand, gently place a finger against the side of your nose to close the opposite nostril.
4) Insert the tip of the bottle or aerosol into the open nostril. Point the tip toward the back and outer side of the nostril once inside.
5) After releasing the spray, close your mouth, sniff deeply, hold your breath for a few seconds, then breathe out through your mouth.
6) Tilt your head back slightly for a few seconds to allow the drug to spread to the back of your nose.
7) Repeat the same procedure for the other nostril.
8) If using more than one spray in each nostril, wait five minutes between sprays.

BRAND NAME: Nasalide

GENERIC NAME: flunisolide

GENERIC FORM AVAILABLE: No

THERAPEUTIC CLASS: Steroid nasal spray

DOSAGE FORMS: 25-micrograms-per-spray nasal solution

MAIN USES: Nasal allergies

USUAL DOSE: one to two sprays in each nostril two to three times daily

AVERAGE PRICE: $38.62 for 25 mL

SIDE EFFECTS: Most common: nasal burning, dryness, irritation, and sneezing (all of these are usually mild). Less common: crusting inside the nose, bloody nose, headache, sore throat, nasal congestion, and hoarseness.

DRUG INTERACTIONS: Caution should be used when taking this drug with other corticosteroids such as prednisone.

ALLERGIES: Individuals allergic to flunisolide or other nasal steroids (such as those listed under "Other Drugs in the Same Therapeutic Class") should discuss this with their doctor or pharmacist before taking this drug.

PREGNANCY/BREAST-FEEDING: Category C—Risk cannot be ruled out. Human studies are lacking, and animal studies are either positive for fetal risk or lacking as well. However, potential benefits may justify the potential risk in using the drug. It is not known whether the drug is excreted in the breast milk; therefore, caution should be used when breast-feeding.

OTHER BRAND NAMES: None

OTHER DRUGS IN THE SAME THERAPEUTIC CLASS: Beconase, Beconase AQ, Dexacort, Flonase, Nasacort, Rhinocort, Vancenase, and Vancenase AQ

IMPORTANT INFORMATION TO REMEMBER: The drug is not intended to provide immediate relief of nasal allergies. To receive the full benefits of the drug, use it on a regular basis as a maintenance medication. If some improvements are not seen in seven days, the individual needs to be reassessed by a doctor. The drug may take up to three weeks before the full benefits are seen. Never exceed the prescribed dosage unless directed to do so by a doctor—excessive use beyond the prescribed dosage is potentially dangerous. This drug should not be used by individuals with fungal, bacterial, systemic viral, or respiratory tract infections; unhealed wounds inside the nose; or tuberculosis.

When using the nasal spray, use the following procedure:

1) Blow your nose gently to clear your nostrils, if necessary.
2) Hold the spray bottle with your thumb at the bottom and your index and middle finger on the shoulder attached to the neck of the bottle (top of the canister for the aerosol).

3) With your other hand, gently place a finger against the side of your nose to close the opposite nostril.
4) Insert the tip of the bottle or aerosol into the open nostril. Point the tip toward the back and outer side of the nostril once inside.
5) After releasing the spray, close your mouth, sniff deeply, hold your breath for a few seconds, then breathe out through your mouth.
6) Tilt your head back slightly for a few seconds to allow the drug to spread to the back of your nose.
7) Repeat the same procedure for the other nostril.
8) If using more than one spray in each nostril, wait five minutes between sprays.

BRAND NAME: Natalins Rx

GENERIC NAME: prenatal Rx (prenatal multivitamin)

GENERIC FORM AVAILABLE: Yes

THERAPEUTIC CLASS: Prenatal vitamin supplement

DOSAGE FORMS: multivitamin tablet

MAIN USES: Nutritional supplement during pregnancy and breast-feeding

USUAL DOSE: one tablet daily

AVERAGE PRICE: $30.03 (B)/$12.59 (G)

SIDE EFFECTS: Most common: none. Less common: diarrhea, gas, and stomach upset.

DRUG INTERACTIONS: The B vitamins in the drug may increase the effect of Larodopa.

ALLERGIES: Individuals allergic to multivitamins or any of their derivatives should discuss this with their doctor or pharmacist before using this drug.

PREGNANCY/BREAST FEEDING: Category B—No evidence of risk in humans. Either animal findings show risk, but human findings do not; or, if no adequate human studies have been done, animal findings show no risk. The drug is safe to use during pregnancy. It is not known whether the drug is excreted in the breast milk; therefore, caution should be used when breast-feeding.

OTHER BRAND NAMES: None

OTHER DRUGS IN THE SAME THERAPEUTIC CLASS: Materna, Prenate 90, Stuartnatal Plus, and Zenate

IMPORTANT INFORMATION TO REMEMBER: Only take the drug exactly as directed by your physician. Do not discontinue the drug without first consulting your physician. If stomach upset occurs, the drug may be taken with food or milk.

BRAND NAME: Navane

GENERIC NAME: thiothixene

GENERIC FORM AVAILABLE: Yes

THERAPEUTIC CLASS: Thioxanthene antipsychotic

DOSAGE FORMS: 1-mg, 2-mg, 5-mg, 10-mg, and 20-mg capsules; and 5 mg/mL oral concentrate

MAIN USES: Psychotic disorders

USUAL DOSE: 2 mg to 5 mg three times daily for mild conditions or 5 mg to 20 mg three times daily for more severe conditions

AVERAGE PRICE: $53.53 (B)/$17.58 (G) for 1 mg; $72.19 (B)/$21.51 (G) for 2 mg; $112.88 (B)/$27.01 (G) for 5 mg; $146.33 (B)/$41.56 (G) for 10 mg

SIDE EFFECTS: Most common: drowsiness, severe restlessness, need to keep moving, difficulty in swallowing, inability to move the eyes, muscle spasms, unusual twisting movements of the body, Parkinson's-like symptoms, lip smacking or puckering, wormlike movements of the tongue, uncontrolled movements of the arms and legs, constipation, increased sweating, increased salivation, dry mouth, increased appetite, weight gain, increased sensitivity to sunburn, and lightheadedness. Less common: changes in menstrual period, decreased sexual ability, swelling of the breasts, unusual secretion of milk, rash, difficulty urinating, blurred vision, low blood pressure, and skin discoloration.

DRUG INTERACTIONS: Alcohol, anxiety medications, and narcotic painkillers may intensify the drowsiness effect of the drug. The drug may decrease the effects of Larodopa. The drug, when taken with Quinidex or Quinaglute, may cause additional cardiovascular side effects.

ALLERGIES: Individuals allergic to thiothixene or any of its derivatives should discuss this with their doctor or pharmacist before using this drug.

PREGNANCY/BREAST-FEEDING: Category C—Risk cannot be ruled out. Human studies are lacking, and animal studies are either positive for fetal risk or lacking as well. However, potential benefits may justify the potential risk in using the drug. It is not known whether the drug is excreted in the breast milk; therefore, caution should be used when breast-feeding.

OTHER BRAND NAMES: None

OTHER DRUGS IN THE SAME THERAPEUTIC CLASS: None

IMPORTANT INFORMATION TO REMEMBER: This drug does cause drowsiness. Individuals should use caution when driving, operating machinery, or performing any task where mental alertness is required. Alcohol, anxiety medications, and narcotic painkillers may intensify the drowsiness effect of the drug. Do not increase the dose or discontinue taking the drug without first consulting with your physician. The drug may require several weeks of treatment before its desired effects are seen. This drug may also increase the sensitivity of the skin to sunburn in some individuals; therefore, a sunscreen is recommended during periods of prolonged exposure to the sun. The drug also decreases an individual's tolerance to hot weather. Individuals should get up slowly from a sitting or lying-down position; otherwise dizziness may occur.

BRAND NAME: Nembutal

GENERIC NAME: pentobarbital

GENERIC FORM AVAILABLE: No

THERAPEUTIC CLASS: Barbiturate sedative

DOSAGE FORMS: 50-mg and 100-mg capsules; and 30-mg, 60-mg, 120-mg, and 200-mg suppositories

MAIN USES: Insomnia and as a sedative

USUAL DOSE: 50 mg to 100 mg at bedtime

AVERAGE PRICE: $48.25 for 50 mg and $75.57 for 100 mg (capsules); $60.06 for 30-mg suppositories (12 each); $70.49 for 60-mg suppositories (12 each); $78.61 for 120-mg suppositories (12 each); $96.64 for 200-mg suppositories (12 each)

SIDE EFFECTS: drowsiness 33%, agitation 1%, confusion 1%, weakness 1%, nervousness 1%, nightmares 1%, anxiety 1%, hallucinations 1%, dizziness 1%, abnormal thinking 1%, low blood pressure 1%, trouble breathing 1%, slow heartbeat 1%, nausea 1%, vomiting 1%, headache 1%, and constipation 1%.

DRUG INTERACTIONS: Alcohol, anxiety medications, and narcotic painkillers will intensify the drowsiness effect of the drug. The drug may decrease the blood levels of Aristocort, Coumadin, Decadron, Deltasone, Medrol, prednisone, Tegretol, and Vibramycin. The drug may also decrease the effectiveness of birth control pills. Depakene and Depakote may increase the blood levels of the drug. The drug should be used with caution by patients taking Dilantin.

ALLERGIES: Individuals allergic to pentobarbital or other barbiturates (such as those listed under "Other Drugs in the Same Therapeutic Class") should discuss this with their doctor or pharmacist before taking this drug.

PREGNANCY/BREAST-FEEDING: Category D—Positive evidence of risk. Human studies show risk to the fetus. Nevertheless, potential benefits may possibly outweigh the potential risks. This drug should not be taken by nursing mothers.

OTHER BRAND NAMES: None

OTHER DRUGS IN THE SAME THERAPEUTIC CLASS: Amytal, Butisol, Mebaral, phenobarbital, Seconal, and Tuinal

IMPORTANT INFORMATION TO REMEMBER: This drug does cause drowsiness. Individuals should use caution when driving, operating machinery, or performing any task where mental alertness is required. Alcohol, anxiety medications, and narcotic painkillers may intensify the drowsiness effect of the drug. This medication is a controlled substance and may be habit-forming. Only take the drug exactly as directed by your physician. Do not increase the dose without first consulting with your physician. Women taking birth control pills should use another form of contraception while taking the drug and for the rest of the current menstrual cycle.

BRAND NAME: Neosporin Ophthalmic

GENERIC NAME: Combination product containing: polymyxin B, neomycin, and gramicidin (the eye ointment contains bacitracin instead of gramicidin)

GENERIC FORM AVAILABLE: Yes

THERAPEUTIC CLASS: Antibiotic eyedrop

DOSAGE FORMS: 10,000 units polymyxin B/1.75 mg neomycin/ 0.025 mg gramicidin per milliliter solution and 10,000 units polymyxin B/3.5 mg neomycin/400 units bacitracin per gram eye ointment

MAIN USES: Bacterial eye infections

USUAL DOSE: For the eyedrops: one to two drops in the affected eye two to four times daily. For the eye ointment: apply a thin ribbon on the ointment in the affected eye every three to four hours.

AVERAGE PRICE: $29.67 (B)/$17.58 (G) for 10-mL solution

SIDE EFFECTS: Most common: itching, redness, and irritation. Less common: burning, stinging, and temporary blurred vision (eye ointment only).

DRUG INTERACTIONS: None of any clinical significance

ALLERGIES: Individuals allergic to polymyxin B, neomycin, gramicidin, bacitracin, or any of their derivatives should discuss this with their doctor or pharmacist before using this drug.

PREGNANCY/BREAST-FEEDING: Category C—Risk cannot be ruled out. Human studies are lacking, and animal studies are either positive for fetal risk or lacking as well. However, potential benefits may justify the potential risk in using the drug. It is not known whether the drug is excreted in the breast milk; therefore, caution should be used when breast-feeding.

OTHER BRAND NAMES: None

OTHER DRUGS IN THE SAME THERAPEUTIC CLASS: Bleph-10, Isopto Cetamide, Polysporin, Polytrim, and Sulamyd

IMPORTANT INFORMATION TO REMEMBER: Individuals should not use the drug while wearing contact lenses unless directed otherwise by a doctor. Keep the container tightly closed and avoid touching the applicator tip to the eye—this could contaminate the product over time. Also, only administer one drop at a time. After application, keep the eye open for at least 30 seconds, roll the eyeball around, and avoid squinting. If a second drop is required, wait one to two minutes between drops. If another medication is to be used in the eye, wait at least 10 minutes before administering it. If you are using the eye ointment, pull the bottom eyelid down gently; then apply a small, thin ribbon of ointment along the rim of the lower eyelid between the eyelid and the eyeball. After application, close the eye and roll the eyeball around. Your vision may be slightly blurred after application.

BRAND NAME: Neptazane

GENERIC NAME: methazolamide

GENERIC FORM AVAILABLE: Yes

THERAPEUTIC CLASS: Carbonic anhydrase inhibitor

DOSAGE FORMS: 25-mg and 50-mg tablets

MAIN USES: Glaucoma

USUAL DOSE: 50 mg to 100 mg two to three times daily

AVERAGE PRICE: $67.78 (B)/$38.79 (G) for 25 mg and $108.39 (B)/ $53.08 (G) for 50 mg

SIDE EFFECTS: Most common: unusual tiredness or weakness, diarrhea, general feeling of discomfort or illness, loss of appetite, metallic taste in the mouth, nausea, vomiting, and weight loss, and numbness, tingling, or burning feeling in the hands, fingers, feet, toes, mouth, tongue, lips, or anus. Less common: dizziness, drowsiness, mental depression, blood in the urine, pain or burning while urinating, pain in the lower back, and increased frequency of urination.

DRUG INTERACTIONS: The effects of Desoxyn, Dexedrine, Quinaglute, and Quinidex may be increased. The effects of Urised may be reduced.

ALLERGIES: Individuals allergic to methazolamide or any of its derivatives should discuss this with their doctor or pharmacist before using this drug.

PREGNANCY/BREAST-FEEDING: Category C—Risk cannot be ruled out. Human studies are lacking, and animal studies are either positive for fetal risk or lacking as well. However, potential benefits

may justify the potential risk in using the drug. It is not known whether the drug is excreted in the breast milk; therefore, caution should be used when breast-feeding.

OTHER BRAND NAMES: None

OTHER DRUGS IN THE SAME THERAPEUTIC CLASS: Daranide and Diamox

IMPORTANT INFORMATION TO REMEMBER: This drug does cause some drowsiness. Individuals should use caution when driving, operating machinery, or performing any task where mental alertness is required. Alcohol, anxiety medications, and narcotic painkillers may intensify the drowsiness effect of the drug. The drug may lower levels of potassium in the body; caution should be used by individuals with low potassium levels. Only take the drug exactly as directed by your physician. Do not discontinue the drug without first consulting your physician.

BRAND NAME: Neupogen

GENERIC NAME: filgrastim

GENERIC FORM AVAILABLE: No

THERAPEUTIC CLASS: White blood cell stimulator

DOSAGE FORMS: 300 micrograms/mL for IV infusion or injection under the skin

MAIN USES: Decrease incidence of infection in patients during chemotherapy

USUAL DOSE: 5 micrograms to 10 micrograms per kilogram of body weight in a single injection or IV infusion (1 kilogram = 2.2 pounds)

AVERAGE PRICE: $243.68 for 1-mL vial

SIDE EFFECTS: Most common: pain in the joints or muscles, hair loss, diarrhea, fever, lower back pain, pain in the pelvis, headache, rash, and itching. Less common: difficulty breathing, constipation, excessive production of white blood cells, pain in the arms and legs, and pain or redness at the injection site.

DRUG INTERACTIONS: Eskalith and Lithobid should be used with caution.

ALLERGIES: Individuals allergic to filgrastim or any of its derivatives should discuss this with their doctor or pharmacist before using this drug.

PREGNANCY/BREAST-FEEDING: Category C—Risk cannot be ruled out. Human studies are lacking, and animal studies are either positive for fetal risk or lacking as well. However, potential benefits may justify the potential risk in using the drug. It is not known whether the drug is excreted in the breast milk; therefore, caution should be used when breast-feeding.

OTHER BRAND NAMES: None

OTHER DRUGS IN THE SAME THERAPEUTIC CLASS: None

IMPORTANT INFORMATION TO REMEMBER: Use proper injection technique if you are giving yourself the injections. Only use the drug exactly as directed by your physician and do not increase the dose without first consulting with your physician. This drug should be stored in the refrigerator. Do not shake the bottle before use—this may destroy the active ingredients inside the vial. If the solution is discolored or contains lumps, or particles can be seen, do not use the solution. At the first sign of infection—sore throat, fever, or chills—contact your physician immediately.

BRAND NAME: **Neurontin**

GENERIC NAME: gabapentin

GENERIC FORM AVAILABLE: No

THERAPEUTIC CLASS: Anticonvulsant

DOSAGE FORMS: 100-mg, 300-mg, and 400-mg capsules

MAIN USES: Epilepsy and seizures

USUAL DOSE: 300 mg to 600 mg three times daily

AVERAGE PRICE: $52.92 for 100 mg; $132.30 for 300 mg; $158.76 for 400 mg

SIDE EFFECTS: drowsiness 19%, dizziness 17%, tiredness 11%, tremors 7%, double vision 6%, runny nose 4%, nervousness 3%, weight gain 3%, back pain 2%, swelling 2%, dry mouth 2%, cough 2%, muscle pain 2%, amnesia 2%, depression 2%, abnormal thinking 2%, constipation 2%, dental abnormalities 2%, increased appetite 1%, twitching 1%, itching 1%, and impotence 1%.

DRUG INTERACTIONS: Antacids may decrease the absorption of the drug.

ALLERGIES: Individuals allergic to gabapentin or any of its derivatives should discuss this with their doctor or pharmacist before using this drug.

PREGNANCY/BREAST-FEEDING: Category C—Risk cannot be ruled out. Human studies are lacking, and animal studies are either positive for fetal risk or lacking as well. However, potential benefits may justify the potential risk in using the drug. It is not known whether the drug is excreted in the breast milk; therefore, caution should be used when breast-feeding.

OTHER BRAND NAMES: None

OTHER DRUGS IN THE SAME THERAPEUTIC CLASS: None

IMPORTANT INFORMATION TO REMEMBER: This drug does cause drowsiness. Individuals should use caution when driving, operating machinery, or performing any task where mental alertness is required. Alcohol, anxiety medications, and narcotic painkillers may intensify the drowsiness effect of the drug. Avoid drinking alcohol while taking this drug. Only take the drug exactly as directed by your physician. Do not discontinue the drug without first consulting your physician. Also, do not increase the dose without first consulting with your physician. Before taking over-the-counter medications, consult your physician or pharmacist.

BRAND NAME: Nicoderm

GENERIC NAME: nicotine transdermal

GENERIC FORM AVAILABLE: No

THERAPEUTIC CLASS: Smoking cessation aid

DOSAGE FORMS: 7-mg, 14-mg, and 21-mg per day transdermal patches

MAIN USES: Aid to help quit smoking

USUAL DOSE: 21-mg patch daily for four to eight weeks, then 14-mg patch daily for two to four weeks, and then 7-mg patch daily for two to four weeks

AVERAGE PRICE: $69.38 for 7 mg (14 patches); $74.92 for 14 mg (14 patches); $81.64 for 21 mg (14 patches)

SIDE EFFECTS: slight skin reactions 47%, headache 29%, insomnia 23%, diarrhea 3%–9%, nausea 3%–9%, muscle pain 3%–9%, abnormal dreams 3%–9%, nervousness 3%–9%, sweating 1%–3%, and dry mouth 1%–3%.

DRUG INTERACTIONS: When an individual stops smoking, the blood levels of Darvocet, Darvon, Inderal, insulin, Normodyne, Slo-bid, Theo-Dur, theophylline, Trandate, Uni-Dur, and Uniphyl may increase.

ALLERGIES: Individuals allergic to nicotine or any of its derivatives should discuss this with their doctor or pharmacist before using this drug.

PREGNANCY/BREAST-FEEDING: Category D—Positive evidence of risk. Human studies show risk to the fetus. Nevertheless, potential benefits may possibly outweigh the potential risks. This drug should not be taken by nursing mothers.

OTHER BRAND NAMES: Nicoderm CQ (over-the-counter)

OTHER DRUGS IN THE SAME THERAPEUTIC CLASS: Habitrol, Nicorette, Nicotrol, Nicotrol NS, and Prostep

IMPORTANT INFORMATION TO REMEMBER: Use the drug exactly as directed by your physician and stop smoking immediately. Do not discontinue the drug without first consulting your physician. Caution should be used by patients with high blood pressure, heart disease, or any other heart or blood vessel disease. Individuals who smoke while using the patch may experience severe cardiovascular side effects. The drug is available over-the-counter (OTC) without a prescription under the brand name Nicoderm CQ.

When using the patches:

1) Do not cut or fold the patch in half. This may cause the medication inside to leak out. Peel off the adhesive liner.
2) Apply the patch to a clean, dry skin area on the upper body or upper arm. This area should be free of hair, cuts, scars, or irritation. Avoid the waistline, since tight clothes may rub or remove the patch.
3) Leave the patch on even during swimming, showering, and exercising. If the patch falls off, replace the patch with a new one.
4) When it's time to apply a new patch, use a different site on the skin. Rotate the sites where you apply the patches every time.

5) Get into the habit of applying the patch at the same time each day.
6) Dispose of used patches properly and keep out of reach of children.

BRAND NAME: Nicorette and Nicorette DS

GENERIC NAME: nicotine polacrilex

GENERIC FORM AVAILABLE: No

THERAPEUTIC CLASS: Smoking cessation aid

DOSAGE FORMS: 2-mg and 4-mg gum

MAIN USES: Aid to help quit smoking

USUAL DOSE: Chew one piece of gum very slowly when there is an urge to smoke. Maximum is 30 pieces per day for Nicorette and 20 pieces per day for Nicorette DS.

AVERAGE PRICE: $56.01 for 2 mg (one box) and $94.13 for 4 mg (one box)

SIDE EFFECTS: nausea 10%–12%, inflammation inside the mouth 5%, tooth disorders 4%, hiccups 3%–9%, prickling or tingling feeling on the skin 3%–9%, increased salivation 3%–9%, inflammation of the tongue 3%, diarrhea 1%–3%, dry mouth 1%–3%, muscle pain 1%–3%, sweating 1%–3%, tongue sores 1%, sores inside the mouth 1%, and gum bleeding 1%.

DRUG INTERACTIONS: When an individual stops smoking, the blood levels of Darvocet, Darvon, Inderal, insulin, Normodyne, Slo-bid, Theo-Dur, theophylline, Trandate, Uni-Dur, and Uniphyl may increase.

ALLERGIES: Individuals allergic to nicotine or any of its derivatives should discuss this with their doctor or pharmacist before using this drug.

PREGNANCY/BREAST-FEEDING: Category C—Risk cannot be ruled out. Human studies are lacking, and animal studies are either positive for fetal risk or lacking as well. However, potential benefits may justify the potential risk in using the drug. The drug is excreted in the breast milk; therefore, extreme caution should be used when breast-feeding.

OTHER BRAND NAMES: None

OTHER DRUGS IN THE SAME THERAPEUTIC CLASS: Habitrol, Nicoderm, Nicotrol, Nicotrol NS, and Prostep

IMPORTANT INFORMATION TO REMEMBER: Use the drug exactly as directed by your physician and stop smoking immediately. Chew one piece of gum very slowly when there is an urge to smoke. Stop chewing when a tingling sensation is felt or when the gum taste becomes apparent. Keep the gum in your mouth and begin chewing again when the taste disappears. Each piece should last about 30 minutes. Caution should be used by patients with high blood pressure, heart disease, or any other heart or blood vessel disease. Individuals who smoke while chewing the gum may experience severe cardiovascular side effects. This drug is now available over-the-counter (OTC) without a prescription.

BRAND NAME: Nicotrol NS

GENERIC NAME: nicotine nasal spray

GENERIC FORM AVAILABLE: No

THERAPEUTIC CLASS: Smoking cessation aid

DOSAGE FORMS: 10 mg/mL nasal spray

MAIN USES: Aid to help quit smoking

USUAL DOSE: one to four sprays per hour (maximum of 10 sprays per hour or 80 sprays per day)

AVERAGE PRICE: $42.68

SIDE EFFECTS: headache 18%, back pain 6%, trouble breathing 5%, nausea 5%, joint pain 5%, menstrual problems (such as missed periods) 4%, pounding heartbeat 4%, gas 4%, tooth problems 4%, gum problems 4%, muscle pain 3%, stomach pain 3%, confusion 3%, acne 3%, menstrual cramps 3%, and itching 2%.

DRUG INTERACTIONS: When an individual stops smoking, the blood levels of Darvocet, Darvon, Inderal, insulin, Normodyne, Slo-bid, Theo-Dur, theophylline, Trandate, Uni-Dur, and Uniphyl may increase.

ALLERGIES: Individuals allergic to nicotine or any of its derivatives should discuss this with their doctor or pharmacist before using this drug.

PREGNANCY/BREAST-FEEDING: Category D—Positive evidence of risk. Human studies show risk to the fetus. Nevertheless, potential benefits may possibly outweigh the potential risks. This drug should not be taken by nursing mothers.

OTHER BRAND NAMES: None

OTHER DRUGS IN THE SAME THERAPEUTIC CLASS: Habitrol, Nicoderm, Nicorette, Nicotrol, and Prostep

IMPORTANT INFORMATION TO REMEMBER: Use the drug exactly as directed by your physician and stop smoking immediately. The head should be tilted back when using the spray. Do not sniff, swallow, or inhale through the nose as the drug is being sprayed into the nose. Caution should be used by patients with high blood pressure, heart disease, or any other cardiovascular or blood vessel disease. Individuals who smoke while using the spray may experience severe cardiovascular side effects.

BRAND NAME: Nicotrol Patches

GENERIC NAME: nicotine

The drug is very similar to Nicoderm. See entry for Nicoderm.

BRAND NAME: Nitro-Bid

GENERIC NAME: nitroglycerin

GENERIC FORM AVAILABLE: Yes

THERAPEUTIC CLASS: Nitrate anti-anginal

DOSAGE FORMS: 2.5-mg, 6.5-mg, and 9-mg capsules

MAIN USES: Prevention of angina

USUAL DOSE: 2.5 mg to 9 mg every 8 to 12 hours

AVERAGE PRICE: $12.74 (G) for 2.5 mg; $19.25 (G) for 6.5 mg; $13.95 (G) for 9 mg. The brand name is not manufactured anymore.

SIDE EFFECTS: Most common: flushing of the neck and face, headache, nausea, vomiting, dizziness when getting up from a sitting or lying-down position, restlessness, and fast heartbeat. Less common: blurred vision and dry mouth.

DRUG INTERACTIONS: Alcohol and the drug may produce low blood pressure. Vasodilan, Apresoline, Loniten, and the drug may also produce low blood pressure.

ALLERGIES: Individuals allergic to nitroglycerin or any of its derivatives should discuss this with their doctor or pharmacist before using this drug.

PREGNANCY/BREAST-FEEDING: Category C—Risk cannot be ruled out. Human studies are lacking, and animal studies are either positive for fetal risk or lacking as well. However, potential benefits may justify the potential risk in using the drug. It is not known whether the drug is excreted in the breast milk; therefore, caution should be used when breast-feeding.

OTHER BRAND NAMES: None

OTHER DRUGS IN THE SAME THERAPEUTIC CLASS: Nitrocap T.D., Nitrogard SR, and Nitrong SR

IMPORTANT INFORMATION TO REMEMBER: This drug is a sustained-release capsule and will not relieve angina attacks; it only prevents them. Take the drug only exactly as directed by your physician. Do not discontinue the drug or increase the dose without first consulting your physician. Do not crush the pellets inside the sustained-release capsules—this will destroy the mechanism that delays the release of the medication. The contents may, however, be sprinkled on soft food (such as applesauce) and swallowed without chewing. Do not drink alcohol while taking this drug. The headache that is common with this drug usually goes away with continued use; if it does not, contact your doctor. Before taking over-the-counter cold and allergy preparations, consult your doctor or pharmacist. This drug is no longer available in the brand-name form; only the generic is available.

BRAND NAME: **Nitrodisc**

GENERIC NAME: nitroglycerin

See entry for Nitro-Dur

BRAND NAME: **Nitro-Dur**

GENERIC NAME: nitroglycerin

GENERIC FORM AVAILABLE: No

THERAPEUTIC CLASS: Anti-anginal patch

DOSAGE FORMS: 0.1 mg/hr, 0.2 mg/hr, 0.3 mg/hr, 0.4 mg/hr, 0.6 mg/hr, and 0.8 mg/hr patches

MAIN USES: Prevention of angina

USUAL DOSE: Apply one patch every morning and remove after 12 hours. Other doses may be individualized according to the patient's needs.

AVERAGE PRICE: $57.03 for 0.1 mg (30 patches); $57.89 for 0.2 mg (30 patches); $64.89 for 0.3 mg and 0.4 mg (30 patches); $70.36 for 0.6 mg and 0.8 mg (30 patches)

SIDE EFFECTS: headache 63%, lightheadedness 6%, low blood pressure 4%, dizziness 4%, increased angina 2%, and some minor skin irritation at the application site.

DRUG INTERACTIONS: Alcohol and the drug may produce low blood pressure. Vasodilan, Apresoline, Loniten, and the drug may also produce low blood pressure.

ALLERGIES: Individuals allergic to nitroglycerin or any of its derivatives should discuss this with their doctor or pharmacist before using this drug.

PREGNANCY/BREAST-FEEDING: Category C—Risk cannot be ruled out. Human studies are lacking, and animal studies are either positive for fetal risk or lacking as well. However, potential benefits may justify the potential risk in using the drug. It is not known whether the drug is excreted in the breast milk; therefore, caution should be used when breast-feeding.

OTHER BRAND NAMES: Deponit, Minitran, Nitrodisc, and Transderm-Nitro

OTHER DRUGS IN THE SAME THERAPEUTIC CLASS: Deponit, Minitran, Nitrodisc, and Transderm-Nitro

IMPORTANT INFORMATION TO REMEMBER: This drug will not relieve angina attacks—it only prevents them. Use the drug only exactly as directed by your physician. Do not discontinue the drug without first consulting your physician. Also, do not increase the dose without first consulting with your physician. Do not drink alcohol while taking this drug. The headache that is common with this drug usually goes away with continued use; if it does not, contact your doctor. Before taking over-the-counter cold and allergy preparations, consult your doctor or pharmacist.

When using the patches:

1) Do not cut or fold the patch in half. This may cause the medication inside to leak out. Peel off the adhesive liner.
2) Apply the patch to a clean, dry skin area on the upper body or upper arm. This area should be free of hair, cuts, scars, or irritation. Avoid the waistline since tight clothes may rub or remove the patch. Also, do not apply the patch below the knee or elbow.
3) Leave the patch on even during swimming, showering, and exercising. If the patch falls off, replace the patch with a new one.
4) When it's time to apply a new patch, use a different site on the skin. Rotate the sites where you apply the patches every time.
5) Get into the habit of applying the patch at the same time each day.
6) Dispose of used patches properly and keep out of reach of children.

BRAND NAME: Nitroglycerin capsules

(sustained-release) by various manufacturers

GENERIC NAME: nitroglycerin

See entry for Nitro-Bid

BRAND NAME: Nitrolingual Spray

GENERIC NAME: nitroglycerin

GENERIC FORM AVAILABLE: No

THERAPEUTIC CLASS: Nitrate anti-anginal

DOSAGE FORMS: 0.4-mg-per-spray lingual aerosol spray

MAIN USES: Acute attacks of angina

USUAL DOSE: One to two sprays onto or under tongue at the beginning of an attack (maximum of three sprays in 15 minutes). Also, one spray 5-10 minutes before activities that trigger an angina attack.

AVERAGE PRICE: $36.48

SIDE EFFECTS: Most common: flushing of the neck and face, headache, nausea, vomiting, dizziness when getting up from a sitting or lying-down position, restlessness, and fast heartbeat. Less common: blurred vision and dry mouth.

DRUG INTERACTIONS: Alcohol and the drug may produce low blood pressure. Apresoline, Dilatrate-SR, Ismo, Imdur, Isordil, Loniten, Nitro-Bid, Nitro-Dur, Sorbitrate, or Vasodilan and the drug may also produce low blood pressure.

ALLERGIES: Individuals allergic to nitroglyercin or any of its derivatives should discuss this with their doctor or pharmacist before using this drug.

PREGNANCY/BREAST-FEEDING: Category C—Risk cannot be ruled out. Human studies are lacking, and animal studies are either positive for fetal risk or lacking as well. However, potential benefits may justify the potential risk in using the drug. It is not known whether the drug is excreted in the breast milk; therefore, caution should be used when breast-feeding.

OTHER BRAND NAMES: None

OTHER DRUGS IN THE SAME THERAPEUTIC CLASS: Nitrostat

IMPORTANT INFORMATION TO REMEMBER: Only use the drug exactly as directed by your physician. Also, do not increase the dose without first consulting with your physician. Do not drink alcohol while taking this drug. The headache that is common with this drug usually goes away with continued use; if it does not, contact your doctor. Before taking over-the-counter cold and allergy preparations, consult your doctor or pharmacist. Use the spray at the first sign of an angina attack; do not wait until the angina attack is severe. Do not shake the spray before using it. Close your mouth after each spray and do not swallow immediately. If pain continues or increases after using the prescribed amount of spray, notify your physician immediately or get to the nearest hospital emergency room for help.

BRAND NAME: Nitrostat

GENERIC NAME: nitroglycerin

GENERIC FORM AVAILABLE: No

THERAPEUTIC CLASS: Nitrate anti-anginal

DOSAGE FORMS: 0.15-mg, 0.3-mg, 0.4-mg, and 0.6-mg sublingual tablets

MAIN USES: Acute attacks of angina

USUAL DOSE: Dissolve one tablet under the tongue at the first sign of an attack. Individuals may repeat the same dose every five minutes for three doses (maximum is three tablets in 15 minutes). Also, take one tablet 5–10 minutes before activities that trigger an angina attack.

AVERAGE PRICE: $10.47 for 0.3-mg, 0.4-mg, and 0.6-mg tablets

SIDE EFFECTS: Most common: flushing of the neck and face, headache, nausea, vomiting, dizziness when getting up from a sitting or lying-down position, restlessness, and fast heartbeat. Less common: blurred vision, increased sweating, and dry mouth.

DRUG INTERACTIONS: Alcohol and the drug may produce low blood pressure. Apresoline, Dilatrate-SR, Ismo, Imdur, Isordil, Loniten, Nitro-Bid, Nitro-Dur, Sorbitrate, or Vasodilan and the drug may also produce low blood pressure.

ALLERGIES: Individuals allergic to nitroglyercin or any of its derivatives should discuss this with their doctor or pharmacist before using this drug.

PREGNANCY/BREAST-FEEDING: Category C—Risk cannot ruled out. Human studies are lacking, and animal studies are either positive for fetal risk or lacking as well. However, potential benefits may justify the potential risk in using the drug. It is not known whether the drug is excreted in the breast milk; therefore, caution should be used when breast-feeding.

OTHER BRAND NAMES: None

OTHER DRUGS IN THE SAME THERAPEUTIC CLASS: Nitrolingual Spray

IMPORTANT INFORMATION TO REMEMBER: Only use the drug exactly as directed by your physician. Also, do not increase the dose without first consulting with your physician. Do not drink alcohol while taking this drug. The headache that is common with this drug usually goes away with continued use; if it does not, contact your doctor. Before taking over-the-counter cold and allergy preparations, consult your doctor or pharmacist. Keep the tablets in the original container with the lid tightly closed. Exposure to the air will destroy the potency of the tablets; for this reason, the tablets should be replaced every six months. The tablets should taste bitter or produce a slight tingling sensation upon use. If they do not, they may be too old and need to be replaced.

When using the sublingual tablets for acute angina attacks:

1) Dissolve the tablet under the tongue (do not swallow) at the first sign of an angina attack; do not wait until the attack is severe.
2) If the angina is not relieved within five minutes after placing the first tablet under the tongue, dissolve a second tablet, and then a third if necessary.
3) If the pain continues or increases, notify your doctor or go to the nearest emergency room immediately.

BRAND NAME: Nizoral

GENERIC NAME: ketoconazole

GENERIC FORM AVAILABLE: No

THERAPEUTIC CLASS: Imidazole antifungal

DOSAGE FORMS: 200-mg tablets, 2% cream, and 2% shampoo

MAIN USES: Fungal infections

USUAL DOSE: For the tablets: 200 mg to 400 mg once daily. For the cream: apply to affected areas once or twice daily. For the shampoo: shampoo twice weekly.

AVERAGE PRICE: $394.10 for 200 mg; $32.92 for 2% cream (30 g); $24.20 for 2% shampoo (120 mL)

SIDE EFFECTS: For the cream and shampoo: Most common: none. Less common: irritation, itching, and burning. For the tablets: nausea 3%, vomiting 3%, itching 2%, and stomach pain 1%.

DRUG INTERACTIONS: *Warning:* This drug should never be taken with Hismanal, Seldane, or Seldane-D—this may cause severe and even life-threatening heart disorders. Antacids, Axid, Carafate,

Pepcid, Prevacid, Prilosec, Tagamet, Videx, and Zantac may decrease the absorption of the drug. The drug may increase the blood levels of Dilantin and Sandimmune. Isoniazid or rifampin may decrease the blood levels of the drug. The drug may increase the effects of Coumadin. Alcohol may increase the toxic effects of the drug on the liver and/or produce a severe disulfiram reaction (intense flushing, stomach pain, vomiting, etc.). Propulsid and the drug may cause dangerous irregular heartbeats when taken together.

ALLERGIES: Individuals allergic to ketoconazole, other antifungals, or any of their derivatives should discuss this with their doctor or pharmacist before using this drug.

PREGNANCY/BREAST-FEEDING: Category C—Risk cannot be ruled out. Human studies are lacking, and animal studies are either positive for fetal risk or lacking as well. However, potential benefits may justify the potential risk in using the drug. The drug is excreted in the breast milk; therefore, extreme caution should be used when breast-feeding.

OTHER BRAND NAMES: None

OTHER DRUGS IN THE SAME THERAPEUTIC CLASS: For the cream: Lotrimin, Monistat-Derm, Oxistat, and Spectazole. For the tablets: Dilfucan and Sporanox.

IMPORTANT INFORMATION TO REMEMBER: For the cream: the drug may stain clothing. The drug is for external use only. Apply and gently rub in enough of the cream to cover the affected area and surrounding areas. Never cover the skin after application with a bandage or wrapping unless directed to do so by a doctor. Discontinue use if irritation occurs. For the tablets: this drug should be taken with food or milk to reduce the potential for stomach upset and increase its absorption. Take the drug at the same time every day. Also, take the drug until all the medication prescribed is gone; otherwise the infection may return. Patients with liver disease should discuss this with their doctor before taking this drug. This drug should never be taken with alcohol, Hismanal, Seldane, or Seldane-D. The shampoo may remove the curl from permanently waved hair.

BRAND NAME: Nolamine

GENERIC NAME: Combination product containing: chlorpheniramine, phenindamine, and phenylpropanolamine

GENERIC FORM AVAILABLE: No

THERAPEUTIC CLASS: Antihistamine + decongestant

DOSAGE FORMS: 4-mg chlorpheniramine/24-mg phenindamine/
50-mg phenylpropanolamine sustained-release tablets

MAIN USES: Nasal allergies and congestion

USUAL DOSE: one tablet every 8 to 12 hours

AVERAGE PRICE: $34.51

SIDE EFFECTS: Most common: drowsiness. Less common: nausea,
giddiness, dry mouth, blurred vision, pounding heartbeat, flushing, and increased irritability or excitability (especially in children).

DRUG INTERACTIONS: Blocadren, Cartrol, Corgard, Inderal, Kerlone,
Levatol, Lopressor, Normodyne, Sectral, Tenormin, Toprol-XL,
Trandate, Visken, and Zebeta may increase the effects of the
drug. The drug may also reduce the effects of blood-pressure-lowering drugs. Nardil or Parnate may significantly raised blood pressure when taken with this drug.

ALLERGIES: Individuals allergic to chlorpheniramine, phenindamine, phenylpropanolamine, or any of their derivatives should discuss this with their doctor or pharmacist before using this drug.

PREGNANCY/BREAST-FEEDING: Category C—Risk cannot be ruled
out. Human studies are lacking, and animal studies are either positive for fetal risk or lacking as well. However, potential benefits
may justify the potential risk in using the drug. It is not known
whether the drug is excreted in the breast milk; therefore, caution
should be used when breast-feeding.

OTHER BRAND NAMES: None

OTHER DRUGS IN THE SAME THERAPEUTIC CLASS: Bromfed, Brom-
fed PD, Claritin-D, Comhist LA, Deconamine SR, Fedahist,
Naldecon, Novafed-A, Ornade, Poly-Histine-D, Rondec, Rynatan,
Seldane-D, Semprex-D, Tavist-D, and Trinalin

IMPORTANT INFORMATION TO REMEMBER: This drug does cause
drowsiness. Individuals should use caution when driving, operating machinery, or performing any task where mental alertness is

required. Alcohol, anxiety medications, and narcotic painkillers may intensify the drowsiness effect of the drug. This drug may also cause a dry mouth; sugarless gum or hard candy will help take care of this problem. Patients with glaucoma, high blood pressure, heart conditions, or urinary or prostate problems should consult their doctor before taking this drug.

BRAND NAME: Nolvadex

GENERIC NAME: tamoxifen

GENERIC FORM AVAILABLE: Yes

THERAPEUTIC CLASS: Anti-estrogen, anticancer

DOSAGE FORMS: 10-mg and 20-mg tablets

MAIN USES: Cancer (primarily breast cancer)

USUAL DOSE: 10 mg to 20 mg twice daily

AVERAGE PRICE: $170.92 (B)/$54.54 (G) for 10 mg

SIDE EFFECTS: hot flashes 64%, weight gain 38%, fluid retention 32%, vaginal discharge 30%, nausea 26%, irregular menstrual periods 25%, weight loss 23%, skin changes 19%, diarrhea 11%, increased liver enzymes 5%, vomiting 2%, and blood disorders 1%.

DRUG INTERACTIONS: The drug may increase the effects of Coumadin.

ALLERGIES: Individuals allergic to tamoxifen or any of their derivatives should discuss this with their doctor or pharmacist before using this drug.

PREGNANCY/BREAST-FEEDING: Category D—Positive evidence of risk. Human studies show risk to the fetus. Nevertheless, potential benefits may possibly outweigh the potential risks. This drug should not be taken by nursing mothers.

OTHER BRAND NAMES: None

OTHER DRUGS IN THE SAME THERAPEUTIC CLASS: Arimidex

IMPORTANT INFORMATION TO REMEMBER: It is extremely important to follow the dosing schedule set by your physician—do not deviate from this schedule. Nausea and vomiting may occur while taking this drug. Do not discontinue use unless directed by your physician. If severe weakness, drowsiness, pain or swelling of the legs, blurred vision, or shortness of breath occur, notify your physician.

BRAND NAME: Nordette

GENERIC NAME: Combination product containing: levonorgestrel and ethinyl estradiol

GENERIC FORM AVAILABLE: No

THERAPEUTIC CLASS: Progestin + estrogen contraceptive

DOSAGE FORMS: 0.15-mg levonorgestrel/30-micrograms ethinyl estradiol tablets

MAIN USES: Birth control

USUAL DOSE: Take one tablet daily for 21 or 28 days, beginning on the fifth day of the cycle. Day One of the cycle is the first day of menstrual bleeding.

AVERAGE PRICE: $26.59 for one Pilpak

SIDE EFFECTS: Most common: stomach cramps, bloating, acne, appetite changes, nausea, swelling of the feet and ankles, weight gain, swelling of the breasts, breast tenderness, and unusual tiredness or weakness. Less common: changes in vaginal bleeding, feeling faint, increased blood pressure, depression, stomach pain, vaginal itching, yeast infections, brown and blotchy spots on the skin, diarrhea, dizziness, headaches, migraines, increased body and facial hair, increased sensitivity of the skin to the sun, irritability, some hair loss from the scalp, vomiting, blood clots, weight loss, and changes in sexual desire.

DRUG INTERACTIONS: Antibiotics may decrease the effectiveness of the drug. The drug may interfere with the effectiveness of Parlodel. The drug may reduce the effects of Coumadin. The drug may increase the blood levels of Anafranil, Asendin, Elavil, Endep, Norpramin, Pamelor, Sinequan, Surmontil, Tofranil, and Vivactil when used for long periods of time. Smoking is not recommended while taking this drug due to the increased risk of heart disease, stroke, and high blood pressure.

ALLERGIES: Individuals allergic to levonorgestrel, ethinyl estradiol, or any of their derivatives should discuss this with their doctor or pharmacist before using this drug.

PREGNANCY/BREAST-FEEDING: Category X—Should not be used during pregnancy. Studies in animals and/or humans have shown fetal abnormalities and birth defects. The risks associated with using this drug clearly outweigh the benefits. This drug should never be used by someone who is pregnant or trying to become pregnant. Also, women should never breast-feed while using this drug.

OTHER BRAND NAMES: None

OTHER DRUGS IN THE SAME THERAPEUTIC CLASS: Brevicon, Demulen, Desogen, Loestrin, Lo/Ovral, Modicon, Norinyl, Ortho-Cept, Ortho-Cyclen, Ortho-Novum, Ovcon

IMPORTANT INFORMATION TO REMEMBER: Only take the drug exactly as directed by your physician. It is important to take the drug at the same time every day (bedtime). Do not discontinue the drug without first consulting your physician. The drug should not be used by women with a history of heart disease, stroke, high blood pressure, breast cancer, or other blood vessel diseases. Breakthrough bleeding may occur during the first few months; if this persists, notify your doctor. This drug will not provide protection against the HIV (AIDS) virus. It is important to use a second method of birth control during the first week when treatment has just begun. It may be necessary to use a second form of birth control when antibiotics are being taken. Also, women who smoke run a higher risk of heart disease, stroke, and high blood pressure when taking this drug. If pregnancy is suspected, stop taking the drug immediately.

BRAND NAME: **Norflex**

GENERIC NAME: orphenadrine

GENERIC FORM AVAILABLE: No

THERAPEUTIC CLASS: Anticholinergic muscle relaxant

DOSAGE FORMS: 100-mg sustained-release tablets

MAIN USES: Muscle spasms

USUAL DOSE: 100 mg twice daily

AVERAGE PRICE: $209.91

SIDE EFFECTS: Most common: drowsiness. Less common: decreased urination, eye pain, fast heartbeat, pounding heartbeat, fainting, dry mouth, blurred vision, dizziness, lightheadedness, headache, nervousness, trembling, stomach pain, constipation, nausea, and vomiting.

DRUG INTERACTIONS: Alcohol, anxiety medications, narcotic painkillers, and drugs used for depression may intensify the drowsiness effect of the drug.

ALLERGIES: Individuals allergic to orphenadrine or any of its derivatives should discuss this with their doctor or pharmacist before using this drug.

PREGNANCY/BREAST-FEEDING: Category C—Risk cannot be ruled out. Human studies are lacking, and animal studies are either positive for fetal risk or lacking as well. However, potential benefits may justify the potential risk in using the drug. It is not known whether the drug is excreted in the breast milk; therefore, caution should be used when breast-feeding.

OTHER BRAND NAMES: None

OTHER DRUGS IN THE SAME THERAPEUTIC CLASS: None

IMPORTANT INFORMATION TO REMEMBER: This drug does cause drowsiness. Individuals should use caution when driving, operating machinery, or performing any task where mental alertness is required. Alcohol, anxiety medications, narcotic painkillers, and drugs used to treat depression may intensify the drowsiness effect of the drug. The drug may cause a dry mouth; sugarless gum or hard candy will help this problem. Also, do not increase the dose without first consulting with your physician. Patients with glaucoma, urinary problems, prostate problems, or myasthenia gravis should consult their doctor before taking this drug.

BRAND NAME: Norgesic and Norgesic Forte

GENERIC NAME: Combination product containing: aspirin, caffeine, and orphenadrine

GENERIC FORM AVAILABLE: No

THERAPEUTIC CLASS: Muscle relaxant + analgesic

DOSAGE FORMS: 385-mg aspirin/30-mg caffeine/25-mg orphenadrine tablets (Norgesic); and 770-mg aspirin/60-mg caffeine/50-mg orphenadrine tablets (Norgesic Forte)

MAIN USES: Muscle spasms and associated pain relief

USUAL DOSE: one to two Norgesic tablets or 1/2 to one Norgesic Forte tablets three to four times daily

AVERAGE PRICE: $117.85 for Norgesic and $171.02 for Norgesic Forte

SIDE EFFECTS: Most common: drowsiness. Less common: decreased urination, eye pain, fast heartbeat, pounding heartbeat, fainting, dry mouth, blurred vision, dizziness, lightheadedness, headache, nervousness, trembling, stomach pain, constipation, nausea, and vomiting.

DRUG INTERACTIONS: Alcohol, anxiety medications, narcotic painkillers, and drugs used for depression may intensify the drowsiness effect of the drug. Other NSAIDs (such as Anaprox, Ansaid, Aleve, aspirin, Cataflam, Clinoril, Daypro, Disalcid, Dolobid, Feldene, Indocin, Lodine, Motrin, Nalfon, Naprosyn, Orudis, Oruvail, Relafen, Tolectin, and Voltaren) may decrease the concentration of the drug in the blood. This drug may also decrease the effects of Lasix, Dyazide, HydroDIURIL, Maxzide, and other water pills. The drug may increase the blood levels of Eskalith, Lithobid, and Sandimmune. The drug may increase the blood levels of Depakene and Depakote, as well as potentially cause other blood disorders. The drug may increase the toxic effects of the drug Rheumatrex. Caution should be used when taking the drug with Coumadin.

ALLERGIES: Individuals allergic to aspirin, caffeine, orphenadrine, Norflex, or any of their derivatives should discuss this with their doctor or pharmacist before using this drug.

PREGNANCY/BREAST-FEEDING: Category C—Risk cannot be ruled out. Human studies are lacking, and animal studies are either positive for fetal risk or lacking as well. However, potential benefits may justify the potential risk in using the drug. The drug should not, however, be used during the late stages (last three months) of pregnancy. It is not known whether the drug is excreted in the breast milk; therefore, caution should be used when breast-feeding.

OTHER BRAND NAMES: None

OTHER DRUGS IN THE SAME THERAPEUTIC CLASS: None

IMPORTANT INFORMATION TO REMEMBER: This drug should be taken with food or milk to reduce the potential for injury to the stomach lining and stomach upset. Drinking alcohol while taking this drug may increase its potential to cause ulcers. This drug should only be used under the direct supervision of a doctor by individuals with a bleeding disorder or ulcer, or those who are currently taking Coumadin. Before taking over-the-counter pain relievers, consult your doctor or pharmacist. This drug does cause drowsiness. Individuals should use caution when driving, operating machinery, or performing any task where mental alertness is required. Alcohol, anxiety medications, narcotic painkillers, and drugs used for depression may intensify the drowsiness effect of the drug. The drug may cause a dry mouth; sugarless gum or hard candy will help this problem. Also, do not increase the dose without first consulting with your physician. Patients with glaucoma, urinary problems, prostate problems, or myasthenia gravis should consult their doctor before taking this drug.

BRAND NAME: Norinyl

GENERIC NAME: Combination product containing: norethindrone and ethinyl estradiol

See entry for Ortho-Novum

BRAND NAME: Normodyne

GENERIC NAME: labetalol

GENERIC FORM AVAILABLE: No

THERAPEUTIC CLASS: Noncardioselective beta-blocker

DOSAGE FORMS: 100-mg, 200-mg, and 300-mg tablets

MAIN USES: High blood pressure

USUAL DOSE: 100 mg to 400 mg twice daily

AVERAGE PRICE: $62.21 for 100 mg; $88.25 for 200 mg; $117.37 for 300 mg

SIDE EFFECTS: dizziness 11%, nausea 6%, tiredness 5%, stuffy nose 3%, failure to ejaculate during sex 2%, headache 2%, taste changes 1%, impotence 1%, swelling 1%, rash 1%, and abnormal vision 1%.

DRUG INTERACTIONS: The drug may cause additive effects when used with reserpine. The drug may increase the effects of Calan, Cardene, Cardizem, Catapres, Covera-HS, Dilacor XR, DynaCirc, Isoptin, Lanoxin, Norvasc, Plendil, Procardia, Sular, Tiazac, Verelan, and Wytensin. Diabetic medications, insulin, Slo-bid, Theo-Dur, theophylline, Uni-Dur, and Uniphyl dosages may need to be adjusted when taking this drug. The drug may also interfere with glaucoma screening tests. Tagamet may increase the blood levels of the drug.

ALLERGIES: Individuals allergic to labetalol or other beta-blockers (such as those listed under "Other Drugs in the Same Therapeutic Class") should discuss this with their doctor or pharmacist before taking this drug.

PREGNANCY/BREAST-FEEDING: Category C—Risk cannot be ruled out. Human studies are lacking, and animal studies are either positive for fetal risk or lacking as well. However, potential benefits may justify the potential risk in using the drug. The drug is excreted in the breast milk; therefore, extreme caution should be used when breast-feeding.

OTHER BRAND NAMES: Trandate

OTHER DRUGS IN THE SAME THERAPEUTIC CLASS: Blocadren, Cartrol, Corgard, Inderal, Levatol, Trandate, and Visken

IMPORTANT INFORMATION TO REMEMBER: Only take the drug exactly as directed by your physician. Do not discontinue the drug without first consulting your physician. This drug may cause some tiredness, especially at first. Individuals should use caution when driving, operating machinery, or performing any task where mental alertness is required. Alcohol, anxiety medications, or narcotic painkillers may intensify the tiredness effect of the drug. Before taking over-the-counter cold and allergy precautions, consult your doctor or pharmacist—these products may raise your blood pressure. This drug may mask the symptoms of low blood sugar in diabetics.

BRAND NAME: **Noroxin**

GENERIC NAME: norfloxacin

GENERIC FORM AVAILABLE: No

THERAPEUTIC CLASS: Quinolone antibiotic

DOSAGE FORMS: 400-mg tablets

MAIN USES: Bacterial infections

USUAL DOSE: 400 mg every 12 hours

AVERAGE PRICE: $82.09 (20 tablets)

SIDE EFFECTS: nausea 4%, headache 3%, dizziness 2%, and weakness 1%.

DRUG INTERACTIONS: Antacids, Videx, iron supplements, and Carafate may reduce the absorption of the drug. Choledyl, Slo-Bid, Theo-Dur, theophylline, Uni-Dur, Uniphyl, and aminophylline blood levels may be increased when used with this drug. The drug may also increase the effects of Coumadin.

ALLERGIES: Individuals allergic to norfloxacin or other quinolone antibiotics (such as those listed under "Other Drugs in the Same Therapeutic Class") should discuss this with their doctor or pharmacist before taking this drug.

PREGNANCY/BREAST-FEEDING: Category C—Risk cannot be ruled out. Human studies are lacking, and animal studies are either positive for fetal risk or lacking as well. However, potential benefits may justify the potential risk in using the drug. It is not known whether the drug is excreted in the breast milk; therefore, caution should be used when breast-feeding.

OTHER BRAND NAMES: None

OTHER DRUGS IN THE SAME THERAPEUTIC CLASS: Cipro, Floxin, Maxaquin, and Penetrex

IMPORTANT INFORMATION TO REMEMBER: Take the drug at even intervals around the clock (if twice a day, take every 12 hours). Take the drug until all the medication prescribed is gone; otherwise the infection may return. This drug should be taken with plenty of water (eight ounces is preferred). If stomach upset occurs, take this drug with food. Do not take antacids, milk, or iron supplements within four hours of taking this drug. Individuals should also use a sunscreen to avoid overexposure to the sun; the drug may increase the skin's sensitivity to sunlight, which may cause one to sunburn more easily. This drug may also cause a tear in the tendons of the lower leg. Report any soreness or pain of the lower legs to your physician immediately.

BRAND NAME: Norpace and Norpace CR

GENERIC NAME: disopyramide

GENERIC FORM AVAILABLE: Yes

THERAPEUTIC CLASS: Class I antiarrhythmic

DOSAGE FORMS: 100-mg and 150-mg capsules (Norpace); and 100-mg and 150-mg controlled-release capsules (Norpace CR)

MAIN USES: Irregular heartbeat

USUAL DOSE: 400 mg to 800 mg per day in divided doses

AVERAGE PRICE: $58.83 (B)/$28.58 (G) for 100 mg and $76.98 (B)/$37.38 (G) for 150 mg (Norpace); $88.31 (B)/$47.82 (G) for 100 mg and $99.64 (B)/$55.53 (G) for 150 mg (Norpace CR)

SIDE EFFECTS: dry mouth 32%, difficulty in urinating 14%, constipation 11%, blurred vision 3%–9%, dry throat and eyes 3%–9%, nausea 3%–9%, stomach pain 3%–9%, gas 3%–9%, dizziness 3%–9%, weakness 3%–9%, headache 3%–9%, aches and pains 3%–9%, tiredness 3%–9%, impotence 1%–3%, low blood pressure 1%–3%, swelling 1%–3%, shortness of breath 1%–3%, weight changes 1%–3%, chest pain 1%–3%, diarrhea 1%–3%, vomiting 1%–3%, rash 1%–3%, and nervousness 1%–3%.

DRUG INTERACTIONS: Caution should be used by patients taking other drugs specifically used for irregular heartbeat. Orap and the drug, when taken together, may cause irregular heartbeat.

ALLERGIES: Individuals allergic to disopyramide or any of its derivatives should discuss this with their doctor or pharmacist before using this drug.

PREGNANCY/BREAST-FEEDING: Category C—Risk cannot be ruled out. Human studies are lacking, and animal studies are either positive for fetal risk or lacking as well. However, potential benefits may justify the potential risk in using the drug. It is not known whether the drug is excreted in the breast milk; therefore, caution should be used when breast-feeding.

OTHER BRAND NAMES: None

OTHER DRUGS IN THE SAME THERAPEUTIC CLASS: Cardioquin, Quinaglute, Quinidex, and Tonocard

IMPORTANT INFORMATION TO REMEMBER: This drug may cause some dizziness or tiredness, especially at first. Individuals should use caution when driving, operating machinery, or performing any task where mental alertness is required. Alcohol, anxiety medications, and narcotic painkillers may intensify these effects. Only take the drug exactly as directed by your physician. Do not discontinue the drug without first consulting your physician. Also, do not increase the dose without first consulting with your physician. Caution should be used in hot weather due to decreased tolerance to the heat. The drug may cause a dry mouth; sugarless gum or hard candy will help this problem.

BRAND NAME: Norplant

GENERIC NAME: levonorgestrel

GENERIC FORM AVAILABLE: No

THERAPEUTIC CLASS: Progestin contraceptive

DOSAGE FORMS: 216 mg in six implants (36 mg each)

MAIN USES: Birth control

USUAL DOSE: The implants should be inserted surgically under the skin of the upper arm during the first seven days after the onset of menses.

AVERAGE PRICE: $638.75 for one kit, six implants

SIDE EFFECTS: increase in bleeding days 28%, prolonged bleeding 17%, spotting 17%, abnormal periods 9%, unpredictable menstrual bleeding 8%, frequent menstrual bleeding onsets 7%, removal difficulties 6%, scanty bleeding 5%, pain or itching at the implant site 4%, and infections at the implant site 1%.

DRUG INTERACTIONS: Dilantin, Mesantoin, and Tegretol may reduce the effectiveness of the drug.

ALLERGIES: Individuals allergic to levonorgestrel or any of its derivatives should discuss this with their doctor or pharmacist before using this drug.

PREGNANCY/BREAST-FEEDING: Category X—Should not be used during pregnancy. Studies in animals and/or humans have shown fetal abnormalities and birth defects. The risks associated with using this drug clearly outweigh the benefits. This drug should never be used by someone who is pregnant or trying to become pregnant. Also, women should never breast-feed while using this drug.

OTHER BRAND NAMES: None

OTHER DRUGS IN THE SAME THERAPEUTIC CLASS: Depo-Provera, Micronor, Nor-QD, and Ovrette

IMPORTANT INFORMATION TO REMEMBER: This system of birth control will last approximately five years. The system does have to be surgically implanted under the skin and surgically removed five years later. Women interested in becoming pregnant within a 5-year period should probably use some other form of birth control. However, the system may be removed at any time if you want to try to become pregnant. Breakthrough bleeding may occur during the first few months. If this persists, notify your doctor. This drug will not provide protection against the HIV (AIDS) virus. It is important to use a second method of birth control for one week after treatment has begun. If pregnancy is suspected, contact your doctor immediately.

BRAND NAME: Norpramin

GENERIC NAME: desipramine

GENERIC FORM AVAILABLE: Yes

THERAPEUTIC CLASS: Tricyclic antidepressant

DOSAGE FORMS: 10-mg, 25-mg, 50-mg, 75-mg, 100-mg, and 150-mg tablets

MAIN USES: Depression

USUAL DOSE: 10 mg to 200 mg daily in divided doses or at bedtime

AVERAGE PRICE: $63.78 (B)/$29.46 (G) for 10 mg; $83.80 (B)/ $31.88 (G) for 25 mg; $171.57 (B)/$69.27 (G) for 50 mg; $193.57 (B)/$83.57 (G) for 75 mg; $228.77 (B)/$100.07 (G) for 100 mg

SIDE EFFECTS: Most common: drowsiness, dizziness, dry mouth, headache, increased appetite, nausea, tiredness, weight gain, and unpleasant taste. Less common: diarrhea, excessive sweating, heartburn, insomnia, vomiting, irregular heartbeat, muscle tremors, urinary difficulties, increased sensitivity to sunburn, and impotence.

DRUG INTERACTIONS: The drug should not be taken with Nardil or Parnate. In fact, 14 days are needed between the time of the use of Nardil or Parnate and this drug. Alcohol, anxiety medications, and narcotic painkillers may make the drowsiness caused by the drug much worse. Compazine, Mellaril, Prolixin, Serentil, Stelazine, Thorazine, and Trilafon may increase the blood levels of the drug. Tagamet may increase the blood levels of the drug. The drug may decrease the effects of Catapres and Ismelin. The drug may increase the effects on the heart of decongestants found in cold and allergy products, possibly causing high blood pressure, fast heartbeat, or irregular heartbeats.

ALLERGIES: Individuals allergies to desipramine or other tricylic antidepressants (such as those listed under "Other Drugs in the Same Therapeutic Class") should discuss this with their doctor or pharmacist before taking this drug.

PREGNANCY/BREAST-FEEDING: Category C—Risk cannot be ruled out. Human studies are lacking, and animal studies are either positive for fetal risk or lacking as well. However, potential benefits may justify the potential risk in using the drug. The drug is excreted in the breast milk; therefore, extreme caution should be used when breast-feeding.

OTHER BRAND NAMES: None

OTHER DRUGS IN THE SAME THERAPEUTIC CLASS: Asendin, Endep, Elavil, Pamelor, Sinequan, Surmontil, Tofranil, and Vivactil

IMPORTANT INFORMATION TO REMEMBER: Only take the drug exactly as directed by your physician. Do not discontinue the drug without first consulting your physician. The drug may require one to six weeks of use before improvement may be noticed. This drug does cause drowsiness. Individuals should use caution when driving, operating machinery, or performing any task where mental alertness is required. Alcohol, anxiety medications, and narcotic painkillers may intensify the drowsiness effect of the drug. The drug may cause a slight amount of dizziness or lightheadedness when rising from a sitting or lying-down position. Individuals should also use a sunscreen to avoid overexposure to the sun; the drug may increase the skin's sensitivity to sunlight, which may cause one to sunburn more easily.

BRAND NAME: Norvasc

GENERIC NAME: amlodipine

GENERIC FORM AVAILABLE: No

THERAPEUTIC CLASS: Calcium channel blocker

DOSAGE FORMS: 2.5-mg, 5-mg, and 10-mg tablets

MAIN USES: High blood pressure and angina

USUAL DOSE: 2.5 mg to 10 mg daily

AVERAGE PRICE: $170.80 for 2.5 mg and 5 mg; $295.55 for 10 mg

SIDE EFFECTS: headache 7%, swelling 6%–15%, tiredness 5%, nausea 3%, flushing 2%–5%, stomach pain 2%, drowsiness 2%, and pounding heartbeat 1%–3%.

DRUG INTERACTIONS: None of any clinical significance

ALLERGIES: Individuals allergic to amlodipine or any of its derivatives should discuss this with their doctor or pharmacist before using this drug.

PREGNANCY/BREAST-FEEDING: Category C—Risk cannot be ruled out. Human studies are lacking, and animal studies arc either positive for fetal risk or lacking as well. However, potential benefits may justify the potential risk in using the drug. It is not known whether the drug is excreted in the breast milk; therefore, caution should be used when breast-feeding.

OTHER BRAND NAMES: None

OTHER DRUGS IN THE SAME THERAPEUTIC CLASS: Adalat, Adalat CC, Calan, Calan SR, Cardizem, Cardizem SR, Cardizem CD, Cardene, Cardene SR, Covera-HS, Dilacor XR, DynaCirc, Isoptin, Isoptin SR, Plendil, Procardia, Procardia XL, Sular, Vascor, and Verelan

IMPORTANT INFORMATION TO REMEMBER: Only take the drug exactly as directed by your physician. Do not discontinue the drug without first consulting your physician. Before taking over-the-counter cold and allergy preparations, consult your doctor or pharmacist— these products may raise your blood pressure. This drug may cause some tiredness at first. Individuals should use caution when driving, operating machinery, or performing any task where mental alertness is required.

BRAND NAME: Norvir

GENERIC NAME: ritonavir

GENERIC FORM AVAILABLE: No

THERAPEUTIC CLASS: Protease inhibitor

DOSAGE FORMS: 100-mg capsules and 80 mg/mL liquid

MAIN USES: AIDS

USUAL DOSE: 600 mg twice daily

AVERAGE PRICE: $175.58

SIDE EFFECTS: nausea 26%, constipation 18%, vomiting 15%, weakness 14%, stomach pain 7%, headache 6%, numbness 6%, appetite changes 6%, taste changes 5%, diarrhea 5%, fever 4%, gas 3%, dizziness 3%, rash 3%, irritated throat 3%, drowsiness 2%, muscle pain 2%, low blood pressure 1%, insomnia 1%, abnormal thinking 1%, and sweating 1%.

DRUG INTERACTIONS: Dilantin, Mycobutin, phenobarbital, Rifadin, Rimactine, and Tegretol may decrease the blood levels of the drug. The drug may increase the blood levels of Calan, Cardene, Cardizem, Catapres, desipramine, Dilacor XR, DynaCirc, Halcion, Invirase, Isoptin, Norvasc, Plendil, Procardia, Quinaglute, Quinidex, Sular, Tiazac, and Verelan. Nizoral may increase the blood levels of the drug. The drug should never be used with Hismanal, Seldane, or Seldane-D. The liquid should never be used with Antabuse, Flagyl, or MetroGel. The drug may decrease the blood levels of Slo-bid, Theo-Dur, theophylline, Uni-Dur, and Uniphyl.

ALLERGIES: Individuals allergic to ritonavir or any of its derivatives should discuss this with their doctor or pharmacist before using this drug.

PREGNANCY/BREAST-FEEDING: Category B—No evidence of risk in humans. Either animal findings show risk, but human findings do not; or, if no adequate human studies have been done, animal findings show no risk. It is not known whether the drug is excreted in the breast milk; therefore, caution should be used when breast-feeding.

OTHER BRAND NAMES: None

OTHER DRUGS IN THE SAME THERAPEUTIC CLASS: Crixivan and Norvir

IMPORTANT INFORMATION TO REMEMBER: The drug should always be taken with meals if possible. Never take the drug on an empty stomach; food increases the absorption of the drug. Also, take the drug at even intervals around the clock (if two times a day, take every 12 hours). Only take the drug exactly as directed by your physician. Do not stop taking the drug without first consulting with your physician. It is important to have regular blood and liver function tests while taking this drug. Before taking any prescription or over-the-counter drugs, consult your physician or pharmacist. The liquid may be mixed with chocolate milk, Ensure, or Advera within one hour of taking the drug to improve the taste.

BRAND NAME: Novafed-A

GENERIC NAME: Combination product containing: chlorpheniramine and pseudoephedrine

See entry for Deconamine/Deconamine SR

BRAND NAME: Novolin Insulin

GENERIC NAME: insulin (recombinant)

Very similar to Humulin. See entry for Humulin.

BRAND NAME: Nucofed, Nucofed Expectorant, and Nucofed Pediatric Expectorant

GENERIC NAME: Combination product containing: codeine and pseudoephedrine. The expectorant formulations also contain guaifenesin.

GENERIC FORM AVAILABLE: No

THERAPEUTIC CLASS: Cough suppressant + decongestant

DOSAGE FORMS: 20-mg codeine/60-mg pseudoephedrine capsules (Nucofed); 20-mg codeine/60-mg pseudoephedrine/200-mg guaifenesin liquid (Nucofed Expectorant); and 10-mg codeine/30-mg pseudoephedrine/100-mg guaifenesin liquid (Nucofed Pediatric Expectorant)

MAIN USES: Cough and congestion

USUAL DOSE: For Nucofed: one capsule every six hours. For Nucofed Expectorant: one teaspoon every six hours. For Nucofed Pediatric Expectorant: 1/2 to 2 teaspoons every six hours, depending on age.

AVERAGE PRICE: $46.24 for capsules and $17.88 for liquids (120 mL)

SIDE EFFECTS: Most common: drowsiness. Less common: dizziness, headache, vision problems, disorientation, upset stomach, stomach pain, constipation, nausea, vomiting, and nervousness (especially in children).

DRUG INTERACTIONS: Alcohol, anxiety medications, and narcotic painkillers may intensify the drowsiness effect of the drug. Nardil and Parnate may increase the effects of the drug. The drug may also reduce the effects of blood-pressure-lowering drugs.

ALLERGIES: Individuals allergic to codeine, pseudoephedrine, guaifenesin, or any of their derivatives should discuss this with their doctor or pharmacist before using this drug.

PREGNANCY/BREAST-FEEDING: Category C—Risk cannot be ruled out. Human studies are lacking, and animal studies are either positive for fetal risk or lacking as well. However, potential benefits may justify the potential risk in using the drug. The drug is excreted in the breast milk; therefore, extreme caution should be used when breast-feeding.

OTHER BRAND NAMES: None

OTHER DRUGS IN THE SAME THERAPEUTIC CLASS: Hycomine, Novahistine Expectorant, Tussar SF

IMPORTANT INFORMATION TO REMEMBER: This drug does cause drowsiness. Individuals should use caution when driving, operating machinery, or performing any task where mental alertness is required. Alcohol, anxiety medications, and narcotic painkillers

may intensify the drowsiness effect of the drug. The drug should only be taken as needed to control a cough and congestion. This drug should not be used as a long-term therapy. This medication is a controlled substance and may be habit-forming. If stomach upset occurs, the drug may be taken with food or milk.

BRAND NAME: NuLYTELY

GENERIC NAME: Combination product containing: polyethylene glycol, sodium bicarbonate, sodium chloride, and potassium chloride

This drug is very similar to Colyte. See entry for Colyte.

BRAND NAME: Nutracort

GENERIC NAME: hydrocortisone

See entry for Hytone

BRAND NAME: Nystatin (various brand-name manufacturers)

GENERIC NAME: nystatin

See entry for Mycostatin

BRAND NAME: Ocuflox

GENERIC NAME: ofloxacin

GENERIC FORM AVAILABLE: No

THERAPEUTIC CLASS: Quinolone antibiotic

DOSAGE FORMS: 0.3% eyedrop solution

MAIN USES: Bacterial eye infections

USUAL DOSE: one to two drops every two to four hours for two days, then four times daily for up to five more days

AVERAGE PRICE: $27.09

SIDE EFFECTS: Most common: None. Less common: slight burning, stinging, itching, skin rash, and allergic reaction.

DRUG INTERACTIONS: None of any clinical significance

ALLERGIES: Individuals allergic to ofloxacin, Chibroxin, Ciloxan, Floxin, or any of their derivatives should discuss this with their doctor or pharmacist before using this drug.

PREGNANCY/BREAST-FEEDING: Category C—Risk cannot be ruled out. Human studies are lacking, and animal studies are either positive for fetal risk or lacking as well. However, potential benefits may justify the potential risk in using the drug. It is not known whether the drug is excreted in the breast milk; therefore, caution should be used when breast-feeding.

OTHER BRAND NAMES: None

OTHER DRUGS IN THE SAME THERAPEUTIC CLASS: Chibroxin and Ciloxan

IMPORTANT INFORMATION TO REMEMBER: Use the drug for the full course of therapy, even if symptoms disappear; otherwise the infection may return. Use the drug at even intervals around the clock (if four times a day, use every six hours). Keep the container tightly closed and avoid touching the applicator tip to the eye—this could contaminate the product over time. Also, only administer one drop at a time. After application, keep the eye open for at least 30 seconds, roll the eyeball around, and avoid squinting. If a second drop is required, wait one to two minutes between drops. If another medication is to be used in the eye, wait at least 10 minutes before administering it.

BRAND NAME: Ocupress

GENERIC NAME: carteolol

GENERIC FORM AVAILABLE: No

THERAPEUTIC CLASS: Noncardioselective beta-blocker

DOSAGE FORMS: 1% eyedrop solution

MAIN USES: Glaucoma

USUAL DOSE: one drop two times daily

AVERAGE PRICE: $42.70 for 10 mL

SIDE EFFECTS: Most common: redness of the eyes, decreased night vision, stinging of the eye, and irritation. Less common: brow-ache (headache around the eyebrows), increased sensitivity of the eye to light, swelling, droopy upper eyelid, discoloration of the eyeball, blurred vision, and changes in vision.

DRUG INTERACTIONS: The drug may cause widening of the pupil when used with epinephrine. The drug may cause additive effects when used with Blocadren, Cartrol, Corgard, Inderal, Kerlone, Levatol, Lopressor, Normodyne, reserpine, Sectral, Tenormin, Toprol-XL, Trandate, Visken, and Zebeta.

ALLERGIES: Individuals allergic to carteolol or any of its derivatives should discuss this with their doctor or pharmacist before using this drug.

PREGNANCY/BREAST-FEEDING: Category C—Risk cannot be ruled out. Human studies are lacking, and animal studies are either positive for fetal risk or lacking as well. However, potential benefits may justify the potential risk in using the drug. It is not known whether the drug is excreted in the breast milk; therefore, caution should be used when breast-feeding.

OTHER BRAND NAMES: None

OTHER DRUGS IN THE SAME THERAPEUTIC CLASS: Betagan, Betimol, OptiPranolol, Timoptic, and Timoptic XE

IMPORTANT INFORMATION TO REMEMBER: Keep the container tightly closed and avoid touching the applicator tip to the eye—this could contaminate the product over time. Also, only administer one drop at a time. After application, keep the eye open for at least 30 seconds, roll the eyeball around, and avoid squinting. If a second drop is required, wait one to two minutes between drops. If another medication is to be used in the eye, wait at least 10 minutes before administering it. Only use the drug exactly as directed by your physician. Do not discontinue the drug without first consulting your physician.

BRAND NAME: Ogen

GENERIC NAME: estropipate

GENERIC FORM AVAILABLE: Yes

THERAPEUTIC CLASS: Estrogen replacement

DOSAGE FORMS: 0.625-mg, 1.25-mg, and 2.5-mg tablets; 1.5 mg/g vaginal cream

MAIN USES: Menopausal disorders, prevention of osteoporosis, and vaginal atrophy (cream only)

USUAL DOSE: Tablets: 0.5 mg to 2 mg every day or daily for three weeks, then off one week. For the cream: 2 g to 4 g daily for three weeks, then off one week.

AVERAGE PRICE: $76.83 (B)/$61.92 (G) for 0.625 mg; $107.32 (B)/$85.71 (G) for 1.25 mg; $186.81 (B)/$150.88 (G) for 2.5 mg

SIDE EFFECTS: Most common: breast tenderness, breast pain, breast enlargement, swelling of feet and lower legs, stomach cramps, bloating, and nausea. Less common: changes in cervical secretions, yeast infections, headache, diarrhea, vomiting, migraine, depression, weight changes, dizziness, breakthrough bleeding, and changes in sex drive.

DRUG INTERACTIONS: The drug may interfere with the actions of Parlodel. The drug may increase the blood levels of Sandimmune. Liver toxicity may be increased when used with Dantrium.

ALLERGIES: Individuals allergic to estropipate, other estrogens, or any of their derivatives should discuss this with their doctor or pharmacist before using this drug.

PREGNANCY/BREAST-FEEDING: Category X—Should not be used during pregnancy. Studies in animals and/or humans have shown fetal abnormalities and birth defects. The risks associated with using this drug clearly outweigh the benefits. This drug should never be used by someone who is pregnant or trying to become pregnant. Also, women should never breast-feed while using this drug.

OTHER BRAND NAMES: Ortho-Est

OTHER DRUGS IN THE SAME THERAPEUTIC CLASS: Climara, Estinyl, Estrace, ESTRADERM, ESTRATAB, Ortho Dienestrol, Ortho-Est, Premarin, and Tace

IMPORTANT INFORMATION TO REMEMBER: Use the drug exactly as directed by your physician. Do not discontinue the drug without first consulting your physician. Caution should be used by patients with previous or current episodes of cancer, high blood pressure, heart disease, or any other cardiovascular or blood vessel disease. This drug may increase the risk of uterine cancer in women who have been through menopause. Report any abnormal vaginal bleeding to your doctor immediately. If using the vaginal cream, insert the applicator high into the vagina (two-thirds the length of the applicator) and push the plunger to release the cream. Do not use a tampon to hold the cream inside the vagina.

BRAND NAME: Omnipen

GENERIC NAME: ampicillin

GENERIC FORM AVAILABLE: Yes

THERAPEUTIC CLASS: Broad-spectrum penicillin antibiotic

DOSAGE FORMS: 250-mg and 500-mg capsules; and 125 mg/5 mL and 250 mg/5 mL suspension

MAIN USES: Bacterial infections

USUAL DOSE: 250 mg to 500 mg every six hours. Doses for small children may be lower.

AVERAGE PRICE: $11.97 (B)/$9.98 (G) for 250 mg (40 capsules) and $16.79 (B)/$14.58 (G) for 500 mg (40 capsules)

SIDE EFFECTS: Most common: mild diarrhea, nausea, vomiting, headache, and yeast infections. Less common: allergic reactions, itching, and skin rash.

DRUG INTERACTIONS: The drug may decrease the effectiveness of birth control pills. The drug probenecid will decrease elimination of the drug by the kidneys.

ALLERGIES: Individuals allergic to ampicillin or any of its derivatives, including other penicillins and cephalosporins, should discuss this with their doctor or pharmacist before taking this drug.

PREGNANCY/BREAST-FEEDING: Category B—No evidence of risk in humans. Either animal findings show risk, but human findings do not; or, if no adequate human studies have been done, animal findings show no risk. The drug is excreted in the breast milk; therefore, caution should be used when breast-feeding.

OTHER BRAND NAMES: Amcill and Principen

OTHER DRUGS IN THE SAME THERAPEUTIC CLASS: Amoxil, amoxicillin, penicillin, Spectrobid, and Veetids

IMPORTANT INFORMATION TO REMEMBER: If possible, take the drug on an empty stomach—one hour before meals or two hours after meals. Take the drug at even intervals around the clock (if four times a day, take every six hours). Take the drug until all the medication prescribed is gone; otherwise the infection may return. Women taking birth control pills should use another form of contraception while taking the drug and for the rest of the current menstrual cycle. Individuals taking the liquid form should shake it thoroughly before use, store the medication in the refrigerator, and discard any remaining medication after 14 days.

BRAND NAME: OptiPranolol

GENERIC NAME: metipranolol

GENERIC FORM AVAILABLE: No

THERAPEUTIC CLASS: Noncardioselective beta-blocker

DOSAGE FORMS: 0.3% eyedrop solution

MAIN USES: Glaucoma

USUAL DOSE: one drop twice daily

AVERAGE PRICE: $28.76 for 10 mL

SIDE EFFECTS: Most common: stinging of the eye and irritation. Less common: brow-ache (headache around the eyebrows), increased sensitivity of the eyes to light, redness, itching, watering of the eye, rash on the eyelid, blurred vision, and changes in vision.

DRUG INTERACTIONS: The drug may cause widening of the pupil when used with Epifrin. The drug may cause additive effects when used with Blocadren, Cartrol, Corgard, Inderal, Kerlone, Levatol, Lopressor, Normodyne, reserpine, Sectral, Tenormin, Toprol-XL, Trandate, Visken, and Zebeta.

ALLERGIES: Individuals allergic to metipranolol or any of its derivatives should discuss this with their doctor or pharmacist before using this drug.

PREGNANCY/BREAST-FEEDING: Category C—Risk cannot be ruled out. Human studies are lacking, and animal studies are either positive for fetal risk or lacking as well. However, potential benefits may justify the potential risk in using the drug. It is not known whether the drug is excreted in the breast milk; therefore, caution should be used when breast-feeding.

OTHER BRAND NAMES: None

OTHER DRUGS IN THE SAME THERAPEUTIC CLASS: Betagan, Betimol, Ocupress, Timoptic, and Timoptic XE

IMPORTANT INFORMATION TO REMEMBER: Keep the container tightly closed and avoid touching the applicator tip to the eye—this could contaminate the product over time. Also, only administer one drop at a time. After application, keep the eye open for at least 30 seconds, roll the eyeball around, and avoid squinting. If a second drop is required, wait one to two minutes between drops. If another medication is to be used in the eye, wait at least 10 minutes before administering it. Only use the drug exactly as directed by your physician. Do not discontinue taking the drug without first consulting your physician.

BRAND NAME: Oramorph SR

GENERIC NAME: morphine sulfate

See entry for MS Contin

BRAND NAME: Oretic

GENERIC NAME: hydrochlorothiazide

See entry for HydroDIURIL

BRAND NAME: Organidin NR

GENERIC NAME: guaifenesin

GENERIC FORM AVAILABLE: No

THERAPEUTIC CLASS: Expectorant

DOSAGE FORMS: 200-mg tablets and 100 mg/5 mL liquid

MAIN USES: Cough

USUAL DOSE: 200 mg to 400 mg every four hours

AVERAGE PRICE: $38.07 for tablets and $25.36 for liquid (120 mL)

SIDE EFFECTS: Most common: none. Less common: diarrhea, drowsiness, nausea, vomiting, and stomach pain.

DRUG INTERACTIONS: None of any clinical significance

ALLERGIES: Individuals allergic to guaifenesin or any of its derivatives should discuss this with their doctor or pharmacist before using this drug.

PREGNANCY/BREAST-FEEDING: Category C—Risk cannot be ruled out. Human studies are lacking, and animal studies are either positive for fetal risk or lacking as well. However, potential benefits may justify the potential risk in using the drug. It is not known whether the drug is excreted in the breast milk; therefore, caution should be used when breast-feeding.

OTHER BRAND NAMES: None

OTHER DRUGS IN THE SAME THERAPEUTIC CLASS: Humibid LA

IMPORTANT INFORMATION TO REMEMBER: This drug should be taken with plenty of water (eight ounces or more is preferred). This will help thin the thick mucous secretions in the chest and help the cough "break up." Individuals should also drink plenty of liquids throughout the day to aid in this action. Do not take more than 12 tablets or 24 teaspoons in a 24-hour period.

BRAND NAME: Orinase

GENERIC NAME: tolbutamide

GENERIC FORM AVAILABLE: Yes

THERAPEUTIC CLASS: First-generation sulfonylurea anti-diabetic

DOSAGE FORMS: 500 mg tablets

MAIN USES: Diabetes

USUAL DOSE: 250 mg to 3 g daily in divided doses

AVERAGE PRICE: $31.57 (B)/$13.20 (G)

SIDE EFFECTS: Most common: changes in taste, constipation, diarrhea, dizziness, mild drowsiness, headache, heartburn, changes in appetite, nausea, vomiting, stomach pain, fullness, and stomach discomfort. Less common: hives, increased sensitivity to sunburn, skin redness, itching, and rash.

DRUG INTERACTIONS: Alcohol may cause a severe stomach reaction (vomiting, pain, diarrhea, etc.) when used with this drug. Coumadin and the drug, when combined, may initially increase the blood levels of both, followed by a decrease in blood levels of both drugs. Blocadren, Cartrol, Corgard, Inderal, Kerlone, Levatol, Lopressor, Normodyne, Sectral, Tenormin, Toprol-XL, Trandate, Visken, Zebeta, chloramphenicol, Esimil, Ismelin, Nardil, Parnate, high doses of aspirin, Bactrim, Gantanol, Gantrisin, and Septra may cause low blood sugar when used with this drug.

ALLERGIES: Individuals allergic to tolbutamide, sulfa drugs, or any of their derivatives should discuss this with their doctor or pharmacist before using this drug.

PREGNANCY/BREAST-FEEDING: Category C—Risk cannot be ruled out. Human studies are lacking, and animal studies are either positive for fetal risk or lacking as well. However, potential benefits may justify the potential risk in using the drug. It is not known whether the drug is excreted in the breast milk; therefore, caution should be used when breast-feeding.

OTHER BRAND NAMES: None

OTHER DRUGS IN THE SAME THERAPEUTIC CLASS: Diabinese and Tolinase

IMPORTANT INFORMATION TO REMEMBER: If stomach upset occurs, take the drug with food or milk. To receive optimum effect, regular compliance with therapy is essential. This includes compliance with a prescribed diet. Avoid alcohol while taking this drug; alcohol may cause severe stomach reactions (vomiting, pain, diarrhea, etc.). This drug lowers blood sugar. Individuals should be aware of the signs and symptoms of blood sugar that is too low: sweating, tremor, blurred vision, weakness, hunger, and confusion. If two or more of these symptoms are seen, treat with oral glucose (sugar) and/or contact your doctor. This drug may increase the risk of cardiovascular disease. Before taking over-the-counter cold and allergy preparations, consult your doctor or pharmacist—these products may affect your blood sugar.

BRAND NAME: Ornade

GENERIC NAME: Combination product containing: chlorpheniramine and phenylpropanolamine

GENERIC FORM AVAILABLE: Yes

THERAPEUTIC CLASS: Antihistamine + decongestant

DOSAGE FORMS: 12-mg chlorpheniramine/75-mg phenylpropanolamine sustained-release capsules

MAIN USES: Nasal allergies and congestion

USUAL DOSE: one capsule every 12 hours

AVERAGE PRICE: $102.97 (B)/$50.43 (G)

SIDE EFFECTS: Most common: drowsiness. Less common: nausea, giddiness, dry mouth, blurred vision, pounding heartbeat, flushing, and increased irritability or excitability (especially in children).

DRUG INTERACTIONS: Blocadren, Cartrol, Corgard, Inderal, Kerlone, Levatol, Lopressor, Normodyne, Sectral, Tenormin, Toprol-XL, Trandate, Visken, and Zebeta may increase the effects of the drug. The drug may also reduce the effects of blood-pressure-lowering drugs. Nardil or Parnate may significantly raise blood pressure when taken with this drug.

ALLERGIES: Individuals allergic to chlorpheniramine, phenylpropanolamine, or other antihistamine/decongestant combinations (such as those listed under "Other Drugs in the Same Therapeutic Class") should discuss this with their doctor or pharmacist before taking this drug.

PREGNANCY/BREAST-FEEDING: Category B—No evidence of risk in humans. Either animal findings show risk, but human findings do not; or, if no adequate human studies have been done, animal findings show no risk. The drug is excreted in the breast milk; therefore, caution should be used when breast-feeding.

OTHER BRAND NAMES: None

OTHER DRUGS IN THE SAME THERAPEUTIC CLASS: Bromfed, Bromfed PD, Claritin-D, Comhist LA, Deconamine, Deconamine SR, Fedahist, Naldecon, Nolamine, Novafed-A, Ornade, Poly-Histine-D, Rondec, Rynatan, Seldane-D, Semprex-D, Tavist-D, and Trinalin

IMPORTANT INFORMATION TO REMEMBER: This drug does cause drowsiness. Individuals should use caution when driving, operating machinery, or performing any task where mental alertness is required. Alcohol, anxiety medications, and narcotic painkillers may intensify the drowsiness effect of the drug. This drug may also cause a dry mouth; sugarless gum or hard candy will help take care of this problem. Patients with glaucoma, high blood pressure, heart conditions, or urinary or prostate problems should consult their doctor before taking this drug. These capsules should be swallowed whole.

BRAND NAME: Ortho-Cept

GENERIC NAME: Combination product containing: desogestrel and ethinyl estradiol

GENERIC FORM AVAILABLE: No

THERAPEUTIC CLASS: Progestin + estrogen contraceptive

DOSAGE FORMS: 0.15-mg desogestrel/30-microgram ethinyl estradiol tablets

MAIN USES: Birth control

USUAL DOSE: Take one tablet daily for 21 or 28 days, beginning on the fifth day of the cycle. Day One of the cycle is the first day of menstrual bleeding.

AVERAGE PRICE: $26.67

SIDE EFFECTS: Most common: stomach cramps, bloating, acne, appetite changes, nausea, swelling of the feet and ankles, weight gain, swelling of the breasts, breast tenderness, and unusual tiredness or weakness. Less common: changes in vaginal bleeding, feeling faint, increased blood pressure, depression, stomach pain, vaginal itching, yeast infections, brown and blotchy spots on the skin, diarrhea, dizziness, headaches, migraines, increased body and facial hair, increased sensitivity of the skin to the sun, irritability, some hair loss from the scalp, vomiting, blood clots, weight loss, and changes in sexual desire.

DRUG INTERACTIONS: Antibiotics may decrease the effectiveness of the drug. The drug may interfere with the effectiveness of Parlodel. The drug may reduce the effects of Coumadin. The drug may increase the blood levels of Anafranil, Asendin, Elavil, Endep, Norpramin, Pamelor, Sinequan, Surmontil, Tofranil, and Vivactil when used for long periods of time. Smoking is not recommended while taking this drug due to the increased risk of heart disease, stroke, and high blood pressure.

ALLERGIES: Individuals allergic to desogestrel, ethinyl estradiol, or any of their derivatives should discuss this with their doctor or pharmacist before using this drug.

PREGNANCY/BREAST-FEEDING: Category X—Should not be used during pregnancy. Studies in animals and/or humans have shown fetal abnormalities and birth defects. The risks associated with using this drug clearly outweigh the benefits. This drug should never be used by someone who is pregnant or trying to become pregnant. Also, women should never breast-feed while using this drug.

OTHER BRAND NAMES: None

OTHER DRUGS IN THE SAME THERAPEUTIC CLASS: Brevicon, Demulen, Desogen, Loestrin, Lo/Ovral, Modicon, Norinyl, Nordette, Ortho-Cyclen, Ortho-Novum, Ovcon, and Ovral

IMPORTANT INFORMATION TO REMEMBER: Only take the drug exactly as directed by your physician. It is important to take the drug at the same time every day (bedtime). Do not discontinue taking the drug without first consulting your physician. The drug should not be used by women with a history of heart disease, stroke, high blood pressure, breast cancer, or other blood vessel diseases. Breakthrough bleeding may occur during the first few months; if this persists, notify your doctor. This drug will not provide protection against the HIV (AIDS) virus. It is important to use a second method of birth control during the first week when treatment has just begun. It may be necessary to use a second form of birth control when antibiotics are being taken. Also, women who smoke run a higher risk of heart disease, stroke, and high blood pressure when taking this drug. If pregnancy is suspected, stop taking the drug immediately.

BRAND NAME: Ortho-Cyclen

GENERIC NAME: Combination product containing: norgestimate and ethinyl estradiol

Very similar to Ortho Tri-Cyclen. See entry for Ortho Tri-Cyclen.

BRAND NAME: Ortho-Est

GENERIC NAME: estropipate

See entry for Ogen

BRAND NAME: Ortho-Novum 7/7/7, 1/35, 1/50, and 10/11

GENERIC NAME: Combination product containing: norethindrone and ethinyl estradiol

GENERIC FORM AVAILABLE: Yes

THERAPEUTIC CLASS: Progestin + estrogen contraceptive

DOSAGE FORMS: Ortho-Novum 7/7/7: 0.5 mg norethindrone/35 micrograms ethinyl estradiol (first seven tablets), 0.75 mg norethindrone/35 micrograms ethinyl estradiol (second seven tablets), and 1 mg norethindrone/35 micrograms ethinyl estradiol (third seven tablets). Ortho-Novum 1/35: 1 mg norethindrone/35 micrograms ethinyl estradiol. Ortho-Novum 1/50: 1 mg norethindrone/ 50 micrograms ethinyl estradiol. Ortho-Novum 10/11: 0.5 mg norethindrone/35 micrograms ethinyl estradiol (first 10 days), and 1 mg norethindrone/35 micrograms ethinyl estradiol (next 11 days).

MAIN USES: Birth control

USUAL DOSE: Take one tablet daily for 21 or 28 days, beginning on the fifth day of the cycle. Day One of the cycle is the first day of menstrual bleeding.

AVERAGE PRICE: $26.43

SIDE EFFECTS: Most common: stomach cramps, bloating, acne, appetite changes, nausea, swelling of the feet and ankles, weight gain, swelling of the breasts, breast tenderness, and unusual tiredness or weakness. Less common: changes in vaginal bleeding, feeling faint, increased blood pressure, depression, stomach pain, vaginal itching, yeast infections, brown and blotchy spots on the skin, diarrhea, dizziness, headaches, migraines, increased body and facial hair, increased sensitivity of the skin to the sun, irritability, some hair loss from the scalp, vomiting, blood clots, weight loss, and changes in sexual desire.

DRUG INTERACTIONS: Antibiotics may decrease the effectiveness of the drug. The drug may interfere with the effectiveness of Parlodel. The drug may reduce the effects of Coumadin. The drug may increase the blood levels of Anafranil, Asendin, Elavil, Endep, Norpramin, Pamelor, Sinequan, Surmontil, Tofranil, and Vivactil when used for long periods of time. Smoking is not recommended while taking this drug due to the increased risk of heart disease, stroke, and high blood pressure.

ALLERGIES: Individuals allergic to norethindrone, ethinyl estradiol, or any of their derivatives should discuss this with their doctor or pharmacist before using this drug.

PREGNANCY/BREAST-FEEDING: Category X—Should not be used during pregnancy. Studies in animals and/or humans have shown fetal abnormalities and birth defects. The risks associated with using this drug clearly outweigh the benefits. This drug should never be used by someone who is pregnant or trying to become pregnant. Also, women should never breast-feed while using this drug.

OTHER BRAND NAMES: Norinyl

OTHER DRUGS IN THE SAME THERAPEUTIC CLASS: For Ortho-Novum 7/7/7: Estrostep, Ortho Tri-Cyclen, Tri-Levlen, Tri-Norinyl, and Triphasil. For Ortho-Novum: Brevicon, Demulen, Desogen, Loestrin, Lo/Ovral, Modicon, Norinyl, Nordette, Ortho-Cept, Ortho-Cyclen, Ovcon, and Ovral

IMPORTANT INFORMATION TO REMEMBER: Only take the drug exactly as directed by your physician. It is important to take the drug at the same time every day (bedtime). Do not discontinue taking the drug without first consulting your physician. The drug should not be used by women with a history of heart disease, stroke, high blood pressure, breast cancer, or other blood vessel diseases. Breakthrough bleeding may occur during the first few months; if this persists, notify your doctor. This drug will not provide protection against the HIV (AIDS) virus. It is important to use a second method of birth control during the first week when treatment has just begun. It may be necessary to use a second form of birth control when antibiotics are being taken. Also, women who smoke run a higher risk of heart disease, stroke, and high blood pressure when taking this drug. If pregnancy is suspected, stop taking the drug immediately.

BRAND NAME: **Ortho Tri-Cyclen**

GENERIC NAME: Combination product containing: norgestimate and ethinyl estradiol

GENERIC FORM AVAILABLE: No

THERAPEUTIC CLASS: Progestin + estrogen contraceptive

DOSAGE FORMS: 0.18 mg norgestimate/35 micrograms ethinyl estradiol (first seven tablets), 0.215 mg norgestimate/35 micrograms ethinyl estradiol (second seven tablets), and 0.25 mg norgestimate/35 micrograms ethinyl estradiol (third seven tablets)

MAIN USES: Birth control

USUAL DOSE: Take one tablet daily for 21 or 28 days, beginning on the fifth day of the cycle. Day One of the cycle is the first day of menstrual bleeding.

AVERAGE PRICE: $27.01

SIDE EFFECTS: Most common: stomach cramps, bloating, acne, appetite changes, nausea, swelling of the feet and ankles, weight gain, swelling of the breasts, breast tenderness, and unusual tiredness or weakness. Less common: changes in vaginal bleeding, feeling faint, increased blood pressure, depression, stomach pain, vaginal itching, yeast infections, brown and blotchy spots on the skin, diarrhea, dizziness, headaches, migraines, increased body and facial hair, increased sensitivity of the skin to the sun, irritability, some hair loss from the scalp, vomiting, blood clots, weight loss, and changes in sexual desire.

DRUG INTERACTIONS: Antibiotics may decrease the effectiveness of the drug. The drug may interfere with the effectiveness of Parlodel. The drug may reduce the effects of Coumadin. The drug may increase the blood levels of Anafranil, Asendin, Elavil, Endep, Norpramin, Pamelor, Sinequan, Surmontil, Tofranil, and Vivactil when used for long periods of time. Smoking is not recommended while taking this drug due to the increased risk of heart disease, stroke, and high blood pressure.

ALLERGIES: Individuals allergic to norgestimate, ethinyl estradiol, or any of their derivatives should discuss this with their doctor or pharmacist before using this drug.

PREGNANCY/BREAST-FEEDING: Category X—Should not be used during pregnancy. Studies in animals and/or humans have shown fetal abnormalities and birth defects. The risks associated with using this drug clearly outweigh the benefits. This drug should never be used by someone who is pregnant or trying to become pregnant. Also, women should never breast-feed while using this drug.

OTHER BRAND NAMES: None

OTHER DRUGS IN THE SAME THERAPEUTIC CLASS: Estrostep, Ortho-Novum 7/7/7, Tri-Levlen, Tri-Norinyl, and Triphasil

IMPORTANT INFORMATION TO REMEMBER: Only take the drug exactly as directed by your physician. It is important to take the drug at the same time every day (bedtime). Do not discontinue taking the drug without first consulting your physician. The drug should not be used by women with a history of heart disease, stroke, high blood pressure, breast cancer, or other blood vessel diseases. Breakthrough bleeding may occur during the first few months; if this persists, notify your doctor. This drug will not provide protection against the HIV (AIDS) virus. It is important to use a second method of birth control during the first week when treatment has just begun. It may be necessary to use a second form of birth control when antibiotics are being taken. Also, women who smoke run a higher risk of heart disease, stroke, and high blood pressure when taking this drug. If pregnancy is suspected, stop taking the drug immediately.

BRAND NAME: Orudis and Oruvail

GENERIC NAME: ketoprofen

GENERIC FORM AVAILABLE: Yes

THERAPEUTIC CLASS: Nonsteroidal anti-inflammatory drug (NSAID)

DOSAGE FORMS: 25-mg, 50-mg, and 75-mg capsules (Orudis); and 100-mg, 150-mg, and 200-mg extended-release capsules (Oruvail)

MAIN USE: Arthritis, menstrual pain, and general pain relief

USUAL DOSE: For Orudis: 25 mg to 75 mg every six to eight hours as needed. For Oruvail: 200 mg once daily.

AVERAGE PRICE: $106.46 (B)/$67.79 (G) for 25 mg; $130.36 (B)/$81.33 (G) for 50 mg; $145.36 (B)/$86.81 (G) for 75 mg; $329.35 for Oruvail

SIDE EFFECTS: nausea 11%, stomach pain 3%–9%, diarrhea 3%–9%, constipation 3%–9%, gas 3%–9%, headache 3%–9%, nervousness 3%–9%, loss of appetite 1%–3%, vomiting 1%–3%, dizziness 1%–3%, tiredness 1%–3%, depression 1%–3%, ringing in the ears 1%–3%, vision disturbances 1%–3%, rash 1%–3%, swelling 1%–3%, impairment of kidney function 1%–3%, and urinary tract irritation 1%–3%.

DRUG INTERACTIONS: Aspirin will decrease the concentration of this drug in the blood. This drug may also decrease the effects of Lasix, Dyazide, HydroDIURIL, Maxzide, and other water pills. The drug may increase the blood levels of Eskalith, Lithobid, and Sandimmune. The drug may increase the toxic effects of the drug Rheumatrex. Caution should be used when taking the drug with Coumadin. Probenecid may increase the blood levels of the drug.

ALLERGIES: Individuals allergic to ketoprofen or other NSAIDs (such as those listed under "Other Drugs in the Same Therapeutic Class") should discuss this with their doctor or pharmacist before taking this drug.

PREGNANCY/BREAST-FEEDING: Category B—No evidence of risk in humans. Either animal findings show risk, but human findings do not; or, if no adequate human studies have been done, animal findings show no risk. The drug should not, however, be used during the late stages (last three months) of pregnancy. It is not known whether the drug is excreted in the breast milk; therefore, caution should be used when breast-feeding.

OTHER BRAND NAMES: Actron and Orudis KT (over-the-counter)

OTHER DRUGS IN THE SAME THERAPEUTIC CLASS: Anaprox, Ansaid, aspirin, Cataflam, Clinoril, Daypro, Disalcid, Dolobid, Easprin, Feldene, Indocin, Lodine, Lodine XL, Motrin, Nalfon, Naprosyn, Relafen, Tolectin, Toradol, Voltaren, and Voltaren XR

IMPORTANT INFORMATION TO REMEMBER: This drug should be taken with food or milk to reduce the potential for injury to the stomach lining and stomach upset. This drug may take up to two weeks before a noticeable improvement in pain relief associated with arthritis is observed. Drinking alcohol while taking this drug may increase its potential to cause ulcers. This drug should only be used under the direct supervision of a doctor by individuals with a bleeding disorder or ulcer, or those who are currently taking Coumadin. Before taking over-the-counter pain relievers, consult your doctor or pharmacist. No more than one pain reliever should be taken at any one time unless otherwise directed by your doctor. When taking Oruvail, do not crush or chew the capsule contents—this will destroy the mechanism that delays the release of the medications. This drug is now available over-the-counter (OTC) without a prescription in a 25-mg tablet under the brand names Actron and Orudis KT.

BRAND NAME: Ovcon

GENERIC NAME: Combination product containing: norethindrone and ethinyl estradiol

GENERIC FORM AVAILABLE: Yes

THERAPEUTIC CLASS: Progestin + estrogen contraceptive

DOSAGE FORMS: 0.4-mg norethindrone/35-microgram ethinyl estradiol tablets (Ovcon-35); and 1-mg norethindrone/50-microgram ethinyl estradiol tablets (Ovcon-50)

MAIN USES: Birth control

USUAL DOSE: Take one tablet daily for 21 or 28 days, beginning on the fifth day of the cycle. Day One of the cycle is the first day of menstrual bleeding.

AVERAGE PRICE: $26.56 (B)/$22.28 (G)

SIDE EFFECTS: Most common: stomach cramps, bloating, acne, appetite changes, nausea, swelling of the feet and ankles, weight gain, swelling of the breasts, breast tenderness, and unusual tiredness or weakness. Less common: changes in vaginal bleeding, feeling faint, increased blood pressure, depression, stomach pain, vaginal itching, yeast infections, brown and blotchy spots on the skin, diarrhea, dizziness, headaches, migraines, increased body and facial hair, increased sensitivity of the skin to the sun, irritability, some hair loss from the scalp, vomiting, blood clots, weight loss, and changes in sexual desire.

DRUG INTERACTIONS: Antibiotics may decrease the effectiveness of the drug. The drug may interfere with the effectiveness of Parlodel. The drug may reduce the effects of Coumadin. The drug may increase the blood levels of Anafranil, Asendin, Elavil, Endep, Norpramin, Pamelor, Sinequan, Surmontil, Tofranil, and Vivactil when used for long periods of time. Smoking is not recommended while taking this drug due to the increased risk of heart disease, stroke, and high blood pressure.

ALLERGIES: Individuals allergic to norethindrone, ethinyl estradiol, or any of their derivatives should discuss this with their doctor or pharmacist before using this drug.

PREGNANCY/BREAST-FEEDING: Category X—Should not be used during pregnancy. Studies in animals and/or humans have shown fetal abnormalities and birth defects. The risks associated with using this drug clearly outweigh the benefits. This drug should never be used by someone who is pregnant or trying to become pregnant. Also, women should never breast-feed while using this drug.

OTHER BRAND NAMES: None

OTHER DRUGS IN THE SAME THERAPEUTIC CLASS: Brevicon, Demulen, Desogen, Loestrin, Lo/Ovral, Modicon, Norinyl, Nordette, Ortho-Cept, Ortho-Cyclen, Ortho-Novum, and Ovral

IMPORTANT INFORMATION TO REMEMBER: Only take the drug exactly as directed by your physician. It is important to take the drug at the same time every day (bedtime). Do not discontinue taking the drug without first consulting your physician. The drug should not be used by women with a history of heart disease, stroke, high blood pressure, breast cancer, or other blood vessel diseases. Breakthrough bleeding may occur during the first few months. If this persists, notify your doctor. This drug will not provide protection against the HIV (AIDS) virus. It is important to use a second method of birth control during the first week when treatment has just begun. It may be necessary to use a second form of birth control when antibiotics are being taken. Also, women who smoke run a higher risk of heart disease, stroke, and high blood pressure when taking this drug. If pregnancy is suspected, stop taking the drug immediately.

BRAND NAME: Ovral and Lo/Ovral

GENERIC NAME: Combination product containing: norgestrel and ethinyl estradiol

GENERIC FORM AVAILABLE: No

THERAPEUTIC CLASS: Progestin + estrogen contraceptive

DOSAGE FORMS: 0.5-mg norgestrel/50-microgram ethinyl estradiol tablets (Ovral); and 0.3-mg norgestrel/30-microgram ethinyl estradiol tablets (Lo/Ovral)

MAIN USES: Birth control

USUAL DOSE: Take one tablet daily for 21 or 28 days, beginning on the fifth day of the cycle. Day One of the cycle is the first day of menstrual bleeding.

AVERAGE PRICE: $34.29

SIDE EFFECTS: Most common: stomach cramps, bloating, acne, appetite changes, nausea, swelling of the feet and ankles, weight gain, swelling of the breasts, breast tenderness, and unusual tiredness or weakness. Less common: changes in vaginal bleeding, feeling faint, increased blood pressure, depression, stomach pain, vaginal itching, yeast infections, brown and blotchy spots on the skin, diarrhea, dizziness, headaches, migraines, increased body and facial hair, increased sensitivity of the skin to the sun, irritability, some hair loss from the scalp, vomiting, blood clots, weight loss, and changes in sexual desire.

DRUG INTERACTIONS: Antibiotics may decrease the effectiveness of the drug. The drug may interfere with the effectiveness of Parlodel. The drug may reduce the effects of Coumadin. The drug may increase the blood levels of Anafranil, Asendin, Elavil, Endep, Norpramin, Pamelor, Sinequan, Surmontil, Tofranil, and Vivactil when used for long periods of time. Smoking is not recommended while taking this drug due to the increased risk of heart disease, stroke, and high blood pressure.

ALLERGIES: Individuals allergic to norgestrel, ethinyl estradiol, or any of their derivatives should discuss this with their doctor or pharmacist before using this drug.

PREGNANCY/BREAST-FEEDING: Category X—Should not be used during pregnancy. Studies in animals and/or humans have shown fetal abnormalities and birth defects. The risks associated with using this drug clearly outweigh the benefits. This drug should never be used by someone who is pregnant or trying to become pregnant. Also, women should never breast-feed while using this drug.

OTHER BRAND NAMES: None

OTHER DRUGS IN THE SAME THERAPEUTIC CLASS: Brevicon, Demulen, Desogen, Loestrin, Modicon, Norinyl, Nordette, Ortho-Cept, Ortho-Cyclen, Ortho-Novum, and Ovcon

IMPORTANT INFORMATION TO REMEMBER: Only take the drug exactly as directed by your physician. It is important to take the drug at the same time every day (bedtime). Do not discontinue taking the drug without first consulting your physician. The drug should not be used by women with a history of heart disease, stroke, high blood pressure, breast cancer, or other blood vessel diseases. Breakthrough bleeding may occur during the first few months; if this persists, notify your doctor. This drug will not provide protection against the HIV (AIDS) virus. It is important to use a second method of birth control during the first week when treatment has just begun. It may be necessary to use a second form of birth control when antibiotics are being taken. Also, women who smoke run a higher risk of heart disease, stroke, and high blood pressure when taking this drug. If pregnancy is suspected, stop taking the drug immediately.

BRAND NAME: Oxistat

GENERIC NAME: oxiconazole

GENERIC FORM AVAILABLE: No

THERAPEUTIC CLASS: Imidazole antifungal

DOSAGE FORMS: 1% cream and lotion

MAIN USES: Fungal infections (mainly ringworm, jock itch, and athlete's foot)

USUAL DOSE: Apply to affected area once or twice daily.

AVERAGE PRICE: $18.29 for 15-g cream and $31.47 for lotion

SIDE EFFECTS: itching 2%, burning 1%, and irritation 1%.

DRUG INTERACTIONS: None of any clinical significance

ALLERGIES: Individuals allergic to oxiconazole or any of its derivatives should discuss this with their doctor or pharmacist before using this drug.

PREGNANCY/BREAST-FEEDING: Category B—No evidence of risk in humans. Either animal findings show risk, but human findings do not; or, if no adequate human studies have been done, animal findings show no risk. The drug can be excreted in the breast milk in very small quantities; therefore, caution should be used when breast-feeding.

OTHER BRAND NAMES: None

OTHER DRUGS IN THE SAME THERAPEUTIC CLASS: Lotrimin, Monistat-Derm, Nizoral, and Spectazole

IMPORTANT INFORMATION TO REMEMBER: This drug is for external use only. The drug may stain clothing. Apply and gently rub in enough of the cream to cover the affected area and surrounding areas. Use the drug for the full course of treatment or the fungal infection may return. Never cover the skin after application with a bandage or wrapping unless directed to do so by a doctor. Discontinue use if irritation occurs.

BRAND NAME: **Pamelor**

GENERIC NAME: nortriptyline

GENERIC FORM AVAILABLE: Yes

THERAPEUTIC CLASS: Tricyclic antidepressant

DOSAGE FORMS: 10-mg, 25-mg, 50-mg, and 75-mg capsules; and 10 mg/5 mL oral solution

MAIN USES: Depression and {insomnia}

USUAL DOSE: 75 mg to 150 mg daily in single or multiple doses

AVERAGE PRICE: $71.47 (B)/$40.68 (G) for 10 mg; $115.13 (B)/$56.52 (G) for 25 mg; $207.49 (B)/$79.62 (G) for 50 mg; $274.51 (B)/$100.30 (G) for 75 mg

SIDE EFFECTS: Most common: drowsiness, dizziness, dry mouth, headache, increased appetite, nausea, tiredness, weight gain, and unpleasant taste. Less common: diarrhea, excessive sweating, heartburn, insomnia, vomiting, increased sensitivity to sunburn, irregular heartbeat, muscle tremors, urinary difficulties, and impotence.

DRUG INTERACTIONS: The drug should not be taken with Nardil or Parnate. In fact, 14 days are needed between the time of the use Nardil or Parnate and this drug. Alcohol, anxiety medications, and narcotic painkillers may make the drowsiness caused by the drug much worse. Compazine, Mellaril, Prolixin, Serentil, Stelazine, Thorazine, and Trilafon may increase the blood levels of the drug.

Tagamet may increase the blood levels of the drug. The drug may decrease the effects of Catapres and Ismelin. The drug may increase the effects on the heart of decongestants found in cold and allergy products, possibly causing high blood pressure, fast heartbeat, or irregular heartbeats.

ALLERGIES: Individuals allergic to nortriptyline or other tricyclic antidepressants (such as those listed under "Other Drugs in the Same Therapeutic Class") should discuss this with their doctor or pharmacist before taking this drug.

PREGNANCY/BREAST-FEEDING: Category C—Risk cannot be ruled out. Human studies are lacking, and animal studies are either positive for fetal risk or lacking as well. However, potential benefits may justify the potential risk in using the drug. The drug is excreted in the breast milk; therefore, extreme caution should be used when breast-feeding.

OTHER BRAND NAMES: Aventyl

OTHER DRUGS IN THE SAME THERAPEUTIC CLASS: Asendin, Elavil, Endep, Norpramin, Sinequan, Surmontil, Tofranil, and Vivactil

IMPORTANT INFORMATION TO REMEMBER: Only take the drug exactly as directed by your physician. Do not discontinue taking the drug without first consulting your physician. The drug may require one to six weeks of use before improvement may be noticed. This drug does cause drowsiness. Individuals should use caution when driving, operating machinery, or performing any task where mental alertness is required. Alcohol, anxiety medications, and narcotic painkillers may intensify the drowsiness effect of the drug. The drug may cause a slight amount of dizziness or lightheadedness when rising from a sitting or lying-down position. Individuals should also use a sunscreen to avoid overexposure to the sun; the drug may increase the skin's sensitivity to sunlight, which may cause one to sunburn more easily.

BRAND NAME: Pancrease MT

GENERIC NAME: Combination product containing the enzymes: lipase, amylase, and protease

GENERIC FORM AVAILABLE: No

THERAPEUTIC CLASS: Pancreatic enzyme replacement

DOSAGE FORMS: 4,000-unit lipase/12,000-unit amylase/12,000-unit protease enteric coated microtablets in capsules (Pancrease MT 4); 10,000-unit lipase/30,000-unit amylase/30,000-unit protease enteric coated microtablets in capsules (Pancrease MT 10); 16,000-unit lipase/48,000-unit amylase/48,000-unit protease enteric coated microtablets in capsules (Pancrease MT 16); and 20,000-unit lipase/56,000-unit amylase/44,000-unit protease enteric coated microtablets in capsules (Pancrease MT 20)

MAIN USES: Pancreatic enzyme replacement therapy

USUAL DOSE: one or more capsules with meals and snacks

AVERAGE PRICE: $37.58 for MT 4; $93.94 for MT 10; $150.15 for MT 16; and $187.89 for MT 20.

SIDE EFFECTS: Most common: none. Less common: nausea, vomiting, bloating, stomach cramps, diarrhea, and constipation.

DRUG INTERACTIONS: The drug should not be taken with antacids.

ALLERGIES: Individuals allergic to amylase, lipase, pancrelipase, protease, or any of their derivatives should discuss this with their doctor or pharmacist before using this drug.

PREGNANCY/BREAST-FEEDING: Category C—Risk cannot be ruled out. Human studies are lacking, and animal studies are either positive for fetal risk or lacking as well. However, potential benefits may justify the potential risk in using the drug. It is not known whether the drug is excreted in the breast milk; therefore, caution should be used when breast-feeding.

OTHER BRAND NAMES: Ultrase

OTHER DRUGS IN THE SAME THERAPEUTIC CLASS: Cotazym, Creon, KU-ZYME, and Viokase

IMPORTANT INFORMATION TO REMEMBER: This drug should be taken with food or milk. Only take the drug exactly as directed by your physician. Do not discontinue or increase the dose of the drug without first consulting your physician. Do not chew or crush the tiny spheres inside the capsules. Individuals can, however, sprinkle the capsule contents on cool, soft foods (such as applesauce) and then swallow without chewing. This drug should be taken with plenty of water (eight ounces is preferred).

BRAND NAME: **Parafon Forte DSC**

GENERIC NAME: chlorzoxazone

GENERIC FORM AVAILABLE: Yes

THERAPEUTIC CLASS: Muscle relaxant

DOSAGE FORMS: 500-mg tablets

MAIN USES: Muscle spasms

USUAL DOSE: one tablet three to four times daily

AVERAGE PRICE: $122.52 (B)/$62.13 (G)

SIDE EFFECTS: Most common: drowsiness, dizziness, and light-headedness. Less common: headache, nervousness, restlessness, insomnia, stomach pain, constipation, diarrhea, heartburn, nausea, and vomiting.

DRUG INTERACTIONS: The drug should not be used with MAO inhibitors (Nardil and Parnate), Eldepryl, Furoxone, or Matulane. In fact, this drug should not be used until at least 14 days after treatment with any of these drugs has stopped. Alcohol, anxiety medications, and narcotic painkillers may intensify the drowsiness effect of the drug.

ALLERGIES: Individuals allergic to chlorzoxazone or any of its derivatives should discuss this with their doctor or pharmacist before using this drug.

PREGNANCY/BREAST-FEEDING: Category C—Risk cannot be ruled out. Human studies are lacking, and animal studies are either positive for fetal risk or lacking as well. However, potential benefits may justify the potential risk in using the drug. It is not known whether the drug is excreted in the breast milk; therefore, caution should be used when breast-feeding.

OTHER BRAND NAMES: None

OTHER DRUGS IN THE SAME THERAPEUTIC CLASS: Flexeril, Lioresal, Robaxin, Skelaxin, and Soma

IMPORTANT INFORMATION TO REMEMBER: Only take the drug exactly as directed by your physician. Also, do not increase the dose without first consulting with your physician. If stomach upset occurs, take the drug with food or milk. This drug does cause drowsiness. Individuals should use caution when driving, operating machinery, or performing any task where mental alertness is required. Alcohol, anxiety medications, and narcotic painkillers may intensify the drowsiness effect of the drug.

BRAND NAME: **Parlodel**

GENERIC NAME: bromocriptine

GENERIC FORM AVAILABLE: No

THERAPEUTIC CLASS: Dopamine agonist

DOSAGE FORMS: 2.5-mg tablets and 5-mg capsules

MAIN USES: Parkinson's disease and {stopping the production of breast milk}

USUAL DOSE: 1.25 mg to 5 mg once or twice daily

AVERAGE PRICE: $66.67 for 2.5 mg (30 tablets) and $101.43 for 5 mg (30 capsules)

SIDE EFFECTS: Most common: dizziness or lightheadedness, especially when getting up from a sitting or lying-down position, and nausea. Less common: confusion; uncontrolled movements of the face, tongue, arms, hands, head, and upper body; hallucinations; constipation; diarrhea; drowsiness; tiredness; dry mouth; leg cramps at night; loss of appetite; depression; tingling or pain when the fingers or toes are exposed to cold; stomach pain; stuffy nose; and vomiting.

DRUG INTERACTIONS: Alcohol may cause a severe reaction (nausea, vomiting, chest pain, throbbing headache, etc.) if taken with this drug. Cycrin, estrogens, Provera, and birth control pills may interfere with effects of the drug. Hydergine and the drug, when taken together, may cause high blood pressure.

ALLERGIES: Individuals allergic to bromocriptine or any of its derivatives should discuss this with their doctor or pharmacist before using this drug.

PREGNANCY/BREAST-FEEDING: Category D—Positive evidence of risk. Human studies show risk to the fetus. Nevertheless, potential benefits may possibly outweigh the potential risks. This drug should not be taken by nursing mothers.

OTHER BRAND NAMES: None

OTHER DRUGS IN THE SAME THERAPEUTIC CLASS: Permax and Symmetrel

IMPORTANT INFORMATION TO REMEMBER: This drug should be taken with food or milk to reduce the potential for stomach upset. Never drink alcohol while taking this drug. Alcohol may cause a severe reaction (nausea, vomiting, chest pain, throbbing headache, etc.) if taken with this drug. Only take the drug exactly as directed by your physician. Do not discontinue taking the drug without first consulting your physician. This drug may cause some dizziness and drowsiness. Individuals should use caution when driving, operating machinery, or performing any task where mental alertness is required. Alcohol, anxiety medications, and narcotic painkillers may intensify the dizziness and drowsiness effect of the drug. Individuals should get up slowly from a sitting or lying-down position; otherwise dizziness may occur.

BRAND NAME: Parnate

GENERIC NAME: tranylcypromine

GENERIC FORM AVAILABLE: No

THERAPEUTIC CLASS: Monoamine oxidase (MAO) inhibitor antidepressant

DOSAGE FORMS: 10-mg tablets

MAIN USES: Depression and psychotic disorders

USUAL DOSE: 30 mg per day in divided doses

AVERAGE PRICE: $67.34

SIDE EFFECTS: Most common: low blood pressure; severe dizziness or lightheadedness, especially when getting up from a sitting or lying-down position; decreased urine output; blurred vision; insomnia; muscle twitching; restlessness; drowsiness; decreased sexual ability; headache; increased appetite; weight gain; increased sweating; shakiness; and weakness. Less common: chills, constipation, dry mouth, diarrhea, swelling of the feet and legs, nervousness, fast heartbeat, and pounding heartbeat.

DRUG INTERACTIONS: This drug interacts with many prescription and over-the-counter (OTC) medications. Before taking this drug, discuss the medications you are currently taking with your doctor and pharmacist; many of these interactions can be severe.

ALLERGIES: Individuals allergic to tranylcypromine or any of its derivatives should discuss this with their doctor or pharmacist before using this drug.

PREGNANCY/BREAST-FEEDING: Category C—Risk cannot be ruled out. Human studies are lacking, and animal studies are either positive for fetal risk or lacking as well. However, potential benefits may justify the potential risk in using the drug. The drug is excreted in the breast milk; therefore, extreme caution should be used when breast-feeding.

OTHER BRAND NAMES: None

OTHER DRUGS IN THE SAME THERAPEUTIC CLASS: Nardil

IMPORTANT INFORMATION TO REMEMBER: This drug does cause drowsiness. Individuals should use caution when driving, operating machinery, or performing any task where mental alertness is required. Alcohol, anxiety medications, and narcotic painkillers may intensify the drowsiness effect of the drug. Take the drug exactly as directed by your physician. Never suddenly stop taking the drug without first consulting with your physician. Before taking any prescription or over-the-counter (OTC) medications, consult with your doctor or pharmacist. The drug may take three to four weeks before a noticeable improvement is seen. While taking the drug and for at least 14 days after stopping, observe the precautions as given by your physician for 14 days. Individuals should avoid tyramine-containing foods (red wines, sherry, liquors, aged cheese, smoked or pickled meats, sauerkraut, beer, and overripe fruits, including avocados, raisins, and overripe bananas), alcoholic beverages, vitamin supplements containing yeast, and large quantities of caffeine-containing beverages.

BRAND NAME: Pavabid

GENERIC NAME: papaverine

GENERIC FORM AVAILABLE: Yes

THERAPEUTIC CLASS: Increased blood circulation agent

DOSAGE FORMS: 150-mg sustained-release capsules

MAIN USES: Lack of blood flow to the brain and body associated with arterial spasm

USUAL DOSE: 150 mg every 12 hours

AVERAGE PRICE: $36.39 (B)/$13.40 (G)

SIDE EFFECTS: Most common: none. Less common: general discomfort, nausea, vomiting, stomach pain, dizziness, constipation, diarrhea, headache, increased heart rate, hot flashes, and flushing of the face.

DRUG INTERACTIONS: None of any clinical significance

ALLERGIES: Individuals allergic to papaverine or any of its derivatives should discuss this with their doctor or pharmacist before using this drug.

PREGNANCY/BREAST-FEEDING: Category C—Risk cannot be ruled out. Human studies are lacking, and animal studies are either positive for fetal risk or lacking as well. However, potential benefits may justify the potential risk in using the drug. It is not known whether the drug is excreted in the breast milk; therefore, caution should be used when breast-feeding.

OTHER BRAND NAMES: None

OTHER DRUGS IN THE SAME THERAPEUTIC CLASS: None

IMPORTANT INFORMATION TO REMEMBER: If stomach upset occurs, the drug should be taken with food or milk. Only take the drug exactly as directed by your physician. Do not discontinue taking the drug without first consulting your physician. Individuals should get up slowly from a sitting or lying-down position; otherwise dizziness may occur.

BRAND NAME: Paxil

GENERIC NAME: paroxetine

GENERIC FORM AVAILABLE: No

THERAPEUTIC CLASS: Serotonin reuptake inhibitor antidepressant

DOSAGE FORMS: 20-mg and 30-mg tablets

MAIN USES: Depression, panic disorder, and obsessive-compulsive disorder

USUAL DOSE: 20 mg to 50 mg daily

AVERAGE PRICE: $276.59 for 20 mg and $294.51 for 30 mg

SIDE EFFECTS: nausea 26%, drowsiness 23%, dry mouth 18%, headache 18%, weakness 15%, constipation 14%, dizziness 13%, ejaculation problems 13%, insomnia 13%, diarrhea 12%, sweating 11%, tremors 8%, decreased appetite 6%, nervousness 5%, gas 4%, yawning 4%, blurred vision 4%, increased urination 3%, stomach pain 3%, decreased sex drive 3%, muscle pain 2%, vomiting 2%, and taste changes 2%.

DRUG INTERACTIONS: The drug may increase the blood levels of Kemadrin. The drug, when taken with Coumadin, may increase the chance of bleeding. The drug should not be used with tryptophan, because tryptophan can be metabolized to serotonin and too much serotonin may cause severe side effects. The drug should not be taken within 14 days of taking Nardil or Parnate.

ALLERGIES: Individuals allergic to paroxetine or any of its derivatives should discuss this with their doctor or pharmacist before using this drug.

PREGNANCY/BREAST-FEEDING: Category B—No evidence of risk in humans. Either animal findings show risk, but human findings do not; or, if no adequate human studies have been done, animal findings show no risk. The drug is excreted in the breast milk; therefore, extreme caution should be used when breast-feeding.

OTHER BRAND NAMES: None

OTHER DRUGS IN THE SAME THERAPEUTIC CLASS: Luvox, Prozac, and Zoloft

IMPORTANT INFORMATION TO REMEMBER: Only take the drug exactly as directed by your physician. Do not discontinue taking the drug without first consulting your physician. The drug may require two to four weeks or longer of use before improvement may be noticed. This drug does cause drowsiness. Individuals should use caution when driving, operating machinery, or performing any task where mental alertness is required. Alcohol, anxiety medications, and narcotic painkillers may intensify the drowsiness effect of the drug. The drug may cause a slight amount of dizziness or lightheadedness when rising from a sitting or lying-down position.

BRAND NAME: PBZ and PBZ SR

GENERIC NAME: tripelennamine

GENERIC FORM AVAILABLE: No

THERAPEUTIC CLASS: Antihistamine

DOSAGE FORMS: 25-mg and 50-mg tablets (PBZ); and 100-mg extended-release tablets (PBZ-SR)

MAIN USES: Allergies

USUAL DOSE: For PBZ: 25 mg to 50 mg every four to six hours. For PBZ-SR: one 100-mg extended-release tablet twice daily.

AVERAGE PRICE: $23.76 for 25 mg; $36.06 for 50 mg; and $59.39 for 100 mg (PBZ-SR)

SIDE EFFECTS: Most common: drowsiness, thickening of mucus, and dry mouth. Less common: blurred vision, difficult or painful urination, dizziness, fast heartbeat, increased sweating, increased appetite, and nausea.

DRUG INTERACTIONS: Alcohol, anxiety medications, and narcotic painkillers may intensify the drowsiness effect of the drug. Individuals should not take Nardil or Parnate while taking this drug. The drug should also not be used with Akineton, Artane, Cogentin, and Kemadrin.

ALLERGIES: Individuals allergic to tripelennamine or other antihistamines (such as those listed under "Other Drugs in the Same Therapeutic Class") should discuss this with their doctor or pharmacist before taking this drug.

PREGNANCY/BREAST-FEEDING: Category C—Risk cannot be ruled out. Human studies are lacking, and animal studies are either positive for fetal risk or lacking as well. However, potential benefits may justify the potential risk in using the drug. It is not known whether the drug is excreted in the breast milk; therefore, caution should be used when breast-feeding.

OTHER BRAND NAMES: None

OTHER DRUGS IN THE SAME THERAPEUTIC CLASS: Atarax, Benadryl, Periactin, Tavist, and Vistaril

IMPORTANT INFORMATION TO REMEMBER: This drug does cause drowsiness. Individuals should use caution when driving, operating machinery, or performing any task where mental alertness is

required. Alcohol, anxiety medications, or narcotic painkillers may intensify the drowsiness effect of the drug. This drug may also cause a dry mouth; sugarless gum or hard candy will help take care of this problem. Patients with glaucoma or urinary or prostate problems should consult their doctor before taking this drug.

BRAND NAME: PCE

GENERIC NAME: erythromycin

GENERIC FORM AVAILABLE: No

THERAPEUTIC CLASS: Macrolide antibiotic

DOSAGE FORMS: 333-mg and 500-mg tablets

MAIN USES: Bacterial infections

USUAL DOSE: 333 mg every 8 hours or 500 mg every 12 hours

AVERAGE PRICE: $49.19 for 333 mg (30 tablets) and $64.81 for 500 mg (30 tablets)

SIDE EFFECTS: Most common: nausea, vomiting, stomach pain, diarrhea, and appetite changes. Less common: dizziness, headache, abnormal taste, and confusion.

DRUG INTERACTIONS: *Warning:* This drug should not be used with Hismanal, Seldane, or Seldane-D. The drug may increase the blood levels of these drugs to extremely toxic and possibly life-threatening levels. The drug may also increase the blood levels of Coumadin, Retrovir, rifabutin, Sandimmune, Slo-bid, Theo-Dur, theophylline, Uni-Dur, Uniphyl, and Tegretol. Propulsid and the drug may cause dangerous irregular heartbeats when taken together.

ALLERGIES: Individuals allergic to erythromycin or other macrolide antibiotics (such as those listed under "Other Drugs in the Same Therapeutic Class") should discuss this with their doctor or pharmacist before taking this drug.

PREGNANCY/BREAST-FEEDING: Category B—No evidence of risk in humans. Either animal findings show risk, but human findings do not; or, if no adequate human studies have been done, animal findings show no risk. The drug is excreted in the breast milk; therefore, extreme caution should be used when breast-feeding.

OTHER BRAND NAMES: None

OTHER DRUGS IN THE SAME THERAPEUTIC CLASS: Biaxin, Dynabac, E.E.S., E-Mycin, ERYC, EryPed, ERY-TAB, Erythrocin, Ilosone, TAO, and Zithromax

IMPORTANT INFORMATION TO REMEMBER: If stomach upset occurs, take the drug with food or milk. Also, take the drug at even intervals around the clock (if three times a day, take every eight hours). Take the drug until all the medication prescribed is gone; otherwise the infection may return. If severe diarrhea occurs while taking this drug, notify your doctor immediately. Never take the drug with Hismanal, Seldane, or Seldane-D. (see "Drug Interactions").

BRAND NAME: Pediapred

GENERIC NAME: prednisolone

GENERIC FORM AVAILABLE: No

THERAPEUTIC CLASS: Glucocorticoid steroid

DOSAGE FORMS: 5 mg/5 mL solution

MAIN USES: Endocrine disorders and {multiple uses for its ability to reduce inflammation in various parts of the body, including asthma}

USUAL DOSE: 1 teaspoon to 12 teaspoons daily

AVERAGE PRICE: $21.68 for 120 mL

SIDE EFFECTS: Short-term use of the tablets: Most common: none. Less common: diarrhea, nausea, dizziness, insomnia, nervousness, headache, and stomach pain. Long-term use of the tablets: high blood pressure, muscle weakness, peptic ulcer, hemorrhage, thin fragile skin, facial swelling, weight gain, menstrual irregularities, glaucoma, and many others. Long-term use of the drug should be avoided if possible.

DRUG INTERACTIONS: Antacids may decrease the absorption of the drug. Amytal, Butisol, Dilantin, Mebaral, Mesantoin, Nembutal, Rifadin, Rifamate, Rifater, Seconal, and Tuinal may decrease the effects of the drug. The drug may increase blood glucose levels. Patients taking drugs for diabetes, including insulin, may need to adjust their dose. The drug may decrease the effects of water pills used to treat high blood pressure and potassium supplements such as K-Dur, Klor-Con, K-Lyte, K-Tab, Micro-K, and Slow-K.

ALLERGIES: Individuals allergic to prednisolone, prednisone, or other steroids (such as those listed under "Other Drugs in the Same Therapeutic Class") should discuss this with their doctor or pharmacist before taking this drug.

PREGNANCY/BREAST-FEEDING: Category C—Risk cannot be ruled out. Human studies are lacking, and animal studies are either positive for fetal risk or lacking as well. However, potential benefits may justify the potential risk in using the drug. The drug is excreted in the breast milk; therefore, extreme caution should be used when breast-feeding.

OTHER BRAND NAMES: None

OTHER DRUGS IN THE SAME THERAPEUTIC CLASS: Aristocort, Celestone, Decadron, Deltasone, Medrol, prednisone, and Prelone

IMPORTANT INFORMATION TO REMEMBER: This drug should be taken with food or milk to reduce the potential for injury to the stomach lining and stomach upset. Drinking alcohol while taking this drug may increase its potential to cause ulcers. Use exactly as directed by your physician. Never suddenly stop taking the drug without first consulting with your physician—this can be very dangerous. The drug may also cause some weight gain when used for long periods of time.

<u>BRAND NAME:</u> Pediazole

GENERIC NAME: Combination product containing: erythromycin ethylsuccinate and sulfisoxazole

GENERIC FORM AVAILABLE: Yes

THERAPEUTIC CLASS: Macrolide + sulfonamide antibiotic

DOSAGE FORMS: 200 mg erythromycin ethylsuccinate/600 mg sulfisoxazole per 5 mL oral suspension

MAIN USES: Bacterial infections

USUAL DOSE: $1/2$ to 2 teaspoons three or four times daily

AVERAGE PRICE: $34.63 (B)/$19.34 (G)

SIDE EFFECTS: Most common: nausea, vomiting, stomach pain, diarrhea, and appetite changes. Less common: dizziness, headache, abnormal taste, confusion, rash, itching, and increased sensitivity to sunburn.

DRUG INTERACTIONS: *Warning:* This drug should not be used with Hismanal, Seldane, or Seldane-D. The drug may increase the blood levels of these drugs to extremely toxic and possibly life-threatening levels. The drug may also increase the blood levels of Coumadin, Retrovir, Rifabutin, Sandimmune, Slo-bid, Theo-Dur, theophylline, Uni-Dur, Uniphyl, and Tegretol. The drug may increase the blood levels of Rheumatrex. The drug may increase the effects of diabetes drugs.

ALLERGIES: Individuals allergic to erythromycin, sulfisoxazole, other sulfa drugs, or any of their derivatives should discuss this with their doctor or pharmacist before using this drug.

PREGNANCY/BREAST-FEEDING: Category C—Risk cannot be ruled out. Human studies are lacking, and animal studies are either positive for fetal risk or lacking as well. However, potential benefits may justify the potential risk in using the drug. The drug is excreted in the breast milk; therefore, extreme caution should be used when breast-feeding.

OTHER BRAND NAMES: None

OTHER DRUGS IN THE SAME THERAPEUTIC CLASS: None

IMPORTANT INFORMATION TO REMEMBER: If stomach upset occurs, take the drug with food or milk. Also, take the drug at even intervals around the clock (if three times a day, take every eight hours). Take the drug until all the medication prescribed is gone; otherwise the infection may return. Individuals taking the liquid form should shake it thoroughly before use, store the medication in the refrigerator, and discard any remaining medication after 14 days. If severe diarrhea occurs while taking this drug, notify your doctor immediately. Never take the drug with Hismanal, Seldane, or Seldane-D. (see "Drug Interactions"). Individuals should also use a sunscreen to avoid overexposure to the sun; the drug may increase the skin's sensitivity to sunlight, which may cause one to sunburn more easily.

BRAND NAME: PediOtic

GENERIC NAME: Combination product containing: polymyxin B, neomycin, and hydrocortisone

See entry for Cortisporin Otic

BRAND NAME: Penetrex

GENERIC NAME: enoxacin

GENERIC FORM AVAILABLE: No

THERAPEUTIC CLASS: Quinolone antibiotic

DOSAGE FORMS: 200-mg and 400-mg tablets

MAIN USES: Bacterial infections

USUAL DOSE: 200 mg to 400 mg every 12 hours

AVERAGE PRICE: $76.44 for 200 mg (20 tablets) and $84.25 for 400 mg (20 tablets)

SIDE EFFECTS: nausea 8%, dizziness 3%, headache 2%, diarrhea 2%, stomach pain 2%, insomnia 1%, rash 1%, nervousness 1%, unusual taste 1%, and itching 1%.

DRUG INTERACTIONS: Antacids, Carafate, iron supplements, and Videx may reduce the absorption of the drug. Choledyl, Slo-bid, Theo-Dur, theophylline, Uni-Dur, Uniphyl, and aminophylline blood levels may be increased when used with this drug. The drug may also increase the effects of Coumadin.

ALLERGIES: Individuals allergic to enoxacin or other quinolone antibiotics (such as those listed under "Other Drugs in the Same Therapeutic Class") should discuss this with their doctor or pharmacist before taking this drug.

PREGNANCY/BREAST-FEEDING: Category C—Risk cannot be ruled out. Human studies are lacking, and animal studies are either positive for fetal risk or lacking as well. However, potential benefits may justify the potential risk in using the drug. It is not known whether the drug is excreted in the breast milk; therefore, caution should be used when breast-feeding.

OTHER BRAND NAMES: None

OTHER DRUGS IN THE SAME THERAPEUTIC CLASS: Cipro, Floxin, Maxaquin, and Noroxin

IMPORTANT INFORMATION TO REMEMBER: Take the drug at even intervals around the clock (if twice a day, take every 12 hours). Take the drug until all the medication prescribed is gone; otherwise the infection may return. This drug should be taken with plenty of water (eight ounces is preferred). If stomach upset occurs, take with food. Do not take antacids, milk, or iron supplements within four hours of taking this drug. Individuals should also use a sunscreen to avoid overexposure to the sun; the drug may increase the skin's sensitivity to sunlight, which may cause one to sunburn more easily. This drug may also cause a tear in the tendons of the lower leg. Report any soreness or pain of the lower legs to your physician immediately.

BRAND NAME: Pentasa

GENERIC NAME: mesalamine

GENERIC FORM AVAILABLE: No

THERAPEUTIC CLASS: Salicylate

DOSAGE FORMS: 250-mg controlled-release capsules

MAIN USES: Mildly to moderately active ulcerative colitis

USUAL DOSE: 1000 mg four times daily

AVERAGE PRICE: $49.09

SIDE EFFECTS: diarrhea 4%, nausea 3%, headache 2%, stomach pain 1%, bloody diarrhea 1%, rash 1%, appetite changes 1%, fever 1%, and vomiting 1%.

DRUG INTERACTIONS: None of any clinical significance

ALLERGIES: Patients allergic to mesalamine, aspirin, or aspirin derivatives should consult their doctor or pharmacist before taking this drug.

PREGNANCY/BREAST-FEEDING: Category B—No evidence of risk in humans. Either animal findings show risk, but human findings do not; or, if no adequate human studies have been done, animal findings show no risk. The drug is excreted in the breast milk; therefore, caution should be used when breast-feeding.

OTHER BRAND NAMES: None

OTHER DRUGS IN THE SAME THERAPEUTIC CLASS: Asacol, Azulfidine, Dipentum, and Rowasa

IMPORTANT INFORMATION TO REMEMBER: If the capsules are too big to swallow, the contents may be sprinkled on soft food (such as applesauce) and swallowed without chewing. Colitis symptoms may become worse in 3% of those taking the drug.

BRAND NAME: Pen•Vee K

GENERIC NAME: penicillin V potassium

See entry for Veetids

BRAND NAME: Pepcid

GENERIC NAME: famotidine

GENERIC FORM AVAILABLE: No

THERAPEUTIC CLASS: Stomach acid blocker

DOSAGE FORMS: 20-mg and 40-mg tablets; and 40 mg/5 mL suspension

MAIN USES: Active stomach ulcers, active duodenal ulcers (ulcers of the upper part of the small intestine, also called peptic ulcers), maintenance of healed duodenal ulcers, and the treatment of gastroesophageal reflux disease (GERD)

USUAL DOSE: 20 mg twice daily or 20 mg to 40 mg at bedtime

AVERAGE PRICE: $183.78 for 20 mg and $345.41 for 40 mg

SIDE EFFECTS: headache 5%, diarrhea 2%, dizziness 1%, and constipation 1%.

DRUG INTERACTIONS: The drug may increase the blood levels of Coumadin.

ALLERGIES: Individuals allergic to famotidine or other stomach acid blockers (such as those listed under "Other Drugs in the Same Therapeutic Class") should discuss this with their doctor or pharmacist before taking this drug.

PREGNANCY/BREAST-FEEDING: Category B—No evidence of risk in humans. Either animal findings show risk, but human findings do not; or, if no adequate human studies have been done, animal findings show no risk. The drug is excreted in the breast milk; therefore, caution should be used when breast-feeding.

OTHER BRAND NAMES: Pepcid AC and Mylanta AR (over-the-counter)

OTHER DRUGS IN THE SAME THERAPEUTIC CLASS: Axid, Tagamet, and Zantac

IMPORTANT INFORMATION TO REMEMBER: Always complete the full course of therapy, and take the drug only as directed. Individuals may take antacids occasionally for heartburn or temporary flare-ups, but antacids should be taken at least one hour before or two hours after taking the drug. Individuals using the liquid should shake it well before use and throw away any medication remaining after 30 days. The drug is now available over-the-counter (OTC) without a prescription in a 10-mg tablet under the brand names Pepcid AC and Mylanta AR.

BRAND NAME: Percocet

GENERIC NAME: Combination product containing: acetaminophen and oxycodone

GENERIC FORM AVAILABLE: Yes

THERAPEUTIC CLASS: Narcotic analgesic + pain reliever

DOSAGE FORMS: 325-mg acetaminophen/5-mg oxycodone tablets

MAIN USES: Moderate to severe pain

USUAL DOSE: one tablet every six hours as needed

AVERAGE PRICE: $82.04 (B)/$18.66 (G)

SIDE EFFECTS: Most common: drowsiness, dizziness, tiredness, nausea, and vomiting. Less common: confusion, decreased urination, dry mouth, constipation, stomach pain, skin rash, headache, weakness, minor vision disturbances, histamine release (symptoms include decreased blood pressure, sweating, fast heartbeat, flushing, and wheezing), and hallucinations.

DRUG INTERACTIONS: Alcohol, anxiety medications, and other narcotic painkillers may intensify the drowsiness effect of the drug. Liver toxicity may occur with long-term use of this drug with Anturane, Dilantin, and Mesantoin. This drug and Nardil or Parnate may cause severe and sometimes fatal reactions.

ALLERGIES: Individuals allergic to acetaminophen, oxycodone, other pain relievers, or any of their derivatives should discuss this with their doctor or pharmacist before using this drug.

PREGNANCY/BREAST-FEEDING: Category C—Risk cannot be ruled out. Human studies are lacking, and animal studies are either positive for fetal risk or lacking as well. However, potential benefits

may justify the potential risk in using the drug. It is not known whether the drug is excreted in the breast milk; therefore, caution should be used when breast-feeding.

OTHER BRAND NAMES: None

OTHER DRUGS IN THE SAME THERAPEUTIC CLASS: Bancap-HC, Darvocet-N 50, Darvocet-N 100, Darvon, Darvon Compound, DHCplus, Empirin #3, Empirin #4, Hydrocet, Lorcet 10/650, Lorcet Plus, Lortab, Percodan, Phenaphen w/Codeine, Synalgos DC, Talacen, Tylenol #2, Tylenol #3, Tylenol #4, Tylox, Vicodin, and Zydone

IMPORTANT INFORMATION TO REMEMBER: This drug does cause drowsiness. Individuals should use caution when driving, operating machinery, or performing any task where mental alertness is required. Alcohol, anxiety medications, and other narcotic painkillers may intensify the drowsiness effect of the drug. If stomach upset occurs, take the drug with food or milk. Do not increase the dose without first consulting with your physician. This prescription cannot be refilled; a new written prescription must be obtained each time. This medication is a controlled substance and may be habit-forming. The potential for abuse with this medication is high.

BRAND NAME: Percodan and Percodan-Demi

GENERIC NAME: Combination product containing: aspirin and oxycodone

GENERIC FORM AVAILABLE: Yes

THERAPEUTIC CLASS: Narcotic analgesic + pain reliever

DOSAGE FORMS: 325-mg aspirin/2.25-mg oxycodone/0.19-mg oxycodone terephthalate tablets (Percodan-Demi); and 325-mg aspirin/4.5-mg oxycodone/0.38-mg oxycodone terephthalate tablets (Percodan)

MAIN USES: Moderate to severe pain

USUAL DOSE: one to two Percodan-Demi tablets or one Percodan tablet every six hours as needed

AVERAGE PRICE: $102.83 (B)/$25.83 (G) for Percodan; $75.68 for Percodan-Demi

SIDE EFFECTS: Most common: drowsiness, dizziness, tiredness, nausea, and vomiting. Less common: confusion, decreased urination, dry mouth, constipation, stomach pain, skin rash, headache, weakness, minor vision disturbances, histamine release (symptoms include decreased blood pressure, sweating, fast heartbeat, flushing, and wheezing), ringing in the ears, and hallucinations.

DRUG INTERACTIONS: Alcohol, anxiety medications, and other narcotic painkillers may intensify the drowsiness effect of the drug. Liver toxicity may occur with long-term use of this drug with Anturane, Dilantin, and Mesantoin. This drug and Nardil or Parnate may cause severe and sometimes fatal reactions. Other NSAIDs (such as Anaprox, Ansaid, Aleve, aspirin, Cataflam, Clinoril, Daypro, Disalcid, Dolobid, Feldene, Indocin, Lodine, Mortrin, Nalfon, Naprosyn, Orudis, Oruvail, Relafen, Tolectin, and Voltaren) may decrease the concentration of the drug in the blood. This drug may also decrease the effects of Lasix, Dyazide, Hydro-DIURIL, Maxzide, and other water pills. The drug may increase the blood levels of Eskalith, Lithobid, and Sandimmune. The drug may increase the blood levels of Depakene and Depakote, as well as potentially cause other blood disorders. The drug may increase the toxic effects of the drug Rheumatrex. Caution should be used when taking the drug with Coumadin.

ALLERGIES: Individuals allergic to aspirin, oxycodone, other pain relievers, or any of their derivatives should discuss this with their doctor or pharmacist before using this drug.

PREGNANCY/BREAST-FEEDING: Category C—Risk cannot be ruled out. Human studies are lacking, and animal studies are either positive for fetal risk or lacking as well. However, potential benefits may justify the potential risk in using the drug. It is not known whether the drug is excreted in the breast milk; therefore, caution should be used when breast-feeding.

OTHER BRAND NAMES: None

OTHER DRUGS IN THE SAME THERAPEUTIC CLASS: Bancap-HC, Darvocet, Darvon, Darvon Compound, DHCplus, Empirin #3, Empirin #4, Hydrocet, Lorcet 10/650, Lorcet Plus, Lortab, Percocet, Phenaphen w/Codeine, Synalgos DC, Talacen, Tylenol #2, Tylenol #3, Tylenol #4, Tylox, Vicodin, and Zydone

IMPORTANT INFORMATION TO REMEMBER: This drug does cause drowsiness. Individuals should use caution when driving, operating machinery, or performing any task where mental alertness is required. Alcohol, anxiety medications, and other narcotic painkillers may intensify the drowsiness effect of the drug. If stomach upset occurs, take the drug with food or milk. Do not increase the dose without first consulting with your physician. Drinking alcohol while taking this drug may increase its potential to cause ulcers. This drug should only be used under the direct supervision of a doctor by individuals with a bleeding disorder or ulcer, or those who are currently taking Coumadin. This prescription cannot be refilled; a new written prescription must be obtained each time. This medication is a controlled substance and may be habit-forming. The potential for abuse with this medication is high.

BRAND NAME: Periactin

GENERIC NAME: cyproheptadine

GENERIC FORM AVAILABLE: Yes

THERAPEUTIC CLASS: Antihistamine

DOSAGE FORMS: 4-mg tablets and 2 mg/5 mL syrup

MAIN USES: Allergies, allergic reactions, and {headaches}, and {to increase appetite}

USUAL DOSE: 4 mg to 8 mg three times daily

AVERAGE PRICE: $55.95 (B)/$16.26 (G) for 4 mg

SIDE EFFECTS: Most common: drowsiness, thickening of mucus, and dry mouth. Less common: blurred vision, difficult or painful urination, dizziness, fast heartbeat, increased sweating, increased appetite, and nausea.

DRUG INTERACTIONS: Alcohol, anxiety medications, and narcotic painkillers may intensify the drowsiness effect of the drug. Individuals should not take Nardil or Parnate while taking this drug. The drug should also not be used with Akineton, Artane, Cogentin, and Kemadrin.

ALLERGIES: Individuals allergic to cyproheptadine or any of its derivatives should discuss this with their doctor or pharmacist before using this drug.

PREGNANCY/BREAST-FEEDING: Category B—No evidence of risk in humans. Either animal findings show risk, but human findings do not; or, if no adequate human studies have been done, animal findings show no risk. It is not known whether the drug is excreted in the breast milk; therefore, caution should be used when breast-feeding.

OTHER BRAND NAMES: None

OTHER DRUGS IN THE SAME THERAPEUTIC CLASS: Atarax, Benadryl, PBZ, Tavist, Temaril, and Vistaril

IMPORTANT INFORMATION TO REMEMBER: This drug does cause drowsiness. Individuals should use caution when driving, operating machinery, or performing any task where mental alertness is required. Alcohol, anxiety medications, or narcotic painkillers may intensify the drowsiness effect of the drug. This drug may also cause a dry mouth; sugarless gum or hard candy will help take care of this problem. Patients with glaucoma or urinary or prostate problems should consult their doctor before taking this drug.

BRAND NAME: Peridex

GENERIC NAME: chlorhexidine gluconate

GENERIC FORM AVAILABLE: Yes

THERAPEUTIC CLASS: Antibacterial dental rinse

DOSAGE FORMS: 0.12% oral rinse

MAIN USES: For use between visits for treatment of gingivitis

USUAL DOSE: Use twice daily, morning and evening, after brushing teeth, rinsing with 1/2 ounce for 30 seconds.

AVERAGE PRICE: $19.89 (B)/$16.64 (G) for 480 mL

SIDE EFFECTS: Most common: change in taste, increased tartar on the teeth, and staining of the teeth, dentures, fillings, or other mouth appliances. Less common: swollen glands on the sides of the face, mouth irritation, and irritation of the tip of the tongue.

DRUG INTERACTIONS: None of any clinical significance

ALLERGIES: Individuals allergic to chlorhexidine gluconate or any of its derivatives should discuss this with their doctor or pharmacist before using this drug.

PREGNANCY/BREAST-FEEDING: Category B—No evidence of risk in humans. Either animal findings show risk, but human findings do not; or, if no adequate human studies have been done, animal findings show no risk. It is not known whether the drug is excreted in the breast milk; therefore, caution should be used when breast-feeding.

OTHER BRAND NAMES: None

OTHER DRUGS IN THE SAME THERAPEUTIC CLASS: None

IMPORTANT INFORMATION TO REMEMBER: The drug should be used after brushing and flossing. Swish the drug around in the mouth for the full 30 seconds and spit it out. Do not swallow the solution after use. Do not rinse your mouth with water after use. The drug may stain fillings, dentures, braces, and teeth.

BRAND NAME: Permax

GENERIC NAME: pergolide

GENERIC FORM AVAILABLE: No

THERAPEUTIC CLASS: Dopamine agonist

DOSAGE FORMS: 0.05-mg, 0.25-mg, and 1-mg tablets

MAIN USES: Parkinson's disease

USUAL DOSE: Take three times daily: 0.05 mg/day for first two days, then gradually increase the dose to 0.1 mg/day or 0.15 mg/day every third day over the next 12 days, and then increases of 0.25 mg/day every third day as needed. The average daily dose is 3 mg/day.

AVERAGE PRICE: $62.21 for 0.05 mg, $129.29 for 0.25 mg, and $467.91 for 1 mg

SIDE EFFECTS: dyskinesias (impairment of movements, jerky movements, etc.) 62%, nausea 24%, dizziness 19%, hallucinations 14%, runny nose 12%, confusion 11%, constipation 11%, drowsiness 10%, low blood pressure when rising from a sitting or lying-down position 9%, insomnia 8%, pain 7%, swelling 7%, abnormal vision 6%, diarrhea 6%, stomach pain 6%, nervousness 6%, trouble breathing 5%, loss of appetite 5%, headache 5%, dry mouth 4%, weakness 4%, chest pain 4%, tremor 4%, flu-like symptoms 3%, vomiting 3%, back pain 2%, pounding heartbeat 2%, low blood pressure 2%, dizziness 2%, muscle pain 2%, and taste changes 2%.

DRUG INTERACTIONS: None of any clinical significance

ALLERGIES: Individuals allergic to pergolide or any of its derivatives should discuss this with their doctor or pharmacist before using this drug.

PREGNANCY/BREAST-FEEDING: Category B—No evidence of risk in humans. Either animal findings show risk, but human findings do not; or, if no adequate human studies have been done, animal findings show no risk. It is not known whether the drug is excreted in the breast milk; therefore, caution should be used when breast-feeding.

OTHER BRAND NAMES: None

OTHER DRUGS IN THE SAME THERAPEUTIC CLASS: Parlodel and Symmetrel

IMPORTANT INFORMATION TO REMEMBER: Do not discontinue the drug without first consulting your physician and only take the drug exactly as directed. This drug may cause some dizziness and drowsiness. Individuals should use caution when driving, operating machinery, or performing any task where mental alertness is required. Alcohol, anxiety medications, and narcotic painkillers may intensify the dizziness and drowsiness effect of the drug. Individuals should get up slowly from a sitting or lying-down position; otherwise dizziness may occur.

BRAND NAME: Persantine

GENERIC NAME: dipyridamole

GENERIC FORM AVAILABLE: Yes

THERAPEUTIC CLASS: Antiplatelet

DOSAGE FORMS: 25-mg, 50-mg, and 75-mg tablets

MAIN USES: Increase blood circulation

USUAL DOSE: 25 mg to 75 mg taken three to four times daily

AVERAGE PRICE: $40.13 (B)/$9.77 (G) for 25 mg; $53.11 (B)/$11.64 (G) for 50 mg; $73.68 (B)/$16.70 (G) for 75 mg

SIDE EFFECTS: dizziness 14%, stomach irritation 6%, nausea 5%, headache 2%, and rash 2%.

DRUG INTERACTIONS: None of any clinical significance

ALLERGIES: Individuals allergic to dipyridamole or any of its derivatives should discuss this with their doctor or pharmacist before using this drug.

PREGNANCY/BREAST-FEEDING: Category B—No evidence of risk in humans. Either animal findings show risk, but human findings do not; or, if no adequate human studies have been done, animal findings show no risk. It is not known whether the drug is excreted in the breast milk; therefore, caution should be used when breast-feeding.

OTHER BRAND NAMES: None

OTHER DRUGS IN THE SAME THERAPEUTIC CLASS: Aspirin and Ticlid

IMPORTANT INFORMATION TO REMEMBER: Do not use aspirin unless it is prescribed by your physician. Only take the drug exactly as directed by your physician. Do not discontinue taking the drug unless directed to do so by your physician.

BRAND NAME: Phenergan and Phenergan VC

GENERIC NAME: promethazine

GENERIC FORM AVAILABLE: Yes (tablets and syrup only)

THERAPEUTIC CLASS: Phenothiazine antihistamine

DOSAGE FORMS: 12.5-mg, 25-mg, and 50-mg tablets; 6.25 mg/5 mL syrup; 25 mg/6 mL syrup (Phenergan Fortis); 12.5-mg, 25-mg, and 50-mg suppositories; and 6.25 mg promethazine/5 mg phenylephrine per 5 mL syrup (Phenergan VC)

MAIN USES: Allergies, allergic reactions, cough, nausea, vomiting, and motion sickness

USUAL DOSE: For allergies: 6.25 mg to 12.5 mg in the tablet form three to four times daily, or 25 mg at bedtime. For nausea and vomiting: 12.5 mg to 25 mg every four to six hours. For cough: one teaspoon every four to six hours.

AVERAGE PRICE: $27.16 (brand name only) for 12.5-mg tablets; $47.98 (B)/$10.54 (G) for 25-mg tablets; $73.54 (B)/$19.23 (G) for 50-mg tablets; $40.81 for 12.5-mg suppositories (box of 12);

$46.84 for 25-mg suppositories (box of 12); $59.97 for 50-mg suppositories (box of 12); and $12.45 (B)/$7.91 (G) for syrups (120 mL)

SIDE EFFECTS: Most common: drowsiness, thickening of mucus, and dry mouth. Less common: blurred vision, difficult or painful urination, dizziness, fast heartbeat, increased sweating, and increased appetite.

DRUG INTERACTIONS: Alcohol, anxiety medications, and narcotic painkillers may intensify the drowsiness effect of the drug. Individuals should not take Nardil or Parnate while taking this drug. The drug should also not be used with Akineton, Artane, Cogentin, and Kemadrin.

ALLERGIES: Individuals allergic to promethazine or any of its derivatives should discuss this with their doctor or pharmacist before using this drug.

PREGNANCY/BREAST-FEEDING: Category C—Risk cannot be ruled out. Human studies are lacking, and animal studies are either positive for fetal risk or lacking as well. However, potential benefits may justify the potential risk in using the drug. It is not known whether the drug is excreted in the breast milk; therefore, caution should be used when breast-feeding.

OTHER BRAND NAMES: None

OTHER DRUGS IN THE SAME THERAPEUTIC CLASS: Temaril

IMPORTANT INFORMATION TO REMEMBER: This drug may cause drowsiness. Individuals should use caution when driving, operating machinery, or performing any task where mental alertness is required. Alcohol, anxiety medications, and narcotic painkillers may intensify the drowsiness effect of the drug. This drug may also cause a dry mouth; sugarless gum or hard candy will help take care of this problem. Patients with glaucoma or urinary or prostate problems should consult their doctor before taking this drug.

For the suppository:

Remove the foil wrapper before inserting the suppository. Store in a cool place to avoid melting, preferably the refrigerator. When inserting, lie on one side and bend the top leg slightly. Then insert suppository into rectum about one inch with one finger. Wash hands thoroughly before and after use. Individuals may want to use a finger cot to cover finger when inserting a suppository.

BRAND NAME: Phenergan with Codeine

GENERIC NAME: Combination product containing: promethazine and codeine

GENERIC FORM AVAILABLE: Yes

THERAPEUTIC CLASS: Antihistamine + cough suppressant

DOSAGE FORMS: 6.25 mg promethazine/10 mg codeine phosphate per 5 mL

MAIN USES: Coughs and upper respiratory symptoms associated with allergies

USUAL DOSE: one teaspoon every four to six hours as needed

AVERAGE PRICE: $9.78 (B)/$6.82 (G)

SIDE EFFECTS: Most common: drowsiness, thickening of mucus, and dry mouth. Less common: blurred vision, difficult or painful urination, constipation, dizziness, fast heartbeat, and increased sweating.

DRUG INTERACTIONS: Alcohol, anxiety medications, and narcotic painkillers may intensify the drowsiness effect of the drug. Individuals should not take Nardil or Parnate while taking this drug. The drug should also not be used with Akineton, Artane, Cogentin, and Kemadrin.

ALLERGIES: Individuals allergic to promethazine, codeine, or any of their derivatives should discuss this with their doctor or pharmacist before using this drug.

PREGNANCY/BREAST-FEEDING: Category C—Risk cannot be ruled out. Human studies are lacking, and animal studies are either positive for fetal risk or lacking as well. However, potential benefits may justify the potential risk in using the drug. It is not known whether the drug is excreted in the breast milk; therefore, caution should be used when breast-feeding.

OTHER BRAND NAMES: None

OTHER DRUGS IN THE SAME THERAPEUTIC CLASS: Tussionex

IMPORTANT INFORMATION TO REMEMBER: This drug does cause drowsiness. Individuals should use caution when driving, operating machinery, or performing any task where mental alertness is required. Alcohol, anxiety medications, and narcotic painkillers may intensify the drowsiness effect of the drug. The drug should only be taken as needed to control a cough and congestion; this drug should not be used as a long-term therapy. This medication is a controlled substance and may be habit-forming. If stomach upset occurs, the drug may be taken with food or milk.

BRAND NAME: **Phenobarbital** (various brand-name manufacturers)

GENERIC NAME: phenobarbital

GENERIC FORM AVAILABLE: Yes

THERAPEUTIC CLASS: Barbiturate sedative

DOSAGE FORMS: 15-mg, 30-mg, 60-mg, and 100-mg tablets; and 20 mg/5 mL elixir

MAIN USES: Sedation, convulsions, and seizure control

USUAL DOSE: For sedation: 30 mg to 120 mg daily in two or three divided doses. For convulsions: 60 mg to 200 mg two to three times daily.

AVERAGE PRICE: $6.99 for 15 mg; $10.57 for 30 mg; $14.41 for 60 mg; and $19.93 for 100 mg

SIDE EFFECTS: Most common: drowsiness, clumsiness, unsteadiness, dizziness, lightheadedness, and feeling of a hangover. Less common: nervousness, anxiety, constipation, feeling faint, headache, irritability, nausea, vomiting, nightmares, depression, and insomnia.

DRUG INTERACTIONS: Alcohol, anxiety medications, and narcotic painkillers will intensify the drowsiness effect of the drug. The drug may decrease the blood levels of Aristocort, Coumadin, Decadron, Deltasone, Medrol, prednisone, and Tegretol. The drug may also decrease the effectiveness of birth control pills. The drug may interfere with the absorption of Fulvicin P/G, Grifulvin V, Gris-PEG, and Grisactin. The drug may decrease the blood levels of Vibramycin.

ALLERGIES: Individuals allergic to phenobarbital or other barbiturates (such as those listed under "Other Drugs in the Same Therapeutic Class") should discuss this with their doctor or pharmacist before taking this drug.

PREGNANCY/BREAST-FEEDING: Category D—Positive evidence of risk. Human studies show risk to the fetus. Nevertheless, potential benefits may possibly outweigh the potential risks. This drug should not be taken by nursing mothers.

OTHER BRAND NAMES: None

OTHER DRUGS IN THE SAME THERAPEUTIC CLASS: Amytal, Butisol, Mebaral, Nembutal, Seconal, and Tuinal

IMPORTANT INFORMATION TO REMEMBER: This drug does cause drowsiness. Individuals should use caution when driving, operating machinery, or performing any task where mental alertness is required. Alcohol, anxiety medications, or narcotic painkillers may intensify the drowsiness effect of the drug. This medication is a controlled substance and may be habit-forming. Only take the drug exactly as directed by your physician. Do not increase the dose without first consulting with your physician. Women taking birth control pills should use another form of contraception while taking the drug and for the rest of the current menstrual cycle.

BRAND NAME: Phrenilin and Phrenilin Forte

GENERIC NAME: Combination products containing: butalbital and acetaminophen

GENERIC FORM AVAILABLE: No

THERAPEUTIC CLASS: Barbiturate sedative + analgesic

DOSAGE FORMS: 50-mg butalbital/325-mg acetaminophen tablets (Phrenilin); and 50-mg butalbital/650-mg acetaminophen tablets (Phrenilin Forte)

MAIN USES: Tension headache

USUAL DOSE: One to two tablets every four hours as needed (Phrenilin) or one capsule every four hours as needed (Phrenilin Forte). Maximum is six tablets or capsules per day.

AVERAGE PRICE: $31.50 for Phrenilin and $36.33 for Phrenilin Forte

SIDE EFFECTS: Most common: drowsiness, lightheadedness, dizziness, sedation, shortness of breath, nausea, vomiting, stomach pain, and drunken feeling. Less common: headache, shaky feeling, dry mouth, gas, constipation, heartburn, muscle fatigue, leg pain, skin rash, stuffy nose, fever, agitation, heavy eyelids, mental confusion, hot flashes, fast heartbeat, and euphoria.

DRUG INTERACTIONS: Nardil and Parnate may enhance the effects of the drug. Alcohol, anxiety medications, and other narcotic painkillers may intensify the drowsiness effect of the drug. The drug may decrease the effects of Aristocort, Blocadren, Coumadin, Cartrol, Corgard, Decadron, Deltasone, estrogens, Fulvicin P/G, Grifulvin V, Grisactin, Gris-PEG, Inderal, Kerlone, Levatol, Lopressor, Medrol, Normodyne, prednisone, Sectral, Slo-bid, Tenormin, Theo-Dur, theophylline, Toprol-XL, Trandate, Uni-Dur, Uniphyl, Vibramycin, Visken, and Zebeta.

ALLERGIES: Individuals allergic to butalbital, acetaminophen, or any of their derivatives should discuss this with their doctor or pharmacist before using this drug.

PREGNANCY/BREAST-FEEDING: Category C—Risk cannot be ruled out. Human studies are lacking, and animal studies are either positive for fetal risk or lacking as well. However, potential benefits may justify the potential risk in using the drug. The drug is excreted in the breast milk; therefore, extreme caution should be used when breast-feeding.

OTHER BRAND NAMES: None

OTHER DRUGS IN THE SAME THERAPEUTIC CLASS: Axocet, Esgic, Esgic-Plus, Fioricet, and Fiorinal

IMPORTANT INFORMATION TO REMEMBER: This drug does cause drowsiness. Individuals should use caution when driving, operating machinery, or performing any task where mental alertness is required. Alcohol, anxiety medications, and narcotic painkillers may intensify the drowsiness effect of the drug. If stomach upset occurs, take the drug with food or milk. Do not increase the dose without first consulting with your physician. Before taking over-the-counter pain relievers, consult your doctor or pharmacist. This drug may be habit-forming.

BRAND NAME: Pilocar

GENERIC NAME: pilocarpine

See entry for Isopto Carpine

BRAND NAME: Pilopine HS

GENERIC NAME: pilocarpine

GENERIC FORM AVAILABLE: No

THERAPEUTIC CLASS: Miotic anti-glaucoma

DOSAGE FORMS: 4% eye gel

MAIN USES: Glaucoma

USUAL DOSE: Apply ½-inch ribbon in lower eyelid at bedtime.

AVERAGE PRICE: $32.38

SIDE EFFECTS: Most common: blurred vision, changes in near or far vision, and decrease in night vision. Less common: eye irritation, headache, eyebrow ache, and eye pain.

DRUG INTERACTIONS: None of any clinical significance

ALLERGIES: Individuals allergic to pilocarpine or any of its derivatives should discuss this with their doctor or pharmacist before using this drug.

PREGNANCY/BREAST-FEEDING: Category C—Risk cannot be ruled out. Human studies are lacking, and animal studies are either positive for fetal risk or lacking as well. However, potential benefits may justify the potential risk in using the drug. It is not known whether the drug is excreted in the breast milk; therefore, caution should be used when breast-feeding.

OTHER BRAND NAMES: None

OTHER DRUGS IN THE SAME THERAPEUTIC CLASS: Isopto Carbachol, Isopto Carpine, Ocusert Pilo, and Pilocar

IMPORTANT INFORMATION TO REMEMBER: Caution should be used when driving or doing other activities at night or in dim light. Changes in near or distance vision can occur with this drug. When using the drug, pull the bottom eyelid down gently. Then apply a small, thin ribbon of ointment along the rim of the lower eyelid between the eyelid and the eyeball. After application, close the eye and roll the eyeball around. Your vision may be slightly blurred after application. If another medication is to be used in the eye, wait at least 10 minutes before administering it. Do not discontinue the drug without first consulting your physician and use exactly as directed.

BRAND NAME: Plaquenil

GENERIC NAME: hydroxychloroquine

GENERIC FORM AVAILABLE: Yes

THERAPEUTIC CLASS: Aminoquinolone

DOSAGE FORMS: 200-mg tablets

MAIN USES: Malaria, lupus, and arthritis

USUAL DOSE: For prevention of malaria: 400 mg taken once weekly, beginning two weeks prior to exposure and continuing for eight weeks after leaving the area. For treatment of malaria: 800 mg initially, followed by 400 mg in six hours, followed by 400 mg daily for two more days. For arthritis: 200 mg to 600 mg daily. For lupus: 200 mg to 400 mg once or twice daily.

AVERAGE PRICE: $170.43 (B)/$154.78 (G)

SIDE EFFECTS: Most common: difficulty in reading (ciliary muscle dysfunction), diarrhea, nausea, loss of appetite, stomach pain, vomiting, headache, and itching (especially in African-American patients). Less common: bleaching of the hair; hair loss; blue-black discoloration of the skin, fingernails, or inside of the mouth; dizziness; nervousness; rash; blurred vision; changes in vision; and blood disorders (which are usually rare).

DRUG INTERACTIONS: None of any clinical significance

ALLERGIES: Individuals allergic to hydroxychloroquine or any of its derivatives should discuss this with their doctor or pharmacist before using this drug.

PREGNANCY/BREAST-FEEDING: Category C—Risk cannot be ruled out. Human studies are lacking, and animal studies are either positive for fetal risk or lacking as well. However, potential benefits may justify the potential risk in using the drug. The drug is excreted in the breast milk; therefore, extreme caution should be used when breast-feeding.

OTHER BRAND NAMES: None

OTHER DRUGS IN THE SAME THERAPEUTIC CLASS: Aralen and Lariam (for malaria only)

IMPORTANT INFORMATION TO REMEMBER: Take the drug exactly as directed by your physician. The drug should be taken with food or milk to reduce the potential for stomach upset. For malaria, take the drug for the full course of treatment. Regular blood tests and vision exams should be conducted if the drug is to be taken for a long time. If flu-like symptoms; aches; soreness of the mouth, gums, throat, or joints; vision problems; or unusual bleeding/bruising occur, notify your physician.

BRAND NAME: Plendil

GENERIC NAME: felodipine

GENERIC FORM AVAILABLE: No

THERAPEUTIC CLASS: Calcium channel blocker

DOSAGE FORMS: 2.5-mg, 5-mg, and 10-mg extended-release tablets

MAIN USES: High blood pressure

USUAL DOSE: 2.5 mg to 10 mg once daily

AVERAGE PRICE: $119.51 for 2.5 mg; $135.54 for 5 mg; and $225.43 for 10 mg

SIDE EFFECTS: swelling 14%–20%, headache 11%–19%, flushing 3%–8%, dizziness 1%, pounding heartbeat 1%, and some drowsiness at first.

DRUG INTERACTIONS: The effects of Blocadren, Cartrol, Corgard, Inderal, Kerlone, Levatol, Lopressor, Minipress, Normodyne, Sectral, Tenormin, Toprol-XL, Trandate, Visken, and Zebeta may be increased when taken with this drug. The drug may increase the blood levels of Lanoxin. Tagamet may increase the blood levels of the drug. Drugs used for seizures and epilepsy may decrease the blood levels of the drug significantly.

ALLERGIES: Individuals allergic to felodipine or any of its derivatives should discuss this with their doctor or pharmacist before using this drug.

PREGNANCY/BREAST-FEEDING: Category C—Risk cannot be ruled out. Human studies are lacking, and animal studies are either positive for fetal risk or lacking as well. However, potential benefits may justify the potential risk in using the drug. It is not known whether the drug is excreted in the breast milk; therefore, caution should be used when breast-feeding.

OTHER BRAND NAMES: None

OTHER DRUGS IN THE SAME THERAPEUTIC CLASS: Adalat, Adalat CC, Calan, Calan SR, Cardene, Cardene SR, Cardizem, Cardizem CD, Cardizem SR, Covera-HS, Dilacor XR, DynaCirc, Isoptin, Isoptin SR, Norvasc, Procardia, Procardia XL, Sular, Vascor, and Verelan

IMPORTANT INFORMATION TO REMEMBER: Only take the drug exactly as directed by your physician. Do not discontinue taking the drug without first consulting your physician. The drug should not be taken with grapefruit juice. Before taking over-the-counter cold and allergy preparations, consult your doctor or pharmacist—these products may raise your blood pressure. This drug may cause some drowsiness at first. Individuals should use caution when driving, operating machinery, or performing any task where mental alertness is required.

BRAND NAME: Poly-Histine CS and Poly-Histine DM

GENERIC NAME: Combination products containing: codeine, brompheniramine, dextromethorphan (instead of codeine in Poly-Histine DM), and phenylpropanolamine

GENERIC FORM AVAILABLE: Yes

THERAPEUTIC CLASS: Antihistamine + cough suppressant + decongestant

DOSAGE FORMS: 10 mg codeine/2 mg brompheniramine/12.5 mg phenylpropanolamine per 5 mL syrup (Poly-Histine CS); and 10 mg dextromethorphan/2 mg brompheniramine/12.5 mg phenylpropanolamine per 5 mL syrup (Poly-Histine DM)

MAIN USES: Cough, congestion, and runny nose

USUAL DOSE: One to two teaspoons every four hours as needed. Doses for children may be less.

AVERAGE PRICE: $17.03 (B)/$13.26 (G) for Poly-Histine CS (120 mL); and $16.94 (B)/$12.96 (G) for Poly-Histine DM (120 mL)

SIDE EFFECTS: Most common: drowsiness and dizziness. Less common: headache, visual disturbances, disorientation, upset stomach, stomach pain, constipation, nausea, vomiting, and nervousness (especially in children).

DRUG INTERACTIONS: Alcohol, anxiety medications, and narcotic painkillers may intensify the drowsiness effect of the drug. Nardil or Parnate may increase the effects of the drug. The drug may also reduce the effects of blood-pressure-lowering drugs.

ALLERGIES: Individuals allergic to codeine, brompheniramine, dextromethorphan, phenylpropanolamine, or any of their derivatives should discuss this with their doctor or pharmacist before using this drug.

PREGNANCY/BREAST-FEEDING: Category C—Risk cannot be ruled out. Human studies are lacking, and animal studies are either positive for fetal risk or lacking as well. However, potential benefits may justify the potential risk in using the drug. The drug is excreted in the breast milk; therefore, extreme caution should be used when breast-feeding.

OTHER BRAND NAMES: None

OTHER DRUGS IN THE SAME THERAPEUTIC CLASS: Actifed w/Codeine, Bromfed-DM, Dimetane-DX, Rondec-DM, and Ru-Tuss w/Hydrocodone

IMPORTANT INFORMATION TO REMEMBER: This drug does cause drowsiness. Individuals should use caution when driving, operating machinery, or performing any task where mental alertness is required. Alcohol, anxiety medications, and narcotic painkillers may intensify the drowsiness effect of the drug. The drug should only be taken as needed to control a cough and congestion. This drug should not be used as a long-term therapy. This medication is a controlled substance and may be habit-forming (Poly-Histine CS only). If stomach upset occurs, the drug may be taken with food or milk.

BRAND NAME: Poly-Histine-D

GENERIC NAME: Combination product containing: pheniramine, pyrilamine, phenyltoloxamine, and phenylpropanolamine

GENERIC FORM AVAILABLE: Yes

THERAPEUTIC CLASS: Antihistamine + decongestant

DOSAGE FORMS: 16-mg pheniramine/16-mg pyrilamine/16-mg phenyltoloxamine/50-mg phenylpropanolamine extended-release capsules (Poly-Histine-D); 8-mg pheniramine/8-mg pyrilamine/8-mg phenyltoloxamine/25-mg phenylpropanolamine extended-release capsules (Poly-Histine-D Ped Caps); and 4 mg pheniramine/4 mg pyrilamine/4 mg phenyltoloxamine/12.5 mg phenylpropanolamine per 5 mL syrup (Poly-Histine-D Elixir)

MAIN USES: Allergies and congestion

USUAL DOSE: One capsule every 8 to 12 hours. Doses for children may be less.

AVERAGE PRICE: $104.94 (B)/$41.82 (G) for Poly-Histine-D capsules; and $14.69 (B)/$11.09 (G) for Poly-Histine-D Elixir (120 mL)

SIDE EFFECTS: Most common: drowsiness. Less common: nausea, giddiness, dry mouth, blurred vision, pounding heartbeat, flushing, and increased irritability or excitability (especially in children).

DRUG INTERACTIONS: Blocadren, Cartrol, Corgard, Inderal, Kerlone, Levatol, Lopressor, Normodyne, Sectral, Tenormin, Toprol-XL, Trandate, Visken, and Zebeta may increase the effects of the drug. The drug may also reduce the effects of blood-pressure-lowering drugs. Nardil or Parnate may significantly raise blood pressure when taken with this drug.

ALLERGIES: Individuals allergic to pheniramine, pyrilamine, phenyltoloxamine, phenylpropanolamine, or any of their derivatives should discuss this with their doctor or pharmacist before using this drug.

PREGNANCY/BREAST-FEEDING: Category C—Risk cannot be ruled out. Human studies are lacking, and animal studies are either positive for fetal risk or lacking as well. However, potential benefits may justify the potential risk in using the drug. It is not known whether the drug is excreted in the breast milk; therefore, caution should be used when breast-feeding.

OTHER BRAND NAMES: None

OTHER DRUGS IN THE SAME THERAPEUTIC CLASS: Bromfed, Bromfed PD, Claritin-D, Comhist LA, Deconamine SR, Fedahist, Naldecon, Novafed-A, Nucofed, Ornade, Rondec, Rynatan, Seldane-D, Semprex-D, Tavist-D, and Trinalin

IMPORTANT INFORMATION TO REMEMBER: This drug does cause drowsiness. Individuals should use caution when driving, operating machinery, or performing any task where mental alertness is required. Alcohol, anxiety medications, and narcotic painkillers

may intensify the drowsiness effect of the drug. This drug may also cause a dry mouth; sugarless gum or hard candy will help take care of this problem. Patients with glaucoma, high blood pressure, heart conditions, or urinary or prostrate problems should consult their doctor before taking this drug.

BRAND NAME: Polytrim

GENERIC NAME: Combination product containing: trimethoprim and polymyxin B

GENERIC FORM AVAILABLE: No

THERAPEUTIC CLASS: Antibiotic eyedrop

DOSAGE FORMS: 1 mg trimethoprim/10,000 units polymyxin B per mL eyedrop solution

MAIN USES: Bacterial eye infections

USUAL DOSE: one drop every three hours (maximum of six doses per day)

AVERAGE PRICE: $24.44

SIDE EFFECTS: Most common: itching, redness, and irritation. Less common: burning, tearing, and stinging.

DRUG INTERACTIONS: None of any clinical significance

ALLERGIES: Individuals allergic to polymyxin B, trimethoprim, or any of their derivatives should discuss this with their doctor or pharmacist before using this drug.

PREGNANCY/BREAST-FEEDING: Category C—Risk cannot be ruled out. Human studies are lacking, and animal studies are either positive for fetal risk or lacking as well. However, potential benefits may justify the potential risk in using the drug. It is not known whether the drug is excreted in the breast milk; therefore, caution should be used when breast-feeding.

OTHER BRAND NAMES: None

OTHER DRUGS IN THE SAME THERAPEUTIC CLASS: Bleph-10, Isopto Cetamide, Polysporin, Neosporin, and Sulamyd

IMPORTANT INFORMATION TO REMEMBER: Individuals should not use the drug while wearing contact lenses unless directed otherwise by a doctor. Keep the container tightly closed and avoid touching the applicator tip to the eye—this could contaminate the product over time. Also, only administer one drop at a time. After application, keep the eye open for at least 30 seconds, roll the eyeball around, and avoid squinting. If a second drop is required, wait one to two minutes between drops. If another medication is to be used in the eye, wait at least 10 minutes before administering it.

BRAND NAME: Ponstel

GENERIC NAME: mefenamic acid

GENERIC FORM AVAILABLE: No

THERAPEUTIC CLASS: Nonsteroidal anti-inflammatory drug (NSAID)

DOSAGE FORMS: 250-mg capsules

MAIN USES: Arthritis, pain relief, and menstrual pain

USUAL DOSE: initially 500 mg, followed by 250 mg every six hours

AVERAGE PRICE: $134.51

SIDE EFFECTS: stomach pain 3%–9%, diarrhea 3%–9%, nausea 3%–9%, skin rash 1%–3%, anemia 1%–3%, bloated feeling 1%–3%, gas 1%–3%, constipation 1%–3%, heartburn 1%–3%, and indigestion 1%–3%.

DRUG INTERACTIONS: Aspirin will decrease the concentration of this drug in the blood. This drug may also decrease the effects of Dyazide, HydroDIURIL, Lasix, Maxzide, and other water pills. The drug may increase the blood levels of Eskalith, Lithobid, and Sandimmune. The drug may increase the toxic effects of the drug Rheumatrex. Caution should be used when taking the drug with Coumadin.

ALLERGIES: Individuals allergic to mefenamic acid or other NSAIDs (such as those listed under "Other Drugs in the Same Therapeutic Class") should discuss this with their doctor or pharmacist before taking this drug.

PREGNANCY/BREAST-FEEDING: Category C—Risk cannot be ruled out. Human studies are lacking, and animal studies are either positive for fetal risk or lacking as well. However, potential benefits may justify the potential risk in using the drug. The drug should not, however, be used during the late stages (last three months) of pregnancy. The drug is excreted in the breast milk; therefore, extreme caution should be used when breast-feeding.

OTHER BRAND NAMES: None

OTHER DRUGS IN THE SAME THERAPEUTIC CLASS: Anaprox, Ansaid, aspirin, Cataflam, Clinoril, Daypro, Disalcid, Dolobid, Easprin, Feldene, Indocin, Lodine, Motrin, Nalfon, Naprosyn, Orudis, Oruvail, Relafen, Tolectin, and Voltaren

IMPORTANT INFORMATION TO REMEMBER: This drug should be taken with food or milk to reduce the potential for injury to the stomach lining and stomach upset. This drug may take up to two weeks before a noticeable improvement in pain relief associated with arthritis is observed. Drinking alcohol while taking this drug may increase its potential to cause ulcers. This drug should only be used under the direct supervision of a doctor by individuals with a bleeding disorder or ulcer, or those who are currently taking Coumadin. Before taking over-the-counter pain relievers, consult your doctor or pharmacist. No more than one pain reliever should be taken at any one time unless otherwise directed by your doctor.

BRAND NAME: Pravachol

GENERIC NAME: pravastatin

GENERIC FORM AVAILABLE: No

THERAPEUTIC CLASS: Cholesterol-lowering agent

DOSAGE FORMS: 10-mg, 20-mg, and 40-mg tablets

MAIN USES: High cholesterol

USUAL DOSE: 10 mg to 40 mg daily at bedtime

AVERAGE PRICE: $210.63 for 10 mg; $269.37 for 20 mg; and $447.34 for 40 mg

SIDE EFFECTS: nausea 3%, gas 3%, constipation 2%, heartburn 2%, tiredness 2%, headache 2%, diarrhea 2%, stomach pain 2%, rash 1%, muscle pain 1%, and urinary problems 1%.

DRUG INTERACTIONS: Lopid, niacin and Sandimmune may cause kidney problems when taken with the drug. Prilosec, Tagamet, and Zantac may increase the blood levels of the drug. The drug may increase the effects of Coumadin. Lopid and the drug, when taken together, may increase the risk of developing rhabdomyolysis (destruction and death of muscle tissue). Symptoms are muscle pain and dark, red-brown colored urine.

ALLERGIES: Individuals allergic to pravastatin, Lescol, Mevacor, Zocor, or any of their derivatives should discuss this with their doctor or pharmacist before using this drug.

PREGNANCY/BREAST-FEEDING: Category X—Should not be used during pregnancy. Studies in animals and/or humans have shown fetal abnormalities and birth defects. The risks associated with using this drug clearly outweigh benefits. This drug should never be used by someone who is pregnant or trying to become pregnant. Also, women should never breast-feed while using this drug.

OTHER BRAND NAMES: None

OTHER DRUGS IN THE SAME THERAPEUTIC CLASS: Lescol, Lipitor, Mevacor, and Zocor

IMPORTANT INFORMATION TO REMEMBER: If stomach upset occurs, take the drug with food or milk. Only take the drug exactly as directed by your physician. It is also important to follow the prescribed low cholesterol diet. Report any sign of unexplained muscle pain or tenderness to your doctor, especially it if is accompanied by tiredness or fever.

BRAND NAME: Precose

GENERIC NAME: acarbose

GENERIC FORM AVAILABLE: No

THERAPEUTIC CLASS: Alpha-glucosidase inhibitor

DOSAGE FORMS: 50-mg and 100-mg tablets

MAIN USES: Diabetes

USUAL DOSE: 25 mg to 100 mg three times daily

AVERAGE PRICE: $64.85 for 50 mg and $82.90 for 100 mg

SIDE EFFECTS: gas 77%, diarrhea 33%, and stomach pain 21%.

DRUG INTERACTIONS: None of any clinical significance

ALLERGIES: Individuals allergic to acarbose or any of its derivatives should discuss this with their doctor or pharmacist before using this drug.

PREGNANCY/BREAST-FEEDING: Category B—No evidence of risk in humans. Either animal findings show risk, but human findings do not; or, if no adequate human studies have been done, animal findings show no risk. The drug is excreted in the breast milk; therefore, extreme caution should be used when breast-feeding.

OTHER BRAND NAMES: None

OTHER DRUGS IN THE SAME THERAPEUTIC CLASS: None

IMPORTANT INFORMATION TO REMEMBER: This drug should be taken exactly as directed by your physician. Do not increase the dose or stop taking the drug without first consulting your physician. It is very important to take this drug at the beginning (first bite) of each meal for it to work properly.

BRAND NAME: Pred Mild and Pred Forte

GENERIC NAME: prednisolone acetate

GENERIC FORM AVAILABLE: No

THERAPEUTIC CLASS: Steroid eyedrop

DOSAGE FORMS: 0.12% prednisolone acetate eyedrop suspension (Pred Mild) and 1% prednisolone acetate eyedrop suspension (Pred Forte)

MAIN USES: Inflammation of the eye

USUAL DOSE: one to two drops two to four times daily

AVERAGE PRICE: $29.23 for 10 mL Pred Mild and $34.84 for 10 mL Pred Forte

SIDE EFFECTS: Most common: temporary, mild blurred vision. Less common: burning, itching, redness, watering of the eyes, and eye pain.

DRUG INTERACTIONS: The drug may decrease the effects of other eyedrops used to treat glaucoma.

ALLERGIES: Individuals allergic to prednisolone acetate or any of its derivations should discuss this with their doctor or pharmacist before using this drug.

PREGNANCY/BREAST-FEEDING: Category C—Risk cannot be ruled out. Human studies are lacking, and animal studies are either positive for fetal risk or lacking as well. However, potential benefits may justify the potential risk in using the drug. It is not known whether the drug is excreted in the breast milk; therefore, caution should be used when breast-feeding.

OTHER BRAND NAMES: None

OTHER DRUGS IN THE SAME THERAPEUTIC CLASS: Decadron, Econopred, Flarex, FML, FML Forte, HMS, Inflamase Forte, Inflamase Mild, Maxidex, and Vexol

IMPORTANT INFORMATION TO REMEMBER: Individuals should not use the drug while wearing contact lenses unless directed otherwise by a physician. Keep the container tightly closed and avoid touching the applicator tip to the eye—this could contaminate the product over time. Also, only administer one drop at a time. After application, keep the eye open for at least 30 seconds, roll the eyeball around, and avoid squinting. If a second drop is required, wait one to two minutes between drops. If another medication is to be used in the eye, wait at least 10 minutes before administering it. Shake the medication well before using.

BRAND NAME: Prelone

GENERIC NAME: prednisolone

Very similar to Pediapred. See entry for Pediapred.

BRAND NAME: Premarin

GENERIC NAME: conjugated estrogens

GENERIC FORM AVAILABLE: No

THERAPEUTIC CLASS: Estrogen replacement

DOSAGE FORMS: 0.3-mg, 0.625-mg, 0.9-mg, 1.25-mg, and 2.5-mg tablets; and 0.625 mg per gram vaginal cream

MAIN USES: Menopausal disorders, prevention of osteoporosis, and vaginal atrophy (cream only)

USUAL DOSE: For the tablets: 0.3 mg to 2.5 mg every day, or on three weeks and off one week. For the cream: 0.5 g to 2 g of cream every day, or on three weeks and off one week. For osteoporosis: 0.625 mg daily for three weeks, then off for one week as a regular cycle.

AVERAGE PRICE: $42.18 for 0.3 mg; $58.77 for 0.625 mg; $69.59 for 0.9 mg; $80.41 for 1.25 mg; $139.27 for 2.5 mg; $48.35 for 0.625-mg vaginal cream with applicator (42.5 g)

SIDE EFFECTS: Most common: breast tenderness, breast pain, breast enlargement, swelling of feet and lower legs, stomach cramps, bloating, and nausea. Less common: changes in cervical secretions, yeast infections, headache, diarrhea, vomiting, migraine, loss of scalp hair, increased facial hair, depression, weight changes, dizziness, breakthrough bleeding, and changes in sex drive.

DRUG INTERACTIONS: The drug may interfere with the actions of Parlodel. The drug may increase the blood levels of Sandimmune. Liver toxicity may be increased when used with Dantrium.

ALLERGIES: Individuals allergic to conjugated estrogens, other estrogens, or any of their derivatives should discuss this with their doctor or pharmacist before using this drug.

PREGNANCY/BREAST-FEEDING: Category X—Should not be used during pregnancy. Studies in animals and/or humans have shown fetal abnormalities and birth defects. The risks associated with using this drug clearly outweigh the benefits. This drug should never be used by someone who is pregnant or trying to become pregnant. Also, women should never breast-feed while using this drug.

OTHER BRAND NAMES: None

OTHER DRUGS IN THE SAME THERAPEUTIC CLASS: Climara, Estinyl, Estrace, ESTRADERM, ESTRATAB, Ortho Dienestrol, Ogen, Ortho-Est, and Tace

IMPORTANT INFORMATION TO REMEMBER: Use the drug exactly as directed by your physician. Do not discontinue the drug without first consulting your physician. Caution should be used by patients with previous or current episodes of cancer, high blood pressure, heart disease, or any other cardiovascular or blood vessel disease. This drug may increase the risk of uterine cancer in women who have been through menopause. Report any abnormal vaginal bleeding to your doctor immediately. If using the vaginal cream, insert the applicator high into the vagina (two-thirds the length of the applicator) and push the plunger to release the cream. Do not use a tampon to hold the cream inside the vagina.

BRAND NAME: Prempro and Premphase

GENERIC NAME: Combination product containing: conjugated estrogens and medroxyprogesterone

See individual entries for Premarin and Provera

BRAND NAME: Prenate 90

GENERIC NAME: prenatal multivitamin with docusate sodium

GENERIC FORM AVAILABLE: No

THERAPEUTIC CLASS: Prenatal vitamin supplement + stool softener

DOSAGE FORMS: multivitamin tablets

MAIN USES: Nutritional supplement during pregnancy and breast-feeding

USUAL DOSE: one tablet daily

AVERAGE PRICE: $48.29 (B)/$28.39 (G)

SIDE EFFECTS: Most common: none. Less common: diarrhea, gas, and stomach upset.

DRUG INTERACTIONS: The B vitamins in the drug may increase the effect of Larodopa.

ALLERGIES: Individuals allergic to multivitamins or any of their derivatives should discuss this with their doctor or pharmacist before using this drug.

PREGNANCY/BREAST-FEEDING: Category B—No evidence of risk in humans. Either animal findings show risk, but human findings do not; or, if no adequate human studies have been done, animal findings show no risk. It is not known whether the drug is excreted in the breast milk; therefore, caution should be used when breast-feeding. This drug is safe to use during pregnancy.

OTHER BRAND NAMES: None

OTHER DRUGS IN THE SAME THERAPEUTIC CLASS: Materna, Natal-ins Rx, Stuartnatal Plus, and Zenate

IMPORTANT INFORMATION TO REMEMBER: Only take the drug exactly as directed by your physician. Do not discontinue taking the drug without first consulting your physician. If stomach upset occurs, the drug may be taken with food or milk.

BRAND NAME: Prevacid

GENERIC NAME: lansoprazole

GENERIC FORM AVAILABLE: No

THERAPEUTIC CLASS: Acid pump inhibitor

DOSAGE FORMS: 15-mg and 30-mg enteric coated granules in capsules

MAIN USES: Ulcers, gastroesophageal reflux disease (GERD), and Zollinger-Ellison syndrome

USUAL DOSE: 15 mg to 30 mg once daily before eating

AVERAGE PRICE: $141.05 for 15 mg (30 capsules) and $149.74 for 30 mg (30 capsules)

SIDE EFFECTS: diarrhea 4%, stomach pain 2%, and nausea 1%.

DRUG INTERACTIONS: Carafate may decrease the absorption of the drug. The drug may decrease the absorption of Nizoral.

ALLERGIES: Individuals allergic to lansoprazole or any of its derivatives should discuss this with their doctor or pharmacist before using this drug.

PREGNANCY/BREAST-FEEDING: Category B—No evidence of risk in humans. Either animal findings show risk, but human findings do not; or, if no adequate human studies have been done, animal findings show no risk. It is not known whether the drug is excreted in the breast milk; therefore, caution should be used when breast-feeding

OTHER BRAND NAMES: None

OTHER DRUGS IN THE SAME THERAPEUTIC CLASS: Prilosec

IMPORTANT INFORMATION TO REMEMBER: Only take the drug exactly as directed by your physician. Also, do not increase the dose without first consulting with your physician. The drug should be taken 30 minutes before eating. Antacids may be taken at the same time for short-term relief of stomach acid and heartburn. The capsules should be swallowed whole. The capsules may, however, be sprinkled on soft food (such as applesauce) and swallowed without chewing.

BRAND NAME: Prilosec

GENERIC NAME: omeprazole

GENERIC FORM AVAILABLE: No

THERAPEUTIC CLASS: Acid pump inhibitor

DOSAGE FORMS: 10-mg and 20-mg enteric coated granules in capsules

MAIN USES: Ulcers, gastroesophageal reflux disease (GERD), and Zollinger-Ellison syndrome

USUAL DOSE: 20 mg daily

AVERAGE PRICE: $136.58 for 30 capsules

SIDE EFFECTS: headache 7%, diarrhea 3%, stomach pain 2%, nausea 2%, dizziness 2%, vomiting 2%, rash 2%, constipation 1%, weakness 1%, and back pain 1%.

DRUG INTERACTIONS: The drug may decrease the absorption of Nizoral. The drug may increase the blood levels of Coumadin, Dilantin, and Valium.

ALLERGIES: Individuals allergic to omeprazole or any of its derivatives should discuss this with their doctor or pharmacist before using this drug.

PREGNANCY/BREAST-FEEDING: Category C—Risk cannot be ruled out. Human studies are lacking, and animal studies are either positive for fetal risk or lacking as well. However, potential benefits may justify the potential risk in using the drug. It is not known whether the drug is excreted in the breast milk; therefore, caution should be used when breast-feeding.

OTHER BRAND NAMES: None

OTHER DRUGS IN THE SAME THERAPEUTIC CLASS: Prevacid

IMPORTANT INFORMATION TO REMEMBER: Only take the drug exactly as directed by your physician. Also, do not increase the dose without first consulting with your physician. The drug should be taken 30 minutes before eating. Antacids may be taken at the same time for short-term relief of stomach acid and heartburn. The capsules should be swallowed whole. The capsules may, however, be sprinkled on soft food (such as applesauce) and swallowed without chewing.

BRAND NAME: Principen

GENERIC NAME: ampicillin

See entry for Omnipen

BRAND NAME: Prinivil

GENERIC NAME: lisinopril

See entry for Zestril

BRAND NAME: Prinzide

GENERIC NAME: Combination product containing: lisinopril and hydrochlorothiazide

See individual entries for HydroDIURIL and Zestril

BRAND NAME: Pro-Banthīne

GENERIC NAME: propantheline

GENERIC FORM AVAILABLE: Yes

THERAPEUTIC CLASS: Anticholinergic

DOSAGE FORMS: 7.5-mg and 15-mg tablets

MAIN USES: Peptic ulcer and {irritable bowel syndrome}

USUAL DOSE: 7.5 mg to 15 mg taken 30 minutes before each meal and at bedtime

AVERAGE PRICE: $59.72 for 7.5 mg and $90.98 (B)/$25.91 (G) for 15 mg

SIDE EFFECTS: Most common: constipation, decreased sweating, and dry mouth. Less common: drowsiness, blurred vision, difficulty in urinating, difficulty in swallowing, pounding heartbeat, insomnia, decreased saliva, and decreased flow of breast milk.

DRUG INTERACTIONS: Antacids and antidiarrheal drugs may decrease the absorption of the drug. The drug may decrease the absorption of Nizoral. The drug may cause additive adverse effects when used with Compazine, Haldol, Mellaril, Nardil, Parnate, Prolixin, Serentil, Stelazine, Thorazine, and Trilafon.

ALLERGIES: Individuals allergic to propantheline or any of its derivatives should discuss this with their doctor or pharmacist before using this drug.

PREGNANCY/BREAST-FEEDING: Category C—Risk cannot be ruled out. Human studies are lacking, and animal studies are either positive for fetal risks or lacking as well. However, potential benefits may justify the potential risk in using the drug. The drug is excreted in the breast milk; therefore, extreme caution should be used when breast-feeding.

OTHER BRAND NAMES: None

OTHER DRUGS IN THE SAME THERAPEUTIC CLASS: Bentyl, Cantil, Levsin, Robinul, and Spacol

IMPORTANT INFORMATION TO REMEMBER: This drug should be taken 30 minutes before meals. This drug may cause drowsiness or blurred vision. Individuals should use caution when driving, operating machinery, or performing any task where mental alertness is required. Alcohol, anxiety medications, and narcotic painkillers may intensify the blurred vision or drowsiness effects of the drug. This drug may also cause a dry mouth; sugarless gum or hard candy will help take care of this problem. Patients with glaucoma, urinary or prostrate problems, bowel obstructions, or severe ulcerative colitis should consult their doctor before taking this drug. Caution should be used during hot weather due to decreased tolerance to the heat.

BRAND NAME: Probenecid (various brand-name manufacturers)

GENERIC NAME: probenecid

See entry for Benemid

BRAND NAME: Procan SR and Procanbid

GENERIC NAME: procainamide

GENERIC FORM AVAILABLE: Yes

THERAPEUTIC CLASS: Class IA antiarrhythmic

DOSAGE FORMS: 250-mg, 500-mg., 750-mg, and 1000-mg sustained-release tablets (Procan SR); and 500-mg and 1000-mg extended-release tablets (Procanbid)

MAIN USES: Irregular heartbeat

USUAL DOSE: 250 mg to 1000 mg every six hours for Procan SR; 500 mg to 2500 mg twice daily for Procanbid

AVERAGE PRICE: For Procan SR: $73.35 (B)/$22.53 (G) for 500 mg; $127.58 (B)/$54.54 (G) for 750 mg; and $181.56 (B)/$89.90 (G). For Procanbid: $81.80 for 500 mg; and $179.39 for 1000 mg

SIDE EFFECTS: Most common: diarrhea and loss of appetite. Less common: allergic reaction, nausea, vomiting, systemic-lupus-erythematosus-like symptoms (fever, chills, joint paint or swelling, pains with breathing, skin rash, or itching), dizziness, and lightheadedness.

DRUG INTERACTIONS: Caution should be used by patients taking other drugs specifically used for irregular heartbeat. Orap and the drug, when taken together, may cause irregular heartbeats. The drug may increase the effects of neuromuscular-blocking agents commonly used before surgery. Medications for high blood pressure and the drug may cause low blood pressure when taken together.

ALLERGIES: Individuals allergic to procainamide or any of its derivatives should discuss this with their doctor or pharmacist before using this drug.

PREGNANCY/BREAST-FEEDING: Category C—Risk cannot be ruled out. Human studies are lacking, and animal studies are either positive for fetal risk or lacking as well. However, potential benefits may justify the potential risk in using the drug. The drug is excreted in the breast milk; therefore, extreme caution should be used when breast-feeding.

OTHER BRAND NAMES: None

OTHER DRUGS IN THE SAME THERAPEUTIC CLASS: None

IMPORTANT INFORMATION TO REMEMBER: This drug may cause some dizziness or tiredness, especially at first. Individuals should use caution when driving, operating machinery, or performing any task where mental alertness is required. Alcohol, anxiety medications, and narcotic painkillers may intensify these effects. Only take the drug exactly as directed by your physician. Do not discontinue taking the drug without first consulting your physician, and do not increase the dose without first consulting with your physician. Do not crush the tablets—this will destroy the mechanism that delays the release of the drug. They may, however, be cut in half for easier swallowing. If stomach upset occurs, the drug may be taken with food or milk.

BRAND NAME: Procardia and Procardia XL

GENERIC NAME: nifedipine

GENERIC FORM AVAILABLE: Yes (not for Procardia XL)

THERAPEUTIC CLASS: Calcium channel blocker

DOSAGE FORMS: 10-mg and 20-mg capsules (Procardia); and 30-mg, 60-mg, and 90-mg sustained-release tablets (Procardia XL)

MAIN USES: Angina and high blood pressure

USUAL DOSE: For Procardia: 10 mg to 20 mg three times daily. For Procardia XL: 30 mg to 90 mg once daily.

AVERAGE PRICE: $62.13 (B)/$38.48 (G) for 10 mg; $107.89 (B)/$46.18 (G) for 20 mg; $178.48 for 30 mg (Procardia XL); $308.85 for 60 mg (Procardia XL); $356.35 for 90 mg (Procardia XL)

SIDE EFFECTS: For Procardia: dizziness 27%, flushing 25%, headache 23%, weakness 12%, nausea 11%, muscle cramps 8%, tremor 8%, nervousness 7%, swelling 7%, pounding heartbeat 7%, trouble breathing 6%, and stuffy nose 6%. For Procardia XL: headache 16%, tiredness 6%, dizziness 4%, constipation 3%, and nausea 3%.

DRUG INTERACTIONS: The effects of Blocadren, Cartrol, Corgard, Inderal, Kerlone, Levatol, Lopressor, Minipress, Normodyne, Norpace, Sectral, Tenormin, Toprol-XL, Trandate, Visken, and Zebeta may be increased when taken with this drug. The drug may increase the blood levels of Tegretol, Sandimmune, Lanoxin, Quinidex, Quinaglute, and Procan. Tagamet may increase the blood levels of the drug.

ALLERGIES: Individuals allergic to nifedipine or any of its derivatives should discuss this with their doctor or pharmacist before using this drug.

PREGNANCY/BREAST-FEEDING: Category C—Risk cannot be ruled out. Human studies are lacking, and animal studies are either positive for fetal risk or lacking as well. However, potential benefits may justify the potential risk in using the drug. The drug is excreted in the breast milk; therefore, extreme caution should be used when breast-feeding.

OTHER BRAND NAMES: Adalat and Adalat CC

OTHER DRUGS IN THE SAME THERAPEUTIC CLASS: Adalat, Adalat CC, Calan, Calan SR, Cardizem, Cardizem CD, Cardizem SR, Cardene, Cardene SR, Covera-HS, Dilacor XR, DynaCirc, Isoptin, Isoptin SR, Norvasc, Plendil, Sular, Vascor, and Verelan

IMPORTANT INFORMATION TO REMEMBER: Only take the drug exactly as directed by your physician. Do not discontinue taking the drug without first consulting your physician. Before taking over-the-counter cold and allergy preparations, consult your doctor or pharmacist—these products may raise your blood pressure. This drug may cause some tiredness at first. Individuals should use caution when driving, operating machinery, or performing any task where mental alertness is required. Do not crush or cut the Procardia XL tablets—this will destroy the mechanism that delays the release of the drug. Individuals taking Procardia XL may notice a yellow-colored empty shell in the stool, which is left over after the medication is absorbed.

BRAND NAME: Procrit

GENERIC NAME: epoetin alfa

See entry for Epogen

BRAND NAME: Prolixin

GENERIC NAME: fluphenazine

GENERIC FORM AVAILABLE: Yes

THERAPEUTIC CLASS: Piperidine phenothiazine antipsychotic

DOSAGE FORMS: 1-mg, 2.5-mg, 5-mg, and 10-mg tablets; and 0.5 mg/mL elixir

MAIN USES: Psychotic disorders

USUAL DOSE: 2.5 mg to 10 mg daily in divided doses

AVERAGE PRICE: $105.36 (B)/$25.28 (G) for 1 mg; $146.27 (B)/$67.06 (G) for 2.5 mg; $184.75 (B)/$96.77 (G) for 5 mg; $235.36 (B)/$107.45 (G) for 10 mg

SIDE EFFECTS: Most common: drowsiness, restlessness, blurred vision, blurred vision, Parkinson's-like symptoms, low blood pressure, stuffy nose, dry mouth, constipation, and dizziness. Less common: increased sensitivity to sunburn, difficulty in urinating, nausea, vomiting, stomach pain, and trembling of fingers and hands, stomach pain, changes in menstrual period, decreased sexual ability, swelling and/or pain in the breasts, weight gain, and secretion of milk from the breasts.

DRUG INTERACTIONS: Drugs used to treat depression and Prolixin may increase the severity and frequency of side effects. Alcohol, anxiety medications, and narcotic painkillers may intensify the drowsiness effect of the drug. Eskalith and Lithobid may decrease the absorption of the drug. Eskalith or Lithobid and the drug may cause disorientation and for one to black out. The drug may decrease the effects of Larodopa. Medications for high blood pressure and the drug may cause low blood pressure when taken together.

ALLERGIES: Individuals allergic to fluphenazine or any of its derivatives should discuss this with their doctor or pharmacist before using this drug.

PREGNANCY/BREAST-FEEDING: Category D—Positive evidence of risk. Human studies show risk to the fetus. Nevertheless, potential benefits may possibly outweigh the potential risks. This drug should not be taken by nursing mothers.

OTHER BRAND NAMES: None

OTHER DRUGS IN THE SAME THERAPEUTIC CLASS: Compazine, Mellaril, Serentil, Stelazine, Thorazine, and Trilafon

IMPORTANT INFORMATION TO REMEMBER: This drug does cause drowsiness. Individuals should use caution when driving, operating machinery, or performing any task where mental alertness is required. Alcohol, anxiety medications, and narcotic painkillers may intensify the drowsiness effect of the drug. Do not increase the dose or stop taking the drug without first consulting with your physician. Individuals should report any involuntary movements of the tongue, arms, or legs to their physician. This drug may also increase the sensitivity of the skin to sunburn in some individuals; therefore, a sunscreen is recommended during periods of prolonged exposure to the sun. Caution should be used during hot weather due to decreased tolerance to the heat.

BRAND NAME: Proloprim

GENERIC NAME: trimethoprim

GENERIC FORM AVAILABLE: Yes

THERAPEUTIC CLASS: Folic acid inhibitor antibiotic

DOSAGE FORMS: 100-mg and 200-mg tablets

MAIN USES: Bacterial infections

USUAL DOSE: 100 mg every 12 hours or 200 mg daily

AVERAGE PRICE: $110.47 (B)/$33.53 (G) for 100 mg and $220.97 (B)/$50.66 (G) for 200 mg

SIDE EFFECTS: Most common: None. Less common: diarrhea, loss of appetite, nausea, vomiting, stomach pain, itching, rash, and headache.

DRUG INTERACTIONS: The drug should not be used with Rheumatrex.

ALLERGIES: Individuals allergic to trimethoprim or any of its derivatives should discuss this with their doctor or pharmacist before using this drug.

PREGNANCY/BREAST-FEEDING: Category C—Risk cannot be ruled out. Human studies are lacking, and animal studies are either positive for fetal risk or lacking as well. However, potential benefits may justify the potential risk in using the drug. The drug is excreted in the breast milk; therefore, extreme caution should be used when breast-feeding.

OTHER BRAND NAMES: Trimpex

OTHER DRUGS IN THE SAME THERAPEUTIC CLASS: Trimpex

IMPORTANT INFORMATION TO REMEMBER: Take the drug at even intervals around the clock (if two times a day, take every 12 hours). Take the drug until all the medication prescribed is gone; otherwise the infection may return. If stomach upset occurs, take the drug with food or milk.

BRAND NAME: Propine

GENERIC NAME: dipivefrin

GENERIC FORM AVAILABLE: Yes

THERAPEUTIC CLASS: Sympathomimetic anti-glaucoma

DOSAGE FORMS: 0.1% eyedrop solution

MAIN USES: Glaucoma

USUAL DOSE: one drop in affected eye(s) every 12 hours

AVERAGE PRICE: $40.74 (B)/$34.50 (G) for 10 mL

SIDE EFFECTS: Most common: none. Less common: burning, sting-ing, eye irritation, and increase sensitivity of the eyes to sunlight.

DRUG INTERACTIONS: None of any clinical significance

ALLERGIES: Individuals allergic to dipivefrin or any of its deriva-tives should discuss this with their doctor or pharmacist before using this drug.

PREGNANCY/BREAST-FEEDING: Category B—No evidence of risk in humans. Either animal findings show risk, but human findings do not; or, if no adequate human studies have been done, animal find-ings show no risk. It is not known whether the drug is excreted in the breast milk; therefore, caution should be used when breast-feeding.

OTHER BRAND NAMES: None

OTHER DRUGS IN THE SAME THERAPEUTIC CLASS: Epifrin

IMPORTANT INFORMATION TO REMEMBER: Keep the container tightly closed and avoid touching the applicator tip to the eye—this could contaminate the product over time. Also, only adminis-ter one drop at a time. After application, keep the eye open for at least 30 seconds, roll the eyeball around, and avoid squinting. If a second drop is required, wait one to two minutes between drops. If another medication is to be used in the eye, wait at least 10 min-utes before administering it. Only use the drug exactly as directed by your physician. Do not discontinue using the drug without first consulting your physician.

BRAND NAME: Propulsid

GENERIC NAME: cisapride

GENERIC FORM AVAILABLE: No

THERAPEUTIC CLASS: Anti-heartburn

DOSAGE FORMS: 10-mg and 20-mg tablets; and 1 mg/mL suspension

MAIN USES: Nighttime heartburn due to gastroesophogeal reflux disease (GERD)

USUAL DOSE: 10 mg to 20 mg four times daily at least 15 minutes before meals and bedtime

AVERAGE PRICE: $100.71 for 10 mg and $177.60 for 20 mg

SIDE EFFECTS: headache 19%, diarrhea 14%, stomach pain 10%, nausea 8%, constipation 7%, running nose 7%, gas 4%, body pain 3%, cough 2%, insomnia 2%, rash 2%, nervousness 1%, muscle pain 1%, vaginal infections 1%, and abnormal vision 1%.

DRUG INTERACTIONS: The increased rate of stomach emptying could affect the absorption rate of other drugs. The drug may cause irregular heartbeats when taken with Biaxin, erythromycin, Diflucan, Mycelex, Nizoral, PCE, Sporanox, and TAO. The drug may increase the effects of Coumadin.

FOOD INTERACTIONS: This drug should be taken 15 minutes before meals and bedtime.

ALLERGIES: Individuals allergic to cisapride or any of its derivatives should discuss this with their doctor or pharmacist before using this drug.

PREGNANCY/BREAST-FEEDING: Category C—Risk cannot be ruled out. Human studies are lacking, and animal studies are either positive for fetal risk or lacking as well. However, potential benefits may justify the potential risk in using the drug. The drug is excreted in the breast milk; therefore, caution should be used when breast-feeding.

OTHER BRAND NAMES: None

OTHER DRUGS IN THE SAME THERAPEUTIC CLASS: Reglan

IMPORTANT INFORMATION TO REMEMBER: The drug should be taken 15 minutes before meals and bedtime. Only take the drug exactly as directed by your physician and do not increase the dose without first consulting with your physician. Individuals using the suspension should shake it well before use.

BRAND NAME: Proscar

GENERIC NAME: finasteride

GENERIC FORM AVAILABLE: No

THERAPEUTIC CLASS: Prostate reducer

DOSAGE FORMS: 5-mg tablets

MAIN USES: Prostate disorders (BPH)

USUAL DOSE: 5 mg taken once daily

AVERAGE PRICE: $82.09 for 30 tablets

SIDE EFFECTS: impotence 4%, decreased sex drive 3%, and decreased volume of ejaculation 3%.

DRUG INTERACTIONS: The drug may decrease the blood levels of Slo-bid, Theo-Dur, theophylline, Uni-Dur, and Uniphyl.

ALLERGIES: Individuals allergic to finasteride or any of its derivatives should discuss this with their doctor or pharmacist before using this drug.

PREGNANCY/BREAST-FEEDING: Category X—Should not be used during pregnancy. Studies in animals and/or humans have shown fetal abnormalities and birth defects. The risks associated with using this drug clearly outweigh the benefits. This drug should never be used by someone who is pregnant or trying to become pregnant. Also, women should never breast-feed while using this drug.

OTHER BRAND NAMES: None

OTHER DRUGS IN THE SAME THERAPEUTIC CLASS: None

IMPORTANT INFORMATION TO REMEMBER: Only take the drug exactly as directed by your physician. The drug may take several weeks or even months before noticeable improvement is seen. Women who are or plan to become pregnant should not handle the Proscar tablets; some of the drug could be absorbed through the skin and possibly cause birth defects.

BRAND NAME: ProSom

GENERIC NAME: estazolam

GENERIC FORM AVAILABLE: No

THERAPEUTIC CLASS: Benzodiazepine sedative

DOSAGE FORMS: 1-mg and 2-mg tablets

MAIN USES: Insomnia

USUAL DOSE: 1 mg to 2 mg at bedtime

AVERAGE PRICE: $123.11 for 1 mg and $138.09 for 2 mg

SIDE EFFECTS: drowsiness 42%, headache 16%, weakness 11%, nervousness 8%, dizziness 7%, tiredness 5%, coordination problems 4%, nausea 4%, hangover feeling 3%, body pain 2%–3%, confusion 2%, abnormal dreams 2%, and itching 1%.

DRUG INTERACTIONS: Central nervous system (CNS) depression may be increased when used with alcohol, narcotic painkillers, or other anxiety medications.

ALLERGIES: Individuals allergic to estazolam, benzodiazepines, or other sleeping medications (such as those listed under "Other Drugs in the Same Therapeutic Class") should discuss this with their doctor or pharmacist before taking this drug.

PREGNANCY/BREAST-FEEDING: Category X—Should not be used during pregnancy. Studies in animals and/or humans have shown fetal abnormalities and birth defects. The risks associated with using this drug clearly outweigh the benefits. This drug should never be used by someone who is pregnant or trying to become pregnant. Also, women should never breast-feed while using this drug.

OTHER BRAND NAMES: None

OTHER DRUGS IN THE SAME THERAPEUTIC CLASS: Dalmane, Doral, Halcion, and Restoril

IMPORTANT INFORMATION TO REMEMBER: This drug will cause drowsiness. Individuals should use caution when driving, operating machinery, or performing any task where mental alertness is required. The drug may take two to three days before maximum effect is seen. The incidence of drowsiness and unsteadiness increases with age. Alcohol, anxiety medications, and narcotic painkillers may intensify the drowsiness effect of the drug. This medication is a controlled substance and may be habit-forming. Do not increase the dose of medication without consulting with your doctor; only take the amount prescribed by your doctor.

BRAND NAME: Prostep

GENERIC NAME: nicotine patch

Very similar to Nicoderm. See entry for Nicoderm.

BRAND NAME: Protostat

GENERIC NAME: metronidazole

See entry for Flagyl

BRAND NAME: Proventil and Proventil HFD

GENERIC NAME: albuterol

GENERIC FORM AVAILABLE: Yes

THERAPEUTIC CLASS: Beta-2-agonist bronchodilator

DOSAGE FORMS: 2-mg and 4-mg tablets; 4-mg sustained-release tablets (Proventil Repetabs); 2 mg/5 mL syrup; 90-micrograms-per-inhalation aerosol inhaler (Proventil and Proventil HFD); 0.5% concentrated solution for inhalation; and 0.083% unit dose (mixed with normal saline) solution for inhalation

MAIN USES: Asthma, chronic bronchitis, emphysema, and {other breathing disorders}

USUAL DOSE: Proventil tablets and syrup: 2 mg to 4 mg three to four times daily. Proventil Repetabs: 4 mg to 8 mg twice a day. Proventil inhaler: one to two inhalations every four to six hours. Inhalation solution: 2.5 mg three to four times daily, given by a breathing machine (nebulizer). Doses for children may be less.

AVERAGE PRICE: $49.47 (B)/$24.13 (G) for 2 mg; $77.42 (B)/$37.93 (G) for 4 mg; $16.37 (B)/$11.86 (G) for syrup; $33.72 (G)/$27.98 (B) for aerosol inhaler (17 g); $22.72 (B)/$19.53 (G) for 5 mg/mL solution (20 mL); and $95.98 for the 4-mg Proventil Repetabs

SIDE EFFECTS: For the tablets and syrup: nervousness 20%, tremor 20%, headache 7%, fast heartbeat 5%, palpitations 5%, muscle cramps 3%, insomnia 2%, irritability 2%, nausea 2%, and chest discomfort 2%. For the inhaler and inhaled solutions: tremors 10%–20%, dizziness 7%, nervousness 4%, nausea 4%, headache 3%, insomnia 3%, cough 3%, trouble breathing 2%, tiredness 2%, and fast heartbeat 1%.

DRUG INTERACTIONS: Anafranil, Asendin, Elavil, Nardil, Norpramin, Pamelor, Parnate, Sinequan, Surmontil, Tofranil, and

Vivactil, and cough, cold, and allergy medications with decongestants may increase the toxicity of this medication. Blocadren, Cartrol, Corgard, Inderal, Levatol, Normodyne, Trandate, and Visken may decrease the effectiveness of the drug.

ALLERGIES: Individuals allergic to albuterol, Ventolin, or any of their derivatives should discuss this with their doctor or pharmacist before using this drug.

PREGNANCY/BREAST-FEEDING: Category C—Risk cannot be ruled out. Human studies are lacking, and animal studies are either positive for fetal risk or lacking as well. However, potential benefits may justify the potential risk in using the drug. It is not known whether the drug is excreted in the breast milk; therefore, caution should be used when breast-feeding.

OTHER BRAND NAMES: Ventolin

OTHER DRUGS IN THE SAME THERAPEUTIC CLASS: Alupent, Brethine, Brethaire, Bricanyl, Bronkometer, Maxair, Metaprel, Serevent, Tornalate, Ventolin, and Volmax

IMPORTANT INFORMATION TO REMEMBER: Only take the drug exactly as directed by your physician. Never increase the dose of the drug without consulting with your physician. Prolonged use of the drug may cause tolerance to its effects to develop. If stomach upset occurs, take the drug with food or milk.

When using the inhaler, use the following procedure:

1) Shake the canister well.
2) Place the mouthpiece close to the mouth, but not touching the lips.
3) Exhale deeply.
4) Inhale slowly and deeply as you press the top of the canister to release the medication.
5) Hold your breath for a few seconds before exhaling.
6) Wait five minutes between puffs.
7) Be sure to wash the inhaler device (mouthpiece) regularly with warm soapy water to avoid bacterial contamination.

BRAND NAME: Provera

GENERIC NAME: medroxprogesterone

GENERIC FORM AVAILABLE: Yes

THERAPEUTIC CLASS: Progestin

DOSAGE FORMS: 2.5-mg, 5-mg, and 10-mg tablets

MAIN USES: Abnormal uterine bleeding, secondary ammenorhea, and hormonal imbalance

USUAL DOSE: For abnormal uterine bleeding and secondary amenorrhea: 5 mg to 10 mg daily for 5 to 10 days. For hormone replacement: 2.5 mg to 10 mg daily for 7, 10, or 30 days per month, depending on each individual patient.

AVERAGE PRICE: $48.05 (B)/$32.90 (G) for 2.5 mg; $72.14 (B)/$46.06 (G) for 5 mg; $81.93 (B)/$29.46 (G) for 10 mg

SIDE EFFECTS: Most common: changes in vaginal bleeding pattern, irregular cycle time, spotting, breakthrough bleeding, complete lack of bleeding, changes in appetite, changes in weight, swelling of the ankles and feet, and unusual tiredness or weakness. Less common: headache, blood clots, acne, fever, increased body and facial hair, increased breast tenderness, brown or blotchy spots on exposed skin, nausea, insomnia, liver enzyme changes, and some loss of scalp hair.

DRUG INTERACTIONS: The drug may interfere with the effects of Parlodel.

ALLERGIES: Individuals allergic to medroxyprogesterone, other progestins, or any of their derivatives should discuss this with their doctor or pharmacist before using this drug.

PREGNANCY/BREAST-FEEDING: Category X—Should not be used during pregnancy. Studies in animals and/or humans have shown fetal abnormalities and birth defects. The risks associated with using this drug clearly outweigh the benefits. This drug should never be used by someone who is pregnant or trying to become pregnant. Also, women should never breast-feed while using this drug.

OTHER BRAND NAMES: Amen and Cycrin

OTHER DRUGS IN THE SAME THERAPEUTIC CLASS: Amen, Aygestin, and Cycrin

IMPORTANT INFORMATION TO REMEMBER: Only take the drug exactly as directed by your physician. If the drug is to be taken only during certain days of the month, follow that dosing schedule closely. If stomach upset occurs, take the drug with food or milk. Diabetics should be aware that the drug may affect blood sugar levels.

BRAND NAME: Prozac

GENERIC NAME: fluoxetine

GENERIC FORM AVAILABLE: No

THERAPEUTIC CLASS: Serotonin reuptake inhibitor antidepressant

DOSAGE FORMS: 10-mg and 20-mg tablets; and 20 mg/5 mL liquid

MAIN USES: Depression, bulimia, and obsessive-compulsive disorder

USUAL DOSE: For depression and obsessive-compulsive disorder: 10 mg to 20 mg daily; doses over 20 mg/day should be taken in two divided doses (in the morning and at noon). For bulimia: 60 mg once daily in the morning.

AVERAGE PRICE: $283.91 for 10 mg and $308.35 for 20 mg

SIDE EFFECTS: nausea 21%, headache 20%, nervousness 15%, insomnia 14%, diarrhea 12%, drowsiness 12%, dry mouth 10%, appetite changes 9%, anxiety 9%, excessive sweating 8%, tremor 8%, dizziness 6%, constipation 5%, tiredness 4%, stomach pain 3%, vomiting 2%, taste changes 2%, gas 2%, itching 2%, rash 2%, decreased sex drive 2%, lightheadedness 2%, and decreased concentration 2%.

DRUG INTERACTIONS: The drug may increase the blood levels of other drugs used to treat depression. The drug may increase the blood levels of Dilantin. The drug, when taken with Coumadin, may increase the chance of bleeding. The drug should not be used with tryptophan, because tryptophan can be metabolized to serotonin and too much serotonin may cause severe side effects. The drug should not be taken within 14 days of taking Nardil or Parnate. Central nervous system (CNS) depression may be increased when used with alcohol, narcotic painkillers, or other anxiety medications.

ALLERGIES: Individuals allergic to fluoxetine or any of its derivatives should discuss this with their doctor or pharmacist before using this drug.

PREGNANCY/BREAST-FEEDING: Category B—No evidence of risk in humans. Either animal findings show risk, but human findings do not; or, if no adequate human studies have been done, animal findings show no risk. The drug is excreted in the breast milk; therefore, extreme caution should be used when breast-feeding.

OTHER BRAND NAMES: None

OTHER DRUGS IN THE SAME THERAPEUTIC CLASS: Luvox, Paxil, and Zoloft

IMPORTANT INFORMATION TO REMEMBER: Only take the drug exactly as directed by your physician. Do not discontinue taking the drug without first consulting your physician. The drug may require two to four weeks or longer of use before improvement may be noticed. This drug does cause drowsiness. Individuals should use caution when driving, operating machinery, or performing any task where mental alertness is required. Alcohol, anxiety medications, and narcotic painkillers may intensify the drowsiness effect of the drug. The drug may cause a slight amount of dizziness or lightheadedness when rising from a sitting or lying-down position.

BRAND NAME: Psorcon

GENERIC NAME: diflorasone

GENERIC FORM AVAILABLE: No

THERAPEUTIC CLASS: Topical corticosteroid

DOSAGE FORMS: 0.05% cream and ointment

MAIN USES: Skin rashes, swelling, itching, and psoriasis

USUAL DOSE: Apply thin film one to three times daily.

AVERAGE PRICE: $43.72 for 30 g

SIDE EFFECTS: Most common: none. Less common: burning, itching, irritation, dry skin, rash, and soreness of the skin.

DRUG INTERACTIONS: None of any clinical significance

ALLERGIES: Individuals allergic to diflorasone or any or its derivatives should discuss this with their doctor or pharmacist before using this drug.

PREGNANCY/BEAST-FEEDING: Category C—Risk cannot be ruled out. Human studies are lacking, and animal studies are either positive for fetal risk or lacking as well. However, potential benefits may justify the potential risk in using the drug. It is not known whether the drug is excreted in the breast milk; therefore, caution should be used when breast-feeding.

OTHER BRAND NAMES: None

OTHER DRUGS IN THE SAME THERAPEUTIC CLASS: Aclovate, Aristocort, Cordran, Cordran SP, Cutivate, Cyclocort, DesOwen, Diprolene, Diprolene AF, Elocon, Florone, Florone E, Halog, Hytone, Kenalog, Lidex, Lidex-E, Synalar, Temovate, Topicort, Tridesilon, Ultravate, and Westcort

IMPORTANT INFORMATION TO REMEMBER: This drug is for external use only. Apply only a thin film of drug to skin and rub it in well. Never cover the skin after application with a bandage or wrapping unless directed to do so by a doctor. Never apply to damaged skin or open wounds unless directed to do so by a doctor. Discontinue use if irritation occurs.

BRAND NAME: Pulmozyme

GENERIC NAME: dornase alfa

GENERIC FORM AVAILABLE: No

THERAPEUTIC CLASS: Anti-cystic-fibrotic

DOSAGE FORMS: 1 mg/mL solution for inhalation in 2.5-mL ampules

MAIN USES: Cystic fibrosis

USUAL DOSE: one 2.5-mL ampule inhaled once daily using a nebulizer

AVERAGE PRICE: $653.52 for 14 ampules

SIDE EFFECTS: pharyngitis 36%, chest pain 18%, voice changes 12%, rash 10%, and eye redness and/or infections 4%.

DRUG INTERACTIONS: Drug interaction studies have not been performed.

ALLERGIES: Individuals allergic to dornase alfa or any of its derivatives should discuss this with their doctor or pharmacist before using this drug.

PREGNANCY/BREAST-FEEDING: Category B—No evidence of risk in humans. Either animal findings show risk, but human findings do not; or, if no adequate human studies have been done, animal findings show no risk. The drug is excreted in the breast milk; therefore, caution should be used when breast-feeding.

OTHER BRAND NAMES: None

OTHER DRUGS IN THE SAME THERAPEUTIC CLASS: None

IMPORTANT INFORMATION TO REMEMBER: The drug should be used only as directed. Each ampule should only be used once. Never use an ampule that has been previously opened. The drug must be used with a nebulizer and used only with a mouthpiece, not a face mask. The drug should be used at the same time every day. For some patients, the drug may require weeks or months before benefits are seen. The ampules should be kept in the refrigerator in the foil pouches at all times.

BRAND NAME: Pyridium

GENERIC NAME: phenazopyridine

GENERIC FORM AVAILABLE: Yes

THERAPEUTIC CLASS: Urinary tract pain reliever

DOSAGE FORMS: 100-mg and 200-mg tablets

MAIN USES: Relief of pain, burning, urgency, frequency, and other symptoms associated with a urinary tract infection

USUAL DOSE: 100 mg to 200 mg three times daily, following meals as needed

AVERAGE PRICE: $17.84 (B)/$9.91 (G) for 100 mg (20 tablets); and $32.53 (B)/$12.92 (G) for 200 mg (20 tablets)

SIDE EFFECTS: Most common: none. Less common: dizziness, itching, discolored contact lens, headache, indigestion, stomach pain, rash, and discolored urine.

DRUG INTERACTIONS: None of any clinical significance

ALLERGIES: Individuals allergic to phenazopyridine or any of its derivatives should discuss this with their doctor or pharmacist before using this drug.

PREGNANCY/BREAST-FEEDING: Category B—No evidence of risk in humans. Either animal findings show risk, but human findings do not; or, if no adequate human studies have been done, animal findings show no risk. It is not known whether the drug is excreted in the breast milk; therefore, caution should be used when breast-feeding.

OTHER BRAND NAMES: None

OTHER DRUGS IN THE SAME THERAPEUTIC CLASS: None

IMPORTANT INFORMATION TO REMEMBER: This drug will not cure urinary tract infections; it only helps relieve the symptoms associated with the infection. The drug should be taken with food or milk. The drug may cause the urine to turn reddish-orange in color, which may stain fabric and clothes. This color change of the urine is nothing to be alarmed about and is normal.

BRAND NAME: Questran and Questran Light

GENERIC NAME: cholestyramine

GENERIC FORM AVAILABLE: Yes

THERAPEUTIC CLASS: Cholesterol binder

DOSAGE FORMS: 378-g can or 9-g-unit dose packets. Questran Light contains Nutrasweet instead of sugar.

MAIN USES: High cholesterol

USUAL DOSE: one to two scoopfuls or packets once or twice daily

AVERAGE PRICE: $115.62 (B)/$95.49 (G) for 60 packets and $50.63 (B)/$41.99 (G) for one can

SIDE EFFECTS: Most common: constipation, heartburn, indigestion, nausea, vomiting, and stomach pain. Less common: belching, bloating, diarrhea, gas, dizziness, and headache.

DRUG INTERACTIONS: The drug may affect the blood levels of Coumadin. This drug can interfere with the absorption of several drugs including Lanoxin, diuretics (water pills), penicillin G, Inderal, Sumycin, Cytomel, Levothroid, Levoxyl, Synthroid, and Vancocin. Before taking any prescription drug, talk to your doctor or pharmacist.

ALLERGIES: Individuals allergic to cholestryamine or any of its derivatives should discuss this with their doctor or pharmacist before using this drug.

PREGNANCY/BREAST-FEEDING: Category C—Risk cannot be ruled out. Human studies are lacking, and animal studies are either positive for fetal risk or lacking as well. However, potential benefits may justify the potential risk in using the drug. It is not known whether the drug is excreted in the breast milk; therefore, caution should be used when breast-feeding.

OTHER BRAND NAMES: None

OTHER DRUGS IN THE SAME THERAPEUTIC CLASS: Colestid

IMPORTANT INFORMATION TO REMEMBER: This drug may interfere with the absorption of many prescription drug products; therefore, it's best to take the drug one to two hours before taking other medications or four hours after taking other medications. Only take the drug exactly as directed by your physician. Do not discontinue the drug without first consulting your physician.

How to mix the drug with liquid:

1) The drug needs to be mixed with liquid before it can be taken.
2) The drug may be mixed with water, milk, flavored drink, any fruit juice, cereals, soups (chicken noodle or tomato), and fruits. Most individuals prefer to mix the drug with heavy or pulpy fruit juices to improve taste.
3) Stir until the drug is completely mixed. The drug will not dissolve completely in the liquid.
4) Rinse the glass after drinking with a little more liquid and drink that as well. This ensures all the medication is taken.

BRAND NAME: Quibron SR and Quibron T

GENERIC NAME: theophylline

GENERIC FORM AVAILABLE: Yes

THERAPEUTIC CLASS: Xanthine bronchodilator

DOSAGE FORMS: 300-mg sustained-release tablets (Quibron SR) and 300-mg tablets (Quibron T)

MAIN USES: Asthma, chronic bronchitis, emphysema, and {other breathing disorders}

USUAL DOSE: 200 mg to 900 mg daily in divided doses

AVERAGE PRICE: $52.68 (B)/$16.22 (G) for Quibron SR and $50.49 (B)/$30.59 (G) for Quibron T

SIDE EFFECTS: Most common: nausea, nervousness, and restlessness. Less common: vomiting, diarrhea, stomach pain, headaches, irritability, insomnia, muscle twitching, fast heartbeat, pounding heartbeat, fast breathing, increased urination, flushing, and low blood pressure.

DRUG INTERACTIONS: The drug may inhibit the effects of Blocadren, Cartrol, Corgard, Inderal, Kerlone, Levatol, Lopressor, Normodyne, Sectral, Tenormin, Toprol-XL, Trandate, Visken, and Zebeta. Dilantin, Tegretol, smoking, and nicotine patches may lower the blood levels of this drug. Cipro, Noroxin, Tagamet, Zantac, erythromycin, and TAO may increase blood levels of the drug. Individuals who stop smoking while taking the drug may have increased levels of the drug in the blood.

ALLERGIES: Individuals allergic to cholestyramine or any of its derivatives should discuss this with their doctor or pharmacist before using this drug.

PREGNANCY/BREAST-FEEDING: Category C—Risk cannot be ruled out. Human studies are lacking, and animal studies are either positive for fetal risk or lacking as well. However, potential benefits may justify the potential risk in using the drug. The drug is excreted in the breast milk; therefore, extreme caution should be used when breast-feeding.

OTHER BRAND NAMES: None

OTHER DRUGS IN THE SAME THERAPEUTIC CLASS: aminophylline, Choledyl, Elixophyllin, Lufyllin, Respbid, Slo-bid, Slo-Phyllin, Theo-24, Theo-Dur, Theo-X, Uni-Dur, and Uniphyl

IMPORTANT INFORMATION TO REMEMBER: Only take the drug exactly as directed by your physician. Do not discontinue the drug or increase the dose without first consulting your physician. This drug should be taken with plenty of water (eight ounces is preferred). Do not crush the sustained-release (labeled SR) tablets—this will destroy the mechanism that slowly releases the drug into the bloodstream. The tablets may, however, be cut on the scored lines marked on the tablet. If stomach upset occurs, take with food or milk. Do not change between brand and generic once you are stabilized on one or the other.

BRAND NAME: Quinaglute Dura-Tabs

GENERIC NAME: quinidine gluconate

GENERIC FORM AVAILABLE: Yes

THERAPEUTIC CLASS: Class I antiarrhythmic

DOSAGE FORMS: 324-mg sustained-release tablets

MAIN USES: Irregular heartbeat

USUAL DOSE: one to two tablets every 8 to 12 hours

AVERAGE PRICE: $61.25 (B)/$23.85 (G)

SIDE EFFECTS: Most common: bitter taste, diarrhea, flushing of the skin, itching, loss of appetite, nausea, vomiting, and stomach pain. Less common: confusion, allergic reaction, skin rash, blurred vision, low blood pressure, dizziness, headache, fever, rash, abnormal EKG, and fainting.

DRUG INTERACTIONS: Caution should be used by patients taking other drugs specifically used for irregular heartbeat. Orap and the drug, when taken together, may cause irregular heartbeat. The drug may increase the effects and the blood levels of Coumadin. The drug may increase the blood levels of Lanoxin.

ALLERGIES: Individuals allergic to quinidine gluconate, quinidine, or any of their derivatives should discuss this with their doctor or pharmacist before using this drug.

PREGNANCY/BREAST-FEEDING: Category C—Risk cannot be ruled out. Human studies are lacking, and animal studies are either positive for fetal risk or lacking as well. However, potential benefits may justify the potential risk in using the drug. The drug is excreted in the breast milk; therefore, extreme caution should be used when breast-feeding.

OTHER BRAND NAMES: None

OTHER DRUGS IN THE SAME THERAPEUTIC CLASS: Cardioquin, Norpace, Norpace CR, Quinidex, and Tonocard

IMPORTANT INFORMATION TO REMEMBER: This drug may cause some dizziness or tiredness, especially at first. Individuals should use caution when driving, operating machinery, or performing any task where mental alertness is required. Alcohol, anxiety medications, and narcotic painkillers may intensify these effects. Only take the drug exactly as directed by your physician. Do not discontinue taking the drug without first consulting your physician; also, do not increase the dose without first consulting with your physician. If stomach upset occurs, take the drug with food or milk. Do not crush or chew the tablets—this will destroy the mechanism, that slowly releases the drug into the bloodstream. Swallow the tablets whole. Report any of the following symptoms to your physician: ringing in the ears, visual disturbances, confusion, or headache.

BRAND NAME: Quinidex Extentabs

GENERIC NAME: quinidine sulfate

GENERIC FORM AVAILABLE: No

THERAPEUTIC CLASS: Class I antiarrhythmic

DOSAGE FORMS: 300-mg extended-release tablets

MAIN USES: Irregular heartbeat

USUAL DOSE: one to two tablets every 8 to 12 hours

AVERAGE PRICE: $155.93

SIDE EFFECTS: Most common: bitter taste, diarrhea, flushing of the skin, itching, loss of appetite, nausea, vomiting, and stomach pain. Less common: confusion, allergic reaction, fever, skin rash, blurred vision, low blood pressure, dizziness, headache, and fainting.

DRUG INTERACTIONS: Caution should be used by patients taking other drugs specifically used for irregular heartbeat. Orap and the drug, when taken together, may cause irregular heartbeat. The drug may increase the effects and the blood levels of Coumadin. The drug may increase the blood levels of Lanoxin.

ALLERGIES: Individuals allergic to quinidine sulfate, quinidine, or any of their derivatives should discuss this with their doctor or pharmacist before using this drug.

PREGNANCY/BREAST-FEEDING: Category C—Risk cannot be ruled out. Human studies are lacking, and animal studies are either positive for fetal risk or lacking as well. However, potential benefits may justify the potential risk in using the drug. The drug is excreted in the breast milk; therefore, extreme caution should be used when breast-feeding.

OTHER BRAND NAMES: None

OTHER DRUGS IN THE SAME THERAPEUTIC CLASS: Cardioquin, Norpace, Norpace CR, Quinaglute, and Tonocard

IMPORTANT INFORMATION TO REMEMBER: This drug may cause some dizziness or tiredness, especially at first. Individuals should use caution when driving, operating machinery, or performing any task where mental alertness is required. Alcohol, anxiety medications, and narcotic painkillers may intensify these effects. Only take the drug exactly as directed by your physician. Do not discontinue taking the drug without first consulting your physician; also, do not increase the dose without first consulting with your physician. If stomach upset occurs, take the drug with food or milk. Do not crush or chew the tablets—this will destroy the mechanism that slowly releases the drug into the bloodstream. Swallow the tablets whole. Report any of the following symptoms to your physician: ringing in the ears, visual disturbances, confusion, or headache.

BRAND NAME: Reglan

GENERIC NAME: metoclopramide

GENERIC FORM AVAILABLE: Yes

THERAPEUTIC CLASS: Antinausea, anti-heartburn

DOSAGE FORMS: 5-mg and 10-mg tablets; and 5 mg/5 mL syrup

MAIN USES: Nausea, vomiting, and gastroesophogeal reflux disease (GERD)

USUAL DOSE: 5 mg to 15 mg taken 30 minutes before each meal and at bedtime, up to four times daily

AVERAGE PRICE: $62.83 (B)/$37.37 (G) for 5 mg; $97.86 (B)/$43.37 (G) for 10 mg; $20.88 (B)/$9.30 (G) for syrup

SIDE EFFECTS: Most common: drowsiness, restlessness, unusual tiredness or weakness, and diarrhea. Less common: breast tenderness and swelling, changes in menstruation, constipation, depression, dizziness, headache, increased flow of breast milk, insomnia, dry mouth, and unusual irritability.

DRUG INTERACTIONS: Central nervous system (CNS) depression may be increased when used with alcohol, narcotic painkillers, or other anxiety medications. The drug may increase the absorption of Sandimmune.

ALLERGIES: Individuals allergic to metoclopramide or any of its derivatives should discuss this with their doctor or pharmacist before using this drug.

PREGNANCY/BREAST-FEEDING: Category B—No evidence of risk in humans. Either animal findings show risk, but human findings do not; or, if no adequate human studies have been done, animal findings show no risk. It is not known whether the drug is excreted in the breast milk; therefore, caution should be used when breast-feeding.

OTHER BRAND NAMES: None

OTHER DRUGS IN THE SAME THERAPEUTIC CLASS: Propulsid

IMPORTANT INFORMATION TO REMEMBER: The drug should be taken 30 minutes before meals. This drug may cause drowsiness. Individuals should use caution when driving, operating machinery, or performing any task where mental alertness is required. The incidence of drowsiness and unsteadiness increases with age. Alcohol, anxiety medications, and narcotic painkillers may intensify the drowsiness effect of the drug. Only take the amount prescribed by your doctor. The drug should be used with caution by patients with Parkinson's disease.

BRAND NAME: Relafen

GENERIC NAME: nabumetone

GENERIC FORM AVAILABLE: No

THERAPEUTIC CLASS: Nonsteroidal anti-inflammatory drug (NSAID)

DOSAGE FORMS: 500-mg and 750-mg tablets

MAIN USES: Arthritis and pain relief

USUAL DOSE: 500 mg to 2000 mg taken once or twice daily

AVERAGE PRICE: $152.82 for 500 mg and $178.84 for 750 mg

SIDE EFFECTS: diarrhea 14%, upset stomach 13%, stomach pain 12%, constipation 3%–9%, gas 3%–9%, dizziness 3%–9%, headache 3%–9%, itching 3%–9%, rash 3%–9%, ringing in the ears 3%–9%, swelling 3%–9%, dry mouth 1%–3%, vomiting 1%–3%, tiredness 1%–3%, increased sweating 1%–3%, insomnia 1%–3%, nervousness 1%–3%, and weakness 1%–3%.

DRUG INTERACTIONS: Aspirin will decrease the concentration of this drug in the blood. This drug may also decrease the effects of Dyazide, HydroDIURIL, Lasix, Maxzide, and other water pills. The drug may increase the blood levels of Eskalith, Lithobid, and Sandimmune. The drug may increase the toxic effects of the drug Rheuma-trex. Caution should be used when taking the drug with Coumadin.

ALLERGIES: Individuals allergic to nambumetone or other NSAIDs (such as those listed under "Other Drugs in the Same Therapeutic Class") should discuss this with their doctor or pharmacist before taking this drug.

PREGNANCY/BREAST-FEEDING: Category C—Risk cannot be ruled out. Human studies are lacking, and animal studies are either positive for fetal risk or lacking as well. However, potential benefits may justify the potential risk in using the drug. The drug should not, however, be used during the late stages (last three months) of pregnancy. It is not known whether the drug is excreted in the breast milk; therefore, caution should be used when breast-feeding.

OTHER BRAND NAMES: None

OTHER DRUGS IN THE SAME THERAPEUTIC CLASS: Anaprox, Ansaid, aspirin, Cataflam, Clinoril, Daypro, Disalcid, Dolobid, Easprin, Feldene, Indocin, Lodine, Lodine XL, Motrin, Nalfon, Naprosyn, Orudis, Oruvail, Tolectin, Toradol, Voltaren, and Voltaren XR

IMPORTANT INFORMATION TO REMEMBER: This drug should be taken with food or milk to reduce the potential for injury to the stomach lining and stomach upset. This drug may take up to two weeks before a noticeable improvement in pain relief associated with arthritis is observed. Drinking alcohol while taking this drug may increase its potential to cause ulcers. This drug should only be used under the direct supervision of a doctor by individuals with a bleeding disorder or ulcer, or those who are currently taking Coumadin. Before taking over-the-counter pain relievers, consult your doctor or pharmacist. No more than one pain reliever should be taken at any one time unless otherwise directed by your doctor.

BRAND NAME: Renova

GENERIC NAME: tretinoin

GENERIC FORM AVAILABLE: No

THERAPEUTIC CLASS: Vitamin A derivative

DOSAGE FORMS: 0.05% cream

MAIN USES: Fine wrinkles, roughness of the face skin, and mottled complexion of the face

USUAL DOSAGE: Apply once daily at bedtime, using enough to cover the affected areas lightly.

AVERAGE PRICE: $59.51 for 40 g

SIDE EFFECTS: Most common: none. Less common: redness, blistering, peeling, feeling of warmth, mild stinging, swelling of the skin, burning sensation, crusty skin, increased sensitivity of the skin to sunburn, and skin irritation.

DRUG INTERACTIONS: Other acne drugs and soaps applied at the same time may increase the effects of the drug.

ALLERGIES: Individuals allergic to tretinoin, Retin-A, or any of their derivatives should discuss this with their doctor or pharmacist before using this drug.

PREGNANCY/BREAST-FEEDING: Category C—Risk cannot be ruled out. Human studies are lacking, and animal studies are either positive for fetal risk or lacking as well. However, potential benefits may justify the potential risk in using the drug. It is not known whether the drug is excreted in the breast milk; therefore, caution should be used when breast-feeding.

OTHER BRAND NAMES: None

OTHER DRUGS IN THE SAME THERAPEUTIC CLASS: None

IMPORTANT INFORMATION TO REMEMBER: The drug should be applied at bedtime 20–30 minutes after thorough washing and drying of the skin. Keep the medication away from the corners of the nose, mouth, and any open wounds or sores. There may be some minor discomfort or peeling during the first few days of treatment. If these symptoms continue or become worse, contact your doctor. The drug should be stored below 80°F. This drug should not be used during the day or during suntanning due to the increased risk of severe sunburn. A sunscreen should be used even if the medication is applied at bedtime. The drug may make the face more sensitive to wind and cold. The drug *does not* completely eliminate wrinkles, repair sun-damaged skin, reverse the aging process caused by the sun, or restore the skin of the face to a more youthful-looking appearance. The percentage of individuals that observed benefits from the drug was less than 50%. The drug should not be used as a long-term therapy.

BRAND NAME: Restoril

GENERIC NAME: temazepam

GENERIC FORM AVAILABLE: Yes

THERAPEUTIC CLASS: Benzodiazepine sedative

DOSAGE FORMS: 7.5-mg, 15-mg, and 30-mg capsules

MAIN USES: Insomnia

USUAL DOSE: 7.5 mg to 30 mg at bedtime

AVERAGE PRICE: $99.61 (B)/$41.75 (G) for 15 mg and $112.81 (B)/ $47.26 (G) for 30 mg

SIDE EFFECTS: daytime drowsiness 9%, headache 9%, tiredness 5%, nervousness 5%, dizziness 5%, nausea 3%, hangover feeling 3%, depression 2%, dry mouth 2%, diarrhea 2%, stomach discomfort 2%, euphoria 2%, weakness 1%, confusion 1%, blurred vision 1%, dizziness and nightmares 1%.

DRUG INTERACTIONS: Central nervous system (CNS) depression may be increased when used with alcohol, narcotic painkillers, or other anxiety medications.

ALLERGIES: Individuals allergic to temazepam, benzodiazepines, or other sleeping medications (such as those listed under "Other Drugs in the Same Therapeutic Class") should discuss this with their doctor or pharmacist before taking this drug.

PREGNANCY/BREAST-FEEDING: Category X—Should not be used during pregnancy. Studies in animals and/or humans have shown fetal abnormalities and birth defects. The risks associated with using this drug clearly outweigh the benefits. This drug should never be used by someone who is pregnant or trying to become pregnant. Also, women should never breast-feed while using this drug.

OTHER BRAND NAMES: None

OTHER DRUGS IN THE SAME THERAPEUTIC CLASS: Dalmane, Doral, Halcion, and ProSom

IMPORTANT INFORMATION TO REMEMBER: This drug will cause drowsiness. Individuals should use caution when driving, operating machinery, or performing any task where mental alertness is required. The drug may take two to three days before maximum effect is seen. The incidence of drowsiness and unsteadiness increases with age. Alcohol, anxiety medications, and narcotic painkillers may intensify the drowsiness effect of the drug. This medication is a controlled substance and may be habit-forming. Do not increase the dose of medication without consulting with your doctor. Only take the amount prescribed by your doctor.

BRAND NAME: Retin-A and Retin-A Micro

GENERIC NAME: tretinoin

GENERIC FORM AVAILABLE: No

THERAPEUTIC CLASS: Retinoic acid derivative

DOSAGE FORMS: 0.025%, 0.05%, and 0.1% cream; 0.025% and 0.01% gel; and 0.05% liquid

MAIN USES: Acne

USUAL DOSE: Apply once daily at bedtime, using enough to cover the affected area lightly.

AVERAGE PRICE: $37.96 for 0.025% cream (20 g); $39.39 for 0.05% cream (20 g); $45.94 for 0.1% cream (20 g); and $31.57 for 0.01% gel (15 g)

SIDE EFFECTS: Most common: none. Less common: redness, blistering, peeling, feeling of warmth, mild stinging, swelling of the skin, burning sensation, crusty skin, and skin irritation.

DRUG INTERACTIONS: Other acne drugs and soaps applied at the same time may increase the effects of the drug.

ALLERGIES: Individuals allergic to tretinoin or any of its derivatives should discuss this with their doctor or pharmacist before using this drug.

PREGNANCY/BREAST-FEEDING: Category C—Risk cannot be ruled out. Human studies are lacking, and animal studies are either positive for fetal risk or lacking as well. However, potential benefits may justify the potential risk in using the drug. It is not known whether the drug is excreted in the breast milk; therefore, caution should be used when breast-feeding.

OTHER BRAND NAMES: None

OTHER DRUGS IN THE SAME THERAPEUTIC CLASS: Differin

IMPORTANT INFORMATION TO REMEMBER: The drug should be applied at bedtime 20–30 minutes after thoroughly washing and drying of the skin. Keep the medication away from the corners of the nose, mouth, and any open wounds or sores. There may be some minor discomfort or peeling during the first few days of treatment. If these symptoms continue or become worse, contact your doctor. The drug should be stored below 80°F. This drug should not be used during the day or during suntanning due to the increased risk of severe sunburn. A sunscreen should be used even if the medication is applied at bedtime. The drug may make the face more sensitive to wind and cold. After three to six weeks of therapy, some new areas of acne may appear; this is normal and only temporary. Individuals should continue using the medication.

BRAND NAME: Retrovir

GENERIC NAME: zidovudine

GENERIC FORM AVAILABLE: No

THERAPEUTIC CLASS: AIDS antiviral

DOSAGE FORMS: 100-mg capsules; 300-mg tablets; and 50 mg/5 mL syrup

MAIN USES: AIDS

USUAL DOSE: 100 mg to 200 mg every four hours

AVERAGE PRICE: $216.72 for 100 mg; and $456.49 for 300 mg

SIDE EFFECTS: headache 58%–63%, tiredness 53%–56%, nausea 51%–57%, loss of appetite 19%–20%, dizziness 18%–20%, diarrhea 12%, muscle weakness 9%–10%, and constipation 6%–8%. Blood disorders and anemia also occur fairly frequently.

DRUG INTERACTIONS: There are numerous drugs that can cause peripheral neuropathy (unusual nerve sensations and damage in the arms, legs, fingers, and toes) when taken with this drug. Some of these are: alcohol, Aldomet, Apresoline, Bactrim, Biaxin, cisplatin, Clinoril, Cytovene, dapsone, Depakene, Depakote, Dilantin, diuretics (water pills), Doryx, Dynabac, erythromycin, Eskalith, estrogens, Flagyl, isoniazid, Lasix, Lithobid, Macrobid, Macrodantin, pentamidine, Septra, Sumycin, Vibramycin, vincristine, and ZERIT. Bactrim, Diflucan, probenecid, and Septra may increase the blood levels of the drug. Biaxim may decrease the blood levels of the drug. Before taking any prescription drug, discuss it with your doctor.

ALLERGIES: Individuals allergic to zidovudine or any of its derivatives should discuss this with their doctor or pharmacist before using this drug.

PREGNANCY/BREAST-FEEDING: Category C—Risk cannot be ruled out. Human studies are lacking, and animal studies are either positive for fetal risk or lacking as well. However, potential benefits may justify the potential risk in using the drug. It is not known whether the drug is excreted in the breast milk; therefore, caution should be used when breast-feeding.

OTHER BRAND NAMES: None

OTHER DRUGS IN THE SAME THERAPEUTIC CLASS: Epivir, HIVID, Videx, and ZERIT

IMPORTANT INFORMATION TO REMEMBER: If stomach upset occurs, take the drug with food or milk. Also, take the drug at even intervals around the clock (if six times a day, take every four hours). Only take the drug exactly as directed by your physician. Do not stop taking the drug without first consulting with your physician. It is important to have regular blood and liver function tests while taking this drug. Before taking any prescription or over-the-counter (OTC) drugs, consult your doctor or pharmacist.

BRAND NAME: ReVia

GENERIC NAME: naltrexone

GENERIC FORM AVAILABLE: No

THERAPEUTIC CLASS: Anti-drug-dependence compound

DOSAGE FORMS: 50-mg tablets

MAIN USES: Narcotic or alcohol dependence

USUAL DOSE: 25 mg to 50 mg daily

AVERAGE PRICE: $318.61 for 50 tablets

SIDE EFFECTS: Most common: stomach pain, nervousness, restlessness, insomnia, headache, joint or muscle pain, nausea, vomiting, and unusual tiredness. Less common: chills, constipation, cough, hoarseness, runny nose, stuffy nose, sneezing, sore throat, diarrhea, dizziness, fast heartbeat, increased thirst, irritability, loss of appetite, and sexual problems in males.

DRUG INTERACTIONS: The drug should not be taken with narcotic painkillers or alcohol.

ALLERGIES: Individuals allergic to naltrexone or any of its derivatives should discuss this with their doctor or pharmacist before using this drug.

PREGNANCY/BREAST-FEEDING: Category C—Risk cannot be ruled out. Human studies are lacking, and animal studies are either positive for fetal risk or lacking as well. However, potential benefits may justify the potential risk in using the drug. It is not known whether the drug is excreted in the breast milk; therefore, caution should be used when breast-feeding.

OTHER BRAND NAMES: None

OTHER DRUGS IN THE SAME THERAPEUTIC CLASS: Revex

IMPORTANT INFORMATION TO REMEMBER: Only take the drug exactly as directed by your physician. Do not discontinue taking the drug without first consulting your physician; also, do not increase the dose without first consulting with your physician. If stomach upset occurs, take the drug with food or milk. Regular liver tests may be needed to detect possible toxic effects to the liver. Individuals should carry an identification card indicating use of the drug. The drug is only intended as an aid to other treatments such as counseling sessions and/or support group meetings.

BRAND NAME: Rezulin

GENERIC NAME: troglitazone

GENERIC FORM AVAILABLE: No

THERAPEUTIC CLASS: Anti-diabetic

DOSAGE FORMS: 200-mg and 400-mg tablets

MAIN USES: Diabetes

USUAL DOSE: 200 mg to 400 mg once daily

AVERAGE PRICE: $105.67 for 200 mg (30 tablets) and $162.93 for 400 mg (30 tablets)

SIDE EFFECTS: headache 11%, general pain 10%, weakness 6%, dizziness 6%, back pain 6%, nausea 6%, runny nose 5%, diarrhea 5%, swelling in the feet and legs 5%, pharyngitis 5%, decreased blood hemoglobin 5%, and abnormal liver tests 2%.

DRUG INTERACTIONS: Colestid and Questran will decrease the absorption of the drug. The drug may decrease the blood levels of Allegra, Seldane, and Seldane-D. Rezulin and birth control pills may decrease the blood levels of both.

ALLERGIES: Individuals allergic to troglitazone or any of its derivatives should discuss this with their doctor or pharmacist before using this drug.

PREGNANCY/BREAST-FEEDING: Category B—No evidence of risk in humans. Either animal findings show risk, but human findings do not; or, if no adequate human studies have been done, animal findings show no risk. The drug may be excreted in the breast milk; therefore, extreme caution should be used when breast-feeding.

OTHER BRAND NAMES: None

OTHER DRUGS IN THE SAME THERAPEUTIC CLASS: None

IMPORTANT INFORMATION TO REMEMBER: This drug should be taken exactly as directed by your physician. Do not increase the dose or stop taking the drug without first consulting your physician. The drug should be taken with food or milk.

BRAND NAME: Rheumatrex

GENERIC NAME: methotrexate

GENERIC FORM AVAILABLE: Yes

THERAPEUTIC CLASS: Anticancer

DOSAGE FORMS: 2.5-mg tablets and unit-of-use dose packs containing 2.5-mg tablets

MAIN USES: Severe arthritis, cancer, and {psoriasis}

USUAL DOSE: For arthritis: 5 mg to 15 mg one day per week. For cancer: doses will vary based on condition and type of cancer.

AVERAGE PRICE: $41.32 (B)/$33.30 (G) for 2.5-mg dose pack (eight each)

SIDE EFFECTS: Most common: nausea and vomiting. Less common: acne, skin boils, loss of appetite, pale skin, skin rash, itching, loss of hair, stomach ulcers and bleeding, intestinal perforation, blood disorders, bacterial infections, increased sensitivity to sunburn, and sores in the mouth and throat.

DRUG INTERACTIONS: Alcohol may increase the toxic effects of the drug on the liver. The drug should be used with caution in individuals taking NSAIDs (such as Anaprox, Ansaid, Aleve, aspirin, Cataflam, Clinoril, Daypro, Disalcid, Dolobid, Feldene, Indocin, Lodine, Motrin, Nalfon, Naprosyn, Orudis, Oruvail, Relafen, Tolectin, and Voltaren). Probenecid may increase the blood levels of the drug. The drug should be used with caution by individuals taking other drugs to treat cancer or who will be given a live virus vaccine.

ALLERGIES: Individuals allergic to methotrexate or any of its derivatives should discuss this with their doctor or pharmacist before using this drug.

PREGNANCY/BREAST-FEEDING: Category X—Should not be used during pregnancy. Studies in animals and/or humans have shown fetal abnormalities and birth defects. The risks associated with using this drug clearly outweigh the benefits. This drug should never be used by someone who is pregnant or trying to become pregnant. Also, women should never breast-feed while using this drug.

OTHER BRAND NAMES: None

OTHER DRUGS IN THE SAME THERAPEUTIC CLASS: None

IMPORTANT INFORMATION TO REMEMBER: Only take the drug exactly as directed by your physician. Do not discontinue taking the drug and do not increase the dose without first consulting your physician. It is very important to follow the dosing schedule set by your physician exactly. If stomach upset occurs, take the drug with food or milk. Individuals should also avoid alcoholic beverages while taking this drug. This drug may also increase the sensitivity of the skin to sunburn in some individuals; therefore, a sunscreen is recommended during periods of prolonged exposure to the sun.

BRAND NAME: Rhinocort

GENERIC NAME: budesonide

GENERIC FORM AVAILABLE: No

THERAPEUTIC CLASS: Steroid nasal spray

DOSAGE FORMS: 32-micrograms-per-spray nasal inhaler

MAIN USES: Nasal allergies

USUAL DOSE: two sprays in each nostril twice daily in the morning and evening, or four sprays in each nostril in the morning

AVERAGE PRICE: $43.66

SIDE EFFECTS: nasal irritation 3%–9%, pharyngitis 3%–9%, increased cough 3%–9%, bloody nose 3%–9%, dry mouth 1%–3%, and nausea 1%–3%.

DRUG INTERACTIONS: Caution should be used when taking this drug with other oral corticosteroids such as Aristocort, Decadron, Deltasone, Medrol, and prednisone.

ALLERGIES: Individuals allergic to budesonide or other nasal steroids (such as those listed under "Other Drugs in the Same Therapeutic Class") should discuss this with their doctor or pharmacist before taking this drug.

PREGNANCY/BREAST-FEEDING: Category C—Risk cannot be ruled out. Human studies are lacking, and animal studies are either positive for fetal risk or lacking as well. However, potential benefits may justify the potential risk in using the drug. It is not known whether the drug is excreted in the breast milk; therefore, caution should be used when breast-feeding.

OTHER BRAND NAMES: None

OTHER DRUGS IN THE SAME THERAPEUTIC CLASS: Beconase, Beconase AQ, Dexacort, Flonase, Nasacort, Nasalide, Vancenase, and Vancenase AQ

IMPORTANT INFORMATION TO REMEMBER: The drug is not intended to provide immediate relief of nasal allergies. To receive the full benefits of the drug, use it on a regular basis as a maintenance medication. If some improvements are not seen in seven days, the individual needs to be reassessed by a doctor. The drug may take up to three weeks before the full benefits are seen. Never exceed the prescribed dosage unless directed to do so by a doctor; excessive use beyond the prescribed dosage is potentially dangerous. This drug should not be used by individuals with fungal, bacterial, systemic viral, or respiratory tract infections; unhealed wounds inside the nose; or tuberculosis.

When using the nasal spray, use the following procedure:

1) Blow your nose gently to clear your nostrils, if necessary.
2) With your other hand, gently place a finger against the side of your nose to close the opposite nostril.
3) Insert the tip of the bottle or aerosol into the open nostril. Point the tip toward the back and outer side of the nostril once inside.
4) After releasing the spray, close your mouth, sniff deeply, hold your breath for a few seconds, then breathe out through your mouth.
5) Tilt your head back slightly for a few seconds to allow the drug to spread to the back of your nose.
6) Repeat the same procedure for the other nostril.
7) If using more than one spray in each nostril, wait five minutes between sprays.

BRAND NAME: Ridaura

GENERIC NAME: auranofin

GENERIC FORM AVAILABLE: No

THERAPEUTIC CLASS: Gold salt antiarthritic

DOSAGE FORMS: 3-mg capsules

MAIN USES: Arthritis

USUAL DOSE: 6 mg daily in one or two divided doses

AVERAGE PRICE: $102.46 for 60 capsules

SIDE EFFECTS: diarrhea 47%, rash 24%, itching 17%, stomach pain 14%, sores in the mouth and throat 13%, nausea 10%, gas 3%–9%, loss of appetite 3%–9%, eye redness 3%–9%, protein in the urine 3%–9%, constipation 1%–3%, hair loss 1%–3%, anemia 1%–3%, and other blood disorders 1%–3%.

DRUG INTERACTIONS: Cuprimine or Depen and the drug, when used together, may increase the risk of serious blood disorders. The drug may increase the blood levels of Dilantin.

ALLERGIES: Individuals allergic to auranofin, other gold salts, or any of their derivatives should discuss this with their doctor or pharmacist before using this drug.

PREGNANCY/BREAST-FEEDING: Category C—Risk cannot be ruled out. Human studies are lacking, and animal studies are either positive for fetal risk or lacking as well. However, potential benefits may justify the potential risk in using the drug. It is not known whether the drug is excreted in the breast milk; therefore, caution should be used when breast-feeding.

OTHER BRAND NAMES: None

OTHER DRUGS IN THE SAME THERAPEUTIC CLASS: Myochrysine and Solganal

IMPORTANT INFORMATION TO REMEMBER: Only take the drug exactly as directed by your physician. Do not discontinue taking the drug without first consulting your physician; also, do not increase the dose without first consulting with your physician. It is important to follow the dosing schedule set by your physician exactly. If stomach upset occurs, take the drug with food or milk. Regular blood and urine tests may be necessary to detect possible adverse effects.

BRAND NAME: Rifamate

GENERIC NAME: Combination product containing: rifampin and isoniazid

GENERIC FORM AVAILABLE: No

THERAPEUTIC CLASS: Antituberculosis

DOSAGE FORMS: 150-mg isoniazid/300-mg rifampin capsules

MAIN USES: Tuberculosis

USUAL DOSE: two capsules daily one hour before meals or two hours after a meal

AVERAGE PRICE: $204.27 for 60 capsules

SIDE EFFECTS: Most common: diarrhea; stomach pain; reddish-orange to reddish-brown discoloration of the urine, feces, sweat, saliva, tears, and sputum; hepatitis; unsteadiness; burning or tingling in the hands and/or feet; nausea; and vomiting. Less common: sores in the mouth or tongue, flu-like syndrome, headache, blood disorders, liver disorders, and itching.

DRUG INTERACTIONS: Alcohol may increase the toxic effects of the drug on the liver. The drug may increase the blood levels of Dilantin and Tegretol. The drug should not be used with Antabuse.

The drug may decrease the blood levels of drugs used to treat irregular heartbeats, diabetes drugs, Aristocort, Calan, Calan SR, Coumadin, Decadron, Deltasone, Dilfucan, Dolophine, estrogens, Isoptin, Isoptin SR, Lanoxin, Medrol, Mycelex, Nizoral, prednisone, Slo-bid, Sporanox, Theo-Dur, theophylline, Uni-Dur, and Uniphyl. The drug may decrease the effectiveness of oral contraceptives (birth control pills).

ALLERGIES: Individuals allergic to rifampin, isoniazid, or any of their derivatives should discuss this with their doctor or pharmacist before using this drug.

PREGNANCY/BREAST-FEEDING: Category C—Risk cannot be ruled out. Human studies are lacking, and animal studies are either positive for fetal risk or lacking as well. However, potential benefits may justify the potential risk in using the drug. The drug is excreted in the breast milk; therefore, extreme caution should be used when breast-feeding.

OTHER BRAND NAMES: None

OTHER DRUGS IN THE SAME THERAPEUTIC CLASS: Rifadin and Rifater

IMPORTANT INFORMATION TO REMEMBER: Only take the drug exactly as directed by your physician. Do not discontinue taking the drug without first consulting your physician. The drug should be taken one hour before meals or two hours after a meal. It is important to complete the full course of therapy, which may take weeks, months, or even years. Individuals should have regular blood and liver tests to detect possible adverse effects of the drug. The drug may cause reddish-orange to reddish-brown discoloration of the urine, feces, sweat, saliva, tears, and sputum; also, individuals taking the drug should not wear contact lenses. Individuals should also avoid alcoholic beverages while taking this drug. Women taking birth control pills should use another form of contraception while taking the drug and for the rest of the current menstrual cycle.

BRAND NAME: Rifater

GENERIC NAME: Combination product containing: rifampin, isoniazid, and pyrazinamide

GENERIC FORM AVAILABLE: No

THERAPEUTIC CLASS: Antituberculosis

DOSAGE FORMS: 120-mg rifampin/50-mg isoniazid/300-mg pyrazinamide tablets

MAIN USES: Tuberculosis

USUAL DOSE: four to six tablets once daily (based on age and weight), one hour before meals or two hours after a meal, with a full glass of water

AVERAGE PRICE: $151.20 for 60 capsules

SIDE EFFECTS: Most common: diarrhea; stomach pain; reddish-orange to reddish-brown discoloration of the urine, feces, sweat, saliva, tears, and sputum; hepatitis; unsteadiness; burning or tingling in the hands and/or feet; nausea; and vomiting. Less common: sores in the mouth or tongue, flu-like syndrome, tightness in the chest, pounding heartbeat, ringing in the ears, blood disorders, liver disorders, and itching.

DRUG INTERACTIONS: Alcohol may increase the toxic effects of the drug on the liver. The drug may increase the blood levels of Dilantin and Tegretol. The drug should not be used with Antabuse. The drug may decrease the blood levels of drugs used to treat irregular heartbeats, diabetes drugs, Aristocort, Calan, Calan SR, Coumadin, Decadron, Deltasone, Dilfucan, Dolophine, estrogens, Isoptin, Isoptin SR, Lanoxin, Medrol, Mycelex, Nizoral, prednisone, Slo-bid, Sporanox, Theo-Dur, theophylline, Uni-Dur, and Uniphyl. The drug may decrease the effectiveness of oral contraceptives (birth control pills).

ALLERGIES: Individuals allergic to rifampin, isoniazid, pyrazinamide, or any of their derivatives should discuss this with their doctor or pharmacist before using this drug.

PREGNANCY/BREAST-FEEDING: Category C—Risk cannot be ruled out. Human studies are lacking, and animal studies are either positive for fetal risk or lacking as well. However, potential benefits may justify the potential risk in using the drug. It is not known whether the drug is excreted in the breast milk; therefore, caution should be used when breast-feeding.

OTHER BRAND NAMES: None

OTHER DRUGS IN THE SAME THERAPEUTIC CLASS: Rifadin and Rifamate

IMPORTANT INFORMATION TO REMEMBER: Only take the drug exactly as directed by your physician. Do not discontinue taking the drug without first consulting your physician. The drug should be taken one hour before meals or two hours after a meal. It is important to complete the full course of therapy, which may take weeks, months, or even years. Individuals should have regular blood and liver tests to detect possible adverse effects of the drug. The drug may cause reddish-orange to reddish-brown discoloration of the urine, feces, sweat, saliva, tears, and sputum; also, individuals taking the drug should not wear contact lenses. Individuals should also avoid alcoholic beverages while taking this drug. Women taking birth control pills should use another form of contraception while taking the drug and for the rest of the current menstrual cycle.

BRAND NAME: Risperdal

GENERIC NAME: risperidone

GENERIC FORM AVAILABLE: No

THERAPEUTIC CLASS: Benzisoxazole antipsychotic

DOSAGE FORMS: 1-mg, 2-mg, 3-mg, and 4-mg tablets; and 1 mg/mL solution

MAIN USES: Psychotic disorders

USUAL DOSE: 1 mg to 3 mg twice daily

AVERAGE PRICE: $265.44 for 1 mg; $441.84 for 2 mg; $552.72 for 3 mg; $735.84 for 4 mg

SIDE EFFECTS: insomnia 26%, agitation 22%, extrapyramidal symptoms (unusual movements of the arms, legs, and tongue) 17%, headache 14%, nervousness 12%, runny nose 10%, constipation 7%, nausea 6%, vomiting 5%, increased sensitivity to sunburn 5%, stomach pain 4%, dizziness 4%, fast heartbeat 3%, coughing 3%, drowsiness 3%, rash 2%, abnormal vision 2%, muscle pain 2%, increased saliva 2%, toothache 2%, and trouble breathing 1%.

DRUG INTERACTIONS: The drug may decrease the effects of Larodopa. Tegretol may decrease the blood levels of the drug. Clozaril may increase the blood levels of the drug.

ALLERGIES: Individuals allergic to risperidone or any of its derivatives should discuss this with their doctor or pharmacist before using this drug.

PREGNANCY/BREAST-FEEDING: Category C—Risk cannot be ruled out. Human studies are lacking, and animal studies are either positive for fetal risk or lacking as well. However, potential benefits may justify the potential risk in using the drug. This drug should not be taken by nursing mothers.

OTHER BRAND NAMES: None

OTHER DRUGS IN THE SAME THERAPEUTIC CLASS: None

IMPORTANT INFORMATION TO REMEMBER: This drug may cause drowsiness. Individuals should use caution when driving, operating machinery, or performing any task where mental alertness is required. Alcohol, anxiety medications, and narcotic painkillers may intensify the drowsiness effect of the drug. Do not increase the dose without first consulting with your physician. Individuals should report any involuntary movements of the tongue and extremities to their physician. If stomach upset occurs, take the drug with food or milk. Individuals should get up slowly from a sitting or lying-down position; otherwise dizziness may occur. This drug may also increase the sensitivity of the skin to sunburn in some individuals; therefore, a sunscreen is recommended during periods of prolonged exposure to the sun. Caution should be used during hot weather due to decreased tolerance to the heat.

BRAND NAME: Ritalin

GENERIC NAME: methylphenidate

GENERIC FORM AVAILABLE: Yes

THERAPEUTIC CLASS: Stimulant

DOSAGE FORMS: 5-mg, 10-mg, and 20-mg tablets; and 20-mg sustained-release tablets

MAIN USES: Treatment of attention deficit disorders with hyperactivity (ADDH) in children six years and older, and treatment of narcolepsy in adults

USUAL DOSE: For attention deficit disorder with hyperactivity (ADDH): 5 mg to 40 mg once or twice daily. For narcolepsy: 10 mg to 60 mg daily in two or three divided doses.

AVERAGE PRICE: $46.04 (B)/$39.55 (G) for 5 mg; $65.70 (B)/ $55.72 (G) for 10 mg; $94.51 (B)/$79.80 (G) for 20 mg; $144.66 (B)/$118.65 (G) for 20 mg sustained-release tablets

SIDE EFFECTS: Most common: nervousness, insomnia, loss of appetite, fast heartbeat, and increased blood pressure. Less common: drowsiness, dizziness, headache, nausea, stomach pain, chest pain, and allergic reaction to the drug (bruising, fever, joint pain, skin rash, or hives).

DRUG INTERACTIONS: Decongestants found in cough, cold, and allergy products may result in additive stimulation and nervousness. The drug should not be taken with Orap. Nardil and Parnate may increase the effects of the drug and may cause very high blood pressure.

ALLERGIES: Individuals allergic to methylphenidate or any of its derivatives should discuss this with their doctor or pharmacist before using this drug.

PREGNANCY/BREAST-FEEDING: Category C—Risk cannot be ruled out. Human studies are lacking, and animal studies are either positive for fetal risk or lacking as well. However, potential benefits may justify the potential risk in using the drug. It is not known whether the drug is excreted in the breast milk; therefore, caution should be used when breast-feeding.

OTHER BRAND NAMES: None

OTHER DRUGS IN THE SAME THERAPEUTIC CLASS: Adderall, Cylert, and Dexedrine

IMPORTANT INFORMATION TO REMEMBER: This drug may cause some drowsiness in children and teens. Individuals should use caution when driving, operating machinery, or performing any task where mental alertness is required. Alcohol, anxiety medications, and narcotic painkillers may intensify the drowsiness effect of the drug. Do not increase the dose of medication without consulting with your doctor. Only take the amount prescribed by your doctor. After long-term use, gradual reduction in dose may be needed if the drug is to be discontinued. This prescription cannot be refilled; a new written prescription must be obtained each time. This medication is a controlled substance and may be habit-forming. The potential for abuse with this medication is high.

BRAND NAME: **Robaxin**

GENERIC NAME: methocarbamol

GENERIC FORM AVAILABLE: Yes

THERAPEUTIC CLASS: Muscle relaxant

DOSAGE FORMS: 500-mg and 750-mg tablets

MAIN USES: Muscle spasms

USUAL DOSE: 500 mg to 1000 mg four times daily

AVERAGE PRICE: $56.85 (B)/$17.17 (G) for 500 mg and $81.16 (B)/$19.44 (G) for 750 mg

SIDE EFFECTS: Most common: blurred vision, drowsiness, and dizziness. Less common: stuffy nose, red eyes, fever, headache, muscle weakness, uncontrolled movements of the eyes, flushing, nausea, rash, itching, and vomiting.

DRUG INTERACTIONS: Alcohol, anxiety medications, and narcotic painkillers may intensify the drowsiness effect of the drug.

ALLERGIES: Individuals allergic to methocarbamol, Robaxisal, or any of their derivatives should discuss this with their doctor or pharmacist before using this drug.

PREGNANCY/BREAST-FEEDING: Category C—Risk cannot be ruled out. Human studies are lacking, and animal studies are either positive for fetal risk or lacking as well. However, potential benefits may justify the potential risk in using the drug. It is not known whether the drug is excreted in the breast milk; therefore, caution should be used when breast-feeding.

OTHER BRAND NAMES: None

OTHER DRUGS IN THE SAME THERAPEUTIC CLASS: Flexeril, Lioresal, Parafon Forte DSC, Skelaxin, and Soma

IMPORTANT INFORMATION TO REMEMBER: Only take the drug exactly as directed by your physician; also, do not increase the dose without first consulting with your physician. If stomach upset occurs, take the drug with food or milk. This drug does cause drowsiness. Individuals should use caution when driving, operating machinery, or performing any task where mental alertness is required. Alcohol, anxiety medications, and narcotic painkillers may intensify the drowsiness effect of the drug.

BRAND NAME: Rocaltrol

GENERIC NAME: calcitriol

GENERIC FORM AVAILABLE: No

THERAPEUTIC CLASS: Vitamin D derivative

DOSAGE FORMS: 0.25-microgram and 0.5-microgram capsules

MAIN USES: Low calcium in chronic renal dialysis and low parathyroid activity

USUAL DOSE: 0.25 micrograms to 1 microgram daily

AVERAGE PRICE: $154.05 for 0.25 micrograms and $246.37 for 0.5 micrograms

SIDE EFFECTS: Most side effects are associated with toxicity (too much of the drug). These symptoms are broken down into early symptoms of toxicity and late symptoms of toxicity. Early symptoms: constipation, diarrhea, dry mouth, continuous headache, increased thirst, increased urination, loss of appetite, metallic taste, nausea, vomiting, and unusual weakness or tiredness. Late symptoms: bone pain, cloudy urine, high blood pressure, irritation of the eyes, increased sensitivity of the eyes to sunlight, irregular heartbeat, itchy skin, muscle pain, psychosis, weight loss, nausea, and vomiting.

DRUG INTERACTIONS: Diuretics (water pills) may cause high levels of calcium in the blood. Antacids may cause high levels of magnesium in the blood. High doses of calcium may cause dangerous levels of calcium in the blood, because the drug increases calcium absorption.

ALLERGIES: Individuals allergic to calcitriol or any of its derivatives should discuss this with their doctor or pharmacist before using this drug.

PREGNANCY/BREAST-FEEDING: Category C—Risk cannot be ruled out. Human studies are lacking, and animal studies are either positive for fetal risk or lacking as well. However, potential benefits may justify the potential risk in using the drug. It is not known whether the drug is excreted in the breast milk; therefore, caution should be used when breast-feeding.

OTHER BRAND NAMES: None

OTHER DRUGS IN THE SAME THERAPEUTIC CLASS: None

IMPORTANT INFORMATION TO REMEMBER: Only take the drug exactly as directed by your physician. Do not discontinue taking the drug without first consulting your physician. If stomach upset occurs, take the drug with food or milk. Do not take large doses of calcium unless directed to do so by your physician.

BRAND NAME: Rogaine

GENERIC NAME: minoxidil

GENERIC FORM AVAILABLE: Yes

THERAPEUTIC CLASS: Hair growth stimulant

DOSAGE FORMS: 2% topical solution

MAIN USES: Male pattern baldness and hair loss or thinning

USUAL DOSE: Apply 1 mL to the affected area twice daily.

AVERAGE PRICE: $67.25 (B)/$37.81 (G)

SIDE EFFECTS: Most common: none. Less common: skin irritation and rash.

DRUG INTERACTIONS: Do not use other medicinal creams, ointments, solutions, and lotions on the scalp while using the drug; this may increase the absorption of the drug into the body.

ALLERGIES: Individuals allergic to minoxidil or any of its derivatives should discuss this with their doctor or pharmacist before using this drug.

PREGNANCY/BREAST-FEEDING: Category C—Risk cannot be ruled out. Human studies are lacking, and animal studies are either positive for fetal risk or lacking as well. However, potential benefits may justify the potential risk in using the drug. It is not known whether the drug is excreted in the breast milk; therefore, caution should be used when breast-feeding.

OTHER BRAND NAMES: None

OTHER DRUGS IN THE SAME THERAPEUTIC CLASS: None

IMPORTANT INFORMATION TO REMEMBER: The drug is for external use only. Avoid contacting the eyes with the solution. Only use the drug exactly as directed by your physician and do not increase the dose. Results may not be noticeable for up to four weeks. This is a treatment, not a cure. The drug must be used forever to sustain hair regrowth. Individuals who stop using the drug will see the new hair fall out within six months. The drug is also available in an over-the-counter 2% solution without a prescription.

BRAND NAME: Rondec, Rondec DM, and Rondec TR

GENERIC NAME: Combination product containing: carbinoxamine, pseudoephedrine, and dextromethorphan (Rondec DM); and carbinoxamine and pseudoephedrine (Rondec and Rondec TR)

GENERIC FORM AVAILABLE: Yes (Rondec DM only)

THERAPEUTIC CLASS: Antihistamine + decongestant (Rondec DM also contains a cough suppressant)

DOSAGE FORMS: Rondec: 4-mg carbinoxamine/60-mg pseudoephedrine tablets and syrup (per 5 mL). Rondec TR: 8-mg carbinoxamine/120-mg pseudoephedrine sustained-release tablets. Rondec Oral Drops: 2 mg carbinoxamine/25 mg pseudoephedrine per mL. Rondec Chewable: 4-mg carbinoxamine/60-mg pseudoephedrine tablets. Rondec DM: 4 mg carbinoxamine/60-mg pseudoephedrine/15 mg dextromethorphan per 5 mL syrup. Rondec DM Oral Drops: 2 mg carbinoxamine/25 mg pseudoephedrine/4 mg dextromethorphan per mL.

MAIN USES: Runny nose, congestion, and cough

USUAL DOSE: For Rondec TR: one tablet twice daily as needed. For Rondec tablets: one tablet four times daily as needed. For Rondec DM and Rondec Syrup: one teaspoon four times daily as needed.

AVERAGE PRICE: $128.99 for Rondec TR tablets; $17.76 (B)/ $9.27 (G) for Rondec DM syrup (120 mL); and $19.78 for Rondec Syrup (120 mL)

SIDE EFFECTS: Most common: drowsiness. Less common: nausea, giddiness, dry mouth, blurred vision, pounding heartbeat, flushing, and increased irritability or excitability (especially in children).

DRUG INTERACTIONS: Blocadren, Cartrol, Corgard, Inderal, Kerlone, Levatol, Lopressor, Normodyne, Sectral, Tenormin, Toprol-

XL, Trandate, Visken, and Zebeta may increase the effects of the drug. The drug may also reduce the effects of blood-pressure-lowering drugs. Nardil or Parnate may significantly raise blood pressure when taken with this drug.

ALLERGIES: Individuals allergic to carbinoxamine, pseudoephedrine, dextromethorphan, or any of their derivatives should discuss this with their doctor or pharmacist before using this drug.

PREGNANCY/BREAST-FEEDING: Category C—Risk cannot be ruled out. Human studies are lacking, and animal studies are either positive for fetal risk or lacking as well. However, potential benefits may justify the potential risk in using the drug. The drug is excreted in the breast milk; therefore, extreme caution should be used when breast-feeding.

OTHER BRAND NAMES: None

OTHER DRUGS IN THE SAME THERAPEUTIC CLASS: For Rondec DM: Actifed w/Codeine, Bromfed-DM, Dimetane-DX, Poly-Histine CS, Poly-Histine DM, and Ru-Tuss w/Hydrocodone. For Rondec and Rondec TR: Bromfed, Bromfed PD, Claritin-D, Comhist LA, Deconamine SR, Fedahist, Naldecon, Novafed-A, Nucofed, Ornade, Poly-Histine-D, Rynatan, Seldane-D, Semprex-D, Tavist-D, and Trinalin

IMPORTANT INFORMATION TO REMEMBER: This drug does cause drowsiness. Individuals should use caution when driving, operating machinery, or performing any task where mental alertness is required. Alcohol, anxiety medications, and narcotic painkillers may intensify the drowsiness effect of the drug. This drug may also cause a dry mouth; sugarless gum or hard candy will help take care of this problem. Patients with glaucoma, high blood pressure, heart conditions, or urinary or prostate problems should consult their doctor before taking this drug. The Rondec TR is a sustained-release formulation; do not crush these tablets. However, they may be cut in half for easier swallowing.

BRAND NAME: Rowasa

GENERIC NAME: mesalamine

GENERIC FORM AVAILABLE: No

THERAPEUTIC CLASS: Salicylate

DOSAGE FORMS: 4 g/60 mL enema and 500-mg rectal suppositories

MAIN USES: Mildly to moderately active ulcerative colitis, proctosigmoiditis, and proctitis

USUAL DOSE: one enema or one suppository once or twice daily

AVERAGE PRICE: $91.65 for seven enemas and $95.70 for 24 suppositories

SIDE EFFECTS: stomach pain/cramps 8%, headache 7%, gas 6%, nausea 6%, tiredness 3%, fever 3%, rash 3%, diarrhea 2%, dizziness 2%, bloating 2%, back pain 1%, itching 1%, rectal pain 1%, hair loss 1%, and swelling 1%.

DRUG INTERACTIONS: None of any clinical significance

ALLERGIES: Patients allergic to mesalamine, aspirin, or aspirin derivatives should consult their doctor or pharmacist before taking this drug.

PREGNANCY/BREAST-FEEDING: Category B—No evidence of risk in humans. Either animal findings show risk, but human findings do not; or, if no adequate human studies have been done, animal findings show no risk. It is not known whether the drug is excreted in the breast milk; therefore, caution should be used when breast-feeding.

OTHER BRAND NAMES: None

OTHER DRUGS IN THE SAME THERAPEUTIC CLASS: Asacol, Azulfidine, Dipentum, and Pentasa

IMPORTANT INFORMATION TO REMEMBER: Colitis symptoms may become worse in 3% of those taking the drug. Only use the drug exactly as directed by your physician and do not increase the dose without first consulting with your physician. For best results, have a bowel movement before using the enema if possible. The enema should be shaken well before use and should be retained in the rectum for eight hours if possible; therefore, it's best to use the enema at bedtime. Keep the suppositories in the refrigerator to avoid melting.

When using the suppositories or enema, individuals should:

1) Lie on the left side with the left leg extended and the right leg bent forward.
2) Remove the suppository from the foil or the cap from the enema.
3) Insert the suppository gently into the rectum about one inch, or

insert the tip of the enema gently into the rectum and steadily squeeze the bottle.
4) Try to retain the medication in the rectum for as long as possible (at least one to three hours or longer for the suppository and eight hours or longer for the enema).

BRAND NAME: Rufen

GENERIC NAME: ibuprofen

See entry for Motrin

BRAND NAME: Ru-Tuss and Ru-Tuss DE

GENERIC NAME: Combination product containing: phenylephrine, phenylpropanolamine, chlorpheniramine, hyoscyamine, atropine, and scopolamine (Ru-Tuss); and pseudoephedrine and guaifenesin (Ru-Tuss DE)

GENERIC FORM AVAILABLE: Yes

THERAPEUTIC CLASS: Antihistamine + decongestant + anticholinergic

DOSAGE FORMS: For Ru-Tuss: 25-mg phenylephrine/50-mg phenylpropanolamine/8-mg chlorpheniramine/0.19-mg hyoscyamine/0.04-mg atropine/0.01-mg scopolamine sustained-release tablets. For Ru-Tuss DE: 120-mg pseudoephedrine/600-mg guaifenesin sustained-release tablets.

MAIN USES: Nasal allergies and congestion (Ru-Tuss); and nasal congestion and cough (Ru-Tuss DE)

USUAL DOSE: one tablet every 12 hours as needed

AVERAGE PRICE: $29.10 (B)/$18.09 (G) for Ru-Tuss and $86.66 (B)/$36.49 (G) for Ru-Tuss DE

SIDE EFFECTS: Most common: drowsiness. Less common: nausea, giddiness, dry mouth, blurred vision, pounding heartbeat, flushing, and increased irritability or excitability (especially in children).

DRUG INTERACTIONS: Blocadren, Cartrol, Corgard, Inderal, Kerlone, Levatol, Lopressor, Normodyne, Sectral, Tenormin, Toprol-XL, Trandate, Visken, and Zebeta may increase the effects of the drug. The drug may also reduce the effects of blood-pressure-lowering drugs. Nardil or Parnate may significantly raise blood pressure when taken with this drug.

ALLERGIES: Individuals allergic to phenylephrine, phenylpropanolamine, chlorpheniramine, pseudoephedrine, hyoscyamine, atropine, scopolamine, antihistamine/decongestant combinations, or any of their derivatives should discuss this with their doctor or pharmacist before using this drug.

PREGNANCY/BREAST-FEEDING: Category C—Risk cannot be ruled out. Human studies are lacking, and animal studies are either positive for fetal risk or lacking as well. However, potential benefits may justify the potential risk in using the drug. The drug is excreted in the breast milk; therefore, extreme caution should be used when breast-feeding.

OTHER BRAND NAMES: Atrohist Plus

OTHER DRUGS IN THE SAME THERAPEUTIC CLASS: For Ru-Tuss: Extendryl JR and Extendryl SR. For Ru-Tuss DE: Deconsal II, Entex, Entex LA, Entex PSE, Exgest LA, and Zephrex LA

IMPORTANT INFORMATION TO REMEMBER: This drug does cause drowsiness. Individuals should use caution when driving, operating machinery, or performing any task where mental alertness is required. Alcohol, anxiety medications, and narcotic painkillers may intensify the drowsiness effect of the drug. This drug may also cause a dry mouth; sugarless gum or hard candy will help take care of this problem. Patients with glaucoma, high blood pressure, heart conditions, or urinary or prostate problems should consult their doctor before taking this drug. These drugs are sustained-release formulations; do not crush the tablets. However, they may be cut in half for easier swallowing. Individuals taking the Ru-Tuss DE should take the drug with a full glass of water; this will help break up the mucus.

BRAND NAME: Rynatan and Rynatan Pediatric Suspension

GENERIC NAME: Combination product containing: chlorpheniramine tannate, pyrilamine tannate, and phenylephrine tannate

GENERIC FORM AVAILABLE: Yes

THERAPEUTIC CLASS: Antihistamine + decongestant

DOSAGE FORMS: 8-mg chlorpheniramine tannate/25-mg pyrilamine tannate/25-mg phenylephrine tannate tablets; and 2-mg chlorpheniramine tannate/12.5-mg pyrilamine tannate/5-mg phenylephrine tannate per 5 mL pediatric suspension

MAIN USES: Nasal allergies and congestion

USUAL DOSE: one or two tablets every 12 hours as needed or $1/2$ to 2 teaspoons every 12 hours as needed

AVERAGE PRICE: $29.22 (B)/$13.83 (G) for Rynatan Pediatric Suspension 120 mL; and $192.05 (B)/$35.36 (G) tablets

SIDE EFFECTS: Most common: drowsiness. Less common: nausea, giddiness, dry mouth, blurred vision, pounding heartbeat, flushing, and increased irritability or excitability (especially in children).

DRUG INTERACTIONS: Blocadren, Cartrol, Corgard, Inderal, Kerlone, Levatol, Lopressor, Normodyne, Sectral, Tenormin, Toprol-XL, Trandate, Visken, and Zebeta may increase the effects of the drug. The drug may also reduce the effects of blood-pressure-lowering drugs. Nardil or Parnate may significantly raise blood pressure when taken with this drug.

ALLERGIES: Individuals allergic to chlorpheniramine tannate, pyrilamine tannate, phenylephrine tannate, or any of their derivatives should discuss this with their doctor or pharmacist before using this drug.

PREGNANCY/BREAST-FEEDING: Category C—Risk cannot be ruled out. Human studies are lacking, and animal studies are either positive for fetal risk or lacking as well. However, potential benefits may justify the potential risk in using the drug. The drug is excreted in the breast milk; therefore, extreme caution should be used when breast-feeding.

OTHER BRAND NAMES: None

OTHER DRUGS IN THE SAME THERAPEUTIC CLASS: Bromfed, Bromfed PD, Claritin-D, Comhist LA, Deconamine SR, Fedahist, Naldecon, Novafed-A, Nucofed, Ornade, Poly-Histine-D, Rynatan, Seldane-D, Semprex-D, Tavist-D, and Trinalin

IMPORTANT INFORMATION TO REMEMBER: This drug does cause drowsiness. Individuals should use caution when driving, operating machinery, or performing any task where mental alertness is

required. Alcohol, anxiety medications, and narcotic painkillers may intensify the drowsiness effect of the drug. This drug may also cause a dry mouth; sugarless gum or hard candy will help take care of this problem. Patients with glaucoma, high blood pressure, heart conditions, or urinary or prostate problems should consult their doctor before taking this drug.

BRAND NAME: Rythmol

GENERIC NAME: propafenone

GENERIC FORM AVAILABLE: No

THERAPEUTIC CLASS: Class IC antiarrhythmic

DOSAGE FORMS: 150-mg, 225-mg, and 300-mg tablets

MAIN USES: Irregular heartbeat

USUAL DOSE: 150 mg to 300 mg every eight hours

AVERAGE PRICE: $117.34 for 150 mg; $167.27 for 225 mg; and $212.91 for 300 mg

SIDE EFFECTS: dizziness 4%–11%, nausea 3%–9%, unusual taste 3%–6%, constipation 2%–5%, tiredness 2%–4%, trouble breathing 2%–4%, angina 2%–3%, headache 2%–3%, blurred vision 1%–3%, fast heartbeat 1%–3%, pounding heartbeat 1%–3%, rash 1%–2%, diarrhea 1%–2%, weakness 1%–2%, dry mouth 1%–2%, chest pain 1%, changes in appetite 1%, slow heartbeat 1%, nervousness 1%, drowsiness 1%, and tremors 1%.

DRUG INTERACTIONS: The drug may increase the blood levels of Coumadin and Lanoxin. Caution should be used by patients taking other drugs specifically used for irregular heartbeat.

ALLERGIES: Individuals allergic to propafenone or any of its derivatives should discuss this with their doctor or pharmacist before using this drug.

PREGNANCY/BREAST-FEEDING: Category C—Risk cannot be ruled out. Human studies are lacking, and animal studies are either positive for fetal risk or lacking as well. However, potential benefits may justify the potential risk in using the drug. It is not known whether the drug is excreted in the breast milk; therefore, caution should be used when breast-feeding.

OTHER BRAND NAMES: None

OTHER DRUGS IN THE SAME THERAPEUTIC CLASS: Tambocor

IMPORTANT INFORMATION TO REMEMBER: This drug may cause some dizziness or tiredness, especially at first. Individuals should use caution when driving, operating machinery, or performing any task where mental alertness is required. Alcohol, anxiety medications, and narcotic painkillers may intensify these effects. Only take the drug exactly as directed by your physician. Do not discontinue taking the drug without first consulting your physician. Also, do not increase the dose without first consulting with your physician.

BRAND NAME: Salflex

GENERIC NAME: salsalate

See entry for Disalcid

BRAND NAME: Sectral

GENERIC NAME: acebutolol

GENERIC FORM AVAILABLE: Yes

THERAPEUTIC CLASS: Cardioselective beta-blocker

DOSAGE FORMS: 200-mg and 400-mg capsules

MAIN USES: High blood pressure and irregular heartbeat

USUAL DOSE: 200 mg to 400 mg once or twice daily

AVERAGE PRICE: $137.45 (B)/$100.98 (G) for 200 mg and $182.74 (B)/$133.98 (G) for 400 mg

SIDE EFFECTS: tiredness 11%, headache 6%, dizziness 6%, constipation 4%, nausea 4%, diarrhea 4%, trouble breathing 4%, gas 3%, increased urination 3%, insomnia 3%, abnormal dreams 2%, rash 2%, chest pain 2%, swelling 2%, depression 2%, muscle pain 2%, runny nose 2%, and abnormal vision 2%.

DRUG INTERACTIONS: The drug may cause additive effects when used with reserpine. The drug may increase the effects of Calan, Cardene, Cardizem, Catapres, Covera-HS, Dilacor XR, DynaCirc, Isoptin, Lanoxin, Norvasc, Plendil, Procardia, Sular, Tiazac, Verelan, and Wytensin. Diabetic medications, insulin, Slo-bid, Theo-Dur, theophylline, Uni-Dur, and Uniphyl dosages may need to be adjusted when taking this drug. The drug may also interfere with glaucoma screening tests.

ALLERGIES: Individuals allergic to acebutolol or other beta-blockers (such as those listed under "Other Drugs in the Same Therapeutic Class") should discuss this with their doctor or pharmacist before taking this drug.

PREGNANCY/BREAST-FEEDING: Category B—No evidence of risk in humans. Either animal findings show risk, but human findings do not; or, if no adequate human studies have been done, animal findings show no risk. The drug is excreted in the breast milk; therefore, extreme caution should be used when breast-feeding.

OTHER BRAND NAMES: None

OTHER DRUGS IN THE SAME THERAPEUTIC CLASS: Kerlone, Lopressor, Tenormin, Toprol-XL, and Zebeta

IMPORTANT INFORMATION TO REMEMBER: Only take the drug exactly as directed by your physician. Do not discontinue taking the drug without first consulting your physician. This drug may cause some tiredness, especially at first. Individuals should use caution when driving, operating machinery, or performing any task where mental alertness is required. Alcohol, anxiety medications, and narcotic painkillers may intensify the tiredness effect of the drug. Before taking over-the-counter cold and allergy preparations, consult your doctor or pharmacist—these products may raise your blood pressure. This drug may mask the symptoms of low blood sugar in diabetics.

BRAND NAME: Seldane and Seldane-D

GENERIC NAME: terfenadine (Seldane-D also contains pseudoephedrine as a decongestant)

GENERIC FORM AVAILABLE: No

THERAPEUTIC CLASS: Nonsedating antihistamine

DOSAGE FORMS: Seldane: 60-mg terfenadine tablets. Seldane-D: 60-mg terfenadine/120-mg pseudoephedrine extended-release tablets

MAIN USES: Allergies and congestion

USUAL DOSE: one tablet twice daily as needed

AVERAGE PRICE: $131.54 for Seldane and $148.26 for Seldane-D

SIDE EFFECTS: headache 16%, slight drowsiness 9%, nausea 8%, dry mouth/nose/throat 5%, tiredness 5%, cough 3%, sore throat 3%, rash 2%, dizziness 1%, nervousness 1%, and bloody nose 1%.

DRUG INTERACTIONS: Warning: This drug should never be used with Biaxin, E.E.S., ERYC, ERY-TABS, Erythrocin, erythromycin, Diflucan, Dynabac, Nizoral, Sporanox, TAO, or Zithromax—this may cause dangerous irregular heartbeats and fast heartbeat. The drug should not be taken with Serzone.

ALLERGIES: Individuals allergic to terfenadine, pseudoephedrine, or any of their derivatives should discuss this with their doctor or pharmacist before using this drug.

PREGNANCY/BREAST-FEEDING: Category C—Risk cannot be ruled out. Human studies are lacking, and animal studies are either positive for fetal risk or lacking as well. However, potential benefits may justify the potential risk in using the drug. It is not known whether the drug is excreted in the breast milk; therefore, caution should be used when breast-feeding.

OTHER BRAND NAMES: None

OTHER DRUGS IN THE SAME THERAPEUTIC CLASS: Allegra, Claritin, Claritin-D, Hismanal, and Zyrtec

IMPORTANT INFORMATION TO REMEMBER: Do not take Seldane or Seldane-D more frequently than every 12 hours. Unless otherwise directed by a physician, take only as needed for relief of allergies. Warning: This drug should never be used with Biaxin, E.E.S., ERYC, ERY-TABS, Erythrocin, erythromycin, Diflucan, Dynabac, Nizoral, Sporanox, TAO, or Zithromax—this may cause dangerous irregular heartbeats and fast heartbeat. If a pounding heartbeat or fainting occurs, report this to your physician immediately. Do not crush or cut Seldane-D tablets; this will destroy the mechanism that slowly releases the pseudoephedrine component of the drug.

BRAND NAME: Seldane-D

GENERIC NAME: Combination product containing: terfenadine and pseudoephedrine

See entry for Seldane

BRAND NAME: **Selsun Blue**

GENERIC NAME: selenium sulfide

GENERIC FORM AVAILABLE: Yes

THERAPEUTIC CLASS: Antiseborrheic/antifungal

DOSAGE FORMS: 2.5% lotion

MAIN USES: Dandruff and tinea versicolor

USUAL DOSE: Use twice weekly as needed.

AVERAGE PRICE: $16.78 (B)/$8.83 (G)

SIDE EFFECTS: Most common: unusual dryness or oiliness of the hair or scalp. Less common: increase in normal hair loss and skin irritation.

DRUG INTERACTIONS: None of any clinical significance

ALLERGIES: Individuals allergic to selenium sulfide, any selenium-containing shampoos, or any of their derivatives should discuss this with their doctor or pharmacist before using this drug.

PREGNANCY/BREAST-FEEDING: Category C—Risk cannot be ruled out. Human studies are lacking, and animal studies are either positive for fetal risk or lacking as well. However, potential benefits may justify the potential risk in using the drug. It is not known whether the drug is excreted in the breast milk; therefore, caution should be used when breast-feeding.

OTHER BRAND NAMES: None

OTHER DRUGS IN THE SAME THERAPEUTIC CLASS: Capitrol

IMPORTANT INFORMATION TO REMEMBER: This drug is for external use only. Do not use the drug on broken or damaged skin, and avoid contact with eyes.

When using the drug for dandruff:

1) Shake the bottle well before use.
2) Massage one to two teaspoons into wet scalp.
3) Allow the drug to remain on the scalp for two to three minutes.
4) Rinse scalp thoroughly.
5) Repeat application and rinse thoroughly.
6) Repeat treatments as directed by your physician.

BRAND NAME: Semprex-D

GENERIC NAME: Combination product containing: acrivastine and pseudoephedrine

GENERIC FORM AVAILABLE: No

THERAPEUTIC CLASS: Antihistamine + decongestant

DOSAGE FORMS: 8-mg acrivastine/60-mg pseudoephedrine capsules

MAIN USES: Nasal allergies and congestion

USUAL DOSE: one capsule every four to six hours, up to a maximum of four capsules per day

AVERAGE PRICE: $69.65

SIDE EFFECTS: headache 19%, drowsiness 12%, dry mouth 7%, insomnia 4%, dizziness 3%, nervousness 3%, nausea 2%, and abnormal menstrual periods 2%.

DRUG INTERACTIONS: Blocadren, Cartrol, Corgard, Inderal, Kerlone, Levatol, Lopressor, Normodyne, Sectral, Tenormin, Toprol-XL, Trandate, Visken, and Zebeta may increase the effects of the drug. The drug may also reduce the effects of blood-pressure-lowering drugs. Nardil or Parnate may significantly raise blood pressure when taken with this drug.

ALLERGIES: Individuals allergic to acrivastine, pseudoephedrine, or other antihistamine/decongestant combinations (such as those listed under "Other Drugs in the Same Therapeutic Class") should discuss this with their doctor or pharmacist before taking this drug.

PREGNANCY/BREAST-FEEDING: Category B—No evidence of risk in humans. Either animal findings show risk, but human findings do not; or, if no adequate human studies have been done, animal findings show no risk. The drug is excreted in the breast milk; therefore, caution should be used when breast-feeding.

OTHER BRAND NAMES: None

OTHER DRUGS IN THE SAME THERAPEUTIC CLASS: Bromfed, Bromfed PD, Claritin-D, Comhist LA, Deconamine, Deconamine SR, Fedahist, Naldecon, Nolamine, Novafed-A, Ornade, Poly-Histine-D, Rondec, Rynatan, Seldane-D, Tavist-D, and Trinalin

IMPORTANT INFORMATION TO REMEMBER: This drug does cause drowsiness. Individuals should use caution when driving, operating machinery, or performing any task where mental alertness is required. Alcohol, anxiety medications, and narcotic painkillers may intensify the drowsiness effect of the drug. This drug may also cause a dry mouth; sugarless gum or hard candy will help take care of this problem. Patients with glaucoma, high blood pressure, heart conditions, or urinary or prostate problems should consult their doctor before taking this drug.

BRAND NAME: Septra and Septra DS

GENERIC NAME: Combination product containing: sulfamethoxazole and trimethoprim

See entry for Bactrim and Bactrim DS

BRAND NAME: Ser-Ap-Es

GENERIC NAME: Combination product containing: reserpine, hydralazine, hydrochlorothiazide

GENERIC FORM AVAILABLE: Yes

THERAPEUTIC CLASS: Blood vessel dilator + diuretic (water pill)

DOSAGE FORMS: 0.1-mg reserpine/25-mg hydralazine/1-mg hydrochlorothiazide tablets

MAIN USES: High blood pressure

USUAL DOSE: one or two tablets three times daily

AVERAGE PRICE: $72.44 (B)/$13.75 (G)

SIDE EFFECTS: Most common: weakness and dizziness. Less common: depression, low blood pressure, low potassium, headache, restlessness, impotence, decreased sex drive, diarrhea, drowsiness, stomach pain, vomiting, dry mouth, stuffy nose, bloody nose, appetite changes, muscle spasms, muscle cramps, irritability, and slow heartbeat.

DRUG INTERACTIONS: The drug may cause low blood pressure when used with alcohol, anxiety medications, narcotic painkillers, Amytal, Butisol, Mebaral, Nembutal, phenobarbital, Seconal, and Tuinal. The drug may require dosage adjustments to diabetic and gout medications. The drug may increase the effects of Equagesic, Flexeril, Lioresal, Norflex, Norgesic, Parafon Forte DSC, Robaxin,

Robaxisal, Skelaxin, and Soma. The drug may increase the blood levels of Eskalith and Lithobid. The drug may cause irregular heartbeats when used with Lanoxin, Quinaglute, and Quinidex. The drug should not be used with Nardil or Parnate. Blocadren, Cartrol, Corgard, Inderal, Kerlone, Levatol, Lopressor, Normodyne, Sectral, Tenormin, Toprol-XL, Trandate, Visken, or Zebeta may increase the effects of the drug.

ALLERGIES: Individuals allergic to reserpine, hydralazine, hydrochlorothiazide, sulfa drugs, or any of their derivatives should discuss this with their doctor or pharmacist before using this drug.

PREGNANCY/BREAST-FEEDING: Category C—Risk cannot be ruled out. Human studies are lacking, and animal studies are either positive for fetal risk or lacking as well. However, potential benefits may justify the potential risk in using the drug. The drug is excreted in the breast milk; therefore, extreme caution should be used when breast-feeding.

OTHER BRAND NAMES: None

OTHER DRUGS IN THE SAME THERAPEUTIC CLASS: None

IMPORTANT INFORMATION TO REMEMBER: This drug may cause some drowsiness and tiredness. Individuals should use caution when driving, operating machinery, or performing any task where mental alertness is required. Alcohol, anxiety medications, and narcotic painkillers may intensify these effects of the drug. The drug may also cause dizziness when suddenly rising from a sitting or lying-down position. If depression or sleep changes occur, notify your physician immediately. If stomach upset occurs, the drug may be taken with food or milk. Before taking over-the-counter cold and allergy preparations, consult your doctor or pharmacist— these products may raise your blood pressure. The drug may cause the elimination of potassium from the body. It is therefore a good idea to eat a banana or drink orange, grapefruit, or apple juice every day to replace lost potassium.

BRAND NAME: Serax

GENERIC NAME: oxazepam

GENERIC FORM AVAILABLE: Yes

THERAPEUTIC CLASS: Benzodiazepine antianxiety

DOSAGE FORMS: 10-mg, 15-mg, and 30-mg capsules; and 15-mg tablets

MAIN USES: Anxiety and alcohol withdrawal

USUAL DOSE: 10 mg to 30 mg three to four times daily

AVERAGE PRICE: $80.48 (B)/$25.94 (G) for 10 mg; $103.49 (B)/$30.34 (G) for 15 mg; $142.65 (B)/$39.80 (G) for 30 mg

SIDE EFFECTS: Most common: drowsiness, clumsiness, and dizziness. Less common: confusion, depression, stomach cramps, nausea, vomiting, dry mouth, changes in sex drive, sleep disturbances, and fast heartbeat.

DRUG INTERACTIONS: Central nervous system (CNS) depression may be increased when used with alcohol, narcotic painkillers, or other anxiety medications.

ALLERGIES: Individuals allergic to oxazepam or other benzodiazepines (such as those listed under "Other Drugs in the Same Therapeutic Class") should discuss this with their doctor or pharmacist before taking this drug.

PREGNANCY/BREAST-FEEDING: Category D—Positive evidence of risk. Human studies show risk to the fetus. Nevertheless, potential benefits may possibly outweigh the potential risk. This drug should not be taken by nursing mothers.

OTHER BRAND NAMES: None

OTHER DRUGS IN THE SAME THERAPEUTIC CLASS: Ativan, Librium, Tranxene, Valium, and Xanax

IMPORTANT INFORMATION TO REMEMBER: This drug may cause drowsiness. Individuals should use caution when driving, operating machinery, or performing any task where mental alertness is required. The incidence of drowsiness and unsteadiness increases with age. Alcohol, anxiety medications, or narcotic painkillers may intensify the drowsiness effect of the drug. This medication is a controlled substance and may be habit-forming. Do not increase the dose of medication without consulting with your doctor. Take only the amount prescribed by your doctor.

BRAND NAME: Serentil

GENERIC NAME: mesoridazine

GENERIC FORM AVAILABLE: No

THERAPEUTIC CLASS: Piperidine phenothiazine antipsychotic

DOSAGE FORMS: 10-mg, 25-mg, 50-mg, and 100-mg tablets

MAIN USES: Psychotic disorders

USUAL DOSE: 100 mg to 400 mg daily divided into several doses

AVERAGE PRICE: $77.88 for 10 mg; $104.41 for 25 mg; $117.76 for 50 mg; and $144.23 for 100 mg

SIDE EFFECTS: Most common: drowsiness, restlessness, blurred vision, Parkinson's-like symptoms, low blood pressure, stuffy nose, dry mouth, constipation, and dizziness. Less common: increased sensitivity to sunburn, difficulty in urinating, nausea, vomiting, stomach pain, and trembling of fingers and hands, stomach pain, changes in menstrual period, decreased sexual ability, swelling and/or pain in the breasts, weight gain, and secretion of milk from the breasts.

DRUG INTERACTIONS: Drugs used to treat depression and Serentil may increase the severity and frequency of side effects. Alcohol, anxiety medications, and narcotic painkillers may intensify the drowsiness effect of the drug. Eskalith and Lithobid may decrease the absorption of the drug. Eskalith or Lithobid and the drug may cause disorientation and one to black out. The drug may decrease the effects of Larodopa. Medications for high blood pressure and the drug may cause low blood pressure when taken together.

ALLERGIES: Individuals allergic to mesoridazine or any of its derivatives should discuss this with their doctor or pharmacist before using this drug.

PREGNANCY/BREAST-FEEDING: Category C—Risk cannot be ruled out. Human studies are lacking, and animal studies are either positive for fetal risk or lacking as well. However, potential benefits may justify the potential risk in using the drug. It is not known whether the drug is excreted in the breast milk; therefore, caution should be used when breast-feeding.

OTHER BRAND NAMES: None

OTHER DRUGS IN THE SAME THERAPEUTIC CLASS: Compazine, Prolixin, Mellaril, Stelazine, Thorazine, and Trilafon

IMPORTANT INFORMATION TO REMEMBER: This drug does cause drowsiness. Individuals should use caution when driving, operating machinery, or performing any task where mental alertness is required. Alcohol, anxiety medications, and narcotic painkillers may intensify the drowsiness effect of the drug. Do not increase the dose or stop taking the drug without first consulting with your physician. Individuals should report any involuntary movements of the tongue, arms, or legs to their physician. This drug may also increase the sensitivity of the skin to sunburn in some individuals; therefore, a sunscreen is recommended during periods of prolonged exposure to the sun. Caution should be used during hot weather due to decreased tolerance to the heat.

BRAND NAME: Serevent

GENERIC NAME: salmeterol

GENERIC FORM AVAILABLE: No

THERAPEUTIC CLASS: Beta-2-agonist bronchodilator

DOSAGE FORMS: 21-micrograms-per-inhalation metered-dose inhaler

MAIN USES: Asthma and {other breathing disorders}

USUAL DOSE: two inhalations every 12 hours (morning and evening)

AVERAGE PRICE: $70.42

SIDE EFFECTS: cough 7%, sinus headache 4%, stomach pain 4%, tremor 4%, lower respiratory infection 4%, fast heartbeat 1%–3%, pounding heartbeat 1%–3%, runny nose 1%–3%, nausea 1%–3%, vomiting 1%–3%, diarrhea 1%–3%, allergic reaction 1%–3%, muscle and joint pain 1%–3%, nervousness 1%–3%, tooth pain 1%–3%, and tiredness 1%–3%.

DRUG INTERACTIONS: Anafranil, Asendin, Elavil, Nardil, Norpramin, Pamelor, Parnate, Sinequan, Surmontil, Tofranil, and Vivactil, and cough, cold, and allergy medications with decongestants may increase the toxicity of this medication. Blocadren, Cartrol, Corgard, Inderal, Levatol, Normodyne, Trandate, and Visken may decrease the effectiveness of the drug.

ALLERGIES: Individuals allergic to salmeterol or any of its derivatives should discuss this with their doctor or pharmacist before using this drug.

PREGNANCY/BREAST-FEEDING: Category C—Risk cannot be ruled out. Human studies are lacking, and animal studies are either positive for fetal risk or lacking as well. However, potential benefits may justify the potential risk in using the drug. It is not known whether the drug is excreted in the breast milk; therefore, caution should be used when breast-feeding.

OTHER BRAND NAMES: None

OTHER DRUGS IN THE SAME THERAPEUTIC CLASS: Alupent, Brethaire, Bricanyl, Bronkometer, Maxair, Metaprel, Proventil, Tornalate, Ventolin, and Volmax

IMPORTANT INFORMATION TO REMEMBER: Only take the drug exactly as directed by your physician. Never increase the dose of the drug without consulting with your physician. This drug should not be used to provide immediate relief from an asthma attack in progress. Prolonged use of the drug may cause tolerance to its effects to develop.

When using the inhaler, use the following procedure:

1) Shake the canister well.
2) Place the mouthpiece close to the mouth, but not touching the lips.
3) Exhale deeply.
4) Inhale slowly and deeply as you press the top of the canister to release the medication.
5) Hold your breath for a few seconds before exhaling.
6) Wait five minutes between puffs.
7) Be sure to wash the inhaler device (mouthpiece) regularly with warm soapy water to avoid bacterial contamination.

BRAND NAME: Serophene

GENERIC NAME: clomiphene

GENERIC FORM AVAILABLE: No

THERAPEUTIC CLASS: Fertility drug

DOSAGE FORMS: 50-mg tablets

MAIN USES: Stimulation of ovulation

USUAL DOSE: 50 mg daily for five days, beginning on the fifth day of menstrual cycle

AVERAGE PRICE: $92.19 for 10 tablets

SIDE EFFECTS: enlargement of the ovaries 15%, hot flashes 10%, birth of twins 10%, stomach pain 7%, breast tenderness 2%, nausea 2%, vomiting 2%, nervousness 2%, insomnia 2%, vision disturbances 2%, and birth of triplets or more 1%.

DRUG INTERACTIONS: None of any clinical significance

ALLERGIES: Individuals allergic to clomiphene or any of its derivatives should discuss this with their doctor or pharmacist before using this drug.

PREGNANCY/BREAST-FEEDING: If pregnancy is suspected, the drug should be stopped immediately. Patients should not breast-feed when taking this medication.

OTHER BRAND NAMES: Clomid

OTHER DRUGS IN THE SAME THERAPEUTIC CLASS: Clomid

IMPORTANT INFORMATION TO REMEMBER: Only take the drug exactly as directed by your physician. It is very important to follow the dosing schedule set by your physician. If pregnancy is suspected, inform your physician and stop taking the drug immediately. The drug may cause multiple births in approximately 10% of the women taking it.

BRAND NAME: Serzone

GENERIC NAME: nefazodone

GENERIC FORM AVAILABLE: No

THERAPEUTIC CLASS: Neurotransmitter reuptake inhibitor antidepressant

DOSAGE FORMS: 100-mg, 150-mg, 200-mg, and 250-mg tablets

MAIN USES: Depression

USUAL DOSE: 100 mg to 300 mg twice daily

AVERAGE PRICE: $112.92 for 100 mg; $125.47 for 150 mg; $134.61 for 200 mg; and $141.28 for 250 mg

SIDE EFFECTS: headache 36%, dry mouth 25%, drowsiness 25%, nausea 22%, dizziness 17%, constipation 14%, muscle weakness 11%, lightheadedness 10%, blurred vision 9%, abnormal vision 7%, confusion 7%, and low blood pressure 4%.

DRUG INTERACTIONS: The drug should not be taken with Hismanal, Nardil, Parnate, Seldane, or Seldane-D. The drug may increase the blood levels of Ativan, Halcion, Haldol, Lanoxin, Restoril, Valium, and Xanax.

ALLERGIES: Individuals allergic to nefazodone or any of its derivatives should discuss this with their doctor or pharmacist before using this drug.

PREGNANCY/BREAST-FEEDING: Category C—Risk cannot be ruled out. Human studies are lacking, and animal studies are either positive for fetal risk or lacking as well. However, potential benefits may justify the potential risk in using the drug. It is not known whether the drug is excreted in the breast milk; therefore, caution should be used when breast-feeding.

OTHER BRAND NAMES: None

OTHER DRUGS IN THE SAME THERAPEUTIC CLASS: Effexor

IMPORTANT INFORMATION TO REMEMBER: Only take the drug exactly as directed by your physician. Do not discontinue the drug without first consulting your physician. This drug does cause drowsiness. Individuals should use caution when driving, operating machinery, or performing any task where mental alertness is required. Alcohol, anxiety medications, and narcotic painkillers may intensify the drowsiness effect of the drug. If stomach upset occurs, take the drug with food or milk. The full effects of the medication may not be seen for several weeks.

BRAND NAME: Silvadene

GENERIC NAME: silver sulfadiazine

GENERIC FORM AVAILABLE: Yes

THERAPEUTIC CLASS: Topical antibacterial

DOSAGE FORMS: 1% cream

MAIN USES: Prevention and treatment of bacterial infections in second- and third-degree burns

USUAL DOSE: Apply one to two times daily, approximately 1/16 inch in depth, to cleansed and debrided burns.

AVERAGE PRICE: $14.68 (B)/$10.13 (G) for 1% cream (50 g)

SIDE EFFECTS: Most common: burning feeling on treated areas. Less common: itching, skin rash, and brownish-gray discoloration of the skin.

DRUG INTERACTIONS: The drug may inactivate other creams used for severe burns such as collagenase, papain, and sutilain.

ALLERGIES: Individuals allergic to silver sulfadiazine or any of its derivatives should discuss this with their doctor or pharmacist before using this drug.

PREGNANCY/BREAST-FEEDING: Category B—No evidence of risk in humans. Either animal findings show risk, but human findings do not; or, if no adequate human studies have been done, animal findings show no risk. It is not known whether the drug is excreted in the breast milk; therefore, caution should be used when breast-feeding.

OTHER BRAND NAMES: SSD

OTHER DRUGS IN THE SAME THERAPEUTIC CLASS: SSD

IMPORTANT INFORMATION TO REMEMBER: The drug is for external use only. Apply the cream after the burn has been cleaned and debrided. The drug should be applied in a thin layer (approximately 1/16 of an inch). If the cream is rubbed off through activity or rubbing, the cream may be reapplied. Use the cream for as long as directed by your physician. The drug may stain the skin brownish-gray and may stain clothing as well.

BRAND NAME: Sinemet and Sinemet CR

GENERIC NAME: Combination product containing: carbidopa and levodopa

GENERIC FORM AVAILABLE: Yes (Sinemet only)

THERAPEUTIC CLASS: Anti-Parkinson's combination compound

DOSAGE FORMS: 10-mg carbidopa/100-mg levodopa, 25-mg carbidopa/100-mg levodopa, and 25-mg carbidopa/250-mg levodopa tablets (Sinemet); and 25-mg carbidopa/100-mg levodopa and

50-mg carbidopa/200-mg levodopa sustained-release tablets (Sinemet CR)

MAIN USES: Parkinson's disease

USUAL DOSE: Sinemet 10 mg/100 mg to Sinemet 25 mg/250 mg tablets three times daily or one Sinemet CR tablet twice daily. Doses may be higher is severe cases.

AVERAGE PRICE: For Sinemet: $75.09 (B)/$54.92 (G) for 10 mg/100 mg; $82.88 (B)/$62.77 (G) for 25 mg/100 mg; $107.70 (B)/$76.64 (G) for 25 mg/250 mg. For Sinemet CR: $106.41 for 25 mg/100 mg and $220.13 for 50 mg/200 mg

SIDE EFFECTS: Most common: dizziness, difficulty in urinating, dizziness when getting up suddenly, irregular heartbeat, nausea, diarrhea, aggressive behavior, unusual or uncontrolled body movements, nervousness, and confusion. Less common: loss of appetite, diarrhea, dry mouth, blurred vision, constipation, darkening in color of urine or sweat, headache, diarrhea, spasm or closing of eyelids, flushing, muscle twitching, and muscle weakness.

DRUG INTERACTIONS: Compazine, Dilantin, Haldol, Mellaril, Prolixin, Serentil, Stelazine, Thorazine, and Trilafon may decrease the effects of the drug. The drug should not be used with Nardil or Parnate. Eldepryl and the drug should be used together with caution.

ALLERGIES: Individuals allergic to carbidopa, levodopa, or any of their derivatives should discuss this with their doctor or pharmacist before using this drug.

PREGNANCY/BREAST-FEEDING: Category C—Risk cannot be ruled out. Human studies are lacking, and animal studies are either positive for fetal risk or lacking as well. However, potential benefits may justify the potential risk in using the drug. The drug is excreted in the breast milk; therefore, extreme caution should be used when breast-feeding.

OTHER BRAND NAMES: None

OTHER DRUGS IN THE SAME THERAPEUTIC CLASS: None

IMPORTANT INFORMATION TO REMEMBER: Only take the drug exactly as directed by your physician and do not stop taking the drug without first consulting with your physician. This drug should be taken with food or milk to reduce the potential for stomach upset.

Individuals should avoid vitamin supplements containing large amounts of vitamin B_6. Individuals with glaucoma or urinary problems should discuss this with their physician before taking this drug. Individuals should get up slowly from a sitting or lying-down position; otherwise dizziness may occur. The drug may take several weeks before noticeable improvements are seen. Do not crush the Sinemet CR tablets—this will destroy the mechanism that delays the release of the medication. Sinemet CR, however, may be cut in half for easier swallowing.

BRAND NAME: Sinequan

GENERIC NAME: doxepin

GENERIC FORM AVAILABLE: Yes

THERAPEUTIC CLASS: Tricyclic antidepressant

DOSAGE FORMS: 10-mg, 25-mg, 50-mg, 75-mg, 100-mg, and 150-mg capsules

MAIN USES: Depression and anxiety (nerves)

USUAL DOSE: 10 mg to 15 mg once daily or 30 mg to 300 mg daily in divided doses

AVERAGE PRICE: $51.65 (B)/$20.86 (G) for 10 mg; $63.75 (B)/$28.25 (G) for 25 mg; $80.17 (B)/$35.07 (G) for 50 mg; $106.23 (B)/$50.25 (G) for 75 mg; $138.74 (B)/$59.25 (G) for 100 mg; $219.13 (B)/$79.79 (G) for 150 mg

SIDE EFFECTS: Most common: drowsiness, dizziness, dry mouth, headache, increased appetite, nausea, tiredness, weight gain, and unpleasant taste. Less common: diarrhea, excessive sweating, heartburn, insomnia, vomiting, irregular heartbeat, muscle tremors, urinary difficulties, and impotence.

DRUG INTERACTIONS: The drug should not be taken with Nardil or Parnate. In fact, 14 days are needed between the time of the use of Nardil or Parnate and this drug. Alcohol, anxiety medications, and narcotic painkillers may make the drowsiness caused by the drug much worse. Compazine, Mellaril, Prolixin, Serentil, Stelazine, Thorazine, and Trilafon may increase the blood levels of the drug. Tagamet may increase the blood levels of the drug. The drug may decrease the effects of Catapres and Ismelin. The drug may increase the effects of decongestants in cold, cough, and allergy products on the heart, possibly causing high blood pressure, fast heartbeat, or irregular heartbeat.

ALLERGIES: Individuals allergic to doxepin or other tricylic antidepressants (such as those listed under "Other Drugs in the Same Therapeutic Class") should discuss this with their doctor or pharmacist before taking this drug.

PREGNANCY/BREAST-FEEDING: Category C—Risk cannot be ruled out. Human studies are lacking, and animal studies are either positive for fetal risk or lacking as well. However, potential benefits may justify the potential risk in using the drug. The drug is excreted in the breast milk; therefore, extreme caution should be used when breast-feeding.

OTHER BRAND NAMES: Adapin

OTHER DRUGS IN THE SAME THERAPEUTIC CLASS: Asendin, Elavil, Endep, Norpramin, Pamelor, Surmontil, Tofranil, and Vivactil

IMPORTANT INFORMATION TO REMEMBER: Only take the drug exactly as directed by your physician. Do not discontinue taking the drug without first consulting your physician. The drug may require one to six weeks to use before improvement may be noticed. This drug does cause drowsiness. Individuals should use caution when driving, operating machinery, or performing any task where mental alertness is required. Alcohol, anxiety medications, and nar-, cotic painkillers may intensify the drowsiness effect of the drug. The drug may cause a slight amount of dizziness or lightheadedness when rising from a sitting or lying-down position. Individuals should also use a sunscreen to avoid overexposure to the sun; the drug may increase the skin's sensitivity to sunlight, which may cause one to sunburn more easily.

BRAND NAME: Skelaxin

GENERIC NAME: metaxalone

GENERIC FORM AVAILABLE: No

THERAPEUTIC CLASS: Muscle relaxant

DOSAGE FORMS: 400-mg tablets

MAIN USES: Muscle spasms

USUAL DOSE: 400 mg to 800 mg three to four times daily

AVERAGE PRICE: $58.31

SIDE EFFECTS: Most common: drowsiness, dizziness, lightheadedness, headache, nervousness, restlessness, insomnia, stomach pain, nausea, and vomiting. Less common: muscle weakness and diarrhea.

DRUG INTERACTIONS: Alcohol, anxiety medications, and narcotic painkillers may intensify the drowsiness effect of the drug.

ALLERGIES: Individuals allergic to metaxalone or any of its derivatives should discuss this with their doctor or pharmacist before using this drug.

PREGNANCY/BREAST-FEEDING: None established

OTHER BRAND NAMES: None

OTHER DRUGS IN THE SAME THERAPEUTIC CLASS: Flexeril, Lioresal, Parafon Forte DSC, Robaxin, and Soma

IMPORTANT INFORMATION TO REMEMBER: Only take the drug exactly as directed by your physician; also, do not increase the dose without first consulting with your physician. If stomach upset occurs, take the drug with food or milk. This drug does cause drowsiness. Individuals should use caution when driving, operating machinery, or performing any task where mental alertness is required. Alcohol, anxiety medications, and narcotic painkillers may intensify the drowsiness effect of the drug.

BRAND NAME: Slo-bid

GENERIC NAME: theophylline

GENERIC FORM AVAILABLE: Yes

THERAPEUTIC CLASS: Xanthine bronchodilator

DOSAGE FORMS: 50-mg, 75-mg, 100-mg, 125-mg, 200-mg, and 300-mg extended-release capsules

MAIN USES: Asthma, chronic bronchitis, emphysema, and {other breathing disorders}

USUAL DOSE: 50 mg to 300 mg every 8 to 12 hours

AVERAGE PRICE: $38.45 (B)/$29.55 (G) for 50 mg; $48.34 (B)/$35.84 (G) for 100 mg; 52.33 (B)/$42.53 (G) for 200 mg; $51.80 (B)/$48.16 (G) for 300 mg

SIDE EFFECTS: Most common: nausea, nervousness, and restlessness. Less common: vomiting, diarrhea, stomach pain, headaches, irritability, insomnia, muscle twitching, fast heartbeat, pounding heartbeat, fast breathing, flushing, and low blood pressure.

DRUG INTERACTIONS: The drug may inhibit the effects of Blocadren, Cartrol, Corgard, Inderal, Kerlone, Levatol, Lopressor, Normodyne, Sectral, Tenormin, Toprol-XL, Trandate, Visken, and Zebeta. Dilantin, Tegretol, smoking, and nicotine patches may lower the blood levels of this drug. Cipro, Noroxin, Tagamet, Zantac, erythromycin, and TAO may increase blood levels of the drug. Individuals who stop smoking while taking the drug may have increased levels of the drug in the blood.

ALLERGIES: Individuals allergic to theophylline or other xanthines (such as those listed under "Other Drugs in the Same Therapeutic Class") should discuss this with their doctor or pharmacist before taking this drug.

PREGNANCY/BREAST-FEEDING: Category C—Risk cannot be ruled out. Human studies are lacking, and animal studies are either positive for fetal risk or lacking as well. However, potential benefits may justify the potential risk in using the drug. The drug is excreted in the breast milk; therefore, extreme caution should be used when breast-feeding.

OTHER BRAND NAMES: None

OTHER DRUGS IN THE SAME THERAPEUTIC CLASS: aminophylline, Choledyl, Elixophyllin, Lufyllin, Respbid, Quibron-SR, Quibron-T, Slo-Phyllin, Theo-24, Theo-Dur, Theo-X, Uni-Dur, and Uniphyl

IMPORTANT INFORMATION TO REMEMBER: Only take the drug exactly as directed by your physician. Do not discontinue taking the drug without first consulting your physician. Do not increase the dose without first consulting your physician. This drug should be taken with plenty of water (eight ounces is preferred). Swallow the capsules whole. The contents of the capsules may, however, be sprinkled on soft food (such as applesauce) and swallowed without chewing. If stomach upset occurs, take with food or milk. Do not change between brand and generic once you are stabilized on one or the other.

BRAND NAME: Slo-Phyllin

GENERIC NAME: theophylline

GENERIC FORM AVAILABLE: Yes

THERAPEUTIC CLASS: Xanthine bronchodilator

DOSAGE FORMS: 100-mg and 200-mg tablets; 60-mg, 125-mg, and 250-mg sustained-release capsules; and 80 mg/15 mL syrup

MAIN USES: Asthma, chronic bronchitis, emphysema, and {other breathing disorders}

USUAL DOSE: 60 mg to 250 mg every 8 to 12 hours

AVERAGE PRICE: $28.75 (B)/$16.22 (G) for 100 mg and $38.19 (B)/ $22.89 (G) for 200 mg

SIDE EFFECTS: Most common: nausea, nervousness, and restlessness. Less common: vomiting, diarrhea, stomach pain, headaches, irritability, insomnia, muscle twitching, fast heartbeat, pounding heartbeat, fast breathing, flushing, and low blood pressure.

DRUG INTERACTIONS: The drug may inhibit the effects of Blocadren, Cartrol, Corgard, Inderal, Kerlone, Levatol, Lopressor, Normodyne, Sectral, Tenormin, Toprol-XL, Trandate, Visken, and Zebeta. Dilantin, Tegretol, smoking, and nicotine patches may lower the blood levels of this drug. Cipro, Noroxin, Tagamet, Zantac, erythromycin, and TAO may increase blood levels of the drug. Individuals who stop smoking while taking the drug may have increased levels of the drug in the blood.

ALLERGIES: Individuals allergic to theophylline or other xanthines (such as those listed under "Other Drugs in the Same Therapeutic Class") should discuss this with their doctor or pharmacist before taking this drug.

PREGNANCY/BREAST-FEEDING: Category C—Risk cannot be ruled out. Human studies are lacking, and animal studies are either positive for fetal risk or lacking as well. However, potential benefits may justify the potential risk in using the drug. The drug is excreted in the breast milk; therefore, extreme caution should be used when breast-feeding.

OTHER BRAND NAMES: None

OTHER DRUGS IN THE SAME THERAPEUTIC CLASS: aminophylline, Choledry, Elixophyllin, Lufyllin, Respbid, Quibron-SR, Quibron-T, Slo-bid, Theo-24, Theo-Dur, Theo-X, Uni-Dur, and Uniphyl

IMPORTANT INFORMATION TO REMEMBER: Only take the drug exactly as directed by your physician. Do not discontinue taking the drug without first consulting your physician. Do not increase the dose without first consulting your physician. This drug should be taken with plenty of water (eight ounces is preferred). Swallow the capsules whole. The contents of the capsules may, however, be sprinkled on soft food (such as applesauce) and swallowed without chewing. If stomach upset occurs, take with food or milk. Do not change between brand and generic once you are stabilized on one or the other.

BRAND NAME: Slow-K

GENERIC NAME: potassium chloride

GENERIC FORM AVAILABLE: Yes

THERAPEUTIC CLASS: Potassium supplement

DOSAGE FORMS: 8-mEqL (600-mg) tablets

MAIN USES: Low potassium

USUAL DOSE: one to four tablets per day in one or two divided doses

AVERAGE PRICE: $27.45 (B)/$15.05 (G)

SIDE EFFECTS: Most common: none. Less common: diarrhea, vomiting, gas, nausea, stomach discomfort, and wax matrix of the tablet may be seen in the stool.

DRUG INTERACTIONS: Aldactazide, Aldactone, Dyazide, Dyrenium, Hygroton, Maxzide, Midamor, and Moduretic may cause potassium levels to become too high when taken with this drug. Accupril, Altace, Capoten, Lotensin, Monopril, Prinivil, Univasc, Vasotec, Zestril, and salt substitutes may cause potassium levels to become too high when taken with this drug. Caution should be used by patients taking Lanoxin and this drug.

ALLERGIES: Individuals allergic to potassium, potassium chloride, or any of their derivatives should discuss this with their doctor or pharmacist before using this drug.

PREGNANCY/BREAST-FEEDING: Category C—Risk cannot be ruled out. Human studies are lacking, and animal studies are either positive for fetal risk or lacking as well. However, potential benefits may justify the potential risk in using the drug. It is not known whether the drug is excreted in the breast milk; therefore, caution should be used when breast-feeding.

OTHER BRAND NAMES: None

OTHER DRUGS IN THE SAME THERAPEUTIC CLASS: KAON-CL, Kay Ciel, K-Dur, K-Lor, Klor-Con, Klorvess, Klotrix, K-Lyte, K-Lyte/Cl, K-Norm, K-Tab, and Micro-K

IMPORTANT INFORMATION TO REMEMBER: This drug should be taken with food or milk to reduce the potential for injury to the stomach lining and stomach upset. The drug should also be taken with a full glass of water (eight ounces is preferred). Only take the drug exactly as directed by your doctor; do not increase the dose or discontinue taking the drug without first consulting with your doctor. Swallow the tablets whole. Do not crush or chew the tablets—this will destroy the wax matrix that delays the release of the drug. Individuals should avoid salt substitutes that contain potassium. Individuals may notice a yellow-colored empty shell in the stool that is left over after the medication is absorbed.

BRAND NAME: Soma, Soma Compound, and Soma Compound with Codeine

GENERIC NAME: Combination product containing: various combinations of carisoprodol, aspirin, and codeine

GENERIC FORM AVAILABLE: Yes

THERAPEUTIC CLASS: Muscle relaxant

DOSAGE FORMS: Soma: 350-mg carisoprodol tablets. Soma Compound: 350-mg carisoprodol/325-mg aspirin tablets. Soma Compound w/Codeine: 350-mg carisoprodol/325-mg aspirin/16-mg codeine tablets.

MAIN USES: Muscle spasms

USUAL DOSE: Soma: one tablet three times daily and at bedtime. Soma Compound or Soma Compound w/Codeine: one or two tablets four times daily.

AVERAGE PRICE: $244.24 (B)/$43.31 (G) for Soma; $216.96 (B)/ $59.63 (G) for Soma Compound; $241.80 for Soma Compound w/Codeine

SIDE EFFECTS: Most common: drowsiness and dizziness. Less common: fast heartbeat, fainting, orthostatic hypotension (low blood pressure when getting up), mental depression, hivelike swellings, skin rash, stinging or burning of the eyes, lightheadedness, headache, nervousness, trembling, flushing of the face, nausea, vomiting, and stomach pain.

DRUG INTERACTIONS: Alcohol, anxiety medications, and narcotic painkillers may intensify the drowsiness effect of the drug. For Soma Compound and Soma Compound w/Codeine only: NSAIDs (such as Anaprox, Ansaid, Aleve, aspirin, Cataflam, Clinoril, Daypro, Disalcid, Dolobid, Feldene, Indocin, Lodine, Motrin, Nalfon, Naprosyn, Orudis, Oruvail, Relafen, Tolectin, and Voltaren) may decrease the concentration of the drug in the blood. This drug may also decrease the effects of Lasix, Dyazide, HydroDIURIL, Maxzide, and other water pills. The drug may increase the blood levels of Eskalith, Lithobid, and Sandimmune. The drug may increase the blood levels of Depakene and Depakote as well as potentially cause other blood disorders. The drug may increase the toxic effects of the drug Rheumatrex. Caution should be used when taking the drug with Coumadin.

ALLERGIES: Individuals allergic to carisoprodol, aspirin, codeine, or any of their derivatives should discuss this with their doctor or pharmacist before using this drug.

PREGNANCY/BREAST-FEEDING: Category C—Risk cannot be ruled out. Human studies are lacking, and animal studies are either positive for fetal risk or lacking as well. However, potential benefits may justify the potential risk in using the drug. The drug should not, however, be used during the late stages (last three months) of pregnancy. The drug is excreted in the breast milk; therefore, extreme caution should be used when breast-feeding.

OTHER BRAND NAMES: None

OTHER DRUGS IN THE SAME THERAPEUTIC CLASS: Flexeril, Lioresal, Parafon Forte DSC, Robaxin, and Skelaxin

IMPORTANT INFORMATION TO REMEMBER: Only take the drug exactly as directed by your physician; also, do not increase the dose without first consulting with your physician. If stomach upset occurs, take the drug with food or milk. This drug does cause drowsiness. Individuals should use caution when driving, operating machinery, or performing any task where mental alertness is required. Alcohol, anxiety medications, and narcotic painkillers may intensify the drowsiness effect of the drug. For Soma Compound and Soma Compound w/Codeine: drinking alcohol while taking this drug may increase its potential to cause ulcers. This drug should only be used under the direct supervision of a doctor by individuals with a bleeding disorder or ulcer, or those who are currently taking Coumadin. Before taking over-the-counter pain relievers, consult your doctor or pharmacist. Soma Compound w/Codeine is a controlled substance and may be habit-forming.

BRAND NAME: Soma Compound with Codeine

GENERIC NAME: Combination product containing: carisoprodol, aspirin, and codeine phosphate

See entry for Soma

BRAND NAME: Sorbitrate

GENERIC NAME: isosorbide dinitrate

See entry for Isordil

BRAND NAME: Spectazole

GENERIC NAME: econazole

GENERIC FORM AVAILABLE: No

THERAPEUTIC CLASS: Imidazole antifungal

DOSAGE FORMS: 1% cream

MAIN USES: Fungal infections (mainly ringworm, jock itch, and athlete's foot)

USUAL DOSE: Apply to affected area once or twice daily.

AVERAGE PRICE: $28.30 for 30 g

SIDE EFFECTS: burning 3%, itching 3%, stinging 3%, and redness 3%.

DRUG INTERACTIONS: None of any clinical significance

ALLERGIES: Individuals allergic to econazole or any of its derivatives should discuss this with their doctor or pharmacist before using this drug.

PREGNANCY/BREAST-FEEDING: Category C—Risk cannot be ruled out. Human studies are lacking, and animal studies are either positive for fetal risk or lacking as well. However, potential benefits may justify the potential risk in using the drug. It is not known whether the drug is excreted in the breast milk; therefore, caution should be used when breast-feeding.

OTHER BRAND NAMES: None

OTHER DRUGS IN THE SAME THERAPEUTIC CLASS: Lotrimin, Monistat-Derm, Nizoral, and Oxistat

IMPORTANT INFORMATION TO REMEMBER: This drug is for external use only. The drug may stain clothing. Apply and gently rub in enough of the cream to cover the affected area and surrounding areas. Use the drug for the full course of treatment or the fungal infection may return. Never cover the skin after application with a bandage or wrapping unless directed to do so by a doctor. Discontinue use if irritation occurs.

BRAND NAME: Sporanox

GENERIC NAME: itraconazole

GENERIC FORM AVAILABLE: No

THERAPEUTIC CLASS: Imidazole antifungal

DOSAGE FORMS: 100-mg capsules

MAIN USES: Fungal infections

USUAL DOSE: 100 mg to 200 mg once or twice daily

AVERAGE PRICE: $109.84 for 14 capsules

SIDE EFFECTS: nausea 11%, rash 9%, vomiting 5%, swelling 4%, headache 4%, diarrhea 3%, tiredness 3%, itching 3%, high blood pressure 3%, abnormal liver function 3%, stomach pain 2%, dizziness 2%, changes in appetite 1%, impotence 1%, and decreased sex drive 1%.

DRUG INTERACTIONS: *Warning:* This drug should never be taken with Hismanal, Seldane, or Seldane-D—this may cause severe and even life-threatening heart disorders. Antacids, Axid, Carafate, Pepcid, Prevacid, Prilosec, Tagamet, Videx, and Zantac may decrease the absorption of the drug. The drug may increase the blood levels of Dilantin and Sandimmune. Isoniazid or rifampin may decrease the blood levels of the drug. The drug may increase the effects of Coumadin. Alcohol may increase the toxic effects of the drug on the liver and/or produce a severe disulfiram reaction (intense flushing, stomach pain, vomiting, etc.). Propulsid and the drug may cause dangerous irregular heartbeats when taken together.

ALLERGIES: Individuals allergic to itraconazole, Nizoral, Dilfucan, or any of their derivatives should discuss this with their doctor or pharmacist before using this drug.

PREGNANCY/BREAST-FEEDING: Category C—Risk cannot be ruled out. Human studies are lacking, and animal studies are either positive for fetal risk or lacking as well. However, potential benefits may justify the potential risk in using the drug. The drug is excreted in the breast milk; therefore, extreme caution should be used when breast-feeding.

OTHER BRAND NAMES: None

OTHER DRUGS IN THE SAME THERAPEUTIC CLASS: Dilfucan and Nizoral

IMPORTANT INFORMATION TO REMEMBER: This drug should be taken with food or milk; this will increase the absorption of the drug and help prevent stomach upset. Take the drug at the same time every day. Also, take the drug until all the medication prescribed is gone; otherwise the infection may return. Patients with liver disease should discuss this with their doctor before taking this drug. The drug should never be taken with Hismanal, Seldane, or Seldane-D.

BRAND NAME: SSD

GENERIC NAME: silver sulfadiazine

See entry for Silvadene

BRAND NAME: Stuartnatal Plus

GENERIC NAME: Prenatal Plus (prenatal multivitamin)

GENERIC FORM AVAILABLE: Yes

THERAPEUTIC CLASS: Prenatal vitamin supplement

DOSAGE FORMS: multivitamin tablet

MAIN USES: Nutritional supplement during pregnancy and breast-feeding

USUAL DOSE: one tablet daily

AVERAGE PRICE: $32.21 (B)/$20.19 (G)

SIDE EFFECTS: Most common: none. Less common: diarrhea, gas, and stomach upset.

DRUG INTERACTIONS: The B vitamins in the drug may increase the effect of Larodopa.

ALLERGIES: Individuals allergic to multivitamins or any of their derivatives should discuss this with their doctor or pharmacist before using this drug.

PREGNANCY/BREAST-FEEDING: Category B—No evidence of risk in humans. Either animal findings show risk, but human findings do not; or, if no adequate human studies have been done, animal findings show no risk. It is not known whether the drug is excreted in the breast milk; therefore, caution should be used when breast-feeding. The drug is safe to use during pregnancy.

OTHER BRAND NAMES: None

OTHER DRUGS IN THE SAME THERAPEUTIC CLASS: Materna, Natalins Rx, Prenate 90, and Zenate

IMPORTANT INFORMATION TO REMEMBER: Only take the drug exactly as directed by your physician. Do not discontinue taking the drug without first consulting your physician. If stomach upset occurs, the drug may be taken with food or milk.

BRAND NAME: Sulamyd

GENERIC NAME: sulfacetamide sodium

GENERIC FORM AVAILABLE: Yes

THERAPEUTIC CLASS: Antibiotic eyedrop

DOSAGE FORMS: 10% eyedrop solution, 30% eyedrop solution, and 10% eye ointment

MAIN USES: Bacterial eye infections

USUAL DOSE: one to two drops or a thin ribbon of ointment three to four times daily

AVERAGE PRICE: $26.93 (B)/$8.60 (G) for 10% solution (15 mL); $28.58 (B)/$9.94 (G) for 30% solution (15 mL); $22.05 (B)/$8.66 (G) for 10% ointment (3.5 g)

SIDE EFFECTS: Most common: burning, redness, and irritation. Less common: itching, swelling, and temporary blurred vision (ointment only).

DRUG INTERACTIONS: The drug should not be used with eye preparations that contain silver nitrate or silver salts.

ALLERGIES: Individuals allergic to sulfacetamide, sulfa drugs, or any of their derivatives should discuss this with their doctor or pharmacist before using this drug.

PREGNANCY/BREAST-FEEDING: Category C—Risk cannot be ruled out. Human studies are lacking, and animal studies are either positive for fetal risk or lacking as well. However, potential benefits may justify the potential risk in using the drug. It is not known whether the drug is excreted in the breast milk; therefore, caution should be used when breast-feeding.

OTHER BRAND NAMES: Bleph-10

OTHER DRUGS IN THE SAME THERAPEUTIC CLASS: Bleph-10, Isopto Cetamide, Neosporin, Polysporin, and Polytrim

IMPORTANT INFORMATION TO REMEMBER: Individuals should not use the drug while wearing contact lenses unless directed otherwise by a doctor. Keep the container tightly closed and avoid touching the applicator tip to the eye—this could contaminate the product over time. Also, only administer one drop at a time. After application, keep the eye open for at least 30 seconds, roll the eyeball around, and avoid squinting. If a second drop is required, wait one to two minutes between drops. If another medication is to be used in the eye, wait at least 10 minutes before administering it. If you are using the eye ointment, pull the bottom eyelid down gently. Then apply a small, thin ribbon of ointment along the rim of the lower eyelid between the eyelid and the eyeball. After application, close the eye and roll the eyeball around. Your vision may be slightly blurred after application.

BRAND NAME: Sular

GENERIC NAME: nisoldipine

GENERIC FORM AVAILABLE: No

THERAPEUTIC CLASS: Calcium channel blocker

DOSAGE FORMS: 10-mg, 20-mg, 30-mg, and 40-mg extended-release tablets

MAIN USES: High blood pressure

USUAL DOSE: 10 mg to 40 mg once daily

AVERAGE PRICE: $114.80 for all strengths

SIDE EFFECTS: swelling in the arms and legs 22%, headache 22%, dizziness 5%, pharyngitis 5%, dilation of the blood vessels 4%, sinus problems 3%, pounding heartbeat 3%, chest pain 2%, and nausea 2%.

DRUG INTERACTIONS: Tagamet may increase blood levels of the drug. The drug may increase the blood levels of Lanoxin and Sandimmune. The drug may increase the blood levels of Quinidex and Quinaglute.

ALLERGIES: Individuals allergic to nisoldipine or any of its derivatives should discuss this with their doctor or pharmacist before using this drug.

PREGNANCY/BREAST-FEEDING: Category C—Risk cannot be ruled out. Human studies are lacking, and animal studies are either positive for fetal risk or lacking as well. However, potential benefits may justify the potential risk in using the drug. It is not known whether the drug is excreted in the breast milk; therefore, caution should be used when breast-feeding.

OTHER BRAND NAMES: None

OTHER DRUGS IN THE SAME THERAPEUTIC CLASS: Adalat, Adalat CC, Calan, Calan SR, Cardene, Cardene SR, Cardizem, Cardizem SR, Cardizem CD, Covera-HS, Dilacor XR, DynaCirc, Isoptin, Isoptin SR, Norvasc, Plendil, Procardia, Procardia XL, Vascor, and Verelan

IMPORTANT INFORMATION TO REMEMBER: Only take the drug exactly as directed by your physician. Do not discontinue taking the drug without first consulting your physician. Before taking over-the-counter cold and allergy preparations, consult your doctor or pharmacist—these products may raise your blood pressure. This drug may cause some tiredness at first. Individuals should use caution when driving, operating machinery, or performing any task where mental alertness is required. Meals high in fat and grapefruit juice should be avoided when taking this drug.

BRAND NAME: Sulfacet-R

GENERIC NAME: Combination product containing: sulfacetamide and sulfur

GENERIC FORM AVAILABLE: No

THERAPEUTIC CLASS: Sulfonamide antibiotic + antibacterial drying agent

DOSAGE FORMS: 10% sulfacetamide/5% sulfur lotion

MAIN USES: Acne

USUAL DOSE: Apply thin film one to three times daily and massage in gently.

AVERAGE PRICE: $32.81

SIDE EFFECTS: Most common: none. Less common: irritation.

DRUG INTERACTIONS: None of any clinical significance

ALLERGIES: Individuals allergic to sulfacetamide, sulfur, or any of their derivatives should discuss this with their doctor or pharmacist before using this drug.

PREGNANCY/BREAST-FEEDING: Category C—Risk cannot be ruled out. Human studies are lacking, and animal studies are either positive for fetal risk or lacking as well. However, potential benefits may justify the potential risk in using the drug. It is not known

whether the drug is excreted in the breast milk; therefore, caution should be used when breast-feeding.

OTHER BRAND NAMES: None

OTHER DRUGS IN THE SAME THERAPEUTIC CLASS: None

IMPORTANT INFORMATION TO REMEMBER: This drug is for external use only. Shake the medication well before using it. It is important to use the medication continuously. It may take three to four weeks before a significant improvement may be seen. If no improvement is seen within this time period, contact your doctor. Also, avoid contact with the eyes, nose, and mouth. Before applying, wash acne area thoroughly with warm soapy water to remove dirt and skin oils, pat skin dry, and then apply the drug. If you need to apply another medication for acne, wait at least one hour. Discontinue use if irritation occurs.

BRAND NAME: Sultrin

GENERIC NAME: Combination product containing: sulfathiazole, sulfacetamide, and sulfabenzamide

GENERIC FORM AVAILABLE: Yes

THERAPEUTIC CLASS: Sulfa antibiotic

DOSAGE FORMS: 3.42% sulfathiazole/2.86% sulfacetamide/3.7% sulfabenzamide vaginal cream

MAIN USES: Vaginal bacterial infections

USUAL DOSE: one applicatorful vaginally twice daily

AVERAGE PRICE: $34.70 (B)/$12.86 (G) for 78 g

SIDE EFFECTS: Most common: none. Less common: itching, burning, stinging, redness, swelling, rash, and irritation of the penis of the sexual partner.

DRUG INTERACTIONS: None of any clinical significance

ALLERGIES: Individuals allergic to sulfathiazole, sulfacetamide, sulfabenzamide, sulfa, or any of their derivatives should discuss this with their doctor or pharmacist before using this drug.

PREGNANCY/BREAST FEEDING: Category C—Risk cannot be ruled out. Human studies are lacking, and animal studies are either positive for fetal risk or lacking as well. However, potential benefits

may justify the potential risk in using the drug. The drug is excreted in the breast milk; therefore, extreme caution should be used when breast-feeding.

OTHER BRAND NAMES: None

OTHER DRUGS IN THE SAME THERAPEUTIC CLASS: AVC, Cleocin Vaginal, and MetroGel Vaginal

IMPORTANT INFORMATION TO REMEMBER: This drug is for use only in and around the vagina. Use the drug for the full course of treatment or the infection may return. Discontinue use if severe irritation occurs. When using the vaginal cream, insert the applicator high into the vagina (two-thirds the length of the applicator) and push the plunger to release the cream. Also, do not use a tampon to hold the cream inside the vagina. The cream may stain clothing. Avoid sexual intercourse until therapy is complete.

BRAND NAME: Sumycin

GENERIC NAME: tetracylcine

GENERIC FORM AVAILABLE: Yes

THERAPEUTIC CLASS: Tetracycline antibiotic

DOSAGE FORMS: 250-mg and 500-mg tablets and capsules; and 125 mg/5 mL syrup

MAIN USES: Bacterial infections and severe acne

USUAL DOSE: 250 mg to 500 mg two to four times a day

AVERAGE PRICE: $12.43 (B)/$9.88 (G) for 250 mg and $14.06 (B)/$13.62 (G) for 500 mg

SIDE EFFECTS: Most common: discoloration on infants and children's teeth, increased sensitivity to sunburn, dizziness, diarrhea, nausea, vomiting, stomach pain, and burning stomach. Less common: sore or darkened tongue, discoloration of the skin and mucous membranes, and fungal overgrowth.

DRUG INTERACTIONS: Antacids, calcium supplements, iron supplements, magnesium laxatives, and other mineral supplements may bind to the drug in the stomach and intestines and prevent its absorption by the body. The drug may decrease the effectiveness of birth control pills.

ALLERGIES: Individuals allergic to tetracycline or other tetracylcine-like drugs (such as those listed under "Other Drugs in the Same Therapeutic Class") should discuss this with their doctor or pharmacist before taking this drug.

PREGNANCY/BREAST-FEEDING: Category D—Positive evidence of risk. Human studies show risk to the fetus. Nevertheless, potential benefits may possibly outweigh the potential risk. This drug should not be taken by nursing mothers.

OTHER BRAND NAMES: None

OTHER DRUGS IN THE SAME THERAPEUTIC CLASS: Achromycin-V, Doryx, Minocin, Monodox, Vibramycin, and Vibratabs

IMPORTANT INFORMATION TO REMEMBER: This drug should be taken on an empty stomach—preferably one hour before or two hours after meals. Also, take the drug at even intervals around the clock (if four times a day, take every six hours). Take the drug until all the medication prescribed is gone; otherwise the infection may return. Avoid taking antacids, calcium supplements, iron supplements, magnesium laxatives, and other mineral supplements within two hours of taking the drug. Women taking birth control pills should use another form of contraception while taking the drug and for the rest of the current menstrual cycle. Individuals should also use a sunscreen to avoid overexposure to the sun; the drug may increase the skin's sensitivity to sunlight, which may cause one to sunburn more easily. The drug should not be used by children under eight years of age due to the potential of permanent tooth staining.

BRAND NAME: Suprax

GENERIC NAME: cefixime

GENERIC FORM AVAILABLE: No

THERAPEUTIC CLASS: Cephalosporin antibiotic

DOSAGE FORMS: 200-mg and 400-mg tablets; and 100 mg/5 mL oral suspension

MAIN USES: Bacterial infections

USUAL DOSE: 400 mg daily in a single dose

AVERAGE PRICE: $45.10 for 200 mg (10 tablets) and $90.21 for 400 mg (10 tablets)

SIDE EFFECTS: diarrhea 16%, nausea 7%, loose and frequent stools 6%, gas 4%, and stomach pain 3%.

DRUG INTERACTIONS: The drug may decrease the effectiveness of oral contraceptives used for birth control. Women may become pregnant while taking Suprax and oral contraceptives. Probenecid will decrease elimination of the drug by the kidneys.

ALLERGIES: Individuals allergic to cefixime, penicillins (including amoxicillin and ampicillin), or other cephalosporins (such as those listed under "Other Drugs in the Same Therapeutic Class") should discuss this with their doctor or pharmacist before taking this drug.

PREGNANCY/BREAST-FEEDING: Category B—No evidence of risk in humans. Either animal findings show risk, but human findings do not; or, if no adequate human studies have been done, animal findings show no risk. It is not known whether the drug is excreted in the breast milk; therefore, caution should be used when breast-feeding.

OTHER BRAND NAMES: None

OTHER DRUGS IN THE SAME THERAPEUTIC CLASS: Ceclor, Cedax, Ceftin, Cefzil, Duricef, Keflex, Keftab, Ultracef, Vantin, and Velosef

IMPORTANT INFORMATION TO REMEMBER: If stomach upset occurs, take the drug with food or milk. Take the drug at the same time every day. Also, take the drug until all the medication prescribed is gone; otherwise the infection may return. Women taking birth control pills should use another form of contraception while taking the drug and for the rest of the current menstrual cycle. Individuals taking the liquid form should shake it thoroughly before use and throw away any remaining medication after 14 days. This liquid medication, unlike other antibiotics, does not need to be refrigerated. The drug may produce a false positive for some glucose and protein urine tests or a false negative for blood glucose tests using ferricyanide.

BRAND NAME: Surmontil

GENERIC NAME: trimipramine

GENERIC FORM AVAILABLE: No

THERAPEUTIC CLASS: Tricyclic antidepressant

DOSAGE FORMS: 25-mg, 50-mg, and 100-mg capsules

MAIN USES: Depression

USUAL DOSE: 50 mg to 150 mg daily in divided doses

AVERAGE PRICE: $92.51 for 25 mg; $151.31 for 50 mg; and $220.08 for 100 mg

SIDE EFFECTS: Most common: drowsiness, dizziness, dry mouth, headache, increased appetite, nausea, tiredness, weight gain, and unpleasant taste. Less common: diarrhea, excessive sweating, heartburn, insomnia, vomiting, increased sensitivity to sunburn, irregular heartbeat, muscle tremors, urinary difficulties, and impotence.

DRUG INTERACTIONS: The drug should not be taken with Nardil or Parnate. In fact, 14 days are needed between the time of the use of this drug and Nardil or Parnate. Alcohol, anxiety medications, and narcotic painkillers may make the drowsiness caused by the drug much worse. Compazine, Mellaril, Prolixin, Serentil, Stelazine, Thorazine, and Trilafon may increase the blood levels of the drug. Tagamet may increase the blood levels of the drug. The drug may decrease the effects of Catapres and Ismelin. The drug may increase the effects of decongestants found in cold and allergy products on the heart, possibly causing high blood pressure, fast heartbeat, or irregular heartbeat.

ALLERGIES: Individuals allergic to trimipramine or other tricyclic antidepressants (such as those listed under "Other Drugs in the Same Therapeutic Class") should discuss this with their doctor or pharmacist before taking this drug.

PREGNANCY/BREAST-FEEDING: Category C—Risk cannot be ruled out. Human studies are lacking, and animal studies are either positive for fetal risk or lacking as well. However, potential benefits may justify the potential risk in using the drug. The drug is excreted in the breast milk; therefore, extreme caution should be used when breast-feeding.

OTHER BRAND NAMES: None

OTHER DRUGS IN THE SAME THERAPEUTIC CLASS: Asendin, Elavil, Endep, Norpramin, Pamelor, Sinequan, Tofranil, and Vivactil

IMPORTANT INFORMATION TO REMEMBER: Only take the drug exactly as directed by your physician. Do not discontinue taking the drug without first consulting your physician. The drug may require one to six weeks of use before improvement may be noticed. This drug does cause drowsiness. Individuals should use caution when driving, operating machinery, or performing any task where mental alertness is required. Alcohol, anxiety medications, and narcotic painkillers may intensify the drowsiness effect of the drug. The drug may cause a slight amount of dizziness or lightheadedness when rising from a sitting or lying-down position. Individuals should also use a sunscreen to avoid overexposure to the sun; the drug may increase the skin's sensitivity to sunlight, which may cause one to sunburn more easily.

BRAND NAME: Symmetrel

GENERIC NAME: amantadine

GENERIC FORM AVAILABLE: Yes

THERAPEUTIC CLASS: Dopamine anti-Parkinson's compound

DOSAGE FORMS: 100-mg capsules and 50 mg/5 mL syrup

MAIN USES: Parkinson's disease and prevention and treatment of influenza A

USUAL DOSE: 100 mg twice daily

AVERAGE PRICE: $98.98 (B)/$33.70 (G) for 100 mg

SIDE EFFECTS: Most common: dizziness, lightheadedness, headache, insomnia, nervousness, nausea, loss of appetite, and purplish-red, netlike, blotchy spots on the skin. Less common: dry mouth, constipation, blurred vision, confusion, difficulty urinating, and fainting.

DRUG INTERACTIONS: Alcohol, Akineton, Artane, Cogentin, and Kemadrin may increase the severity of side effects associated with taking the drug. The drug may increase the effects of diet pills, Dexadrine, Desoxyn, and Ritalin.

ALLERGIES: Individuals allergic to amantadine or any of its derivatives should discuss this with their doctor or pharmacist before using this drug.

PREGNANCY/BREAST-FEEDING: Category C—Risk cannot be ruled out. Human studies are lacking, and animal studies are either positive for fetal risk or lacking as well. However, potential benefits

may justify the potential risk in using the drug. The drug is excreted in the breast milk; therefore, extreme caution should be used when breast-feeding.

OTHER BRAND NAMES: None

OTHER DRUGS IN THE SAME THERAPEUTIC CLASS: For Parkinson's: Parlodel and Permax. For the flu: Flumadine.

IMPORTANT INFORMATION TO REMEMBER: Take the drug exactly as directed. Do not increase the dose or discontinue taking the drug without first consulting with your physician. This drug may cause some dizziness. Individuals should use caution when driving, operating machinery, or performing any task where mental alertness is required. Alcohol, anxiety medications, and narcotic painkillers may intensify the dizziness effect of the drug. The drug may cause a slight amount of dizziness or lightheadedness when rising from a sitting or lying-down position. Do not drink alcohol while taking this drug.

BRAND NAME: Synacort

GENERIC NAME: hydrocortisone

See entry for Hytone

BRAND NAME: Synalar and Synalar-HP

GENERIC NAME: fluocinolone

GENERIC FORM AVAILABLE: Yes

THERAPEUTIC CLASS: Topical corticosteroid

DOSAGE FORMS: 0.025% cream and ointment; 0.01% solution; and 0.2% cream (Synalar-HP)

MAIN USES: Skin rashes, swelling, and itching.

USUAL DOSE: Apply to the affected area as a thin film two to four times daily.

AVERAGE PRICE: $19.97 (B)/$9.85 (G) for 0.025% cream and ointment (15 g); $25.03 (B)/$13.93 (G) for 0.01% solution (20 mL); $38.24 for 0.2% cream (Synalar-HP, 12 g)

SIDE EFFECTS: Most common: none. Less common: burning, itching, irritation, dry skin, rash, and soreness of the skin.

DRUG INTERACTIONS: None of any clinical significance

ALLERGIES: Individuals allergic to fluocinolone or any of its derivatives should discuss this with their doctor or pharmacist before using this drug.

PREGNANCY/BREAST-FEEDING: Category C—Risk cannot be ruled out. Human studies are lacking, and animal studies are either positive for fetal risk or lacking as well. However, potential benefits may justify the potential risk in using the drug. It is not known whether the drug is excreted in the breast milk; therefore, caution should be used when breast-feeding.

OTHER BRAND NAMES: None

OTHER DRUGS IN THE SAME THERAPEUTIC CLASS: Aclovate, Aristocort, Cordran, Cordran SP, Cutivate, Cyclocort, DesOwen, Diprolene, Diprolene AF, Elocon, Florone, Florone E, Halog, Hytone, Kenalog, Lidex, Lidex-E, Temovate, Topicort, Tridesilon, Ultravate, Valisone, and Westcort

IMPORTANT INFORMATION TO REMEMBER: This drug is for external use only. Apply only a thin film of drug to skin and rub it in well. Never cover the skin after application with a bandage or wrapping unless directed to do so by a doctor. Never apply to damaged skin or open wounds unless directed to do so by a doctor. Discontinue use if irritation occurs.

BRAND NAME: Synarel

GENERIC NAME: nafarelin

GENERIC FORM AVAILABLE: No

THERAPEUTIC CLASS: Pituitary gland hormone analogue

DOSAGE FORMS: 200-micrograms-per-spray intranasal solution

MAIN USES: Endometriosis and central precocious puberty (early puberty)

USUAL DOSE: For endometriosis: start between days Two and Four of menstrual cycle, 400 micrograms daily (one spray in one nostril in the morning and one spray in the other nostril in the evening). For central precocious puberty: 1600 micrograms daily (two sprays in each nostril in the morning and two sprays in each nostril in the evening).

AVERAGE PRICE: $429.58 for 10 mL

SIDE EFFECTS: acne 10%, breast enlargement 8%, vaginal bleeding 8%, emotional changes 6%, increase in pubic hair 5%, body odor 5%, runny nose 5%, oily skin 3%, hot flashes 3%, and white or brown vaginal discharge 3%.

DRUG INTERACTIONS: None of any clinical significance

ALLERGIES: Individuals allergic to nafarelin or any of its derivatives should discuss this with their doctor or pharmacist before using this drug.

PREGNANCY/BREAST-FEEDING: Category X—Should not be used during pregnancy. Studies in animals and/or humans have shown fetal abnormalities and birth defects. The risks associated with using this drug clearly outweigh the benefits. This drug should never be used by someone who is pregnant or trying to become pregnant. Also, women should never breast-feed while using this drug.

OTHER BRAND NAMES: None

OTHER DRUGS IN THE SAME THERAPEUTIC CLASS: Lupron Depot and Zoladex

IMPORTANT INFORMATION TO REMEMBER: Take the drug exactly as directed. Do not increase the dose or discontinue taking the drug without first consulting with your physician.

When using the nasal spray, use the following procedure:

1) Blow your nose gently to clear your nostrils, if necessary.
2) With your other hand, gently place a finger against the side of your nose to close the opposite nostril.
3) Insert the tip of the bottle or aerosol into the open nostril. Point the tip toward the back and outer side of the nostril once inside.
4) After releasing the spray, close your mouth, sniff deeply, hold your breath for a few seconds, then breathe out through your mouth.
5) Tilt your head back slightly for a few seconds to allow the drug to spread to the back of your nose.
6) Repeat the same procedure for the other nostril, if necessary.
7) If using more than one spray in each nostril, wait two minutes between sprays.

BRAND NAME: Synemol

GENERIC NAME: fluocinolone

Very similar to Synalar. See entry for Synalar/Synalar-HP.

BRAND NAME: Synthroid

GENERIC NAME: levothyroxine

GENERIC FORM AVAILABLE: No

THERAPEUTIC CLASS: Thyroid replacement

DOSAGE FORMS: 25-, 50-, 75-, 88-, 100-, 112-, 125-, 150-, 175-, 200-, and 300-microgram tablets

MAIN USES: Thyroid hormone replacement therapy

USUAL DOSE: 25 micrograms to 300 micrograms daily

AVERAGE PRICE: $24.69 for 25 micrograms; $27.97 for 50 micrograms; $30.99 for 75 micrograms; $31.91 for 88 micrograms; $31.75 for 100 micrograms; $37.45 for 112 micrograms; $38.01 for 125 micrograms; $38.22 for 150 micrograms; $46.67 for 150 micrograms; $48.69 for 200 micrograms; $61.90 for 300 micrograms

SIDE EFFECTS: Most common: none. Less common: sensitivity to the heat, sweating, nervousness, fast heartbeat, pounding heartbeat, insomnia, stomach cramps, diarrhea, and weight loss. These side effects are most often caused from taking too much of the drug.

DRUG INTERACTIONS: The drug may increase the effects of Coumadin. The drug may also decrease the effects of diabetes drugs. Climara, Estrace, Estraderm, Ogen, Premarin, and Vivelle may alter the effectiveness of the drug. Colestid and Questran may decrease the absorption of the drug in the stomach if taken with the drug.

ALLERGIES: Individuals allergic to levothyroxine, other thyroid drugs, or any of their derivatives should discuss this with their doctor or pharmacist before using this drug.

PREGNANCY/BREAST-FEEDING: Category A—Controlled studies show no risk. Adequate well-controlled studies in pregnant women have failed to demonstrate risk to the fetus. Women who wish to breast-feed should consult their physician first.

OTHER BRAND NAMES: None

OTHER DRUGS IN THE SAME THERAPEUTIC CLASS: Armour Thyroid, Levothroid, and Levoxyl

IMPORTANT INFORMATION TO REMEMBER: It's best to take the drug on an empty stomach—one hour before or two hours after meals. Do not stop taking the drug without first consulting your physician. It is important to take the drug at the same time every day for consistent effects. Before taking over-the-counter medications, consult with your doctor or pharmacist.

BRAND NAME: Tagamet

GENERIC NAME: cimetidine

GENERIC FORM AVAILABLE: Yes

THERAPEUTIC CLASS: Stomach acid blocker

DOSAGE FORMS: 200-mg, 300-mg, 400-mg, and 800-mg tablets; 300 mg/5 mL liquid

MAIN USES: Active stomach ulcers, active duodenal ulcers (ulcers of the upper part of the small intestine, also called peptic ulcers), maintenance of healed duodenal ulcers, the treatment of gastroesophageal reflux disease, {itching}, and {warts in children}.

USUAL DOSE: 300 mg four times daily, 400 mg twice daily, or 800 mg at bedtime

AVERAGE PRICE: $103.82 (B)/$54.65 (G) for 200 mg; $119.26 (B)/ $61.71 (G) for 300 mg; $133.85 (B)/$69.94 (G) for 400 mg; $266.83 (B)/$116.11 (G) for 800 mg

SIDE EFFECTS: headache 4%, enlarged breasts in males 1%–4%, dizziness 1%, drowsiness 1%, confusion 1%, and diarrhea 1%.

DRUG INTERACTIONS: The drug may increase the blood levels of Coumadin, Dilantin, Flagyl, Inderal, Librium, Procardia, Slo-bid, Theo-Dur, theophylline, Uni-Dur, Uniphyl, and Valium. The drug may also increase the blood levels of Anafranil, Asendin, Elavil, Endep, Norpramin, Pamelor, Sinequan, Surmontil, Tofranil, and Vivactil.

ALLERGIES: Individuals allergic to cimetidine or other stomach acid blockers (such as those listed under "Other Drugs in the Same

Therapeutic Class") should discuss this with their doctor or pharmacist before taking this drug.

PREGNANCY/BREAST-FEEDING: Category B—No evidence of risk in humans. Either animal findings show risk, but human findings do not; or, if no adequate human studies have been done, animal findings show no risk. The drug is excreted in the breast milk; therefore, extreme caution should be used when breast-feeding.

OTHER BRAND NAMES: Tagamet HB 200 (over-the-counter)

OTHER DRUGS IN THE SAME THERAPEUTIC CLASS: Axid, Pepcid, and Zantac

IMPORTANT INFORMATION TO REMEMBER: Always complete the full course of therapy, and take the drug only as directed. Individuals may take antacids occasionally for heartburn or temporary flare-ups, but antacids should be taken at least one hour before or two hours after taking the drug. The drug is now available over-the-counter (OTC) without a prescription in a 200-mg tablet as Tagamet HB 200.

BRAND NAME: Talacen

GENERIC NAME: Combination product containing: pentazocine and acetaminophen

GENERIC FORM AVAILABLE: No

THERAPEUTIC CLASS: Narcotic analgesic + pain reliever

DOSAGE FORMS: 25-mg pentazocine/650-mg acetaminophen caplets

MAIN USES: Mild to moderate pain

USUAL DOSE: one tablet every four hours as needed

AVERAGE PRICE: $105.70

SIDE EFFECTS: Most common: drowsiness, false sense of well-being, tiredness, nausea, and vomiting. Less common: confusion, decreased urination, allergic reaction, fast or slow heartbeat, dry mouth, constipation, stomach pain, skin rash, dizziness, nervousness, nightmares, headache, weakness, minor vision disturbances, histamine release (symptoms include decreased blood pressure, sweating, fast heartbeat, flushing, and wheezing), and hallucinations.

DRUG INTERACTIONS: Alcohol, anxiety medications, and other narcotic painkillers may intensify the drowsiness effect of the drug. This drug and Nardil or Parnate may cause severe and sometimes fatal reactions if taken together.

ALLERGIES: Individuals allergic to pentazocine, acetaminophen, or any of their derivatives should discuss this with their doctor or pharmacist before using this drug.

PREGNANCY/BREAST-FEEDING: Category C—Risk cannot be ruled out. Human studies are lacking, and animal studies are either positive for fetal risk or lacking as well. However, potential benefits may justify the potential risk in using the drug. It is not known whether the drug is excreted in the breast milk; therefore, caution should be used when breast-feeding.

OTHER BRAND NAMES: None

OTHER DRUGS IN THE SAME THERAPEUTIC CLASS: Bancap-HC, Darvocet-N 50, Darvocet-N 100, Darvon, Darvon Compound, DHCplus, Empirin #3, Empirin #4, Hydrocet, Lorcet Plus, Lorcet 10/650, Lortab, Percocet, Percodan, Phenaphen w/Codeine, Synalgos DC, Tylenol #2, Tylenol #3, Tylenol #4, Tylox, Vicodin, and Zydone

IMPORTANT INFORMATION TO REMEMBER: This drug does cause drowsiness. Individuals should use caution when driving, operating machinery, or performing any task where mental alertness is required. Alcohol, anxiety medications, and narcotic painkillers may intensify the drowsiness effect of the drug. If stomach upset occurs, take the drug with food or milk. Do not increase the dose without first consulting with your physician. This medication is a controlled substance and may be habit-forming.

BRAND NAME: Talwin Nx

GENERIC NAME: Combination product containing: pentazocine and naloxone

GENERIC FORM AVAILABLE: No

THERAPEUTIC CLASS: Narcotic analgesic + narcotic antagonist

DOSAGE FORMS: 50-mg pentazocine/0.5-mg naloxone tablets

MAIN USES: Moderate to severe pain

USUAL DOSE: one tablet every three to four hours as needed

AVERAGE PRICE: $119.80

SIDE EFFECTS: Most common: drowsiness, false sense of well-being, tiredness, nausea, and vomiting. Less common: confusion, decreased urination, allergic reaction, fast or slow heartbeat, dry mouth, constipation, stomach pain, skin rash, dizziness, nervousness, nightmares, headache, weakness, minor vision disturbances, histamine release (symptoms include decreased blood pressure, sweating, fast heartbeat, flushing, and wheezing), and hallucinations.

DRUG INTERACTIONS: Alcohol, anxiety medications, and other narcotic painkillers may intensify the drowsiness effect of the drug. This drug and Nardil or Parnate may cause severe and sometimes fatal reactions if taken together.

ALLERGIES: Individuals allergic to pentazocine, naloxone, or any of their derivatives should discuss this with their doctor or pharmacist before using this drug.

PREGNANCY/BREAST-FEEDING: Category C—Risk cannot be ruled out. Human studies are lacking, and animal studies are either positive for fetal risk or lacking as well. However, potential benefits may justify the potential risk in using the drug. It is not known whether the drug is excreted in the breast milk; therefore, caution should be used when breast-feeding.

OTHER BRAND NAMES: None

OTHER DRUGS IN THE SAME THERAPEUTIC CLASS: None

IMPORTANT INFORMATION TO REMEMBER: This drug does cause drowsiness. Individuals should use caution when driving, operating machinery, or performing any task where mental alertness is required. Alcohol, anxiety medications, and narcotic painkillers intensify the drowsiness effect of the drug. If stomach upset occurs, take the drug with food or milk. Do not increase the dose without first consulting with your physician. This medication is a controlled substance and may be habit-forming. Note: the drug originally only contained pentazocine. Back then the drug was melted down and injected by drug addicts when it only contained pentazocine. The naloxone component was then added to counter the effects of the drug if it is injected. Naloxone, if taken orally, is destroyed by stomach acid and has no effects whatsoever.

BRAND NAME: **Tambocor**

GENERIC NAME: flecainide

GENERIC FORM AVAILABLE: No

THERAPEUTIC CLASS: Class IC antiarrhythmic

DOSAGE FORMS: 50-mg, 100-mg, and 150-mg tablets

MAIN USES: Irregular heartbeat

USUAL DOSE: 50 mg to 150 mg every 12 hours

AVERAGE PRICE: $94.08 for 50 mg; $170.85 for 100 mg; and $235.11 for 150 mg

SIDE EFFECTS: dizziness 19%, vision disturbances 16%, trouble breathing 10%, headache 10%, nausea 9%, tiredness 8%, pounding heartbeat 6%, chest pain 5%, muscle weakness 5%, tremor 5%, constipation 4%, swelling 4%, and stomach pain 3%.

DRUG INTERACTIONS: The drug may increase the blood levels of Inderal and Lanoxin. Caution should be used by patients taking other drugs specifically used for irregular heartbeat. Inderal and Tagamet may increase the blood levels of the drug.

ALLERGIES: Individuals allergic to flecainide or any of its derivatives should discuss this with their doctor or pharmacist before using this drug.

PREGNANCY/BREAST-FEEDING: Category C—Risk cannot be ruled out. Human studies are lacking, and animal studies are either positive for fetal risk or lacking as well. However, potential benefits may justify the potential risk in using the drug. The drug is excreted in the breast milk; therefore, extreme caution should be used when breast-feeding.

OTHER BRAND NAMES: None

OTHER DRUGS IN THE SAME THERAPEUTIC CLASS: Rythmol

IMPORTANT INFORMATION TO REMEMBER: This drug may cause some dizziness or tiredness, especially at first. Individuals should use caution when driving, operating machinery, or performing any task where mental alertness is required. Alcohol, anxiety medications, and narcotic painkillers may intensify these effects. Only take the drug exactly as directed by your physician. Do not discontinue taking the drug without first consulting your physician; also, do not increase the dose without first consulting with your physician.

BRAND NAME: Tegison

GENERIC NAME: etretinate

GENERIC FORM AVAILABLE: No

THERAPEUTIC CLASS: Vitamin A derivative, anti-psoriasis

DOSAGE FORMS: 10-mg and 25-mg tablets

MAIN USES: Severe psoriasis

USUAL DOSE: 0.5 mg to 0.75 mg per kg of body weight per day in divided doses (1 kg = 2.2 pounds)

AVERAGE PRICE: $86.04 for 10 mg (30 tablets) and $134.55 for 25 mg (30 tablets)

SIDE EFFECTS: dry nose 75%; chapped lips 75%; loss of hair 75%; peeling of the palms, sole of the foot, or fingertips 75%; thickening of the bone tissue 75%; excessive thirst 50%–75%; sore mouth 50%–75%; dry skin 50%–75%; itching 50%–75%; red, scaly face 50%–75%; bone/joint pain 50%–75%; tiredness 50%–75%; irritation of the eyes 50%–75%; nosebleed 25%–50%; bruising 25%–50%; sunburn 25%–50%; muscle cramps 25%–50%; headache 25%–50%; eyeball pain 25%–50%; eyelid abnormalities 25%–50%; stomach pain 25%–50%; changes in appetite 25%–50%; sore tongue 10%–25%; nail disorders 10%–25%; skin peeling 10%–25%; fever 10%–25%; abnormalities of the eyeball 10%–25%; vision disturbances 10%–25%; and nausea 10%–25%.

DRUG INTERACTIONS: Alcohol and the drug may increase cholesterol levels. Accutane, Differin, Retin-A, Renova, and vitamin A may increase the toxic effects of the drug. Rheumatrex and the drug may increase the toxic effects on the liver. Doryx, Monocin, Monodox, Sumycin, and Vibramycin may increase incidence of pseudotumor cerebri (a dangerous increase in the blood pressure within the brain).

ALLERGIES: Individuals allergic to etretinate or any of its derivatives should discuss this with their doctor or pharmacist before using this drug.

PREGNANCY/BREAST-FEEDING: Category X—Should not be used during pregnancy. Studies in animals and/or humans have shown fetal abnormalities and birth defects. The risks associated with using this drug clearly outweigh the benefits. This drug should never be used by someone who is pregnant or trying to become pregnant. Also, women should never breast-feed while using this drug.

OTHER BRAND NAMES: None

OTHER DRUGS IN THE SAME THERAPEUTIC CLASS: None

IMPORTANT INFORMATION TO REMEMBER: Females should definitely use contraceptive measures while taking this drug to avoid becoming pregnant. If a woman suspects she may be pregnant, she should stop taking the drug immediately. Individuals should also use a sunscreen to avoid overexposure to the sun; the drug may increase the skin's sensitivity to sunlight, which may cause one to sunburn more easily. Headaches, visual disturbances, nausea, and vomiting may be symptoms of pseudotumor cerebri and should be reported to a physician immediately. Finally, take with food or milk to increase absorption of the drug and reduce the potential for stomach upset. Avoid vitamin supplements containing large amounts of vitamin A. The drug may decrease night vision suddenly; caution should therefore be used when driving at night.

BRAND NAME: Tegretol and Tegretol-XR

GENERIC NAME: carbamazepine

GENERIC FORM AVAILABLE: Yes (Tegretol only)

THERAPEUTIC CLASS: Anticonvulsant

DOSAGE FORMS: 100-mg chewable tablets; 200-mg tablets; 100 mg/5 mL suspension; and 100-mg, 200-mg, and 400-mg extended-release tablets

MAIN USES: Seizures, epilepsy, trigeminal neuralgia, {bipolar disorder}, and {alcohol withdrawal}

USUAL DOSE: 200 mg to 1200 mg daily in divided doses

AVERAGE PRICE: $31.74 (B)/$28.91 (G) for 100 mg; $48.25 (B)/$37.99 (G) for 200 mg; $34.67 for 100 mg XR tablets; $48.91 for 200 mg XR tablets; and $84.98 for 400 mg XR tablets

SIDE EFFECTS: Most common: blurred vision, double vision, continuous back-and-forth eye movements, drowsiness, dizziness, lightheadedness, confusion, nausea, vomiting, clumsiness, and unsteadiness. Less common: muscle/joint pain, muscle cramps, loss of hair, loss of appetite, constipation, diarrhea, increased sweating, dry mouth, sore tongue or mouth, increased sensitivity of the skin to sunburn, stomach pain, unusual tiredness, weakness, sexual problems in males, rash, itching, and behavioral changes.

DRUG INTERACTIONS: The drug may decrease the effects of Coumadin. The drug may decrease the blood levels of Amytal, Aristocort, Butisol, Climara, Decadron, Deltasone, Depakene, Depakote, Dilantin, Estrace, Estraderm, Klonopin, Mebaral, Medrol, Mesantoin, Mysoline, Nembutal, Ogen, phenobarbital, prednisone, Premarin, Seconal, Tuinal, Valium, and Vivelle. Drugs used to treat depression may increase the side effects of the drug and decrease its effectiveness. Biaxin, Calan, Cardizem, Darvocet-N, Darvon, Darvon Compound, Dilacor XR, erythromycin, Isoptin, and Tagamet may increase the blood levels of the drug. The drug may decrease the effectiveness of estrogens and birth control pills. Isoniazid and the drug may increase the toxic effects on the liver. The drug should never be taken with Nardil or Parnate. In fact, Nardil or Parnate should be stopped at least 14 days before Tegretol is taken.

ALLERGIES: Individuals allergic to carbamazepine or any of its derivatives should discuss this with their doctor or pharmacist before using this drug.

PREGNANCY/BREAST-FEEDING: Category C—Rick cannot be ruled out. Human studies are lacking, and animal studies are either positive for fetal risk or lacking as well. However, potential benefits may justify the potential risk in using the drug. The drug is excreted in the breast milk; therefore, extreme caution should be used when breast feeding.

OTHER BRAND NAMES: None

OTHER DRUGS IN THE SAME THERAPEUTIC CLASS: None

IMPORTANT INFORMATION TO REMEMBER: The drug should be taken with food or milk. This drug does cause drowsiness. Individuals should use caution when driving, operating machinery, or performing any task where mental alertness is required. Alcohol, anxiety medications, and narcotic painkillers may intensify the drowsiness effect of the drug. Avoid drinking alcohol while taking this drug. Only take the drug exactly as directed by your physician. Do not discontinue taking the drug without first consulting your physician; also, do not increase the dose without first consulting with your physician. Before taking over-the-counter medications, consult your doctor or pharmacist. Birth control pills may be ineffective while taking this drug—another method of birth control is recommended. Individuals may want to use a sunscreen to avoid overexposure to the sun; the drug may increase the skin's sensitivity to sunlight, which may cause one to sunburn more easily. The 100-mg tablets may be swallowed or chewed and should be taken with a full glass of water. Be sure to shake the liquid suspension well before use. Do not change between brand and generic once you are stabilized on one or the other.

BRAND NAME: Temaril

GENERIC NAME: trimeprazine

GENERIC FORM AVAILABLE: No

THERAPEUTIC CLASS: Phenothiazine antihistamine

DOSAGE FORMS: 2.5-mg tablets; 5-mg extended-release capsules; and 2.5 mg/5 mL liquid

MAIN USES: Allergic reactions and itching

USUAL DOSE: 2.5 mg four times daily or one 5-mg extended-release capsule twice daily

AVERAGE PRICE: $91.60 for 2.5-mg tablets

SIDE EFFECTS: Most common: drowsiness and thickening of mucus. Less common: blurred vision, confusion, difficulty in urinating, dizziness, dry mouth, increased sweating, loss of appetite, nightmares, nervousness, fast heartbeat, ringing in the ears, increased sensitivity to sunburn, and skin rash.

DRUG INTERACTIONS: Alcohol, anxiety medications, and other narcotic painkillers may intensify the drowsiness effect of the drug. The drug should not be used with Nardil or Parnate. The drug should also not be used with Akineton, Artane, Cogentin, and Kemadrin. The drug may decrease the effects of Larodopa.

ALLERGIES: Individuals allergic to trimeprazine or any of its derivatives should discuss this with their doctor or pharmacist before using this drug.

PREGNANCY/BREAST-FEEDING: Category D—Positive evidence of risk. Human studies show risk to the fetus. Nevertheless, potential benefits may possibly outweigh the potential risks. This drug should not be taken by nursing mothers.

OTHER BRAND NAMES: None

OTHER DRUGS IN THE SAME THERAPEUTIC CLASS: Phenergan

IMPORTANT INFORMATION TO REMEMBER: This drug may cause drowsiness. Individuals should use caution when driving, operating machinery, or performing any task where mental alertness is required. Alcohol, anxiety medications, and narcotic painkillers may intensify the drowsiness effect of the drug. This drug may also cause a dry mouth; sugarless gum or hard candy will help take care of this problem. Patients with glaucoma or urinary or prostate problems should consult their doctor before taking this drug.

BRAND NAME: Temovate

GENERIC NAME: clobetasol

GENERIC FORM AVAILABLE: Yes

THERAPEUTIC CLASS: Topical corticosteroid

DOSAGE FORMS: 0.05% cream, gel, ointment, scalp application, and emollient cream

MAIN USES: Skin rashes, swelling, and itching

USUAL DOSE: Apply to the affected area as a thin film twice daily.

AVERAGE PRICE: $33.67 (B)/$27.60 (G) for 0.05% cream, gel, ointment, and emollient cream (15 g); and $34.37 (B)/$29.81 (G) for 0.05% for scalp application (25 mL)

SIDE EFFECTS: burning or stinging sensation 1%, itching 1%, and irritation 1%.

DRUG INTERACTIONS: None of any clinical significance

ALLERGIES: Individuals allergic to clobetasol or any of its derivatives should discuss this with their doctor or pharmacist before using this drug.

PREGNANCY/BREAST-FEEDING: Category C—Risk cannot be ruled out. Human studies are lacking, and animal studies are either positive for fetal risk or lacking as well. However, potential benefits may justify the potential risk in using the drug. It is not known whether the drug is excreted in the breast milk; therefore, caution should be used when breast-feeding.

OTHER BRAND NAMES: Cormax (scalp application only)

OTHER DRUGS IN THE SAME THERAPEUTIC CLASS: Aclovate, Aristocort, Cordran, Cordran SP, Cutivate, Cyclocort, DesOwen, Diprolene, Diprolene AF, Elocon, Florone, Florone E, Halog, Hytone, Kenalog, Lidex, Synalar, Topicort, Tridesilon, Ultravate, Valisone, and Westcort

IMPORTANT INFORMATION TO REMEMBER: This drug is for external use only. Apply only a thin film of drug to skin and rub it in well. Never cover the skin after application with a bandage or wrapping unless directed to do so by a doctor. Never apply to damaged skin or open wounds unless directed to do so by a doctor. Discontinue use if irritation occurs.

BRAND NAME: Tenex

GENERIC NAME: guanfacine

GENERIC FORM AVAILABLE: No

THERAPEUTIC CLASS: Central blood vessel dilator

DOSAGE FORMS: 1-mg and 2-mg tablets

MAIN USES: High blood pressure

USUAL DOSE: 1 mg to 2 mg daily at bedtime

AVERAGE PRICE: $121.95 for 1 mg and $167.20 for 2 mg

SIDE EFFECTS: dry mouth 47%, constipation 16%, tiredness 12%, drowsiness 10%–21%, weakness 6%, dizziness 6%, headache 4%, and insomnia 4%.

DRUG INTERACTIONS: Amytal, Butisol, Mebaral, Nembutal, phenobarbital, Seconal, and Tuinal may decrease the blood levels of the drug.

ALLERGIES: Individuals allergic to guanfacine or any of its derivatives should discuss this with their doctor or pharmacist before using this drug.

PREGNANCY/BREAST-FEEDING: Category B—No evidence of risk in humans. Either animal findings show risk, but human findings do not; or, if no adequate human studies have been done, animal findings show no risk. It is not known whether the drug is excreted in the breast milk; therefore, caution should be used when breast-feeding.

OTHER BRAND NAMES: None

OTHER DRUGS IN THE SAME THERAPEUTIC CLASS: Wytensin

IMPORTANT INFORMATION TO REMEMBER: The drug may cause drowsiness and/or dizziness, especially when treatment is begun or daily dosage is increased. Alcohol, anxiety medications, and narcotic painkillers may intensify these effects of the drug. To minimize the drowsiness, the drug should be taken at bedtime. Drowsiness may go away once the body adjusts to the medication. Before taking over-the-counter cold and allergy preparations, consult your doctor or pharmacist—these products may raise your blood pressure. If stomach upset occurs, take with food or milk. Tolerance to the effects of alcohol may be decreased while taking this drug. Do not stop taking the drug suddenly.

BRAND NAME: Tenoretic

GENERIC NAME: Combination product containing: atenolol and chlorthalidone

See individual entries for Tenormin and Hygroton

BRAND NAME: Tenormin

GENERIC NAME: atenolol

GENERIC FORM AVAILABLE: Yes

THERAPEUTIC CLASS: Cardioselective beta-blocker

DOSAGE FORMS: 25-mg, 50-mg, and 100-mg tablets

MAIN USES: High blood pressure and angina

USUAL DOSE: 25 mg to 100 mg once daily

AVERAGE PRICE: $96.60 (B)/$30.26 (G) for 25 mg; $82.76 (B)/$24.37 (G) for 50 mg; $136.55 (B)/$35.54 (G) for 100 mg

SIDE EFFECTS: dizziness 4%, nausea 4%, slow heartbeat 3%, tiredness 3%, low blood pressure 2%, diarrhea 2%, drowsiness 1%, and trouble breathing 1%.

DRUG INTERACTIONS: The drug may cause additive effects when used with reserpine. The drug may increase the effects of Calan, Cardene, Cardizem, Catapres, Covera-HS, Dilacor XR, Dyna-Circ, Isoptin, Lanoxin, Norvasc, Plendil, Procardia, Sular, Tiazac, Verelan, and Wytensin. Diabetic medications, insulin, Slo-bid,

Theo-Dur, theophylline, Uni-Dur, and Uniphyl dosages may need to be adjusted when taking this drug.

ALLERGIES: Individuals allergic to atenolol or other beta-blockers (such as those listed under "Other Drugs in the Same Therapeutic Class") should discuss this with their doctor or pharmacist before taking this drug.

PREGNANCY/BREAST-FEEDING: Category C—Risk cannot be ruled out. Human studies are lacking, and animal studies are either positive for fetal risk or lacking as well. However, potential benefits may justify the potential risk in using the drug. The drug is excreted in the breast milk; therefore, extreme caution should be used when breast-feeding.

OTHER BRAND NAMES: None

OTHER DRUGS IN THE SAME THERAPEUTIC CLASS: Lopressor, Kerlone, Sectral, Toprol-XL, and Zebeta

IMPORTANT INFORMATION TO REMEMBER: Only take the drug exactly as directed by your physician. Do not discontinue taking the drug without first consulting your physician. This drug may cause some tiredness, especially at first. Individuals should use caution when driving, operating machinery, or performing any task where mental alertness is required. Alcohol, anxiety medications, and narcotic painkillers may intensify the tiredness effect of the drug. Before taking over-the-counter cold and allergy preparations, consult your doctor or pharmacist—these products may raise your blood pressure. This drug may mask the symptoms of low blood sugar in diabetics.

BRAND NAME: Terazol

GENERIC NAME: terconazole

GENERIC FORM AVAILABLE: No

THERAPEUTIC CLASS: Antifungal

DOSAGE FORMS: 0.4% cream (Terazol 7), 0.8% cream (Terazol 3), and 80-mg suppository (Terazol 3 Suppositories)

MAIN USES: Vaginal yeast infections

USUAL DOSE: One applicatorful of 0.4% cream administered in the vagina once daily at bedtime for seven consecutive days; or one

80-mg suppository or one applicatorful of 0.8% cream administered in the vagina once daily at bedtime for three consecutive days.

AVERAGE PRICE: $33.85 for all strengths and types

SIDE EFFECTS: headache 21%, menstrual pain 6%, burning 5%–15%, itching 5%, pain in the genital area 4%, body pain 4%, stomach pain 3%, chills 2%, and fever 1%.

DRUG INTERACTIONS: None of any clinical significance

ALLERGIES: Individuals allergic to terconazole or other antifungals (such as those listed under "Other Drugs in the Same Therapeutic Class") should discuss this with their doctor or pharmacist before taking this drug.

PREGNANCY/BREAST-FEEDING: Category C—Risk cannot be ruled out. Human studies are lacking, and animal studies are either positive for fetal risk or lacking as well. Potential benefits may justify the potential risk in using the drug. However, the drug should not be used during the first trimester (first three months) of pregnancy. It is not known whether the drug is excreted in the breast milk; therefore, caution should be used when breast-feeding.

OTHER BRAND NAMES: None

OTHER DRUGS IN THE SAME THERAPEUTIC CLASS: Femstat, Gyne-Lotrimin, Monistat, Mycelex, and Vagistat-1

IMPORTANT INFORMATION TO REMEMBER: Use the drug for the full course of therapy even if symptoms disappear; otherwise the infection may return. Continue using the drug even if your menstrual period begins. When using the vaginal cream, insert the applicator high into the vagina (two-thirds the length of the applicator) and push the plunger to release the cream. Do not use a tampon to hold the cream inside the vagina. It is recommended that your sexual partner use a condom until the infection clears up. If using the suppository, insert it as far into the vagina as possible.

BRAND NAME: Tessalon

GENERIC NAME: benzonatate

GENERIC FORM AVAILABLE: Yes

THERAPEUTIC CLASS: Antitussive

DOSAGE FORMS: 100-mg capsules (perles)

MAIN USES: Cough

USUAL DOSE: 100 mg three times daily as needed

AVERAGE PRICE: $117.16 (B)/$83.14 (G)

SIDE EFFECTS: Most common: none. Less common: drowsiness, dizziness, constipation, nausea, vomiting, skin rash, and stuffy nose.

DRUG INTERACTIONS: None of any clinical significance

ALLERGIES: Individuals allergic to benzonatate or any of its derivatives should discuss this with their doctor or pharmacist before using this drug.

PREGNANCY/BREAST-FEEDING: Category C—Risk cannot be ruled out. Human studies are lacking, and animal studies are either positive for fetal risk or lacking as well. However, potential benefits may justify the potential risk in using the drug. It is not known whether the drug is excreted in the breast milk; therefore, caution should be used when breast-feeding.

OTHER BRAND NAMES: None

OTHER DRUGS IN THE SAME THERAPEUTIC CLASS: None

IMPORTANT INFORMATION TO REMEMBER: This drug may cause some mild drowsiness. Individuals should use caution when driving, operating machinery, or performing any task where mental alertness is required. Alcohol, anxiety medications, and narcotic painkillers may intensify the drowsiness effect of the drug. It is important to swallow the capsules whole—do not chew, crush, or dissolve them in the mouth. Only take the drug exactly as directed by your physician and do not increase the dose without consulting with your physician first. If you have difficulty breathing or swallowing shortly after taking the drug, contact your physician immediately.

BRAND NAME: **Testoderm Patch**

GENERIC NAME: testosterone

GENERIC FORM AVAILABLE: No

THERAPEUTIC CLASS: Testosterone hormone

DOSAGE FORMS: 4 mg/day and 6 mg/day transdermal patches

MAIN USES: Testosterone replacement therapy

USUAL DOSE: one patch every 22–24 hours

AVERAGE PRICE: $100.46 for 30 patches (both strengths)

SIDE EFFECTS: Most common: hair overgrowth in certain areas, enlargement of the breasts in males, male pattern baldness on the head, acne, enlargement of penis, and frequent or persistent erections. Less common: diarrhea, changes in sex drive, insomnia, watery mouth, dizziness, swelling, vomiting, and nausea.

DRUG INTERACTIONS: The drug may increase the effectiveness of Coumadin. The drug may also decrease blood sugar levels, which may decrease the amount of insulin needed.

ALLERGIES: Individuals allergic to testosterone or any of its derivatives should discuss this with their doctor or pharmacist before using this drug.

PREGNANCY/BREAST-FEEDING: Category X—Should not be used during pregnancy. Studies in animals and/or humans have shown fetal abnormalities and birth defects. The risks associated with using this drug clearly outweigh the benefits. This drug should never be used by someone who is pregnant or trying to become pregnant. Also, women should never breast-feed while using this drug.

OTHER BRAND NAMES: None

OTHER DRUGS IN THE SAME THERAPEUTIC CLASS: Androderm, Android, Halotestin, Testred, and Winstrol

IMPORTANT INFORMATION TO REMEMBER: Only use the drug exactly as directed by your physician. Do not discontinue taking the drug without first consulting your physician.

When using the patches:

1) Do not cut or fold the patch in half. This may cause the medication inside to leak out. Peel off the adhesive liner.
2) Apply the patch to a clean, dry skin area on the scrotum. This area should be free of hair, cuts, scars, or irritation.
3) Leave the patch on even during swimming, showering, and exercising. If the patch falls off, replace the patch with a new one.
4) When it's time to apply a new patch, use a different site on the skin. Rotate the sites where you apply the patches every time.
5) Get into the habit of applying the patch at the same time each day.

BRAND NAME: Theo-24

GENERIC NAME: theophylline

Very similar to Theo-Dur. See entry for Theo-Dur.

BRAND NAME: Theo-Dur

GENERIC NAME: theophylline anhydrous

GENERIC FORM AVAILABLE: Yes

THERAPEUTIC CLASS: Xanthine bronchodilator

DOSAGE FORMS: 100-mg, 200-mg, 300-mg, and 450-mg sustained-release tablets; 50-mg, 75-mg, 125-mg, and 200-mg sustained-release sprinkle capsules

MAIN USES: Asthma, chronic bronchitis, emphysema, and other breathing disorders

USUAL DOSE: 100 mg to 450 mg every 12 hours

AVERAGE PRICE: $34.06 (B)/$21.96 (G) for 100 mg; $44.97 (B)/$25.94 (G) for 200 mg; $54.32 (B)/$31.44 (G) for 300 mg; $69.93 (B)/$46.73 (G) for 450 mg

SIDE EFFECTS: Most common: nausea, nervousness, and restlessness. Less common: vomiting, diarrhea, stomach pain, headaches, irritability, insomnia, muscle twitching, fast heartbeat, pounding heartbeat, fast breathing, flushing, and low blood pressure.

DRUG INTERACTIONS: The drug may inhibit the effects of Blocadren, Cartrol, Corgard, Inderal, Kerlone, Levatol, Lopressor, Normodyne, Sectral, Tenormin, Toprol-XL, Trandate, Visken, and Zebeta. Dilantin, Tegretol, smoking, and nicotine patches may lower the blood levels of this drug. Cipro, Noroxin, Tagamet, Zantac, erythromycin, and TAO may increase blood levels of the drug. Individuals who stop smoking while taking the drug may have increased levels of the drug in the blood.

ALLERGIES: Individuals allergic to theophylline or other xanthines (such as those listed under "Other Drugs in the Same Therapeutic Class") should discuss this with their doctor or pharmacist before taking this drug.

PREGNANCY/BREAST-FEEDING: Category C—Risk cannot be ruled out. Human studies are lacking, and animal studies are either positive for fetal risk or lacking as well. However, potential benefits may justify the potential risk in using the drug. The drug is excreted in the breast milk; therefore, extreme caution should be used when breast-feeding.

OTHER BRAND NAMES: None

OTHER DRUGS IN THE SAME THERAPEUTIC CLASS: aminophylline, Choledyl, Elixophyllin, Lufyllin, Respbid, Quibron-SR, Quibron-T, Slo-bid, Slo-Phyllin, Theo-24, Theo-X, Uni-Dur, and Uniphyl

IMPORTANT INFORMATION TO REMEMBER: Only take the drug exactly as directed by your physician. Do not discontinue taking the drug without first consulting your physician. Do not increase the dose without first consulting with your physician. This drug should be taken with plenty of water (eight ounces is preferred). If using the capsules, swallow them whole. The contents of the capsules may, however, be sprinkled on soft food (such as applesauce) and swallowed without chewing. If using the tablets, do not crush them; they may, however, be cut in half for easier swallowing. If stomach upset occurs, take with food or milk. Do not change between brand and generic once you are stabilized on one or the other.

BRAND NAME: Theo-X

GENERIC NAME: theophylline

Very similar to Theo-Dur. See entry for Theo-Dur.

BRAND NAME: Thorazine

GENERIC NAME: chlorpromazine

GENERIC FORM AVAILABLE: Yes (tablets only)

THERAPEUTIC CLASS: Phenothiazine antipsychotic

DOSAGE FORMS: 10-mg, 25-mg, 50-mg, 100-mg, and 200-mg tablets; 30-mg, 75-mg, and 150-mg sustained-release capsules; 10 mg/5mL syrup; and 25-mg and 100-mg suppositories

MAIN USES: Psychotic disorders, nausea, and {hiccups}

USUAL DOSE: 10 mg to 200 mg two to four times daily

AVERAGE PRICE: $56.71 (B)/$21.96 (G) for 10-mg tablets; $70.27 (B)/$25.66 (G) for 25-mg tablets; $85.12 (B)/$31.29 (G) for 50-mg tablets; $105.50 (B)/$39.17 (G) for 100-mg tablets; $182.95 (B)/$46.88 (G) for 200-mg tablets; $145.32 for 30-mg capsules; $195.30 for 75-mg capsules; $263.20 for 150-mg capsules; $55.95 for 25-mg suppositories (box of 12); and $70.50 for 100-mg suppositories (box of 12)

SIDE EFFECTS: Most common: drowsiness, restlessness, blurred vision, Parkinson's-like symptoms, low blood pressure, stuffy nose, dry mouth, constipation, and dizziness. Less common: increased sensitivity to sunburn, difficulty in urinating, nausea, vomiting, stomach pain, and trembling of fingers and hands, stomach pain, changes in menstrual period, decreased sexual ability, swelling and/or pain in the breasts, weight gain, and secretion of milk from the breasts.

DRUG INTERACTIONS: Drugs used to treat depression and Thorazine may increase the severity and frequency of side effects. Alcohol, anxiety medications, and narcotic painkillers may intensify the drowsiness effect of the drug. Eskalith and Lithobid may decrease the absorption of the drug. Eskalith or Lithobid and the drug may cause disorientation and one to black out. The drug may decrease the effects of Larodopa. Inderal may increase the blood levels of the drug.

ALLERGIES: Individuals allergic to chlorpromazine or any of its derivatives should discuss this with their doctor or pharmacist before using this drug.

PREGNANCY/BREAST-FEEDING: Category C—Risk cannot be ruled out. Human studies are lacking, and animal studies are either positive for fetal risk or lacking as well. However, potential benefits may justify the potential risk in using the drug. The drug is excreted in the breast milk; therefore, extreme caution should be used when breast-feeding.

OTHER BRAND NAMES: None

OTHER DRUGS IN THE SAME THERAPEUTIC CLASS: Compazine, Mellaril, Prolixin, Serentil, Stelazine, and Trilafon

IMPORTANT INFORMATION TO REMEMBER: This drug does cause drowsiness. Individuals should use caution when driving, operating machinery, or performing any task where mental alertness is required. Alcohol, anxiety medications, and narcotic painkillers

may intensify the drowsiness effect of the drug. Do not increase the dose or stop taking the drug without first consulting with your physician. Individuals should report any involuntary movements of the tongue, arms, or legs to your physician. This drug may also increase the sensitivity of the skin to sunburn in some individuals; therefore, a sunscreen is recommended during periods of prolonged exposure to the sun. Caution should be used during hot weather due to decreased tolerance to the heat.

BRAND NAME: Ticlid

GENERIC NAME: ticlopidine

GENERIC FORM AVAILABLE: No

THERAPEUTIC CLASS: Antiplatelet

DOSAGE FORMS: 250-mg tablets

MAIN USES: Prevention of stroke

USUAL DOSE: 250 mg twice daily with food

AVERAGE PRICE: $208.79

SIDE EFFECTS: diarrhea 13%, nausea 7%, rash 5%, stomach pain 4%, blood disorders 3%, blood vessel breaking that causes purple patches on the skin 2%, vomiting 2%, gas 2%, nosebleeds 2%, itching 1%, dizziness 1%, appetite changes 1%, and abnormal liver tests 1%.

DRUG INTERACTIONS: Coumadin and aspirin may increase the risk of bleeding disorders. Antacids and Tagamet may decrease the blood levels of the drug. The drug may increase the blood levels of Slo-bid, Theo-Dur, theophylline, Uni-Dur, and Uniphyl.

ALLERGIES: Individuals allergic to ticlopidine or any of its derivatives should discuss this with their doctor or pharmacist before using this drug.

PREGNANCY/BREAST-FEEDING: Category B—No evidence of risk in humans. Either animal findings show risk, but human findings do not; or, if no adequate human studies have been done, animal findings show no risk. It is not known whether the drug is excreted in the breast milk; therefore, caution should be used when breast-feeding.

OTHER BRAND NAMES: None

OTHER DRUGS IN THE SAME THERAPEUTIC CLASS: Persantine

IMPORTANT INFORMATION TO REMEMBER: The drug should be taken with food or milk to increase its absorption and decrease the potential for stomach upset. The drug should be taken only as directed by your physician. Individuals should have regular blood tests to detect potential adverse effects while taking the drug. The drug should be stopped 10–14 days before any surgical procedure, including dental surgery. Individuals should notify their physician immediately if any signs of abnormal bleeding or severe bruising are seen.

BRAND NAME: Tigan

GENERIC NAME: trimethobenzamide

GENERIC FORM AVAILABLE: Yes (250-mg capsules and 100-mg and 200-mg suppositories only)

THERAPEUTIC CLASS: Antiemetic

DOSAGE FORMS: 100-mg and 250-mg capsules; and 100-mg and 200-mg suppositories

MAIN USES: Nausea and vomiting

USUAL DOSE: For the capsules: 100 mg to 250 mg three to four times daily. For the suppositories: 100 mg to 200 mg three to four times daily.

AVERAGE PRICE: $64.05 for 100-mg capsules; $72.16 (B)/$54.25 (G) for 250-mg capsules; $35.79 (B)/$16.70 (G) for 100-mg suppositories (box of 10); $43.96 (B)/$23.41 (G) for 200-mg suppositories (box of 10)

SIDE EFFECTS: Most common: drowsiness. Less common: blurred vision, dizziness, diarrhea, headache, and muscle cramps.

DRUG INTERACTIONS: Alcohol, anxiety medications, and narcotic painkillers may intensify the drowsiness effect of the drug.

ALLERGIES: Individuals allergic to trimethobenzamide or any of its derivatives should discuss this with their doctor or pharmacist before using this drug.

PREGNANCY/BREAST-FEEDING: Category C—Risk cannot be ruled out. Human studies are lacking, and animal studies are either positive for fetal risk or lacking as well. However, potential benefits

may justify the potential risk in using the drug. It is not known whether the drug is excreted in the breast milk; therefore, caution should be used when breast-feeding.

OTHER BRAND NAMES: None

OTHER DRUGS IN THE SAME THERAPEUTIC CLASS: None

IMPORTANT INFORMATION TO REMEMBER: This drug does cause drowsiness. Individuals should use caution when driving, operating machinery, or performing any task where mental alertness is required. Alcohol, anxiety medications, and narcotic painkillers may intensify the drowsiness effect of the drug. Do not increase the dose without first consulting with your physician.

For the suppository:

Store in a cool place to avoid melting, preferably the refrigerator. Remove the foil wrapper before inserting the suppository. When inserting, lie on one side and bend the top leg slightly. Then insert suppository into rectum about one inch with one finger. Wash hands thoroughly before and after use. Individuals may want to use a finger cot to cover finger when inserting a suppository.

BRAND NAME: Tilade

GENERIC NAME: nedocromil

GENERIC FORM AVAILABLE: No

THERAPEUTIC CLASS: Anti-inflammatory inhaler

DOSAGE FORMS: 1.75-mg-per-spray metered-dose inhaler

MAIN USES: Asthma

USUAL DOSE: two inhalations four times daily at regular intervals

AVERAGE PRICE: $37.80 per inhaler

SIDE EFFECTS: unpleasant taste 13%, cough 7%, pharyngitis 6%, headache 6%, runny nose 5%, nausea 4%, chest pain 4%, upper respiratory tract infections 4%, trouble breathing 3%, increased sputum 2%, vomiting 2%, tiredness 1%, bronchitis 1%, diarrhea 1%, and dry mouth 1%.

DRUG INTERACTIONS: None of any clinical significance

ALLERGIES: Individuals allergic to nedocromil or any of its derivatives should discuss this with their doctor or pharmacist before using this drug.

PREGNANCY/BREAST-FEEDING: Category B—No evidence of risk in humans. Either animal findings show risk, but human findings do not; or, if no adequate human studies have been done, animal findings show no risk. It is not known whether the drug is excreted in the breast milk; therefore, caution should be used when breast-feeding.

OTHER BRAND NAMES: None

OTHER DRUGS IN THE SAME THERAPEUTIC CLASS: None

IMPORTANT INFORMATION TO REMEMBER: The drug is not intended to provide immediately relief of a bronchospasm, shortness of breath, or an asthma attack; it is used only for prevention of attacks. To receive the full benefits of the drug, use it on a regular basis as a maintenance medication. The drug may take two to four weeks before noticeable benefits may be seen. Never exceed the prescribed dosage unless directed to do so by a doctor—excessive use beyond the prescribed dosage is potentially dangerous. If another inhaler is also being used at the same time, use the other one a few minutes prior to using Tilade.

When using the inhaler, use the following procedure:

1) Shake the canister well.
2) Place the mouthpiece close to the mouth, but not touching the lips.
3) Exhale deeply.
4) Inhale slowly and deeply as you press the top of the canister to release the medication.
5) Hold your breath for a few seconds before exhaling.
6) Wait five minutes between puffs.
7) Be sure to wash the inhaler device (mouthpiece) regularly with warm soapy water to avoid bacterial contamination.

BRAND NAME: Timolide

GENERIC NAME: Combination product containing timolol and hydrochlorothiazide

See individual entries for Blocadren and HydroDIURIL

BRAND NAME: Timoptic and Timoptic-XE

GENERIC NAME: timolol

GENERIC FORM AVAILABLE: No

THERAPEUTIC CLASS: Noncardioselective beta-blocker

DOSAGE FORMS: 0.25% and 0.5% eyedrop solution (Timoptic); and 0.25% and 0.5% eye gel (Timoptic-XE)

MAIN USES: Glaucoma

USUAL DOSE: For Timoptic: one drop twice daily. For Timoptic-XE: one drop once daily.

AVERAGE PRICE: $42.11 for Timoptic 0.25% (10 mL); $50.02 for Timoptic 0.5% (10 mL); $31.65 for Timoptic-XE 0.25% (5 mL); and $37.61 for Timoptic-XE 0.5% (5 mL)

SIDE EFFECTS: Most common: stinging of the eye and irritation. Less common: browache (headache above the eye), increased sensitivity of the eyes to light, redness, itching, watering of the eye, rash on the eyelid, blurred vision, and changes in vision.

DRUG INTERACTIONS: The drug may cause widening of the pupil when used with Epifrin. The drug may cause additive effects when used with Blocadren, Cartrol, Corgard, Inderal, Kerlone, Levatol, Lopressor, Normodyne, reserpine, Sectral, Tenormin, Toprol-XL, Trandate, Visken, and Zebeta.

ALLERGIES: Individuals allergic to timolol or any of its derivatives should discuss this with their doctor or pharmacist before using this drug.

PREGNANCY/BREAST-FEEDING: Category C—Risk cannot be ruled out. Human studies are lacking, and animal studies are either positive for fetal risk or lacking as well. However, potential benefits may justify the potential risk in using the drug. It is not known whether the drug is excreted in the breast milk; therefore, caution should be used when breast-feeding.

OTHER BRAND NAMES: None

OTHER DRUGS IN THE SAME THERAPEUTIC CLASS: Betagan, Betimol, Ocupress, OptiPranolol

IMPORTANT INFORMATION TO REMEMBER: Keep the container tightly closed and avoid touching the applicator tip to the eye—this could contaminate the product over time. Also, only administer one drop at a time. After application, keep the eye open for at least 30 seconds, roll the eyeball around, and avoid squinting. If a second drop is required, wait one to two minutes between drops. If another medication is to be used in the eye, wait at least 10 minutes before administering it. Use the drug only exactly as directed by your physician. Do not discontinue the drug without first consulting your physician.

BRAND NAME: TobraDex and Tobrex

GENERIC NAME: tobramycin (Tobrex) and tobramycin + dexamethasone (TobraDex)

GENERIC FORM AVAILABLE: Yes (Tobrex only)

THERAPEUTIC CLASS: Antibiotic eyedrop (Tobrex) and antibiotic + steroid eyedrop (TobraDex)

DOSAGE FORMS: For TobraDex: 0.3% tobramycin/0.1% dexamethasone eyedrop suspension and eye ointment. For Tobrex: 0.3% tobramycin eyedrop solution and eye ointment

MAIN USES: Bacterial infections of the eye

USUAL DOSE: For the drops: one to two drops every four to six hours. For the ointment: apply a thin ribbon two to four times daily.

AVERAGE PRICE: $27.57 (B)/$19.78 (G) for Tobrex (5 mL) and $31.23 for TobraDex (5 mL)

SIDE EFFECTS: Most common: temporary, mild blurred vision. Less common: burning, itching, redness, watering of the eyes, and eye pain.

DRUG INTERACTIONS: The drug may decrease the effects of other eyedrops used to treat glaucoma.

ALLERGIES: Individuals allergic to tobramycin, dexamethazone, or any of their derivatives should discuss this with their doctor or pharmacist before using this drug.

PREGNANCY/BREAST-FEEDING: For TobraDex: Category C—Risk cannot be ruled out. Human studies are lacking, and animal studies are either positive for fetal risk or lacking as well. However, potential benefits may justify the potential risk in using the drug. It is not known whether the drug is excreted in the breast milk; therefore, caution should be used when breast-feeding. For Tobrex: Category B—No evidence of risk in humans. Either animal findings show risk, but human findings do not; or, if no adequate human studies have been done, animal findings show no risk. It is not known whether the drug is excreted in the breast milk; therefore, caution should be used when breast-feeding.

OTHER BRAND NAMES: None

OTHER DRUGS IN THE SAME THERAPEUTIC CLASS: For TobraDex: Cortisporin, FML-S, Isopto Cetapred, Maxitrol, Metimyd, Neo-decadron, Poly-Pred, and Vasocidin. For Tobrex: Garamycin.

IMPORTANT INFORMATION TO REMEMBER: Shake the bottle thoroughly before using the eyedrops (TobraDex only). Individuals should not use the drug while wearing contact lenses unless directed otherwise by a doctor. Keep the container tightly closed and avoid touching the applicator tip to the eye—this could contaminate the product over time. Also, only administer one drop at a time. After application, keep the eye open for at least 30 seconds, roll the eyeball around, and avoid squinting. If a second drop is required, wait one to two minutes between drops. If another medication is to be used in the eye, wait at least 10 minutes before administering it. If using the eye ointment, insert a small ribbon of the ointment inside the lower eyelid. Then close the eye and roll the eyeball around in all directions. Do not touch the tip of the ointment tube to the eye if possible. When using the eye ointment, your vision may become temporarily blurred after use. Use the drug for the full duration of treatment; otherwise the infection may return.

BRAND NAME: Tofranil and Tofranil-PM

GENERIC NAME: imipramine

GENERIC FORM AVAILABLE: Yes (Tofranil tablets only)

THERAPEUTIC CLASS: Tricyclic antidepressant

DOSAGE FORMS: 10-mg, 25-mg, and 50-mg tablets (Tofranil); and 75-mg, 100-mg, 125-mg, and 150-mg long-acting capsules (Tofranil-PM)

MAIN USES: Depression and bedwetting

USUAL DOSE: For depression: 75 mg to 150 mg daily in divided doses (fewer doses per day may be needed for the capsules). For bedwetting: 25 mg to 75 mg at bedtime.

AVERAGE PRICE: $40.90 (B)/$10.96 (G) for 10 mg; $65.96 (B)/$13.16 (G) for 25 mg; $86.58 (B)/$14.88 (G) for 50 mg; $150.22 for 75 mg (Tofranil-PM); $197.48 for 100 mg (Tofranil-PM); $246.26 for 125 mg (Tofranil-PM); $280.71 for 150 mg (Tofranil-PM)

SIDE EFFECTS: Most common: drowsiness, dizziness, dry mouth, headache, increased appetite, nausea, tiredness, weight gain, and unpleasant taste. Less common: diarrhea, excessive sweating, heartburn, insomnia, vomiting, increased sensitivity to sunburn, irregular heartbeat, muscle tremors, urinary difficulties, and impotence.

DRUG INTERACTIONS: The drug should not be taken with Nardil or Parnate. In fact, 14 days are needed between the time of the use of Nardil or Parnate and this drug. Alcohol, anxiety medications, and narcotic painkillers may make the drowsiness caused by the drug much worse. Compazine, Mellaril, Prolixin, Serentil, Stelazine, Thorazine, and Trilafon may increase the blood levels of the drug. Tagamet may increase the blood levels of the drug. The drug may decrease the effects of Catapres and Ismelin. The drug may increase the effects of decongestants found in cough, cold, and allergy products on the heart, possibly causing high blood pressure, fast heartbeat, or irregular heartbeats.

ALLERGIES: Individuals allergic to imipramine or other tricylic antidepressants (such as those listed under "Other Drugs in the Same Therapeutic Class") should discuss this with their doctor or pharmacist before taking this drug.

PREGNANCY/BREAST-FEEDING: Category D—Positive evidence of risk. Human studies show risk to the fetus. Nevertheless, potential benefits may possibly outweigh the potential risks. This drug should not be taken by nursing mothers.

OTHER BRAND NAMES: None

OTHER DRUGS IN THE SAME THERAPEUTIC CLASS: Asendin, Elavil, Endep, Norpramin, Pamelor, Surmontil, Tofranil, and Vivactil

IMPORTANT INFORMATION TO REMEMBER: Only take the drug exactly as directed by your physician. Do not discontinue taking the drug without first consulting your physician. The drug may require one to six weeks of use before improvement may be noticed. This drug does cause drowsiness. Individuals should use caution when driving, operating machinery, or performing any task where mental alertness is required. Alcohol, anxiety medications, and narcotic painkillers may intensify the drowsiness effect of the drug. The drug may cause a slight amount of dizziness or lightheadedness when rising from a sitting or lying-down position. Individuals should also use a sunscreen to avoid overexposure to the sun; the drug may increase the skin's sensitivity to sunlight, which may cause one to sunburn more easily.

BRAND NAME: Tolectin 200, Tolectin DS, and Tolectin 600

GENERIC NAME: tolmetin

GENERIC FORM AVAILABLE: Yes

THERAPEUTIC CLASS: Nonsteroidal anti-inflammatory drug (NSAID)

DOSAGE FORMS: 200-mg tablets, 400-mg capsules, and 600-mg tablets

MAIN USES: Arthritis and pain relief

USUAL DOSE: 200 mg to 600 mg three times daily

AVERAGE PRICE: $74.89 (B)/$44.62 (G) for 200 mg; $118.61 (B)/$64.11 (G) for 400 mg; $143.64 (B)/$83.36 (G) for 600 mg

SIDE EFFECTS: nausea 11%, stomach distress 3%–9%, stomach pain 3%–9%, diarrhea 3%–9%, gas 3%–9%, vomiting 3%–9%, headache 3%–9%, muscle weakness 3%–9%, dizziness 3%–9%, swelling 3%–9%, increased blood pressure 3%–9%, weight changes 3%–9%, constipation 1%–3%, peptic ulcer 1%–3%, chest pain 1%–3%, drowsiness 1%–3%, depression 1%–3%, ringing in the ears 1%–3%, and vision disturbances 1%–3%.

DRUG INTERACTIONS: Aspirin will decrease the concentration of this drug in the blood. This drug may also decrease the effects of Dyazide, HydroDIURIL, Lasix, Maxzide, and other water pills. The drug may increase the blood levels of Eskalith, Lithobid, and Sandimmune. The drug may increase the toxic effects of the drug Rheumatrex. Caution should be used when taking the drug with Coumadin.

ALLERGIES: Individuals allergic to tolmetin or other NSAIDs (such as those listed under "Other Drugs in the Same Therapeutic Class") should discuss this with their doctor or pharmacist before taking this drug.

PREGNANCY/BREAST-FEEDING: Category C—Risk cannot be ruled out. Human studies are lacking, and animal studies are either positive for fetal risk or lacking as well. However, potential benefits may justify the potential risk in using the drug. The drug should not, however, be used during the late stages (last three months) of pregnancy. The drug is excreted in the breast milk; therefore, extreme caution should be used when breast-feeding.

OTHER BRAND NAMES: None

OTHER DRUGS IN THE SAME THERAPEUTIC CLASS: Anaprox, Ansaid, aspirin, Cataflam, Clinoril, Daypro, Disalcid, Dolobid, Easprin, Feldene, Indocin, Lodine, Lodine XL, Motrin, Nalfon, Naprosyn, Orudis, Oruvail, Relafen, Toradol, Voltaren, and Voltaren XR

IMPORTANT INFORMATION TO REMEMBER: This drug should be taken with food or milk to reduce the potential for injury to the stomach lining and stomach upset. This drug may take up to two weeks before a noticeable improvement in pain relief associated with arthritis is observed. Drinking alcohol while taking this drug may increase its potential to cause ulcers. This drug should only be used under the direct supervision of a doctor by individuals with a bleeding disorder or ulcer, or those who are currently taking Coumadin. Before taking over-the-counter pain relievers, consult your doctor or pharmacist. No more than one pain reliever should be taken at any one time unless otherwise directed by your doctor.

BRAND NAME: Tolinase

GENERIC NAME: tolazamide

GENERIC FORM AVAILABLE: Yes

THERAPEUTIC CLASS: First-generation sulfonylurea anti-diabetic

DOSAGE FORMS: 100-mg, 250-mg, and 500-mg tablets

MAIN USES: Diabetes

USUAL DOSE: 100 mg to 1000 mg daily

AVERAGE PRICE: $32.98 (B)/$13.45 (G) for 100 mg; $68.40 (B)/$16.92 (G) for 250 mg; $132.92 (B)/$27.04 (G) for 500 mg

SIDE EFFECTS: Most common: constipation, diarrhea, dizziness, mild drowsiness, headache, heartburn, changes in appetite, nausea, vomiting, stomach pain, fullness, and stomach discomfort. Less common: hives, increased sensitivity to sunburn, skin redness, itching, and rash.

DRUG INTERACTIONS: Alcohol may cause a severe stomach reaction (vomiting, pain, diarrhea, etc.) when used with this drug. The blood levels of Coumadin and the drug, when combined, may initially increase, followed by a decrease in blood levels of both. Blocadren, Cartrol, Corgard, Inderal, Kerlone, Levatol, Lopressor, Normodyne, Sectral, Tenormin, Toprol-XL, Trandate, Visken, Zebeta, chloramphenicol, Esimil, Ismelin, Nardil, Parnate, high doses of aspirin, Bactrim, Gantanol, Gantrisin, and Septra may cause low blood sugar when used with this drug.

ALLERGIES: Individuals allergic to tolazamide, sulfa drugs, or any of their derivatives should discuss this with their doctor or pharmacist before using this drug.

PREGNANCY/BREAST-FEEDING: Category C—Risk cannot be ruled out. Human studies are lacking, and animal studies are either positive for fetal risk or lacking as well. However, potential benefits may justify the potential risk in using the drug. It is not known whether the drug is excreted in the breast milk; therefore, caution should be used when breast-feeding.

OTHER BRAND NAMES: None

OTHER DRUGS IN THE SAME THERAPEUTIC CLASS: Diabinese and Orinase

IMPORTANT INFORMATION TO REMEMBER: If stomach upset occurs, take the drug with food or milk. To receive optimum effect, regular compliance with therapy is essential; this includes compliance with a prescribed diet. Avoid alcohol while taking this drug—alcohol may cause severe stomach reactions (vomiting, pain, diarrhea, etc.). This drug lowers blood sugar. Individuals should be aware of the signs and symptoms of blood sugar that is too low: sweating, tremor, blurred vision, weakness, hunger, and confusion. If two or more of these symptoms are seen, treat with oral glucose (sugar) and/or contact your doctor. This drug may increase the risk of cardiovascular disease. Before taking over-the-counter cold and allergy preparations, consult your doctor or pharmacist—these products may affect your blood sugar.

BRAND NAME: **Tonocard**

GENERIC NAME: tocainide

GENERIC FORM AVAILABLE: No

THERAPEUTIC CLASS: Class I antiarrhythmic

DOSAGE FORMS: 400-mg and 600-mg tablets

MAIN USES: Irregular heartbeat

USUAL DOSE: 400 mg every eight hours

AVERAGE PRICE: $112.59 for 400 mg and $143.50 for 600 mg

SIDE EFFECTS: nausea 15%, vomiting 8%, dizziness 8%, increased sweating 5%, numbness 4%, tremor 3%, low blood pressure 3%, slow heartbeat 2%, pounding heartbeat 2%, chest pain 2%, heart conduction disorders 2%, nervousness 2%, altered mood 2%, blurred vision 1%, unsteadiness 1%, and appetite changes 1%.

DRUG INTERACTIONS: Caution should be used by patients taking other drugs specifically used for irregular heartbeat.

ALLERGIES: Individuals allergic to tocainide or any of its derivatives should discuss this with their doctor or pharmacist before using this drug.

PREGNANCY/BREAST-FEEDING: Category C—Risk cannot be ruled out. Human studies are lacking, and animal studies are either positive for fetal risk or lacking as well. However, potential benefits may justify the potential risk in using the drug. It is not known whether the drug is excreted in the breast milk; therefore, caution should be used when breast-feeding.

OTHER BRAND NAMES: None

OTHER DRUGS IN THE SAME THERAPEUTIC CLASS: Cardioquin, Norpace, Norpace CR, Quinaglute, and Quinidex

IMPORTANT INFORMATION TO REMEMBER: This drug may cause some dizziness or tiredness, especially at first. Individuals should use caution when driving, operating machinery, or performing any task where mental alertness is required. Alcohol, anxiety medications, and narcotic painkillers may intensify these effects. Only take the drug exactly as directed by your physician. Do not discontinue taking the drug without first consulting your physician; also, do not increase the dose without first consulting with your physician. If stomach upset occurs, take the drug with food or milk.

BRAND NAME: Topicort

GENERIC NAME: desoximetasone

GENERIC FORM AVAILABLE: Yes

THERAPEUTIC CLASS: Topical corticosteroid

DOSAGE FORMS: 0.25% cream and ointment; 0.05% gel and LP cream

MAIN USES: Skin rashes, swelling, and itching

USUAL DOSE: Apply to the affected area as a thin film two times daily.

AVERAGE PRICE: $25.51 (B)/$14.81 (G) for 0.25% cream, LP cream, and ointment; and 0.05% gel (15 g)

SIDE EFFECTS: Most common: none. Less common: burning, itching, irritation, dry skin, rash, and soreness of the skin.

DRUG INTERACTIONS: None of any clinical significance

ALLERGIES: Individuals allergic to desoximetasone or any of its derivatives should discuss this with their doctor or pharmacist before using this drug.

PREGNANCY/BREAST-FEEDING: Category C—Risk cannot be ruled out. Human studies are lacking, and animal studies are either positive for fetal risk or lacking as well. However, potential benefits may justify the potential risk in using the drug. It is not known whether the drug is excreted in the breast milk; therefore, caution should be used when breast-feeding.

OTHER BRAND NAMES: None

OTHER DRUGS IN THE SAME THERAPEUTIC CLASS: Aclovate, Aristocort, Cordran, Cordran SP, Cutivate, Cyclocort, DesOwen, Diprolene, Diprolene AF, Elocon, Florone, Florone E, Halog, Hytone, Kenalog, Lidex, Synalar, Temovate, Tridesilon, Ultravate, Valisone, and Westcort

IMPORTANT INFORMATION TO REMEMBER: This drug is for external use only. Apply only a thin film of drug to skin and rub it in well. Never cover the skin after application with a bandage or wrapping unless directed to do so by a doctor. Never apply to damaged skin or open wounds unless directed to do so by a doctor. Discontinue use if irritation occurs.

BRAND NAME: Toprol-XL

GENERIC NAME: metoprolol

Very similar to Lopressor. See entry for Lopressor.

BRAND NAME: Toradol

GENERIC NAME: ketorolac

GENERIC FORM AVAILABLE: No

THERAPEUTIC CLASS: Nonsteroidal anti-inflammatory drug (NSAID)

DOSAGE FORMS: 10-mg tablets

MAIN USES: Short-term (five days or less) use for moderate to severe pain

USUAL DOSE: one tablet every four to six hours as needed, for no more than five days

AVERAGE PRICE: $52.46 for 30 tablets

SIDE EFFECTS: headache 17%, stomach pain 13%, nausea 12%, drowsiness 3%–9%, dizziness 3%–9%, swelling 3%–9%, itching 3%–9%, diarrhea 3%–9%, high blood pressure 1%–3%, rash 1%–3%, constipation 1%–3%, gas 1%–3%, sweating 1%–3%, vomiting 1%–3%, and bloated feeling 1%–3%.

DRUG INTERACTIONS: Aspirin will decrease the concentration of this drug in the blood. This drug may also decrease the effects of Dyazide, HydroDIURIL, Lasix, Maxzide, and other water pills. The drug may increase the blood levels of Eskalith, Lithobid, and Sandimmune. The drug may increase the toxic effects of the drug Rheumatrex. Caution should be used when taking the drug with Coumadin.

ALLERGIES: Individuals allergic to ketorolac or other NSAIDs (such as those listed under "Other Drugs in the Same Therapeutic

Class") should discuss this with their doctor or pharmacist before taking this drug.

PREGNANCY/BREAST-FEEDING: Category C—Risk cannot be ruled out. Human studies are lacking, and animal studies are either positive for fetal risk or lacking as well. However, potential benefits may justify the potential risk in using the drug. The drug is excreted in the breast milk; therefore, extreme caution should be used when breast-feeding.

OTHER BRAND NAMES: None

OTHER DRUGS IN THE SAME THERAPEUTIC CLASS: Anaprox, Ansaid, aspirin, Cataflam, Clinoril, Daypro, Disalcid, Dolobid, Easprin, Feldene, Indocin, Lodine, Lodine XL, Motrin, Nalfon, Naprosyn, Orudis, Oruvail, Relafen, Tolectin, Voltaren, and Voltaren XR

IMPORTANT INFORMATION TO REMEMBER: This drug should be taken with food or milk to reduce the potential for injury to the stomach lining and stomach upset. Drinking alcohol while taking this drug may increase its potential to cause ulcers. This drug should only be used under the direct supervision of a doctor by individuals with a bleeding disorder or ulcer, or those who are currently taking Coumadin. Before taking over-the-counter pain relievers, consult your doctor or pharmacist. This drug should not be used for more than five days. This drug may cause drowsiness. Individuals should use caution when driving, operating machinery, or performing any task where mental alertness is required. Alcohol, anxiety medications, and other narcotic painkillers may intensify the drowsiness effect of the drug.

BRAND NAME: Torecan

GENERIC NAME: thiethylperazine

GENERIC FORM AVAILABLE: No

THERAPEUTIC CLASS: Antinausea

DOSAGE FORMS: 10-mg tablets

MAIN USES: Nausea and vomiting

USUAL DOSE: one tablet one to three times daily as needed

AVERAGE PRICE: $76.02

SIDE EFFECTS: Most common: drowsiness and dizziness. Less common: blood disorders, cholestatic jaundice, confusion, swelling, muscle spasms, muscle twitching, Parkinson's-like effects, vision problems, constipation, dry mouth, decreased sweating, fever, headache, faint feeling, nervousness, restlessness, and ringing in the ears.

DRUG INTERACTIONS: Alcohol, anxiety medications, and narcotic painkillers may intensify the drowsiness effect of the drug. The drug may decrease the effects of Larodopa. The drug may increase the cardiac effects of Quinaglute and Quinidex.

ALLERGIES: Individuals allergic to thiethylperazine or any of its derivatives should discuss this with their doctor or pharmacist before using this drug.

PREGNANCY/BREAST-FEEDING: Category X—Should not be used during pregnancy. Studies in animals and/or humans have shown fetal abnormalities and birth defects. The risks associated with using this drug clearly outweigh the benefits. This drug should never be used by someone who is pregnant or trying to become pregnant. Also, women should never breast-feed while using this drug.

OTHER BRAND NAMES: None

OTHER DRUGS IN THE SAME THERAPEUTIC CLASS: Phenergan

IMPORTANT INFORMATION TO REMEMBER: This drug does cause drowsiness and/or blurred vision. Individuals should use caution when driving, operating machinery, or performing any task where mental alertness is required. Alcohol, anxiety medications, and narcotic painkillers may intensify these effects of the drug. Do not increase the dose without first consulting with your physician. Individuals should get up slowly from a sitting or lying-down position; otherwise dizziness may occur.

BRAND NAME: Tornalate

GENERIC NAME: bitolterol

GENERIC FORM AVAILABLE: No

THERAPEUTIC CLASS: Beta-2-agonist bronchodilator

DOSAGE FORMS: 0.37-mg-of-bitolterol-per-inhalation metered-dose inhaler and 0.2% inhalation solution

MAIN USES: Asthma and {other breathing disorders}

USUAL DOSE: two inhalations every eight hours

AVERAGE PRICE: $50.31 for inhaler and $19.94 for 0.2% solution (30 mL)

SIDE EFFECTS: tremors 14%, nervousness 5%, throat irritation 5%, coughing 4%, headache 4%, pounding heartbeat 3%, dizziness 3%, nausea 3%, lightheadedness 3%, insomnia 1%, and chest tightness 1%.

DRUG INTERACTIONS: Anafranil, Asendin, Elavil, Nardil, Norpramin, Pamelor, Parnate, Sinequan, Surmontil, Tofranil, and Vivactil, and cough, cold, and allergy medications with decongestants may increase the toxicity of this medication. Blocadren, Cartrol, Corgard, Inderal, Levatol, Normodyne, Trandate, and Visken may decrease the effectiveness of the drug.

ALLERGIES: Individuals allergic to bitolterol or any of its derivatives should discuss this with their doctor or pharmacist before using this drug.

PREGNANCY/BREAST-FEEDING: Category C—Risk cannot be ruled out. Human studies are lacking, and animal studies are either positive for fetal risk or lacking as well. However, potential benefits may justify the potential risk in using this drug. It is not known whether the drug is excreted in the breast milk; therefore, caution should be used when breast-feeding.

OTHER BRAND NAMES: None

OTHER DRUGS IN THE SAME THERAPEUTIC CLASS: Alupent, Brethaire, Bronkometer, Maxair, Metaprel, Proventil, Serevent, and Ventolin

IMPORTANT INFORMATION TO REMEMBER: Only take the drug exactly as directed by your physician. Never increase the dose of the drug without consulting with your physician. Prolonged use of the drug may cause tolerance to its effects to develop.

When using the inhaler, use the following procedure:

1) Shake the canister well.
2) Place the mouthpiece close to the mouth, but not touching the lips.
3) Exhale deeply.

4) Inhale slowly and deeply as you press the top of the canister to release the medication.
5) Hold your breath for a few seconds before exhaling.
6) Wait five minutes between puffs.
7) Be sure to wash the inhaler device (mouthpiece) regularly with warm soapy water to avoid bacterial contamination.

BRAND NAME: Trandate

GENERIC NAME: labetalol

See entry for Normodyne

BRAND NAME: Transderm-Nitro

GENERIC NAME: nitroglycerin

GENERIC FORM AVAILABLE: No

THERAPEUTIC CLASS: Anti-anginal patch

DOSAGE FORMS: 0.1 mg/hr, 0.2 mg/hr, 0.4 mg/hr, 0.6 mg/hr, and 0.8 mg/hr transdermal patch

MAIN USES: Prevention of angina

USUAL DOSE: Apply one patch every morning and remove after 12 hours. Other doses may be individualized according to the patient's needs.

AVERAGE PRICE: $64.82 for 0.1 mg/hr patch (30 patches); $66.34 for 0.2 mg/hr patch (30 patches); $75.82 for 0.4 mg/hr patch (30 patches); $83.56 for 0.6 mg/hr patch (30 patches); and $91.92 for 0.8 mg/hr patch (30 patches)

SIDE EFFECTS: headache 63%, lightheadedness 6%, low blood pressure 4%, dizziness 4%, increased angina 2%, and some minor skin irritation at the application site.

DRUG INTERACTIONS: Alcohol and the drug may produce low blood pressure. Apresoline, Loniten, Vasodilan, and the drug may also produce low blood pressure.

ALLERGIES: Individuals allergic to nitroglycerin or any of its derivatives should discuss this with their doctor or pharmacist before using this drug.

PREGNANCY/BREAST-FEEDING: Category C—Risk cannot be ruled out. Human studies are lacking, and animal studies are either positive for fetal risk or lacking as well. However, potential benefits may justify the potential risk in using the drug. It is not known whether the drug is excreted in the breast milk; therefore, caution should be used when breast-feeding.

OTHER BRAND NAMES: Deponit, Minitran, Nitrodisc, and Nitro-Dur

OTHER DRUGS IN THE SAME THERAPEUTIC CLASS: Deponit, Minitran, Nitrodisc, and Nitro-Dur

IMPORTANT INFORMATION TO REMEMBER: This drug will not relieve angina attacks; it only prevents them. Only use the drug exactly as directed by your physician. Do not discontinue taking the drug without first consulting your physician; also, do not increase the dose without first consulting with your physician. Do not drink alcohol while taking this drug. The headache that is common with this drug usually goes away with continued use; if it does not, contact your doctor. Before taking over-the-counter cold and allergy preparations, consult your doctor or pharmacist.

When using the patches:

1) Do not cut or fold the patch in half. This may cause the medication inside to leak out. Peel off the adhesive liner.
2) Apply the patch to a clean, dry skin area on the upper body or upper arm. This area should be free of hair, cuts, scars, or irritation. Avoid the waistline since tight clothes may rub or remove the patch. Also, do not apply the patch below the knee or elbow.
3) Leave the patch on even during swimming, showering, and exercising. If the patch falls off, replace the patch with a new one.
4) When it's time to apply a new patch, use a different site on the skin. Rotate the sites where you apply the patches every time.
5) Get into the habit of applying the patch at the same time each day.
6) Dispose of used patches properly and keep out of reach of children.

<u>BRAND NAME:</u> **Tranxene and Tranxene SD**

GENERIC NAME: clorazepate

GENERIC FORM AVAILABLE: Yes (Tranxene only)

THERAPEUTIC CLASS: Benzodiazepine antianxiety

DOSAGE FORMS: 3.75-mg, 7.5-mg, and 15-mg tablets; 11.25-mg and 22.5-mg sustained-release tablets (Tranxene SD)

MAIN USES: Anxiety

USUAL DOSE: 7.5 mg to 60 mg daily in divided doses

AVERAGE PRICE: $164.61 (B)/$52.15 (G) for 3.75 mg; $186.97 (B)/$60.02 (G) for 7.5 mg; $225.78 (B)/$70.01 (G) for 15 mg

SIDE EFFECTS: Most common: drowsiness, clumsiness, and dizziness. Less common: confusion, depression, stomach cramps, nausea, vomiting, dry mouth, changes in sex drive, sleep disturbances, and fast heartbeat.

DRUG INTERACTIONS: Central nervous system (CNS) depression may be increased when used with alcohol, narcotic painkillers, or other anxiety medications.

ALLERGIES: Individuals allergic to clorazepate or other benzodiazepines (such as those listed under "Other Drugs in the Same Therapeutic Class") should discuss this with their doctor or pharmacist before taking this drug.

PREGNANCY/BREAST-FEEDING: Category D—Positive evidence of risk. Human studies show risk to the fetus. Nevertheless, potential benefits may possibly outweigh the potential risks. This drug should not be taken by nursing mothers.

OTHER BRAND NAMES: None

OTHER DRUGS IN THE SAME THERAPEUTIC CLASS: Ativan, Librium, Serax, Valium, and Xanax

IMPORTANT INFORMATION TO REMEMBER: This drug may cause drowsiness. Individuals should use caution when driving, operating machinery, or performing any task where mental alertness is required. The incidence of drowsiness and unsteadiness increases with age. Alcohol, anxiety medications, or narcotic painkillers may intensify the drowsiness effect of the drug. This medication is a controlled substance and may be habit-forming. Do not increase the dose of medication without consulting with your doctor; take only the amount prescribed by your doctor.

BRAND NAME: Trental

GENERIC NAME: pentoxifylline

GENERIC FORM AVAILABLE: No

THERAPEUTIC CLASS: Circulatory agent

DOSAGE FORMS: 400-mg sustained-release tablets

MAIN USES: Intermittent claudication and poor circulation

USUAL DOSE: 400 mg three times daily with food

AVERAGE PRICE: $81.80

SIDE EFFECTS: nausea 3%, dizziness 2%, vomiting 1%, headache 1%, belching 1%, gas 1%, bloating 1%, chest pain 1%, and tremor 1%.

DRUG INTERACTIONS: Individuals taking Coumadin should have their prothrombin times monitored closely.

ALLERGIES: Individuals allergic to pentoxifylline or any of its derivatives should discuss this with their doctor or pharmacist before using this drug.

PREGNANCY/BREAST-FEEDING: Category C—Risk cannot be ruled out. Human studies are lacking, and animal studies are either positive for fetal risk or lacking as well. However, potential benefits may justify the potential risk in using the drug. The drug is excreted in the breast milk; therefore, extreme caution should be used when breast-feeding.

OTHER BRAND NAMES: None

OTHER DRUGS IN THE SAME THERAPEUTIC CLASS: None

IMPORTANT INFORMATION TO REMEMBER: This drug should be taken with food or milk to reduce the potential for injury to the stomach lining and stomach upset. Do not crush, cut, or chew the tablets—this will destroy the mechanism that causes the delayed release of the medication. Take the drug exactly as directed and do not discontinue taking the drug unless directed to do so by your physician.

BRAND NAME: Triavil

GENERIC NAME: Combination product containing: perphenazine and amitriptyline

GENERIC FORM AVAILABLE: Yes

THERAPEUTIC CLASS: Tricyclic antidepressant + antipsychotic

DOSAGE FORMS: 2-mg perphenazine/10-mg amitriptyline; 2-mg perphenazine/25-mg amitriptyline; 4-mg perphenazine/10-mg amitriptyline; 4-mg perphenazine/25-mg amitriptyline; and 4-mg perphenazine/50-mg amitriptyline tablets

MAIN USES: Anxiety (nerves) with depression

USUAL DOSE: one tablet two to four times daily

AVERAGE PRICE: $100.01 (B)/$30.25 (G) for 2 mg perphenazine/10 mg amitriptyline; $127.83 (B)/$39.84 (G) for 2 mg perphenazine/10 mg amitriptyline; $102.25 (B)/$31.05 (G) for 4 mg perphenazine/25 mg amitriptyline; and $154.68 (B)/$46.65 (G) for 4 mg perphenazine/50 mg amitriptyline

SIDE EFFECTS: Most common: drowsiness; dizziness; dry mouth; headache; increased appetite; restlessness; blurred vision; muscle spasms of the face, neck, and back; muscle twitching; fainting; nausea; tiredness; weight gain; and unpleasant taste. Less common: diarrhea, excessive sweating, heartburn, insomnia, vomiting, irregular heartbeat, muscle tremors, urinary difficulties, and impotence.

DRUG INTERACTIONS: The drug should not be taken with Nardil or Parnate. In fact, 14 days are needed between the time of the use of Nardil or Parnate and this drug. Alcohol, anxiety medications, and narcotic painkillers may make the drowsiness caused by the drug much worse. The drug may decrease the effects of Larodopa. Compazine, Mellaril, Prolixin, Serentil, Stelazine, Thorazine, and Trilafon may increase the blood levels of the drug. Tagamet may increase the blood levels of the drug. The drug may decrease the effects of Catapres and Ismelin. The drug may increase the effects of decongestants found in cough, cold, and allergy products on the heart, possibly causing high blood pressure, fast heartbeat, or irregular heartbeats.

ALLERGIES: Individuals allergic to perphenazine, amitriptyline, Elavil, or any of their derivatives should discuss this with their doctor or pharmacist before using this drug.

PREGNANCY/BREAST-FEEDING: Category D—Positive evidence of risk. Human studies show risk to the fetus. Nevertheless, potential benefits may possibly outweigh the potential risk. This drug should not be taken by nursing mothers.

OTHER BRAND NAMES: Etrafon 2-25

OTHER DRUGS IN THE SAME THERAPEUTIC CLASS: Etrafon 2-25

IMPORTANT INFORMATION TO REMEMBER: Only take the drug exactly as directed by your physician. Do not discontinue taking the drug without first consulting your physician. The drug may require four to six weeks of use before improvement may be noticed. This drug does cause drowsiness. Individuals should use caution when driving, operating machinery, or performing any task where mental alertness is required. Alcohol, anxiety medications, and narcotic painkillers may intensify the drowsiness effect of the drug. The drug may cause a slight amount of dizziness or lightheadedness when rising from a sitting or lying-down position. Individuals should also use a sunscreen to avoid overexposure to the sun; the drug may increase the skin's sensitivity to sunlight, which may cause one to sunburn more easily.

BRAND NAME: Tridesilon

GENERIC NAME: desonide

See entry for DesOwen

BRAND NAME: Trilafon

GENERIC NAME: perphenazine

GENERIC FORM AVAILABLE: Yes

THERAPEUTIC CLASS: Piperidine phenothiazine antipsychotic

DOSAGE FORMS: 2-mg, 4-mg, 8-mg, and 16-mg tablets; and 16 mg/5 mL concentrated solution

MAIN USES: Psychotic disorders

USUAL DOSE: 4 mg to 16 mg two to four times daily

AVERAGE PRICE: $86.44 (B)/$43.63 (G) for 2 mg; $138.86 (B)/$52.60 (G) for 4 mg; $172.00 (B)/$81.99 (G) for 8 mg; $186.32 (B)/$107.65 (G) for 16 mg

SIDE EFFECTS: Most common: drowsiness, restlessness, blurred vision, blurred vision, Parkinson's-like symptoms, low blood pressure, stuffy nose, dry mouth, constipation, and dizziness. Less common: increased sensitivity to sunburn, difficulty in urinating, nausea, vomiting, stomach pain, and trembling of fingers and hands, stomach pain, changes in menstrual period, decreased sexual ability, swelling and/or pain in the breasts, weight gain, and secretion of milk from the breasts.

DRUG INTERACTIONS: Drugs used to treat depression and Mellaril may increase the severity and frequency of side effects. Alcohol, anxiety medications, and narcotic painkillers may intensify the drowsiness effect of the drug. Eskalith and Lithobid may decrease the absorption of the drug. Eskalith or Lithobid and the drug may cause disorientation and for one to black out. The drug may decrease the effects of Larodopa. Inderal may increase the blood levels of the drug.

ALLERGIES: Individuals allergic to perphenazine or any of its derivatives should discuss this with their doctor or pharmacist before using this drug.

PREGNANCY/BREAST-FEEDING: Category C—Risk cannot be ruled out. Human studies are lacking, and animal studies are either positive for fetal risk or lacking as well. However, potential benefits may justify the potential risk in using the drug. The drug is excreted in the breast milk; therefore, extreme caution should be used when breast-feeding.

OTHER BRAND NAMES: None

OTHER DRUGS IN THE SAME THERAPEUTIC CLASS: Compazine, Mallaril, Prolixin, Serentil, Stelazine, and Thorazine

IMPORTANT INFORMATION TO REMEMBER: This drug does cause drowsiness. Individuals should use caution when driving, operating machinery, or performing any task where mental alertness is required. Alcohol, anxiety medications, and narcotic painkillers may intensify the drowsiness effect of the drug. Do not increase the dose or stop taking the drug without first consulting with your physician. Individuals should report any involuntary movements of the tongue, arms, or legs to their physician. This drug may also increase the sensitivity of the skin to sunburn in some individuals; therefore, a sunscreen is recommended during periods of prolonged exposure to the sun. Caution should be used during hot weather due to decreased tolerance to the heat.

BRAND NAME: **Tri-Levlen**

GENERIC NAME: Combination product containing: levonorgestrel and ethinyl estradiol

See entry for Triphasil

BRAND NAME: **Trimox**

GENERIC NAME: amoxicillin

See entry for Amoxil

BRAND NAME: **Trimpex**

GENERIC NAME: trimethoprim

See entry for Proloprim

BRAND NAME: **Trinalin**

GENERIC NAME: Combination product containing: pseudoephedrine and azatadine

GENERIC FORM AVAILABLE: No

THERAPEUTIC CLASS: Decongestant + antihistamine

DOSAGE FORMS: 120-mg pseudoephedrine/1-mg azatadine sustained-release tablets

MAIN USES: Nasal allergies and congestion

USUAL DOSE: one tablet every 12 hours

AVERAGE PRICE: $133.14

SIDE EFFECTS: Most common: drowsiness. Less common: nausea, giddiness, dry mouth, blurred vision, pounding heartbeat, flushing, and increased irritability or excitability (especially in children).

DRUG INTERACTIONS: Blocadren, Cartrol, Corgard, Inderal, Kerlone, Levatol, Lopressor, Normodyne, Sectral, Tenormin, Toprol-XL, Trandate, Visken, and Zebeta may increase the effects of the drug. The drug may also reduce the effects of blood-pressure-lowering drugs. Nardil or Parnate may significantly raise blood pressure when taken with this drug.

ALLERGIES: Individuals allergic to azatadine, pseudoephedrine, or other antihistamine/decongestant combinations (such as those listed under "Other Drugs in the Same Therapeutic Class") should discuss this with their doctor or pharmacist before taking this drug.

PREGNANCY/BREAST-FEEDING: Category C—Risk cannot be ruled out. Human studies are lacking, and animal studies are either positive for fetal risk or lacking as well. However, potential benefits may justify the potential risk in using the drug. It is not known whether the drug is excreted in the breast milk; therefore, caution should be used when breast-feeding.

OTHER BRAND NAMES: None

OTHER DRUGS IN THE SAME THERAPEUTIC CLASS: Bromfed, Bromfed PD, Claritin-D, Comhist LA, Deconamine, Deconamine SR, Fedahist, Naldecon, Nolamine, Novafed-A, Ornade, Poly-Histine-D, Rondec, Rynatan, Seldane-D, Semprex-D, and Tavist-D

IMPORTANT INFORMATION TO REMEMBER: This drug does cause drowsiness. Individuals should use caution when driving, operating machinery, or performing any task where mental alertness is required. Alcohol, anxiety medications, or narcotic painkillers may intensify the drowsiness effect of the drug. This drug may also cause a dry mouth; sugarless gum or hard candy will help take care of this problem. Patients with glaucoma, high blood pressure, heart conditions, or urinary or prostate problems should consult their doctor before taking this drug. Do not crush, cut, or chew the tablets—this will destroy the mechanism that causes the delayed release of the medication. The tablets should be swallowed whole.

BRAND NAME: Tri-Norinyl

GENERIC NAME: Combination product containing: norethindrone and ethinyl estradiol

GENERIC FORM AVAILABLE: No

THERAPEUTIC CLASS: Progestin + estrogen contraceptive

DOSAGE FORMS: 0.5 mg norethindrone/35 micrograms ethinyl estradiol (first seven tablets), 1 mg norethindrone/35 micrograms/ethinyl estradiol (next nine tablets), and 0.5 mg norethindrone/35 micrograms/ethinyl estradiol (next five tablets)

MAIN USES: Birth control

USUAL DOSE: Take one tablet daily for 21 or 28 days, beginning on the fifth day of the cycle. Day One of the cycle is the first day of menstrual bleeding.

AVERAGE PRICE: $28.21

SIDE EFFECTS: Most common: stomach cramps, bloating, acne, appetite changes, nausea, swelling of the feet and ankles, weight gain, swelling of the breasts, breast tenderness, and unusual tiredness or weakness. Less common: changes in vaginal bleeding, feeling faint, increased blood pressure, depression, stomach pain, vaginal itching, yeast infections, brown and blotchy spots on the skin, diarrhea, dizziness, headaches, migraines, increased body and facial hair, increased sensitivity of the skin to the sun, irritability, some hair loss from the scalp, vomiting, blood clots, weight loss, and changes in sexual desire.

DRUG INTERACTIONS: Antibiotics may decrease the effectiveness of the drug. The drug may interfere with the effectiveness of Parlodel. The drug may reduce the effects of Coumadin. The drug may increase the blood levels of Anafranil, Asendin, Elavil, Endep, Norpramin, Pamelor, Sinequan, Surmontil, Tofranil, and Vivactil when used for long periods of time. Smoking is not recommended while taking this drug due to the increased risk of heart disease, stroke, and high blood pressure.

ALLERGIES: Individuals allergic to norethindrone and ethinyl estradiol or any of their derivatives should discuss this with their doctor or pharmacist before using this drug.

PREGNANCY/BREAST-FEEDING: Category X—Should not be used during pregnancy. Studies in animals and/or humans have shown fetal abnormalities and birth defects. The risks associated with using this drug clearly outweigh the benefits. This drug should never be used by someone who is pregnant or trying to become pregnant. Also, women should never breast-feed while using this drug.

OTHER BRAND NAMES: None

OTHER DRUGS IN THE SAME THERAPEUTIC CLASS: Estrostep, Ortho-Novum 7/7/7, Ortho Tri-Cylen, Tri-Levlen, and Triphasil

IMPORTANT INFORMATION TO REMEMBER: Only take the drug exactly as directed by your physician. It is important to take the drug at the same time every day (bedtime). Do not discontinue taking the drug without first consulting your physician. The drug should not be used by women with a history of heart disease, stroke, high blood pressure, breast cancer, or other blood vessel diseases. Breakthrough bleeding may occur during the first few months; if this persists, notify your doctor. This drug will not provide protection against the HIV (AIDS) virus. It is important to use a second method of birth control during the first week when treatment has just begun. It may be necessary to use a second form of birth control when antibiotics are being taken. Also, women who smoke run a higher risk of heart disease, stroke, and high blood pressure when taking this drug. If pregnancy is suspected, stop taking the drug immediately.

BRAND NAME: Trinsicon

GENERIC NAME: Combination product containing: iron, vitamin B_{12}, folic acid, vitamin C, and liver–stomach concentrate

GENERIC FORM AVAILABLE: No

THERAPEUTIC CLASS: Hematinic vitamin

DOSAGE FORMS: 110-mg iron/15-microgram vitamin B_{12}/0.5-mg folic acid/75-mg vitamin C/240-mg liver–stomach concentrate capsules

MAIN USES: Anemia and iron deficiency

USUAL DOSE: one capsule twice daily

AVERAGE PRICE: $65.47

SIDE EFFECTS: Most common: stomach pain, stomach cramps, nausea, vomiting, constipation, and diarrhea. Less common: dark urine and heartburn.

DRUG INTERACTIONS: The drug should not be taken within two hours of taking Didronel, Doryx, Minocin, Monodox, Sumycin, and Vibramycin.

ALLERGIES: Individuals allergic to iron, vitamin B_{12}, folic acid, vitamin C, the liver–stomach concentrate in this combination, or any of their derivatives should discuss this with their doctor or pharmacist before using this drug.

PREGNANCY/BREAST-FEEDING: Category C—Risk cannot be ruled out. Human studies are lacking, and animal studies are either positive for fetal risk or lacking as well. However, potential benefits

may justify the potential risk in using the drug. It is not known whether the drug is excreted in the breast milk; therefore, caution should be used when breast-feeding.

OTHER BRAND NAMES: None

OTHER DRUGS IN THE SAME THERAPEUTIC CLASS: Chromagen, Feosol, Fer-In-Sol, Fergon, Fero-Folic-500, Ferro-Sequels, Iberet-Folic-500, and Slow FE

IMPORTANT INFORMATION TO REMEMBER: This drug should be taken with food or milk to reduce the potential for injury to the stomach lining and stomach upset. Take the drug exactly as directed and do not discontinue taking the drug unless directed to do so by your physician. The drug may cause the urine to become dark from the iron component; this is normal and individuals should not become alarmed.

BRAND NAME: Triphasil

GENERIC NAME: Combination product containing: levonorgestrel and ethinyl estradiol

GENERIC FORM AVAILABLE: No

THERAPEUTIC CLASS: Progestin + estrogen contraceptive

DOSAGE FORMS: 0.05 mg levonorgestrol/30 micrograms ethinyl estradiol (first 6 tablets), 0.075 mg levonorgestrol/40 micrograms ethinyl estradiol (second 5 tablets), and 0.125 mg levonorgestrol/30 micrograms ethinyl estradiol (third 10 tablets)

MAIN USES: Birth control

USUAL DOSE: Take one tablet daily for 21 or 28 days, beginning on the fifth day of the cycle. Day One of the cycle is the first day of menstrual bleeding.

AVERAGE PRICE: $34.06

SIDE EFFECTS: Most common: stomach cramps, bloating, acne, appetite changes, nausea, swelling of the feet and ankles, weight gain, swelling of the breasts, breast tenderness, and unusual tiredness or weakness. Less common: changes in vaginal bleeding, feeling faint, increased blood pressure, depression, stomach pain, vaginal itching, yeast infections, brown and blotchy spots on the skin, diarrhea, dizziness, headaches, migraines, increased body and facial hair, increased sensitivity of the skin to the sun, irritability, some hair loss from the scalp, vomiting, blood clots, weight loss, and changes in sexual desire.

DRUG INTERACTIONS: Antibiotics may decrease the effectiveness of the drug. The drug may interfere with the effectiveness of Parlodel. The drug may reduce the effects of Coumadin. The drug may increase the blood levels of Anafranil, Asendin, Elavil, Endep, Norpramin, Pamelor, Sinequan, Surmontil, Tofranil, and Vivactil when used for long periods of time. Smoking is not recommended while taking this drug due to the increased risk of heart disease, stroke, and high blood pressure.

ALLERGIES: Individuals allergic to levonorgestrel, ethinyl estradiol, or any of their derivatives should discuss this with their doctor or pharmacist before using this drug.

PREGNANCY/BREAST-FEEDING: Category X—Should not be used during pregnancy. Studies in animals and/or humans have shown fetal abnormalities and birth defects. The risks associated with using this drug clearly outweigh the benefits. This drug should never be used by someone who is pregnant or trying to become pregnant. Also, women should never breast-feed while using this drug.

OTHER BRAND NAMES: Tri-Levlen

OTHER DRUGS IN THE SAME THERAPEUTIC CLASS: Estrostep, Ortho-Novum 7/7/7, Ortho Tri-Cylen, Tri-Levlen, and Tri-Norinyl

IMPORTANT INFORMATION TO REMEMBER: Only take the drug exactly as directed by your physician. It is important to take the drug at the same time every day (bedtime). Do not discontinue taking the drug without first consulting your physician. The drug should not be used by women with a history of heart disease, stroke, high blood pressure, breast cancer, or other blood vessel diseases. Breakthrough bleeding may occur during the first few months; if this persists, notify your doctor. This drug will not provide protection against the HIV (AIDS) virus. It is important to use a second method of birth control during the first week when treatment has just begun. It may be necessary to use a second form of birth control when antibiotics are being taken. Also, women who smoke run a higher risk of heart disease, stroke, and high blood pressure when taking this drug. If pregnancy is suspected, stop taking the drug immediately.

BRAND NAME: Tritec

GENERIC NAME: ranitidine bismuth citrate

GENERIC FORM AVAILABLE: No

THERAPEUTIC CLASS: Stomach acid blocker + antibacterial

DOSAGE FORMS: 400-mg tablets

MAIN USES: Active stomach ulcers and active duodenal ulcers (ulcers of the upper part of the small intestine, also called peptic ulcers)

USUAL DOSE: 400 mg twice daily for four weeks

AVERAGE PRICE: $94.90 for 60 tablets

SIDE EFFECTS: diarrhea 2%, nausea 1%, vomiting 1%, headache 1%, dizziness 1%, and yeast infections 1%.

DRUG INTERACTIONS: The drug may increase the blood levels of Coumadin. Antacids may decrease the blood levels of the drug.

ALLERGIES: Individuals allergic to ranitidine, Zantac, bismuth, or other H-2 receptor blockers (such as those listed under "Other Drugs in the Same Therapeutic Class") should discuss this with their doctor or pharmacist before taking this drug.

PREGNANCY/BREAST-FEEDING: Category C—Risk cannot be ruled out. Human studies are lacking, and animal studies are either positive for fetal risk or lacking as well. However, potential benefits may justify the potential risk in using the drug. The drug is excreted in the breast milk; therefore, extreme caution should be used when breast-feeding.

OTHER BRAND NAMES: None

OTHER DRUGS IN THE SAME THERAPEUTIC CLASS: None

IMPORTANT INFORMATION TO REMEMBER: Always complete the full course of therapy, and take the drug only as directed. Individuals may take antacids occasionally for heartburn or temporary flare-ups, but antacids should be taken at least one hour before or two hours after taking the drug. The drug is most often taken with Biaxin (500 mg) three times daily for 14 days.

BRAND NAME: Trusopt

GENERIC NAME: dorzolamide

GENERIC FORM AVAILABLE: No

THERAPEUTIC CLASS: Carbonic anhydrase inhibitor, anti-glaucoma

DOSAGE FORMS: 2% eyedrop solution

MAIN USES: Glaucoma

USUAL DOSE: one drop three times daily

AVERAGE PRICE: $29.43 for 5 mL

SIDE EFFECTS: burning, stinging, or discomfort 33%; bitter taste following use 25%; superficial keratitis 10%–15%; allergic reactions in the eye 10%; blurred vision 1%–5%; dryness 1%–5%; tearing 1%–5%; and increased sensitivity of eyes to sunlight 1%–5%.

DRUG INTERACTIONS: None of any clinical significance

ALLERGIES: Individuals allergic to dorzolamide or any of its derivatives should discuss this with their doctor or pharmacist before using this drug.

PREGNANCY/BREAST-FEEDING: Category C—Risk cannot be ruled out. Human studies are lacking, and animal studies are either positive for fetal risk or lacking as well. However, potential benefits may justify the potential risk in using the drug. It is not known whether the drug is excreted in the breast milk; therefore, caution should be used when breast-feeding.

OTHER BRAND NAMES: None

OTHER DRUGS IN THE SAME THERAPEUTIC CLASS: None

IMPORTANT INFORMATION TO REMEMBER: Keep the container tightly closed and avoid touching the applicator tip to the eye—this could contaminate the product over time. Also, only administer one drop at a time. After application, keep the eye open for at least 30 seconds, roll the eyeball around, and avoid squinting. If a second drop is required, wait one to two minutes between drops. If another medication is to be used in the eye, wait at least 10 minutes before administering it. Only use the drug exactly as directed by your physician. Do not discontinue taking the drug without first consulting your physician.

BRAND NAME: T-Stat

GENERIC NAME: erythromycin

See entry for A/T/S

BRAND NAME: Tussionex

GENERIC NAME: Combination product containing: chlorphenira-mine and hydrocodone

GENERIC FORM AVAILABLE: No

THERAPEUTIC CLASS: Antihistamine + cough suppressant

DOSAGE FORMS: 8 mg chlorpheniramine/70 mg hydrocodone per 5 mL extended-release suspension

MAIN USES: Cough, along with allergy and/or cold symptoms

USUAL DOSE: one teaspoon every 12 hours

AVERAGE PRICE: $15.99 for 60 mL

SIDE EFFECTS: Most common: drowsiness, thickening of mucus, and dry mouth. Less common: blurred vision, difficult or painful urination, constipation, dizziness, fast heartbeat, increased sweating, and increased appetite.

DRUG INTERACTIONS: Central nervous system (CNS) depression may be increased when used with alcohol, narcotic painkillers, or other anxiety medications. The drug should not be used with Nardil or Parnate.

ALLERGIES: Individuals allergic to chlorpheniramine, hydroco-done, or any of their derivatives should discuss this with their doctor or pharmacist before using this drug.

PREGNANCY/BREAST-FEEDING: Category C—Risk cannot be ruled out. Human studies are lacking, and animal studies are either positive for fetal risk or lacking as well. However, potential benefits may justify the potential risk in using the drug. It is not known whether the drug is excreted in the breast milk; therefore, caution should be used when breast-feeding.

OTHER BRAND NAMES: None

OTHER DRUGS IN THE SAME THERAPEUTIC CLASS: Phenergan w/Codeine

IMPORTANT INFORMATION TO REMEMBER: This drug does cause drowsiness. Individuals should use caution when driving, operating machinery, or performing any task where mental alertness is required. Alcohol, anxiety medications, and narcotic painkillers may intensify the drowsiness effect of the drug. The drug should only be taken as needed to control a cough; this drug should not be used as a long-term therapy. This medication is a controlled substance and may be habit-forming. If stomach upset occurs, the drug may be taken with food or milk. Be sure to shake the medication well before taking it.

BRAND NAME: Tussi-Organidin NR and Tussi-Organidin DM NR

GENERIC NAME: Combination product containing: codeine and guaifenesin (Tussi-Organidin NR) or dextromethorphan and guaifenesin (Tussi-Organidin DM NR)

GENERIC FORM AVAILABLE: No

THERAPEUTIC CLASS: Cough suppressant + expectorant

DOSAGE FORMS: 10 mg codeine/100 mg guaifenesin per 5 mL liquid (Tussi-Organidin NR) and 10 mg dextromethorphan/100 mg guaifenesin per 5 mL liquid (Tussi-Organidin DM NR)

MAIN USES: Cough

USUAL DOSE: one to two teaspoons every four hours as needed

AVERAGE PRICE: $21.83 for 120 mL

SIDE EFFECTS: Most common: drowsiness, nausea, and vomiting. Less common: blurred vision, headache, constipation, rash, and dizziness.

DRUG INTERACTIONS: Central nervous system (CNS) depression may be increased when used with alcohol, narcotic painkillers, or other anxiety medications.

ALLERGIES: Individuals allergic to codeine, dextromethorphan, guaifenesin, or any of their derivatives should discuss this with their doctor or pharmacist before using this drug.

PREGNANCY/BREAST-FEEDING: Category C—Risk cannot be ruled out. Human studies are lacking, and animal studies are either positive for fetal risk or lacking as well. However, potential benefits

may justify the potential risk in using the drug. The drug is excreted in the breast milk; therefore, extreme caution should be used when breast-feeding.

OTHER BRAND NAMES: None

OTHER DRUGS IN THE SAME THERAPEUTIC CLASS: Robitussin-AC and Vicodin Tuss

IMPORTANT INFORMATION TO REMEMBER: This drug does cause drowsiness. Individuals should use caution when driving, operating machinery, or performing any task where mental alertness is required. Alcohol, anxiety medications, and narcotic painkillers may intensify the drowsiness effect of the drug. The drug should only be taken as needed to control a cough; this drug should not be used as a long-term therapy. This medication is a controlled substance and may be habit-forming (Tussi-Organidin NR only). If stomach upset occurs, the drug may be taken with food or milk. The drug should also be taken with plenty of water to help the guaifenesin thin and to "cough up" mucous secretions in the lungs.

BRAND NAME: Tylenol #2, Tylenol #3, and Tylenol #4

GENERIC NAME: Combination product containing: acetaminophen and codeine

GENERIC FORM AVAILABLE: Yes

THERAPEUTIC CLASS: Narcotic analgesic + pain reliever

DOSAGE FORMS: 300-mg acetaminophen/15-mg codeine tablets (Tylenol #2); 300-mg acetaminophen/30-mg codeine tablets (Tylenol #3); 300-mg acetaminophen/60-mg codeine tablets (Tylenol #4); and 120 mg acetaminophen/12 mg codeine per 5 mL liquid (Tylenol w/Codeine Elixir)

MAIN USES: Mild to moderate pain

USUAL DOSE: one to two tablets every four hours as needed

AVERAGE PRICE: $43.29 (B)/$19.49 (G) for Tylenol #2; $52.38 (B)/$29.95 (G) for Tylenol #3; and $87.49 (B)/$38.29 (G) for Tylenol #4

SIDE EFFECTS: Most common: drowsiness, tiredness, and constipation. Less common: allergic reaction, shortness of breath, irregular heartbeat, restlessness, confusion, decreased blood pressure, increased sweating, flushing of the face, decreased urination, blurred vision, dizziness, dry mouth, headache, general feeling of discomfort or illness, nausea, loss of appetite, weakness, and difficulty urinating.

DRUG INTERACTIONS: Alcohol, anxiety medications, and other narcotic painkillers may intensify the drowsiness effect of the drug. The drug may increase the blood levels of Tegretol. Liver toxicity may occur with long-term use of Anturane, Dilantin, and Mesantoin. This drug and Nardil or Parnate may cause severe and sometimes fatal reactions.

ALLERGIES: Individuals allergic to acetaminophen, codeine, or any of their derivatives should discuss this with their doctor or pharmacist before using this drug.

PREGNANCY/BREAST-FEEDING: Category C—Risk cannot be ruled out. Human studies are lacking, and animal studies are either positive for fetal risk or lacking as well. However, potential benefits may justify the potential risk in using the drug. The drug is excreted in the breast milk; therefore, extreme caution should be used when breast-feeding.

OTHER BRAND NAMES: None

OTHER DRUGS IN THE SAME THERAPEUTIC CLASS: Bancap-HC, DHCplus, Darvocet N-100, Empirin #3, Empirin #4, Hydrocet, Lorcet 10/650, Lorcet Plus, Lortab, Percocet, Percodan, Phenaphen w/Codeine, Synalgos DC, Talacen, Tylox, Vicodin, and Zydone

IMPORTANT INFORMATION TO REMEMBER: This drug does cause drowsiness. Individuals should use caution when driving, operating machinery, or performing any task where mental alertness is required. Alcohol, anxiety medications, and other narcotic painkillers may intensify the drowsiness effect of the drug. Do not increase the dose without first consulting with your physician. This medication is a controlled substance and may be habit-forming. If stomach upset occurs, take the drug with food or milk.

BRAND NAME: Tylox

GENERIC NAME: Combination product containing: acetaminophen and oxycodone

GENERIC FORM AVAILABLE: No

THERAPEUTIC CLASS: Narcotic analgesic + pain reliever

DOSAGE FORMS: 500-mg acetaminophen/5-mg oxycodone capsules

MAIN USES: Moderate to severe pain

USUAL DOSE: one capsule every six hours as needed

AVERAGE PRICE: $103.33

SIDE EFFECTS: Most common: drowsiness, dizziness, tiredness, nausea, and vomiting. Less common: confusion, decreased urination, dry mouth, constipation, stomach pain, skin rash, headache, weakness, minor vision disturbances, histamine release (symptoms include decreased blood pressure, sweating, fast heartbeat, flushing, and wheezing), and hallucinations.

DRUG INTERACTIONS: Alcohol, anxiety medications, and other narcotic painkillers may intensify the drowsiness effect of the drug. The drug may increase the blood levels of Tegretol. Liver toxicity may occur with long-term use of Anturane, Dilantin, and Mesantoin. This drug and Nardil or Parnate may cause severe and sometimes fatal reactions.

ALLERGIES: Individuals allergic to acetaminophen, oxycodone, or any of their derivatives should discuss this with their doctor or pharmacist before using this drug.

PREGNANCY/BREAST-FEEDING: Category C—Risk cannot be ruled out. Human studies are lacking, and animal studies are either positive for fetal risk or lacking as well. However, potential benefits may justify the potential risk in using the drug. It is not known whether the drug is excreted in the breast milk; therefore, caution should be used when breast-feeding.

OTHER BRAND NAMES: None

OTHER DRUGS IN THE SAME THERAPEUTIC CLASS: Bancap-HC, Darvocet-N 50, Darvocet-N 100, Darvon, Darvon Compound, DHC-plus, Empirin #3, Empirin #4, Hydrocet, Lorcet 10/650, Lorcet Plus, Lortab, Percocet, Percodan, Phenaphen w/Codeine, Synalgos DC, Talacen, Tylenol #2, Tylenol #3, Tylenol #4, Vicodin, and Zydone

IMPORTANT INFORMATION TO REMEMBER: This drug does cause drowsiness. Individuals should use caution when driving, operating machinery, or performing any task where mental alertness is

required. Alcohol, anxiety medications, and other narcotic pain-killers may intensify the drowsiness effect of the drug. Do not increase the dose without first consulting with your physician. If stomach upset occurs, take the drug with food or milk. This prescription cannot be refilled; a new written prescription must be obtained each time. This medication is a controlled substance and may be habit-forming. The potential for abuse with this medication is high.

BRAND NAME: Ultracef

GENERIC NAME: cefadroxil

See entry for Duricef

BRAND NAME: Ultram

GENERIC NAME: tramadol

GENERIC FORM AVAILABLE: No

THERAPEUTIC CLASS: Centrally acting pain reliever

DOSAGE FORMS: 50-mg tablets

MAIN USES: Moderate to severe pain

USUAL DOSE: 50 mg to 100 mg every four to six hours as needed

AVERAGE PRICE: $84.03

SIDE EFFECTS: dizziness 26%–33%, nausea 24%–40%, constipation 24%–46%, headache 18%–32%, drowsiness 16%–25%, vomiting 9%–17%, itching 8%–11%, nervousness 7%–14%, weakness 6%–12%, increased sweating 6%–9%, dry mouth 5%–10%, and diarrhea 5%–10%.

DRUG INTERACTIONS: Central nervous system (CNS) depression may be increased when used with alcohol, anxiety medications, other pain medications, Nardil, Parnate, and drugs used to treat depression. Quinaglute and Quinidex may affect the blood levels of the drug. Tegretol may decrease the blood levels of the drug.

ALLERGIES: Individuals allergic to tramadol or any of its derivatives should discuss this with their doctor or pharmacist before using this drug.

PREGNANCY/BREAST-FEEDING: Category C—Risk cannot be ruled out. Human studies are lacking, and animal studies are either positive for fetal risk or lacking as well. However, potential benefits may justify the potential risk in using the drug. The drug is excreted in the breast milk; therefore, extreme caution should be used when breast-feeding.

OTHER BRAND NAMES: None

OTHER DRUGS IN THE SAME THERAPEUTIC CLASS: None

IMPORTANT INFORMATION TO REMEMBER: This drug does cause drowsiness and dizziness. Individuals should use caution when driving, operating machinery, or performing any task where mental alertness is required. Alcohol, anxiety medications, and other narcotic painkillers may intensify the drowsiness effect of the drug. If stomach upset occurs, take the drug with food or milk. Do not increase the dose without first consulting with your physician.

BRAND NAME: Ultrase

GENERIC NAME: Combination product containing: the enzymes lipase, amylase, and protease

See entry for Pancrease MT

BRAND NAME: Ultravate

GENERIC NAME: halobetasol

GENERIC FORM AVAILABLE: No

THERAPEUTIC CLASS: Topical corticosteroid

DOSAGE FORMS: 0.05% cream and ointment

MAIN USES: Skin rashes, swelling, and itching

USUAL DOSE: Apply thin layer one to two times daily.

AVERAGE PRICE: $29.26 for 15 g

SIDE EFFECTS: stinging 4%, burning 4%, and itching 4%.

DRUG INTERACTIONS: None of any clinical significance

ALLERGIES: Individuals allergic to halobetasol or any of their derivatives should discuss this with their doctor or pharmacist before using this drug.

PREGNANCY/BREAST-FEEDING: Category C—Risk cannot be ruled out. Human studies are lacking, and animal studies are either positive for fetal risk or lacking as well. However, potential benefits may justify the potential risk in using the drug. It is not known whether the drug is excreted in the breast milk; therefore, caution should be used when breast-feeding.

OTHER BRAND NAMES: None

OTHER DRUGS IN THE SAME THERAPEUTIC CLASS: Aclovate, Aristocort, Cordran, Cordran SP, Cutivate, Cyclocort, DesOwen, Diprolene, Diprolene AF, Elocon, Florone, Florone E, Halog, Hytone, Kenalog, Lidex, Lidex E, Synalar, Temovate, Topicort, Tridesilon, Valisone, and Westcort

IMPORTANT INFORMATION TO REMEMBER: This drug is for external use only. Apply only a thin film of drug to skin and rub it in well. Never cover the skin after application with a bandage or wrapping unless directed to do so by a doctor. Never apply the drug to damaged skin or open wounds unless directed to do so by a doctor. Discontinue use if irritation occurs.

BRAND NAME: Uniphyl

GENERIC NAME: theophylline

GENERIC FORM AVAILABLE: No

THERAPEUTIC CLASS: Xanthine bronchodilator

DOSAGE FORMS: 400-mg and 600-mg sustained-release tablets

MAIN USES: Asthma, chronic bronchitis, emphysema, and {other breathing disorders}

USUAL DOSE: once daily in the morning or evening with meals

AVERAGE PRICE: $104.89 for 400 mg and $149.62 for 600 mg

SIDE EFFECTS: Most common: nausea, nervousness, and restlessness. Less common: vomiting, diarrhea, stomach pain, headaches, irritability, insomnia, muscle twitching, fast heartbeat, pounding heartbeat, fast breathing, flushing, and low blood pressure.

DRUG INTERACTIONS: The drug may inhibit the effects of Blocadren, Cartrol, Corgard, Inderal, Kerlone, Levatol, Lopressor, Normodyne, Sectral, Tenormin, Toprol-XL, Trandate, Visken, and Zebeta. Dilantin, Tegretol, smoking, and nicotine patches may lower the blood levels of this drug. Cipro, Noroxin, Tagamet, Zantac, erythromycin, and TAO may increase blood levels of the drug. Individuals who stop smoking while taking the drug may have increased levels of the drug in the blood.

ALLERGIES: Individuals allergic to theophylline or other xanthines (such as those listed under "Other Drugs in the Same Therapeutic Class") should discuss this with their doctors or pharmacist before taking this drug.

PREGNANCY/BREAST-FEEDING: Category C—Risk cannot be ruled out. Human studies are lacking, and animal studies are either positive for fetal risk or lacking as well. However, potential benefits may justify the potential risk in using the drug. The drug is excreted in the breast milk; therefore, extreme caution should be used when breast-feeding.

OTHER BRAND NAMES: None

OTHER DRUGS IN THE SAME THERAPEUTIC CLASS: aminophylline, Choledyl, Elixophyllin, Lufyllin, Respbid, Quibron-SR, Quibron-T, Slo-bid, Slo-Phyllin, Theo-24, Theo-Dur, Theo-X, and Uni-Dur

IMPORTANT INFORMATION TO REMEMBER: Only take the drug exactly as directed by your physician. Do not discontinue taking the drug without first consulting your physician. Do not increase the dose without first consulting with your physician. This drug should be taken with plenty of water (eight ounces is preferred). Do not crush or chew the tablets; they may, however, be cut in half for easier swallowing. If stomach upset occurs, take with food or milk. Do not change between brand and generic once you are stabilized on one or the other.

BRAND NAME: Univasc

GENERIC NAME: moexipril

GENERIC FORM AVAILABLE: No

THERAPEUTIC CLASS: ACE inhibitor

DOSAGE FORMS: 7.5-mg and 15-mg tablets

MAIN USES: High blood pressure

USUAL DOSE: 7.5 mg to 30 mg daily in one or two divided doses

AVERAGE PRICE: $69.56 for 7.5 mg and $73.41 for 15 mg

SIDE EFFECTS: increased cough 6%, dizziness 4%, diarrhea 3%, flu-like symptoms 3%, tiredness 2%, pharyngitis 2%, flushing 2%, rash 2%, and muscle pain 1%.

DRUG INTERACTIONS: May decrease the absorption of the antibiotic Sumycin and other tetracycline antibiotics. High potassium levels may occur when used together with Dyrenium and Aldactone, and potassium supplements such as K-Dur, Klor-Con, K-Lyte, and Micro-K, Slow-K. Patients on water pills, especially those recently started on a water pill, may experience low blood pressure. The drug may also increase the toxic effects of Eskalith and Lithobid, especially when taken with a water pill.

ALLERGIES: Individuals allergic to moexipril or other ACE inhibitors (such as those listed under "Other Drugs in the Same Therapeutic Class") should discuss this with their doctor or pharmacist before using this drug.

PREGNANCY/BREAST-FEEDING: Category C (first trimester)—Risk cannot be ruled out. Human studies are lacking, and animal studies are either positive for fetal risk or lacking as well. However, potential benefits may justify the potential risk in using the drug. Category D (second and third trimesters)—Positive evidence of risk. Human studies show risk to the fetus. Nevertheless, potential benefits may possibly outweigh the potential risk. This drug should not be taken by nursing mothers.

OTHER BRAND NAMES: None

OTHER DRUGS IN THE SAME THERAPEUTIC CLASS: Accupril, Altace, Capoten, Lotensin, Mavik, Monopril, Prinivil, Vasotec, and Zestril

IMPORTANT INFORMATION TO REMEMBER: Take this drug regularly and exactly as directed by your physician. Do not stop taking the drug unless otherwise directed by your doctor. Avoid salt substitutes containing potassium. Before taking over-the-counter cold and allergy preparations, consult your doctor or pharmacist—these products may raise your blood pressure. If you experience swelling of the face, lips, or tongue or difficulty in breathing, contact your doctor immediately.

BRAND NAME: Urecholine

GENERIC NAME: bethanechol

GENERIC FORM AVAILABLE: Yes

THERAPEUTIC CLASS: Urinary problem reliever

DOSAGE FORMS: 5-mg, 10-mg, 25-mg, and 50-mg tablets

MAIN USES: Symptomatic relief of urinary problems

USUAL DOSE: 10 mg to 50 mg three or four times daily

AVERAGE PRICE: $50.07 (B)/$14.26 (G) for 5 mg; $90.13 (B)/ $20.18 (G) for 10 mg; $129.11 (B)/$22.27 (G) for 25 mg; $175.48 (B)/$28.91 (G) for 50 mg

SIDE EFFECTS: Most common: none. Less common: belching, blurred vision, diarrhea, and increase in frequency of the urge to urinate.

DRUG INTERACTIONS: None of any clinical significance

ALLERGIES: Individuals allergic to bethanechol or any of its derivatives should discuss this with their doctor or pharmacist before using this drug.

PREGNANCY/BREAST-FEEDING: Category C—Risk cannot be ruled out. Human studies are lacking, and animal studies are either positive for fetal risk or lacking as well. However, potential benefits may justify the potential risk in using the drug. It is not known whether the drug is excreted in the breast milk; therefore, caution should be used when breast-feeding.

OTHER BRAND NAMES: None

OTHER DRUGS IN THE SAME THERAPEUTIC CLASS: None

IMPORTANT INFORMATION TO REMEMBER: Take this drug regularly and exactly as directed by your physician. Do not stop taking the drug unless otherwise directed by your doctor. The drug should be taken on an empty stomach.

BRAND NAME: Urised

GENERIC NAME: Combination product containing: methenamine, phenyl salicylate, methylene blue, benzoic acid, atropine, and hyoscyamine

GENERIC FORM AVAILABLE: Yes

THERAPEUTIC CLASS: Anticholinergic + antibacterial + analgesic

DOSAGE FORMS: 40.8-mg methenamine/18.1-mg phenyl salicylate/5.4-mg methylene blue/4.5-mg benzoic acid/0.03-mg atropine/0.03-mg hyoscyamine tablets

MAIN USES: Urinary tract infections

USUAL DOSE: two tablets four times daily

AVERAGE PRICE: $78.41 (B)/$42.87 (G)

SIDE EFFECTS: Most common: blue or blue-green urine or stool. Less common: difficulty in urinating; dry mouth, nose, or throat; nausea; vomiting; and stomach pain.

DRUG INTERACTIONS: Diuretics (water pills) may make the urine alkaline, which reduces the effectiveness of the drug. Drugs used to treat diarrhea and antacids may reduce the absorption of the drug. The drug may reduce the absorption of Nizoral. The drug may increase the potential damage to the stomach lining from potassium supplements such as K-Dur, Klor-Con, K-Lyte, Micro-K, and Slow-K. Bactrim, Gantanol, Gantrisin, or Septra and the drug may cause insoluble crystals in the urinary tract, which may be dangerous. To prevent this problem, drink about 64 ounces of liquids per day.

ALLERGIES: Individuals allergic to methenamine, phenyl salicylate, methylene blue, benzoic acid, atropine, hyoscyamine, or any of their derivatives should discuss this with their doctor or pharmacist before using this drug.

PREGNANCY/BREAST-FEEDING: Category C—Risk cannot be ruled out. Human studies are lacking, and animal studies are either positive for fetal risk or lacking as well. However, potential benefits may justify the potential risk in using the drug. The drug is excreted in the breast milk; therefore, extreme caution should be used when breast-feeding.

OTHER BRAND NAMES: None

OTHER DRUGS IN THE SAME THERAPEUTIC CLASS: None

IMPORTANT INFORMATION TO REMEMBER: Take the drug at even intervals around the clock (if four times a day, take every six hours). Take the drug until all the medication prescribed is gone; otherwise the infection may return. The drug should also be taken with plenty of water (about 64 ounces per day); this will help flush out the infection from the urinary tract. The drug may cause the urine or stools to turn a blue or blue-green color; this is normal and is no cause for alarm.

BRAND NAME: Urispas

GENERIC NAME: flavoxate

GENERIC FORM AVAILABLE: No

THERAPEUTIC CLASS: Anti-urinary spasmatic

DOSAGE FORMS: 100-mg tablets

MAIN USES: Symptomatic relief of urinary problems

USUAL DOSE: one to two tablets three to four times daily

AVERAGE PRICE: $109.48

SIDE EFFECTS: Most common: drowsiness, dry mouth, and dry throat. Less common: constipation, difficulty in urinating, blurred vision, difficulty concentrating, dizziness, fast heartbeat, headache, increased sweating, nausea, vomiting, stomach pain, and increased sensitivity of the eyes to sunlight.

DRUG INTERACTIONS: None of any clinical significance

ALLERGIES: Individuals allergic to flavoxate or any of their derivatives should discuss this with their doctor or pharmacist before using this drug.

PREGNANCY/BREAST-FEEDING: Category B—No evidence of risk in humans. Either animal findings show risk, but human findings do not; or, if no adequate human studies have been done, animal findings show no risk. It is not known whether the drug is excreted in the breast milk; therefore, caution should be used when breast-feeding.

OTHER BRAND NAMES: None

OTHER DRUGS IN THE SAME THERAPEUTIC CLASS: None

IMPORTANT INFORMATION TO REMEMBER: Take this drug regularly and exactly as directed by your physician. Do not stop taking the drug unless otherwise directed by your doctor. This drug may cause drowsiness or blurred vision. Individuals should use caution when driving, operating machinery, or performing any task where mental alertness is required. Alcohol, anxiety medications, and narcotic painkillers may intensify the drowsiness effect of the drug. The drug may make an individual more sensitive to hot weather and the heat.

BRAND NAME: Vagistat-1

GENERIC NAME: tioconazole

GENERIC FORM AVAILABLE: No

THERAPEUTIC CLASS: Antifungal

DOSAGE FORMS: 6.5% vaginal ointment

MAIN USES: Vaginal yeast infections

USUAL DOSE: one applicatorful vaginally at bedtime as a single dose

AVERAGE PRICE: $33.88

SIDE EFFECTS: burning 6% and itching 5%.

DRUG INTERACTIONS: None of any clinical significance

ALLERGIES: Individuals allergic to tioconazole or other antifungals (such as those listed under "Other Drugs in the Same Therapeutic Class") should discuss this with their doctor or pharmacist before taking this drug.

PREGNANCY/BREAST-FEEDING: Category C—Risk cannot be ruled out. Human studies are lacking, and animal studies are either positive for fetal risk or lacking as well. However, potential benefits may justify the potential risk in using the drug. However, the drug should not be used during the first trimester (first three months) of pregnancy. It is not known whether the drug is excreted in the breast milk; therefore, caution should be used when breast-feeding.

OTHER BRAND NAMES: None

OTHER DRUGS IN THE SAME THERAPEUTIC CLASS: Femstat, Gyne-Lotrimin, Monistat, Mycelex, and Terazol

IMPORTANT INFORMATION TO REMEMBER: Continue using the drug even if your menstrual period begins. When using the drug, insert the applicator high into the vagina (two-thirds the length of the applicator) and push the plunger to release the medication. Do not use a tampon to hold the drug inside the vagina. It is recommended that your sexual partner use a condom until the infection clears up. This drug is now available over-the-counter without a prescription.

BRAND NAME: Valisone

GENERIC NAME: betamethasone valerate

GENERIC FORM AVAILABLE: Yes

THERAPEUTIC CLASS: Topical corticosteroid

DOSAGE FORMS: 0.1% ointment, cream, and lotion

MAIN USES: Skin rashes, swelling, and itching

USUAL DOSE: Apply to affected area(s) one to three times daily.

AVERAGE PRICE: $27.45 (B)/$15.71 (G) for 0.1% cream and ointment (15 g); and $27.91 (B)/$14.52 (G) for 0.1% lotion (60 mL)

SIDE EFFECTS: Most common: none. Less common: burning, itching, stinging, rash, dryness, and skin redness.

DRUG INTERACTIONS: None of any clinical significance

ALLERGIES: Individuals allergic to betamethasone valerate or any of its derivatives should discuss this with their doctor or pharmacist before using this drug.

PREGNANCY/BREAST-FEEDING: Category C—Risk cannot be ruled out. Human studies are lacking, and animal studies are either positive for fetal risk or lacking as well. However, potential benefits may justify the potential risk in using the drug. It is not known whether the drug is excreted in the breast milk; therefore, caution should be used when breast-feeding.

OTHER BRAND NAMES: None

OTHER DRUGS IN THE SAME THERAPEUTIC CLASS: Aclovate, Aristocort, Cordran, Cordran SP, Cutivate, Cyclocort, DesOwen, Diprolene, Diprolene AF, Elocon, Florone, Florone E, Halog, Hytone, Kenalog, Lidex, Lidex E, Synalar, Temovate, Topicort, Tridesilon, Ultravate, and Westcort

IMPORTANT INFORMATION TO REMEMBER: This drug is for external use only. Apply only a thin film of drug to skin and rub it in well. Never cover the skin after application with a bandage or wrapping unless directed to do so by a doctor. Never apply to damaged skin or open wounds unless directed to do so by a doctor. Discontinue use if irritation occurs.

BRAND NAME: Valium

GENERIC NAME: diazepam

GENERIC FORM AVAILABLE: Yes

THERAPEUTIC CLASS: Benzodiazepine antianxiety

DOSAGE FORMS: 2-mg, 5-mg, and 10-mg tablets

MAIN USES: Anxiety, muscle spasms, and seizures

USUAL DOSE: 2 mg to 10 mg two to four times daily

AVERAGE PRICE: $61.17 (B)/$17.46 (G) for 2 mg; $80.89 (B)/$26.54 (G) for 5 mg; and $152.19 (B)/$30.03 (G) for 10 mg

SIDE EFFECTS: Most common: drowsiness, clumsiness, and dizziness. Less common: confusion, depression, stomach cramps, nausea, vomiting, dry mouth, changes in sex drive, sleep disturbances, and fast heartbeat.

DRUG INTERACTIONS: Central nervous system (CNS) depression may be increased when used with alcohol, anxiety medications, and narcotic painkillers.

ALLERGIES: Individuals allergic to diazepam or other benzodiazepines (such as those listed under "Other Drugs in the Same Therapeutic Class") should discuss this with their doctor or pharmacist before taking this drug.

PREGNANCY/BREAST-FEEDING: Category D—Positive evidence of risk. Human studies show risk to the fetus. Nevertheless, potential benefits may possibly outweigh the potential risks. This drug should not be taken by nursing mothers.

OTHER BRAND NAMES: None

OTHER DRUGS IN THE SAME THERAPEUTIC CLASS: Ativan, Librium, Serax, Tranxene, and Xanax

IMPORTANT INFORMATION TO REMEMBER: This drug may cause drowsiness. Individuals should use caution when driving, operating machinery, or performing any task where mental alertness is required. The incidence of drowsiness and unsteadiness increases with age. Alcohol, anxiety medications, or narcotic painkillers may intensify the drowsiness effect of the drug. This medication is a controlled substance and may be habit-forming. Do not increase the dose of medication without consulting with your doctor; take only the amount prescribed by your doctor.

BRAND NAME: **Valtrex**

GENERIC NAME: valacyclovir

GENERIC FORM AVAILABLE: No

THERAPEUTIC CLASS: Antiviral

DOSAGE FORMS: 500-mg caplets

MAIN USES: Shingles and genital herpes

USUAL DOSE: 500 mg to 100 mg one to three times daily

AVERAGE PRICE: $162.28 to 42 caplets

SIDE EFFECTS: nausea 16%, headache 13%, vomiting 7%, diarrhea 5%, constipation 5%, weakness 4%, dizziness 4%, stomach pain 3%, and appetite changes 3%.

DRUG INTERACTIONS: Probenecid and Tagamet may slightly increase the blood levels of the drug.

ALLERGIES: Individuals allergic to valacyclovir, Cytovene, Famvir, Zovirax, or any of their derivatives should discuss this with their doctor or pharmacist before using this drug.

PREGNANCY/BREAST-FEEDING: Category B—No evidence of risk in humans. Either animal findings show risk, but human findings do not; or, if no adequate human studies have been done, animal findings show no risk. The drug is excreted in the breast milk; therefore, extreme caution should be used when breast-feeding.

OTHER BRAND NAMES: None

OTHER DRUGS IN THE SAME THERAPEUTIC CLASS: Cytovene, Famvir, and Zovirax

IMPORTANT INFORMATION TO REMEMBER: Only take the drug exactly as directed by your physician. If stomach upset occurs, take the drug with food or milk. Also, take the drug at even intervals around the clock (if two times a day, take every 12 hours while awake). Take the drug for the full course of therapy; otherwise the infection may return. The drug should be started at the first sign of shingles for maximum effectiveness; the drug is most effective if started within 48 hours of the onset of shingles.

BRAND NAME: **Vancenase, Vancenase AQ, and Vancenase AQ Double Strength**

GENERIC NAME: beclomethasone dipropionate

GENERIC FORM AVAILABLE: No

THERAPEUTIC CLASS: Steroid nasal spray

DOSAGE FORMS: 42-micrograms-per-inhalation aerosol (Vancenase); 42-micrograms-per-spray nasal spray (Vancenase AQ); and 84-micrograms-per-spray nasal spray (Vancenase AQ Double Strength)

MAIN USES: Nasal allergies, {nasal polyps}, and {nasal inflammation}

USUAL DOSE: For Vancenase AQ: one to two sprays in each nostril twice daily. For Vancenase: one inhalation in each nostril two to four times daily. For Vancenase AQ Double Strength: one to two sprays in each nostril once daily.

AVERAGE PRICE: $43.91 for Vancenase; $47.40 for Vancenase AQ; and $49.91 for Vancenase AQ Double Strength

SIDE EFFECTS: For the aerosol: nasal irritation 11%, burning 11%, sneezing attacks 10%, nosebleeds 2%, and runny nose 1%. For the spray: nasal irritation 24%, sneezing attacks 4%, headache less than 5%, lightheadedness less than 5%, nausea less than 5%, nosebleeds less than 3%, stuffy nose less than 3%, and runny nose less than 3%.

DRUG INTERACTIONS: Caution should be used when taking this drug with other oral corticosteroids such as Aristocort, Decadron, Deltasone, Medrol, and prednisone.

ALLERGIES: Individuals allergic to beclomethasone dipropionate or other nasal steroids (such as those listed under "Other Drugs in the Same Therapeutic Class") should discuss this with their doctor or pharmacist before taking this drug.

PREGNANCY/BREAST-FEEDING: Category C—Risk cannot be ruled out. Human studies are lacking, and animal studies are either positive for fetal risk or lacking as well. However, potential benefits may justify the potential risk in using the drug. It is not known whether the drug is excreted in the breast milk; therefore, caution should be used when breast-feeding.

OTHER BRAND NAMES: Vancenase and Vancenase AQ

OTHER DRUGS IN THE SAME THERAPEUTIC CLASS: Dexacort, Flonase, Nasacort, Nasalide, and Rhinocort

IMPORTANT INFORMATION TO REMEMBER: The drug is not intended to provide immediate relief of nasal allergies; to receive the full benefits of the drug, use it on a regular basis as a maintenance medication. The drug may take up to three weeks before noticeable benefits may be seen. Never exceed the prescribed dosage unless directed to do so by a doctor—excessive use beyond the prescribed dosage is potentially dangerous. This drug should not be used by individuals with fungal, bacterial, systemic viral, or respiratory tract infections; unhealed wounds inside the nose; or tuberculosis.

When using the nasal spray or aerosol, use the following procedure:

1) Blow your nose gently to clear your nostrils, if necessary.
2) Hold the spray bottle with your thumb at the bottom and your index and middle finger on the shoulder attached to the neck of the bottle (top of the canister for the aerosol).
3) With your other hand, gently place a finger against the side of your nose to close the opposite nostril.
4) Insert the tip of the bottle or aerosol into the open nostril. Point the tip toward the back and outer side of the nostril once inside.
5) After releasing the spray, close your mouth, sniff deeply, hold your breath for a few seconds, then breathe out through your mouth.
6) Tilt your head back slightly for a few seconds to allow the drug to spread to the back of your nose.
7) Repeat the same procedure for the other nostril.
8) If using more than one spray in each nostril, wait five minutes between sprays.

BRAND NAME: Vanceril

GENERIC NAME: beclomethasone dipropionate

GENERIC FORM AVAILABLE: No

THERAPEUTIC CLASS: Steroid inhaler

DOSAGE FORMS: 42-micrograms-per-inhalation metered-dose inhaler

MAIN USES: Asthma and (other diseases causing inflammation in the lungs)

USUAL DOSE: one to two inhalations three to four times daily or four inhalations twice daily

AVERAGE PRICE: $44.95

SIDE EFFECTS: Most common: cough, dry mouth, hoarseness, and throat irritation. Less common: dry throat, headache, nausea, skin bruising, unpleasant taste, and thrush.

DRUG INTERACTIONS: Caution should be used when taking this drug with other oral corticosteroids such as Aristocort, Decadron, Deltasone, Medrol, and prednisone.

ALLERGIES: Individuals allergic to beclomethasone dipropionate, systemic corticosteroids, or other inhaled steroids (such as those listed under "Other Drugs in the Same Therapeutic Class") should discuss this with their doctor or pharmacist before taking this drug.

PREGNANCY/BREAST-FEEDING: Category C—Risk cannot be ruled out. Human studies are lacking, and animal studies are either positive for fetal risk or lacking as well. However, potential benefits may justify the potential risk in using the drug. It is not known whether the drug is excreted in the breast milk; therefore, caution should be used when breast-feeding.

OTHER BRAND NAMES: Beclovent

OTHER DRUGS IN THE SAME THERAPEUTIC CLASS: Aerobid, Azmacort, Beclovent, and Flovent

IMPORTANT INFORMATION TO REMEMBER: The drug is not intended to provide immediate relief of a bronchospasm, shortness of breath, or an asthma attack. To receive the full benefits of the drug, use it on a regular basis as a maintenance medication. The drug may take up to four weeks before noticeable benefits may be seen. Never exceed the prescribed dosage unless directed to do so by a doctor—excessive use beyond the prescribed dosage is potentially dangerous. If another inhaler is also being used at the same time, use the other one a few minutes prior to using Vanceril.

When using the inhaler, use the following procedure:

1) Shake the canister well.
2) Place the mouthpiece close to the mouth, but not touching the lips.

3) Exhale deeply.
4) Inhale slowly and deeply as you press the top of the canister to release the medication.
5) Hold your breath for a few seconds before exhaling.
6) Wait five minutes between puffs.
7) Rinse your mouth out with water after use; otherwise this drug may cause a fungal infection in the mouth.
8) Be sure to wash the inhaler device (mouthpiece) regularly with warm soapy water to avoid bacterial contamination.

BRAND NAME: Vancocin (oral forms only)

GENERIC NAME: vancomycin

GENERIC FORM AVAILABLE: No

THERAPEUTIC CLASS: GI tract antibiotic

DOSAGE FORMS: 125-mg and 250-mg capsules; and 1-g and 10-g powder for oral solution

MAIN USES: Stomach and intestinal infections

USUAL DOSE: 500 mg to 2000 mg daily in three to four divided doses

AVERAGE PRICE: $132.30 for 125 mg (20 capsules) and $264.61 for 250 mg (20 capsules)

SIDE EFFECTS: Most common: bitter or unpleasant taste, mouth irritation, nausea, and vomiting. Less common: skin rash.

DRUG INTERACTIONS: Colestid and Questran may bind up the drug, which makes it ineffective.

ALLERGIES: Individuals allergic to vancomycin or any of their derivatives should discuss this with their doctor or pharmacist before using this drug.

PREGNANCY/BREAST-FEEDING: Category C—Risk cannot be ruled out. Human studies are lacking, and animal studies are either positive for fetal risk or lacking as well. However, potential benefits may justify the potential risk in using the drug. The drug is excreted in the breast milk; therefore, extreme caution should be used when breast-feeding.

OTHER BRAND NAMES: None

OTHER DRUGS IN THE SAME THERAPEUTIC CLASS: None

IMPORTANT INFORMATION TO REMEMBER: Take the drug at even intervals around the clock (if four times a day, take every six hours). Take the drug until all the medication prescribed is gone; otherwise the infection may return. Check with your pharmacist or physician if diarrhea occurs while taking this drug.

BRAND NAME: Vantin

GENERIC NAME: cefpodoxime

GENERIC FORM AVAILABLE: No

THERAPEUTIC CLASS: Cephalosporin antibiotic

DOSAGE FORMS: 100-mg and 200-mg tablets; 50 mg/5 mL; and 100 mg/5 mL oral suspension

MAIN USES: Bacterial infections

USUAL DOSE: 100 mg and 200 mg every 12 hours

AVERAGE PRICE: $61.74 for 100 mg (20 tablets) and $104.46 for 200 mg (20 tablets)

SIDE EFFECTS: diarrhea 7%, nausea 4%, diaper rash 4%, vaginal yeast infections 3%, stomach pain 2%, rash 1%, headache 1%, and vomiting 1%.

DRUG INTERACTIONS: The drug may decrease the effectiveness of oral contraceptives used for birth control. Women may become pregnant while taking Vantin and oral contraceptives. The drug probenecid will decrease elimination of the drug by the kidneys. Axid, Pepcid, Tagamet, Zantac, and antacids may decrease the absorption of the drug.

ALLERGIES: Individuals allergic to cefpodoxime, penicillins (including amoxicillin and ampicillin), or other cephalosporins (such as those listed under "Other Drugs in the Same Therapeutic Class") should discuss this with their doctor or pharmacist before taking this drug.

PREGNANCY/BREAST-FEEDING: Category B—No evidence of risk in humans. Either animal findings show risk, but human findings do not; or, if no adequate human studies have been done, animal findings show no risk. The drug is excreted in the breast milk; therefore, extreme caution should be used when breast-feeding.

OTHER BRAND NAMES: None

OTHER DRUGS IN THE SAME THERAPEUTIC CLASS: Ceclor, Cedax, Ceftin, Cefzil, Duricef, Keflex, Keftab, Suprax, Ultracef, and Velosef

IMPORTANT INFORMATION TO REMEMBER: The drug should be taken with food or milk to enhance its absorption. Also, take the drug at even intervals around the clock (if two times a day, take every 12 hours). Take the drug until all the medication prescribed is gone; otherwise the infection may return. Women taking birth control pills should use another form of contraception while taking the drug and for the rest of the current menstrual cycle. Individuals taking the liquid form should shake it thoroughly before use, store the medication in the refrigerator, and discard any remaining medication after 14 days.

BRAND NAME: Varivax

GENERIC NAME: varicella virus vaccine live

GENERIC FORM AVAILABLE: No

THERAPEUTIC CLASS: Vaccines

DOSAGE FORMS: 0.5-mL subcutaneous injection

MAIN USES: Chickenpox vaccination

USUAL DOSE: Adults and children 13 years or older: one dose of 0.5-mL injection and a second injection of 0.5 mL four to eight weeks later. Children: Under 12 months not recommended; over 12 months to 13 years old, one 0.5-mL injection.

AVERAGE PRICE: $50 to $60 per injection

SIDE EFFECTS: injection-site complaints (soreness, redness, swelling, itching, rash, or numbness) 24%–32%, fever 10%, and rash (chickenpoxlike) 1%–6%; other side effects may include chills, cough, nervousness, insomnia, diaper rash, diarrhea, vomiting, upper respiratory illness, headache, and tiredness.

DRUG INTERACTIONS: Individuals should not take aspirin or aspirin-containing compounds for at least six weeks after the vaccination.

ALLERGIES: Individuals allergic to the varicella virus, eggs, or any of their derivatives should discuss this with their doctor or pharmacist before using this drug.

PREGNANCY/BREAST-FEEDING: Category C—Risk cannot be ruled out. Human studies are lacking, and animal studies are either positive for fetal risk or lacking as well. However, potential benefits may justify the potential risk in using the drug. It is not known whether the drug is excreted in the breast milk; therefore, caution should be used when breast-feeding.

OTHER BRAND NAMES: None

OTHER DRUGS IN THE SAME THERAPEUTIC CLASS: None

IMPORTANT INFORMATION TO REMEMBER: Discuss previous medical problems with your doctor before the vaccine is given. Individuals with immune system problems should not receive this vaccine.

BRAND NAME: Vascor

GENERIC NAME: bepridil

GENERIC FORM AVAILABLE: No

THERAPEUTIC CLASS: Calcium channel blocker

DOSAGE FORMS: 200-mg, 300-mg, and 400-mg tablets

MAIN USES: Angina

USUAL DOSE: 100 mg to 300 mg once daily

AVERAGE PRICE: $320.89 for 200 mg; $420.18 for 300 mg; and $539.58 for 400 mg

SIDE EFFECTS: dizziness 15%, nausea 12%, headache 11%, weakness 10%, diarrhea 8%, nervousness 7%, tremor 5%, stomach disorders 4%, drowsiness 4%, trouble breathing 4%, dry mouth 3%, appetite changes 3%, stomach pain 3%, hand tremors 3%, constipation 3%, numbness 2%, and flu-like symptoms 2%.

DRUG INTERACTIONS: The effects of Blocadren, Cartrol, Corgard, Inderal, Kerlone, Levatol, Lopressor, Minipress, Normodyne, Norpace, Sectral, Tenormin, Toprol-XL, Trandate, Visken, and Zebeta may be increased when taken with this drug. The drug may increase the blood levels of Tegretol, Sandimmune, Lanoxin, Quinidex, Quinaglute, and Procan. Anafranil, Asendin, Endep, Norpramin, Pamelor, Procan, Quinidex, Quinaglute, Sinequan, Surmontil, Tofranil, and Vivactil may cause potentially serious adverse effects on the heart.

ALLERGIES: Individuals allergic to bepridil or any of its derivatives should discuss this with their doctor or pharmacist before using this drug.

PREGNANCY/BREAST-FEEDING: Category C—Risk cannot be ruled out. Human studies are lacking, and animal studies are either positive for fetal risk or lacking as well. However, potential benefits may justify the potential risk in using the drug. The drug is excreted in the breast milk; therefore, extreme caution should be used when breast-feeding.

OTHER BRAND NAMES: None

OTHER DRUGS IN THE SAME THERAPEUTIC CLASS: Adalat, Adalat CC, Calan, Calan SR, Cardene, Cardene SR, Cardizem, Cardizem CD, Cardizem SR, Covera-HS, Dilacor XR, DynaCirc, Isoptin, Isoptin SR, Norvasc, Plendil, Procardia, Procardia XL, Sular, and Verelan

IMPORTANT INFORMATION TO REMEMBER: Only take the drug actly as directed by your physician. Do not discontinue taking the drug without first consulting your physician. Before taking over-the-counter cold and allergy preparations, consult your doctor or pharmacist—these products may raise your blood pressure. This drug may cause some tiredness at first. Individuals should use caution when driving, operating machinery, or performing any task where mental alertness is required.

BRAND NAME: **Vaseretic**

GENERIC NAME: Combination product containing: enalapril and hydrochlorothiazide

See individual entries for Vasotec and HydroDIURIL

BRAND NAME: **Vasotec**

GENERIC NAME: enalapril

GENERIC FORM AVAILABLE: No

THERAPEUTIC CLASS: ACE inhibitor

DOSAGE FORMS: 2.5-mg, 5-mg, 10-mg, and 20-mg tablets

MAIN USES: High blood pressure and heart failure

USUAL DOSE: 5 mg to 40 mg daily in one or two divided doses

AVERAGE PRICE: $89.73 for 2.5 mg; $114.00 for 5 mg; $119.70 for 10 mg; and $170.28 for 20 mg

SIDE EFFECTS: headache 5%, dizziness 4%, tiredness 3%, weakness 1%, rash 1%, cough 1%, nausea 1%, and low blood pressure 1%.

DRUG INTERACTIONS: May decrease the absorption of the antibiotic Sumycin and other tetracycline antibiotics. High potassium levels may occur when used together with Dyrenium and Aldactone, and potassium supplements such as Micro-K, K-Dur, Klor-Con, K-Lyte, and Slow-K. Patients on water pills, especially those recently started on a water pill, may experience low blood pressure. The drug may also increase the toxic effects of Eskalith and Lithobid, especially when taken with a water pill.

ALLERGIES: Individuals allergic to enalapril or other ACE inhibitors (such as those listed under "Other Drugs in the Same Therapeutic Class") should discuss this with their doctor or pharmacist before using this drug.

PREGNANCY/BREAST-FEEDING: Category C (first trimester)—Risk cannot be ruled out. Human studies are lacking, and animal studies are either positive for fetal risk or lacking as well. However, potential benefits may justify the potential risk in using the drug. Category D (second and third trimesters)—Positive evidence of risk. Human studies show risk to the fetus. Nevertheless, potential benefits may possibly outweigh the potential risk. This drug should not be taken by nursing mothers.

OTHER BRAND NAMES: None

OTHER DRUGS IN THE SAME THERAPEUTIC CLASS: Accupril, Altace, Capoten, Lotensin, Mavik, Monopril, Prinivil, Univasc, and Zestril

IMPORTANT INFORMATION TO REMEMBER: Take this drug regularly and exactly as directed by your physician. Do not stop taking the drug unless otherwise directed by your doctor. Avoid salt substitutes containing potassium. Before taking over-the-counter cold and allergy preparations, consult your doctor or pharmacist—these products may raise your blood pressure. If you experience swelling of the face, lips, or tongue or difficulty in breathing, contact your doctor immediately.

BRAND NAME: V-Cillin-K

GENERIC NAME: penicillin V potassium

See entry for Veetids

BRAND NAME: Veetids

GENERIC NAME: penicillin V potassium

GENERIC FORM AVAILABLE: No

THERAPEUTIC CLASS: Penicillin antibiotic

DOSAGE FORMS: 250-mg and 500-mg tablets; 125 mg/5 mL and 250 mg/5 mL oral solution

MAIN USES: Bacterial infections

USUAL DOSE: 250 mg to 500 mg every six to eight hours. Doses for small children may be less.

AVERAGE PRICE: $13.31 (B)/$9.56 (G) for 250 mg (40 tablets) and $15.51 (B)/$12.34 (G) for 500 mg (40 tablets)

SIDE EFFECTS: Most common: mild diarrhea, nausea, vomiting, headache, and yeast infections. Less common: allergic reactions, itching, and skin rash.

DRUG INTERACTIONS: The drug may decrease the effectiveness of birth control pills. The drug probenecid will decrease elimination of the drug by the kidneys. The drug may increase the blood levels of Rheumatrex.

ALLERGIES: Individuals allergic to penicillin or any of its derivatives—including other penicillins (such as ampicillin and amoxicillin)—and cephalosporins should discuss this with their doctor or pharmacist before taking this drug.

PREGNANCY/BREAST-FEEDING: Category B—No evidence of risk in humans. Either animal findings show risk, but human findings do not; or, if no adequate human studies have been done, animal findings show no risk. The drug is excreted in the breast milk; therefore, extreme caution should be used when breast-feeding.

OTHER BRAND NAMES: Pen•Vee K and V-Cillin-K

OTHER DRUGS IN THE SAME THERAPEUTIC CLASS: Amoxil, Omnipen, and Spectrobid

IMPORTANT INFORMATION TO REMEMBER: If possible, take the drug on an empty stomach—one hour before meals or two hours after meals. Also, take the drug at even intervals around the clock (if four times a day, take every six hours). Take the drug until all the medication prescribed is gone; otherwise the infection may return. Women taking birth control pills should use another form of contraception while taking the drug and for the rest of the current menstrual cycle. Individuals taking the liquid form should shake it thoroughly before use, store the medication in the refrigerator, and discard any remaining medication after 14 days.

BRAND NAME: Ventolin

GENERIC NAME: albuterol

See entry for Proventil/Proventil HFD

BRAND NAME: Verelan

GENERIC NAME: verapamil

GENERIC FORM AVAILABLE: No

THERAPEUTIC CLASS: Calcium channel blocker

DOSAGE FORMS: 120-mg, 180-mg, 240-mg, and 360-mg sustained-release capsules

MAIN USES: High blood pressure

USUAL DOSE: 120 mg to 360 mg as a single dose in the morning

AVERAGE PRICE: $158.11 for 120 mg; $165.60 for 180 mg; $186.91 for 240 mg; and $201.32 for 360 mg

SIDE EFFECTS: constipation 7%, headache 5%, dizziness 4%, tiredness 3%, nausea 3%, rash 1%, ankle swelling 1%, insomnia 1%, and muscle pain 1%.

DRUG INTERACTIONS: The effects of Blocadren, Cartrol, Corgard, Inderal, Kerlone, Levatol, Lopressor, Minipress, Normodyne, Norpace, Sectral, Tenormin, Toprol-XL, Trandate, Visken, and Zebeta may be increased when taken with this drug. The drug may increase the blood levels of Tegretol, Sandimmune, Lanoxin, Quinidex, Quinaglute, and Procan.

ALLERGIES: Individuals allergic to verapamil or any of its derivatives should discuss this with their doctor or pharmacist before using this drug.

PREGNANCY/BREAST-FEEDING: Category C—Risk cannot be ruled out. Human studies are lacking, and animal studies are either positive for fetal risk or lacking as well. However, potential benefits may justify the potential risk in using the drug. The drug is excreted in the breast milk; therefore, extreme caution should be used when breast-feeding.

OTHER BRAND NAMES: None

OTHER DRUGS IN THE SAME THERAPEUTIC CLASS: Adalat, Adalat CC, Calan, Calan SR, Cardene, Cardene SR, Cardizem, Cardizem CD, Cardizem SR, Covera-HS, Dilacor XR, DynaCirc, Isoptin, Isoptin SR, Norvasc, Plendil, Procardia, Procardia XL, Sular, and Vascor

IMPORTANT INFORMATION TO REMEMBER: This drug should be taken with food or milk. Only take the drug exactly as directed by your physician. Do not discontinue taking the drug without first consulting your physician. Before taking over-the-counter cold and allergy preparations, consult your doctor or pharmacist—these products may raise your blood pressure. This drug may cause some tiredness at first. Individuals should use caution when driving, operating machinery, or performing any task where mental alertness is required. Individuals having trouble swallowing the capsules can open them up, sprinkle the contents onto soft food (such as applesauce), and swallow without chewing.

BRAND NAME: Vermox

GENERIC NAME: mebendazole

GENERIC FORM AVAILABLE: No

THERAPEUTIC CLASS: Anti-worm

DOSAGE FORMS: 100-mg chewable tablets

MAIN USES: Pinworm, whipworm, common roundworm, and hookworm (intestinal worms)

USUAL DOSE: For pinworm: one tablet once daily. For all other types of worms: one tablet in the morning and evening for three days.

AVERAGE PRICE: $25.08 for three tablets

SIDE EFFECTS: Most common: none. Less common: stomach pain, nausea, diarrhea, and vomiting.

DRUG INTERACTIONS: Tagamet may increase the blood levels of the drug.

ALLERGIES: Individuals allergic to mebendazole or any of its derivatives should discuss this with their doctor or pharmacist before using this drug.

PREGNANCY/BREAST-FEEDING: Category C—Risk cannot be ruled out. Human studies are lacking, and animal studies are either positive for fetal risk or lacking as well. However, potential benefits may justify the potential risk in using the drug. It is not known whether the drug is excreted in the breast milk; therefore, caution should be used when breast-feeding.

OTHER BRAND NAMES: None

OTHER DRUGS IN THE SAME THERAPEUTIC CLASS: None

IMPORTANT INFORMATION TO REMEMBER: The tablets may be chewed, swallowed whole, crushed, or mixed with food. Take the drug at even intervals around the clock (if two times a day, take every 12 hours). Take the drug until all the medication prescribed is gone; otherwise the worm infection may return. If the individual is not cured within three weeks of treatment, a second course of treatment should be conducted. Individuals with these types of infections should always wash their hands after a bowel movement to avoid reinfection. Due to the easy spread of pinworm infections, it is recommended that all family members or people with close contact to the infected individual be treated.

BRAND NAME: Vexol

GENERIC NAME: rimexolone

GENERIC FORM AVAILABLE: No

THERAPEUTIC CLASS: Steroid eyedrop

DOSAGE FORMS: 1% eyedrop suspension

MAIN USES: Inflammation after eye surgery and anterior uveitis

USUAL DOSE: one to two drops four times daily, starting 24 hours after surgery and continuing for approximately two weeks

AVERAGE PRICE: $22.58 for 5 mL

SIDE EFFECTS: blurred vision 1%–5%, discharge from the eye 1%–5%, discomfort 1%–5%, feeling of a foreign body in the eye 1%–5%, pain 1%–5%, itching 1%–5%, stinging 1%–5%, and increased intraocular pressure 1%–5%.

DRUG INTERACTIONS: The drug may decrease the effects of other eyedrops used to treat glaucoma.

ALLERGIES: Individuals allergic to rimexolone or any of its derivatives should discuss this with their doctor or pharmacist before using this drug.

PREGNANCY/BREAST-FEEDING: Category C—Risk cannot be ruled out. Human studies are lacking, and animal studies are either positive for fetal risk or lacking as well. However, potential benefits may justify the potential risk in using the drug. It is not known whether the drug is excreted in the breast milk; therefore, caution should be used when breast-feeding.

OTHER BRAND NAMES: None

OTHER DRUGS IN THE SAME THERAPEUTIC CLASS: Decadron, Econopred, Flarex, FML, FML Forte, HMS, Inflamase Forte, Inflamase Mild, Maxidex, Pred Mild, and Pred Forte

IMPORTANT INFORMATION TO REMEMBER: Individuals should not use the drug while wearing contact lenses unless directed otherwise by a physician. Keep the container tightly closed and avoid touching the applicator tip to the eye—this could contaminate the product over time. Also, only administer one drop at a time. After application, keep the eye open for at least 30 seconds, roll the eyeball around, and avoid squinting. If a second drop is required, wait one to two minutes between drops. If another medication is to be used in the eye, wait at least 10 minutes before administering it. Shake the medication well before using.

BRAND NAME: Vibramycin and Vibra-Tabs

GENERIC NAME: doxycycline hyclate

GENERIC FORM AVAILABLE: Yes

708   Vibramycin and Vibra-Tabs

THERAPEUTIC CLASS: Tetracycline antibiotic

DOSAGE FORMS: 100-mg tablets (Vibra-Tabs); 50-mg and 100-mg capsules; 50 mg/5 mL syrup; and 25 mg/5 mL oral suspension

MAIN USES: Bacterial infections

USUAL DOSE: 50 mg to 100 mg every 12 hours

AVERAGE PRICE: $57.66 (B)/$13.47 (G) for 50 mg (Vibramycin and Vibra-Tabs) and $90.81 (B)/$18.52 (G) for 100 mg (Vibramycin and Vibra-Tabs)

SIDE EFFECTS: Most common: discoloration on infants' and children's teeth, increased sensitivity to sunburn, dizziness, diarrhea, nausea, vomiting, stomach pain, and burning stomach. Less common: sore or darkened tongue, discoloration of the skin and mucous membranes, and fungal overgrowth.

DRUG INTERACTIONS: Antacids, calcium supplements, iron supplements, magnesium laxatives, and other mineral supplements may bind to the drug in the stomach and intestines and prevent its absorption by the body. The drug may decrease the effectiveness of birth control pills.

ALLERGIES: Individuals allergic to doxycycline or other tetracyclines (such as those listed under "Other Drugs in the Same Therapeutic Class") should discuss this with their doctor or pharmacist before taking this drug.

PREGNANCY/BREAST-FEEDING: Category D—Positive evidence of risk. Human studies show risk to the fetus. Nevertheless, potential benefits may possibly outweigh the potential risks. This drug should not be taken by nursing mothers.

OTHER BRAND NAMES: None

OTHER DRUGS IN THE SAME THERAPEUTIC CLASS: Achromycin V, Doryx, Minocin, Monodox, and Sumycin

IMPORTANT INFORMATION TO REMEMBER: If stomach upset occurs, take the drug with food. Take the drug at the same time every day. Also, take the drug until all the medication prescribed is gone; otherwise the infection may return. Avoid taking antacids, calcium supplements, iron supplements, magnesium laxatives, and other mineral supplements within two hours of taking the drug. Women taking birth control pills should use another form of contraception while taking the drug and for the rest of the current menstrual cycle. Individuals should also use a sunscreen to avoid overexposure to the sun; the drug may increase the skin's sensitivity to sunlight, which may cause one to sunburn more easily. The drug should not be used by children under eight years of age due to the potential of permanent tooth staining.

BRAND NAME: Vicodin, Vicodin ES, and Vicodin HP

GENERIC NAME: Combination product containing: acetaminophen and hydrocodone

GENERIC FORM AVAILABLE: Yes

THERAPEUTIC CLASS: Narcotic analgesic + pain reliever

DOSAGE FORMS: 5-mg hydrocodone/500-mg acetaminophen tablets (Vicodin); and 7.5-mg hydrocodone/750-mg acetaminophen tablets (Vicodin ES); and 10-mg hydrocodone/660-mg acetaminophen tablets (Vicodin HP)

MAIN USES: Moderate to severe pain

USUAL DOSE: one tablet every 4 to 6 hours as needed (maximum of eight Vicodin, five Vicodin ES, or six Vicodin HP tablets every 24 hours)

AVERAGE PRICE: $55.04 (B)/$26.44 (G) for Vicodin; $60.70 (B)/$43.59 (G) for Vicodin ES; and $65.09 for Vicodin HP

SIDE EFFECTS: Most common: drowsiness, dizziness, tiredness, nausea, vomiting, and histamine release (symptoms include decreased blood pressure, sweating, fast heartbeat, flushing, and wheezing). Less common: confusion, decreased urination, dry mouth, constipation, stomach pain, skin rash, headache, weakness, minor vision disturbances, and hallucinations.

DRUG INTERACTIONS: Alcohol, anxiety medications, and other narcotic painkillers may intensify the drowsiness effect of the drug. Liver toxicity may occur with long-term use of Anturane, Dilantin, and Mesantoin. This drug and Nardil or Parnate may cause severe and sometimes fatal reactions.

ALLERGIES: Individuals allergic to acetaminophen, hydrocodone, other pain relievers, or any of their derivatives should discuss this with their doctor or pharmacist before using this drug.

PREGNANCY/BREAST-FEEDING: Category C—Risk cannot be ruled out. Human studies are lacking, and animal studies are either positive for fetal risk or lacking as well. However, potential benefits may justify the potential risk in using the drug. It is not known whether the drug is excreted in the breast milk; therefore, caution should be used when breast-feeding.

OTHER BRAND NAMES: None

OTHER DRUGS IN THE SAME THERAPEUTIC CLASS: Bancap-HC, Darvocet-N 50, Darvocet-N 100, Darvon, Darvon Compound, DHCplus, Empirin #3, Empirin #4, Hydrocet, Lortab, Lorcet Plus, Lorcet 10/650, Percocet, Percodan, Phenaphen w/Codeine, Synalgos DC, Talacen, Tylenol #2, Tylenol #3, Tylenol #4, Tylox, and Zydone

IMPORTANT INFORMATION TO REMEMBER: This drug does cause drowsiness. Individuals should use caution when driving, operating machinery, or performing any task where mental alertness is required. Alcohol, anxiety medications, and other narcotic painkillers may intensify the drowsiness effect of the drug. If stomach upset occurs, take the drug with food or milk. Do not increase the dose without first consulting with your physician. This medication is a controlled substance and may be habit-forming.

BRAND NAME: Videx

GENERIC NAME: didanosine

GENERIC FORM AVAILABLE: No

THERAPEUTIC CLASS: AIDS antiviral

DOSAGE FORMS: 25-mg, 50-mg, 100-mg, and 150-mg buffered, chewable tablets; 100-mg, 167-mg, 250-mg, and 375-mg packets of powder for oral solution; and pediatric powder for oral solution

MAIN USES: AIDS

USUAL DOSE: 125 mg to 200 mg twice daily of the tablets or 167 mg to 250 mg of the buffered powder twice daily. Doses for children may be less.

AVERAGE PRICE: $51.34 for 25 mg; $103.85 for 50 mg; $207.69 for 100 mg; and $311.57 for 150 mg

SIDE EFFECTS: diarrhea 20%–28%; pain, numbness, or unusual sensations in the arms, legs, feet, and hands 17%–20%; chills 9%–12%; stomach pain 7%–10%; headache 7%–10%; rash 7%–9%; pain 7%; pancreatitis 6%–10%; nausea/vomiting 6%–7%; weakness 5%–7%; infection 5%–6%; pneumonia 5%–6%; dry mouth 2%–3%; muscle pain 2%–3%; trouble breathing 2%–3%; convulsions 2%; nervousness 2%; depression 2%; dizziness 1%; constipation 1%; sweating 1%; and blurred vision 1% (blood disorders and anemia also occur fairly frequently).

DRUG INTERACTIONS: There are numerous drugs that can cause peripheral neuropathy (unusual nerve sensations and damage in the arms, legs, fingers, and toes) when taken with this drug. Some of these are: alcohol, Aldomet, Apresoline, Bactrim, Biaxin, cisplatin, Clinoril, Cytovene, dapsone, Depakene, Depakote, Dilantin, diuretics (water pills), Doryx, Dynabac, erythromycin, Eskalith, estrogens, Flagyl, isoniazid, Lasix, Lithobid, Macrobid, Macrodantin, pentamidine, Septra, Sumycin, Vibramycin, vincristine, and ZERIT. Bactrim, probenecid, and Septra may increase the blood levels of the drug. Biaxin may decrease the blood levels of the drug. The drug may decrease the absorption of dapsone, Nizoral, and Sporanox. The drug may decrease the blood levels of Cipro, Doryx, Floxin, Maxaquin, Minocin, Monodox, Noroxin, Penetrex, Sumycin, and Vibramycin. Before taking any medication, discuss it with your doctor.

ALLERGIES: Individuals allergic to didanosine or any of its derivatives should discuss this with their doctor or pharmacist before using this drug.

PREGNANCY/BREAST-FEEDING: Category B—No evidence of risk in humans. Either animal findings show risk, but human findings do not; or, if no adequate human studies have been done, animal findings show no risk. It is not known whether the drug is excreted in the breast milk; therefore, caution should be used when breast-feeding.

OTHER BRAND NAMES: None

OTHER DRUGS IN THE SAME THERAPEUTIC CLASS: Epivir, HIVID, Retrovir, and ZERIT

IMPORTANT INFORMATION TO REMEMBER: It's best to take the drug on an empty stomach—one hour before meals or two hours after meals—if possible. Also, take the drug at even intervals around the clock (if two times a day, take every 12 hours). Only take the drug exactly as directed by your physician. Do not stop taking the drug without first consulting with your doctor. It is important to have regular blood and liver function tests while taking this drug. Before taking any prescription or over-the-counter (OTC) drugs, consult your doctor or pharmacist. The tablets may be thoroughly chewed, manually crushed, or mixed in one ounce of water before taking them. To mix the tablets with water: add two tablets to at least one ounce of water, mix until the liquid looks uniform, and then drink the entire solution immediately. For the powder packets, mix the powder with about four ounces of water. Do not use fruit juice or other acidic liquids, such as soda pop. Stir the mixture for about two to three minutes and then drink the entire solution immediately.

BRAND NAME: Viokase

GENERIC NAME: Combination product containing: the enzymes lipase, protease, and amylase

Very similar to Pancrease MT. See entry for Pancrease MT.

BRAND NAME: Visken

GENERIC NAME: pindolol

GENERIC FORM AVAILABLE: Yes

THERAPEUTIC CLASS: Noncardioselective beta-blocker

DOSAGE FORMS: 5-mg and 10-mg tablets.

MAIN USES: High blood pressure

USUAL DOSE: 5 mg to 10 mg twice daily

AVERAGE PRICE: $115.78 (B)/$79.46 (G) for 5 mg and $155.50 (B)/ $102.98 (G) for 10 mg

SIDE EFFECTS: insomnia 10%, muscle pain 10%, dizziness 9%, tiredness 8%, nervousness 7%, joint pain 7%, swelling 6%, nausea 5%, trouble breathing 5%, multiple dreams 5%, bizarre dreams 5%, stomach pain 4%, weakness 4%, chest pain 3%, muscle cramps 3%, rash 1%, and itching 1%.

DRUG INTERACTIONS: The drug may cause additive effects when used with reserpine. The drug may increase the effects of Calan,

Cardene, Cardizem, Catapres, Covera-HS, Dilacor XR, DynaCirc, Isoptin, Lanoxin, Norvasc, Plendil, Procardia, Sular, Tiazac, Verelan, and Wytensin. Diabetic medications, insulin, Slo-bid, Theo-Dur, theophylline, Uni-Dur, and Uniphyl dosages may need to be adjusted when taking this drug. The drug may also interfere with glaucoma screening tests. The drug may increase the blood levels of Mellaril, and Mellaril may increase the blood levels of the drug as well.

ALLERGIES: Individuals allergic to pindolol or other beta-blockers (such as those listed under "Other Drugs in the Same Therapeutic Class") should discuss this with their doctor or pharmacist before taking this drug.

PREGNANCY/BREAST-FEEDING: Category B—No evidence of risk in humans. Either animal findings show risk, but human findings do not; or, if no adequate human studies have been done, animal findings show no risk. The drug is excreted in the breast milk; therefore, extreme caution should be used when breast-feeding.

OTHER BRAND NAMES: None

OTHER DRUGS IN THE SAME THERAPEUTIC CLASS: Blocadren, Cartrol, Corgard, Inderal, Levatol, Normodyne, and Trandate

IMPORTANT INFORMATION TO REMEMBER: Only take the drug exactly as directed by your physician. Do not discontinue taking the drug without first consulting your physician. This drug may cause some tiredness, especially at first. Individuals should use caution when driving, operating machinery, or performing any task where mental alertness is required. Alcohol, anxiety medications, or narcotic painkillers may intensify the tiredness effect of the drug. Before taking over-the-counter cold and allergy preparations, consult your doctor or pharmacist—these products may raise your blood pressure. This drug may mask the symptoms of low blood sugar in diabetics.

BRAND NAME: Vistaril

GENERIC NAME: hydroxyzine pamoate

GENERIC FORM AVAILABLE: Yes

THERAPEUTIC CLASS: Antihistamine

DOSAGE FORMS: 25-mg, 50-mg, and 100-mg capsules; and 25 mg/5 mL suspension

MAIN USES: Allergic reactions, itching, allergies, anxiety, and as a (sedative)

USUAL DOSE: 50 mg to 100 mg four times daily for anxiety and 25 mg three to four times daily for allergic reactions and itching

AVERAGE PRICE: $100.67 (B)/$21.40 (G) for 25 mg and $142.47 (B)/$28.18 (G) for 50 mg

SIDE EFFECTS: Most common: drowsiness, thickening of mucus, and dry mouth. Less common: blurred vision, difficult or painful urination, dizziness, fast heartbeat, increased sweating, increased appetite, and nausea.

DRUG INTERACTIONS: Central nervous system (CNS) depression may be increased when used with alcohol, anxiety medications, or narcotic painkillers. The drug should not be taken with Nardil and Parnate. The drug should also not be used with Akineton, Artane, Cogentin, or Kemadrin.

ALLERGIES: Individuals allergic to hydroxyzine, Atarax, or any of their derivatives should discuss this with their doctor or pharmacist before using this drug.

PREGNANCY/BREAST-FEEDING: Category C—Risk cannot be ruled out. Human studies are lacking, and animal studies are either positive for fetal risk or lacking as well. However, potential benefits may justify the potential risk in using the drug. It is not known whether the drug is excreted in the breast milk; therefore, caution should be used when breast-feeding.

OTHER BRAND NAMES: None

OTHER DRUGS IN THE SAME THERAPEUTIC CLASS: Atarax, Benadryl, PBZ, Periactin, Tavist, and Temaril

IMPORTANT INFORMATION TO REMEMBER: This drug may cause drowsiness. Individuals should use caution when driving, operating machinery, or performing any task where mental alertness is required. Alcohol, nerve medication, or narcotic painkillers may intensify the drowsiness effect of the drug. This drug may also cause a dry mouth; sugarless gum or hard candy will help take care of this problem. Patients with glaucoma or urinary or prostate problems should consult their doctor before taking this drug.

BRAND NAME: Vivactil

GENERIC NAME: protriptyline

GENERIC FORM AVAILABLE: No

THERAPEUTIC CLASS: Tricyclic antidepressant

DOSAGE FORMS: 5-mg and 10-mg tablets

MAIN USES: Depression

USUAL DOSE: 5 mg to 10 mg three to four times daily

AVERAGE PRICE: $65.08 for 5 mg and $94.30 for 10 mg

SIDE EFFECTS: Most common: drowsiness, dizziness, dry mouth, headache, increased appetite, nausea, tiredness, weight gain, and unpleasant taste. Less common: diarrhea, excessive sweating, heartburn, insomnia, vomiting, irregular heartbeat, muscle tremors, urinary difficulties, and impotence.

DRUG INTERACTIONS: The drug should not be taken with Nardil or Parnate. In fact, 14 days are needed between the time of the use of Nardil or Parnate and this drug. Alcohol, anxiety medications, and narcotic painkillers may make the drowsiness caused by the drug much worse. Compazine, Mellaril, Prolixin, Serentil, Stelazine, Thorazine, and Trilafon may increase the blood levels of the drug. Tagamet may increase the blood levels of the drug. The drug may decrease the effects of Catapres and Ismelin. The drug may increase the effects of decongestants found in cough, cold, and allergy products on the heart, possibly causing high blood pressure, fast heartbeat, or irregular heartbeats.

ALLERGIES: Individuals allergic to protriptyline or other tricyclic antidepressants (such as those listed under "Other Drugs in the Same Therapeutic Class") should discuss this with their doctor or pharmacist before taking this drug.

PREGNANCY/BREAST-FEEDING: Category C—Risk cannot be ruled out. Human studies are lacking, and animal studies are either positive for fetal risk or lacking as well. However, potential benefits may justify the potential risk in using the drug. The drug is excreted in the breast milk; therefore, extreme caution should be used when breast-feeding.

OTHER BRAND NAMES: None

OTHER DRUGS IN THE SAME THERAPEUTIC CLASS: Asendin, Elavil, Endep, Norpramin, Pamelor, Sinequan, Surmontil, and Tofranil

IMPORTANT INFORMATION TO REMEMBER: Only take the drug exactly as directed by your physician. Do not discontinue taking the drug without first consulting your physician. The drug may require one to six weeks of use before improvement may be noticed. This drug does cause drowsiness. Individuals should use caution when driving, operating machinery, or performing any task where mental alertness is required. Alcohol, anxiety medications, and narcotic painkillers may intensify the drowsiness effect of the drug. The drug may cause a slight amount of dizziness or lightheadedness when rising from a sitting or lying-down position. Individuals should also use a sunscreen to avoid overexposure to the sun; the drug may increase the skin's sensitivity to sunlight, which may cause one to sunburn more easily.

BRAND NAME: Volmax

GENERIC NAME: albuterol

GENERIC FORM AVAILABLE: No

THERAPEUTIC CLASS: Beta-2-agonist bronchodilator

DOSAGE FORMS: 4-mg and 8-mg extended-release tablets

MAIN USES: Bronchospasm, {asthma}, and {other breathing disorders}

USUAL DOSE: 4 mg to 8 mg every 12 hours

AVERAGE PRICE: $88.53 for 4 mg and $164.38 for 8 mg

SIDE EFFECTS: tremor 24%, headache 19%, nervousness 9%, nausea 4%, fast heartbeat 3%, muscle cramps 3%, insomnia 2%, dizziness 2%, pounding heartbeat 2%, and drowsiness 1%.

DRUG INTERACTIONS: Decongestants in cough, cold, and allergy products, along with Asendin, Endep, Elavil, Nardil, Norpramin, Pamelor, Parnate, Sinequan, Surmontil, Tofranil, and Vivactil, may increase the toxicity of this drug. Blocadren, Cartrol, Corgard, Inderal, Levatol, Normodyne, reserpine, Trandate, and Visken may decrease the effects of the drug.

ALLERGIES: Individuals allergic to albuterol, Proventil, Ventolin, or any of their derivatives should discuss this with their doctor or pharmacist before using this drug.

PREGNANCY/BREAST-FEEDING: Category C—Risk cannot be ruled out. Human studies are lacking, and animal studies are either positive for fetal risk or lacking as well. However, potential benefits may justify the potential risk in using the drug. It is not known whether the drug is excreted in the breast milk; therefore, caution should be used when breast-feeding.

OTHER BRAND NAMES: None

OTHER DRUGS IN THE SAME THERAPEUTIC CLASS: Alupent, Brethine, Bricanyl, Metaprel, Proventil, and Ventolin

IMPORTANT INFORMATION TO REMEMBER: Only take the drug exactly as directed by your physician. Never increase the dose of the drug without consulting with your physician. Prolonged use of the drug may cause tolerance to its effects to develop. If stomach upset occurs, take the drug with food or milk. Do not crush, cut, or chew the tablets—this will destroy the mechanism that delays the release of the medication. The tablets should be swallowed whole.

BRAND NAME: Voltaren and Voltaren XR

GENERIC NAME: diclofenac sodium

GENERIC FORM AVAILABLE: Yes (Voltaren only)

THERAPEUTIC CLASS: Nonsteroidal anti-inflammatory drug (NSAID)

DOSAGE FORMS: 25-mg, 50-mg, and 75-mg enteric coated tablets; and 100-mg extended-release tablets (Voltaren XR)

MAIN USES: Arthritis, pain relief, and menstrual pain

USUAL DOSE: 25 mg to 50 mg three to four times daily, 75 mg twice daily, or 100 mg once daily (Voltaren XR)

AVERAGE PRICE: $72.57 (B)/$65.91 (G) for 25 mg; $141.07 (B)/$126.02 (G) for 50 mg; $170.85 (B)/$151.85 (G) for 75 mg; and $274.25 for 100 mg (Voltaren XR)

SIDE EFFECTS: headache 7%, stomach pain 3%–9%, upset stomach 3%–9%, diarrhea 3%–9%, indigestion 3%–9%, constipation 3%–9%, peptic ulcer 1%–3%, stomach swelling 1%–3%, gas 1%–3%, rash 1%–3%, dizziness 3%, and ringing in the ears 1%–3%.

DRUG INTERACTIONS: Aspirin will decrease the concentration of this drug in the blood. This drug may also decrease the effects of Lasix, Dyazide, HydroDIURIL, Maxzide, and other water pills. The drug may increase the blood levels of Eskalith, Lithobid, and Sandimmune. The drug may increase the toxic effects of the drug Rheumatrex. Caution should be used when taking the drug with Coumadin.

ALLERGIES: Individuals allergic to diclofenac or other NSAIDs (such as those listed under "Other Drugs in the Same Therapeutic Class") should discuss this with their doctor or pharmacist before taking this drug.

PREGNANCY/BREAST-FEEDING: Category B—No evidence of risk in humans. Either animal findings show risk, but human findings do not; or, if no adequate human studies have been done, animal findings show no risk. The drug should not, however, be used during the late stages (last three months) of pregnancy. The drug is excreted in the breast milk; therefore, extreme caution should be used when breast-feeding.

OTHER BRAND NAMES: None

OTHER DRUGS IN THE SAME THERAPEUTIC CLASS: Anaprox, Ansaid, aspirin, Cataflam, Clinoril, Daypro, Disalcid, Dolobid, Easprin, Feldene, Indocin, Lodine, Motrin, Nalfon, Naprosyn, Orudis, Oruvail, Relafen, Tolectin, and Toradol

IMPORTANT INFORMATION TO REMEMBER: This drug should be taken with food or milk to reduce the potential for injury to the stomach lining and stomach upset. This drug may take up to two weeks before a noticeable improvement in pain relief associated with arthritis is observed. Drinking alcohol while taking this drug may increase its potential to cause ulcers. This drug should only be used under the direct supervision of a doctor by individuals with a bleeding disorder or ulcer, or those who are currently taking Coumadin. Before taking over-the-counter pain relievers, consult your doctor or pharmacist. No more than one pain reliever should be taken at any one time unless otherwise directed by your doctor.

BRAND NAME: Wellbutrin and Wellbutrin SR

GENERIC NAME: bupropion

GENERIC FORM AVAILABLE: No

THERAPEUTIC CLASS: antidepressant

DOSAGE FORMS: 75-mg and 100-mg tablets (Wellbutrin); and 100-mg and 150-mg sustained-release tablets (Wellbutrin SR)

MAIN USES: Depression

USUAL DOSE: 100 mg three times daily (Wellbutrin) or 100 mg to 150 mg once or twice daily (Wellbutrin SR)

AVERAGE PRICE: $78.80 for 75 mg and $105.15 for 100 mg (Wellbutrin); $165.76 for 100 mg and $171.89 for 150 mg (Wellbutrin SR)

SIDE EFFECTS: agitation 32%, dry mouth 28%, headache 26%, constipation 26%, weight loss 23%, nausea 23%, dizziness 22%, tremors 22%, drowsiness 20%, insomnia 19%, loss of appetite 18%, blurred vision 15%, weight gain 14%, fast heartbeat 11%, rash 8%, nervous system problems 8%, confusion 8%, diarrhea 7%, irregular heartbeat 5%, menstrual complaints 5%, hostility 5%, tiredness 5%, hearing disturbances 5%, impaired sleep quality 4%, sensory disturbances 4%, high blood pressure 4%, appetite increase 4%, pounding heartbeat 4%, increased salivation 3%, low blood pressure 3%, impotence 3%, increased urination 3%, decreased concentration 3%, decreased sex drive 3%, muscle disturbances 2%, and dizziness 1%.

DRUG INTERACTIONS: Alcohol, Clozaril, Desyrel, Eskalith, Haldol, Lithobid, Loxitane, Ludiomil, Moban, Navane, and Prozac may make seizures more likely in some individuals. Anafranil, Asendin, Compazine, Elavil, Endep, Mellaril, Norpramin, Pamelor, Prolixin, Serentil, Sinequan, Stelazine, Surmontil, Thorazine, Tofranil, Trilafon, and Vivactil may also promote seizures in some individuals. Therefore, there's an increase in the risk of having a major seizure if the drug is taken with one of the drugs listed above. The drug should not be taken with Nardil or Parnate. In fact, 14 days are needed between the time of the use of Nardil or Parnate and this drug.

ALLERGIES: Individuals allergic to bupropion or any of its derivatives should discuss this with their doctor or pharmacist before using this drug.

PREGNANCY/BREAST-FEEDING: Category B—No evidence of risk in humans. Either animal findings show risk, but human findings do not; or, if no adequate human studies have been done, animal findings show no risk. The drug is excreted in the breast milk; therefore, extreme caution should be used when breast-feeding.

OTHER BRAND NAMES: None

OTHER DRUGS IN THE SAME THERAPEUTIC CLASS: None

IMPORTANT INFORMATION TO REMEMBER: Only take the drug exactly as directed by your physician. Do not discontinue taking the drug without first consulting your physician and do not double dose. The drug may require up to four weeks or longer of use before improvement may be noticed. This drug does cause drowsiness. Individuals should use caution when driving, operating machinery, or performing any task where mental alertness is required. Alcohol, anxiety medications, and narcotic painkillers may intensify the drowsiness effect of the drug. Do not take over-the-counter (OTC) medications without first consulting your physician or pharmacist. If a seizure occurs, notify your physician immediately. This drug should not be used by patients with epilepsy or other seizure disorders.

BRAND NAME: Westcort

GENERIC NAME: hydrocortisone valerate

GENERIC FORM AVAILABLE: No

THERAPEUTIC CLASS: Topical corticosteroid

DOSAGE FORMS: 0.2% cream and ointment

MAIN USES: Skin rashes, swelling, and itching

USUAL DOSE: Apply thin film two to three times daily.

AVERAGE PRICE: $18.99 for 0.2% cream and ointment (15 g)

SIDE EFFECTS: Most common: none. Less common: burning, itching, stinging, rash, dryness, and skin redness.

DRUG INTERACTIONS: None of any clinical significance

ALLERGIES: Individuals allergic to hydrocortisone or any of its derivatives should discuss this with their doctor or pharmacist before using this drug.

PREGNANCY/BREAST-FEEDING: Category C—Risk cannot be ruled out. Human studies are lacking, and animal studies are either positive for fetal risk or lacking as well. However, potential benefits may justify the potential risk in using the drug. It is not known whether the drug is excreted in the breast milk; therefore, caution should be used when breast-feeding.

OTHER BRAND NAMES: None

OTHER DRUGS IN THE SAME THERAPEUTIC CLASS: Aclovate, Aristocort, Cordran, Cordran SP, Cutivate, Cyclocort, DesOwen, Diprolene, Diprolene AF, Elocon, Florone, Florone E, Halog, Hytone, Kenalog, Lidex, Lidex E, Synalar, Temovate, Topicort, Tridesilon, Ultravate, and Valisone

IMPORTANT INFORMATION TO REMEMBER: This drug is for external use only. Apply only a thin film of drug to skin and rub it in well. Never cover the skin after application with a bandage or wrapping unless directed to do so by a doctor. Never apply to damaged skin or open wounds unless directed to do so by a doctor. Discontinue use if irritation occurs.

BRAND NAME: Wigraine

GENERIC NAME: Combination product containing: ergotamine and caffeine

See entry for Cafergot

BRAND NAME: Wygesic

GENERIC NAME: Combination product containing: propoxyphene and acetaminophen

Very similar to Darvocet-N 100. See entry for Darvocet-N.

BRAND NAME: Wymox

GENERIC NAME: amoxicillin

See entry for Amoxil

BRAND NAME: Wytensin

GENERIC NAME: guanabenz

GENERIC FORM AVAILABLE: Yes

THERAPEUTIC CLASS: Centrally acting blood vessel dilator

DOSAGE FORMS: 4-mg and 8-mg tablets

MAIN USES: High blood pressure

USUAL DOSE: 4 mg to 8 mg twice daily

AVERAGE PRICE: $103.05 (B)/$82.12 (G) for 4 mg and $154.71 (B)/$119.73 (G) for 8 mg

SIDE EFFECTS: Most common: dizziness, drowsiness, dry mouth, and weakness. Less common: headache, nausea, and decreased sexual ability.

DRUG INTERACTIONS: The effects of other medications for high blood pressure may be increased when taken with this drug.

ALLERGIES: Individuals allergic to guanabenz or any of its derivatives should discuss this with their doctor or pharmacist before using this drug.

PREGNANCY/BREAST-FEEDING: Category C—Risk cannot be ruled out. Human studies are lacking, and animal studies are either positive for fetal risk or lacking as well. However, potential benefits may justify the potential risk in using the drug. It is not known whether the drug is excreted in the breast milk; therefore, caution should be used when breast-feeding.

OTHER BRAND NAMES: None

OTHER DRUGS IN THE SAME THERAPEUTIC CLASS: Tenex

IMPORTANT INFORMATION TO REMEMBER: The drug may cause drowsiness and/or dizziness, especially when treatment is begun or daily dosage is increased. Alcohol, anxiety medications, and narcotic painkillers may intensify the drowsiness effect of the drug. Drowsiness may go away once the body adjusts to the medication. Before taking over-the-counter cold and allergy preparations, consult your doctor or pharmacist—these products may raise your blood pressure. If stomach upset occurs, take with food or milk. Tolerance to the effects of alcohol may be decreased while taking this drug. Do not stop taking the drug suddenly.

BRAND NAME: Xalatan

GENERIC NAME: latanoprost

GENERIC FORM AVAILABLE: No

THERAPEUTIC CLASS: Prostaglandin agonist, anti-glaucoma

DOSAGE FORMS: 0.005% eyedrop solution

MAIN USES: Glaucoma

USUAL DOSE: one drop once daily in the evening

AVERAGE PRICE: $42.19 for 2.5 mL

SIDE EFFECTS: blurred vision 5%–15%, burning 5%–15%, stinging 5%–15%, itching 5%–15%, color change of the eyes 5%–15%, feeling of something in the eye 5%–15%, cold and flu 4%, dry eyes 1%–4%, excessive tearing 1%–4%, eye pain 1%–4%, eyelid crusting 1%–4%, eyelid swelling 1%–4%, eye pain 1%–4%, increased sensitivity of the eyes to sunlight 1%–4%, allergic skin reactions 1%–2%, and muscle, joint, and back pain 1%-2%.

DRUG INTERACTIONS: None of any clinical significance

ALLERGIES: Individuals allergic to latanoprost or any of its derivatives should discuss this with their doctor or pharmacist before using this drug.

PREGNANCY/BREAST-FEEDING: Category C—Risk cannot be ruled out. Human studies are lacking, and animal studies are either positive for fetal risk or lacking as well. However, potential benefits may justify the potential risk in using the drug. It is not known whether the drug is excreted in the breast milk; therefore, caution should be used when breast-feeding.

OTHER BRAND NAMES: None

OTHER DRUGS IN THE SAME THERAPEUTIC CLASS: None

IMPORTANT INFORMATION TO REMEMBER: The drug may gradually change eye color. The long-term effects of this color change are unknown. Keep the container tightly closed and avoid touching the applicator tip to the eye—this could contaminate the product over time. Also, only administer one drop at a time. After application, keep the eye open for at least 30 seconds, roll the eyeball around, and avoid squinting. If a second drop is required, wait one to two minutes between drops. If another medication is to be used in the eye, wait at least 10 minutes before administering it.

Only use the drug exactly as directed by your physician. Do not discontinue using the drug without first consulting your physician. Do not increase the dose; using more of the medication than prescribed may actually decrease its effectiveness.

BRAND NAME: Xanax

GENERIC NAME: alprazolam

GENERIC FORM AVAILABLE: Yes

THERAPEUTIC CLASS: Benzodiazepine antianxiety

DOSAGE FORMS: 0.25-mg, 0.5-mg, 1-mg, and 2-mg tablets

MAIN USES: Anxiety and panic disorder

USUAL DOSE: 0.25 mg to 0.5 mg three times daily. Doses for panic disorder may be higher.

AVERAGE PRICE: $64.86 (B)/$33.98 (G) for 0.25 mg; $82.01 (B)/$26.93 (G) for 0.5 mg; $116.07 (B)/$50.14 (G) for 1 mg; and $245.56 (B)/$226.61 (G) for 2 mg

SIDE EFFECTS: drowsiness 41%, lightheadedness 21%, dry mouth 15%, depression 14%, headache 13%, nausea 10%, constipation 10%, diarrhea 10%, confusion 10%, insomnia 9%, fast heartbeat 8%, pounding heartbeat 8%, blurred vision 6%, low blood pressure 5%, muscle tremors 4%, allergic reaction 4%, increased salivation 4%, dizziness 3%, and weight changes 3%.

DRUG INTERACTIONS: Central nervous system (CNS) depression may be increased when used with alcohol, anxiety medications, and narcotic painkillers. The drug may increase the blood levels of Norpramin and Tofranil. Tagamet and birth control pills may increase the blood levels of the drug.

ALLERGIES: Individuals allergic to alprazolam or other benzodiazepines (such as those listed under "Other Drugs in the Same Therapeutic Class") should discuss this with their doctor or pharmacist before taking this drug.

PREGNANCY/BREAST-FEEDING: Category D—Positive evidence of risk. Human studies show risk to the fetus. Nevertheless, potential benefits may possibly outweigh the potential risks. This drug should not be taken by nursing mothers.

OTHER BRAND NAMES: None

OTHER DRUGS IN THE SAME THERAPEUTIC CLASS: Ativan, Librium, Serax, Tranxene, and Valium

IMPORTANT INFORMATION TO REMEMBER: This drug may cause drowsiness. Individuals should use caution when driving, operating machinery, or performing any task where mental alertness is required. The incidence of drowsiness and unsteadiness increases with age. Alcohol, anxiety medications, and narcotic painkillers may intensify the drowsiness effect of the drug. This medication is a controlled substance and may be habit-forming. Do not increase the dose of medication without consulting with your doctor; take only the amount prescribed by your doctor.

BRAND NAME: Yocon

GENERIC NAME: yohimbine

GENERIC FORM AVAILABLE: Yes

THERAPEUTIC CLASS: Blood vessel dilator

DOSAGE FORMS: 5.4-mg tablets

MAIN USES: {Impotence}

USUAL DOSE: one tablet three times daily

AVERAGE PRICE: $57.33 (B)/$20.82 (G)

SIDE EFFECTS: Most common: none. Less common: dizziness, headache, increased blood pressure, increased heart rate, irritability, restlessness, and nervousness.

DRUG INTERACTIONS: None of any clinical significance

ALLERGIES: Individuals allergic to yohimbine or any of its derivatives should discuss this with their doctor or pharmacist before using this drug.

PREGNANCY/BREAST-FEEDING: None. The drug is only used by men.

OTHER BRAND NAMES: None

OTHER DRUGS IN THE SAME THERAPEUTIC CLASS: None

IMPORTANT INFORMATION TO REMEMBER: The drug may cause dizziness, especially when treatment is begun or daily dosage is increased. Alcohol, anxiety medications, and narcotic painkillers may intensify the dizziness effect of the drug. The dizziness may go away once the body adjusts to the medication. Before taking over-the-counter cold and allergy preparations, consult your doctor or pharmacist. Do not increase the dose without first consulting with your physician.

BRAND NAME: Zantac

GENERIC NAME: ranitidine

GENERIC FORM AVAILABLE: No

THERAPEUTIC CLASS: Stomach acid blocker

DOSAGE FORMS: 150-mg and 300-mg tablets; 150-mg and 300-mg GELdose capsules; 150-mg EFFERdose granules and tablets; and 15 mg/mL syrup

MAIN USES: Active stomach ulcers, active duodenal ulcers (ulcers of the upper part of the small intestine, also called peptic ulcers), maintenance of healed duodenal ulcers, and the treatment of gastroesophageal reflux disease (GERD).

USUAL DOSE: 150 mg twice daily or 150 mg to 300 mg at bedtime

AVERAGE PRICE: $231.46 for 150 mg; $126.07 for 300 mg (30 tablets); $237.50 for 150 mg GELdose; and $129.40 for 300 mg GELdose (30 capsules)

SIDE EFFECTS: headache 2%, blurred vision 1%–2%, diarrhea 1%–2%, dizziness 1%–2%, drowsiness 1%–2%, nausea 1%–2%, and skin rash 1%–2%.

DRUG INTERACTIONS: The drug may increase the blood levels of Coumadin.

ALLERGIES: Individuals allergic to ranitidine or other stomach acid blockers (such as those listed under "Other Drugs in the Same Therapeutic Class") should discuss this with their doctor or pharmacist before taking this drug.

PREGNANCY/BREAST-FEEDING: Category B—No evidence of risk in humans. Either animal findings show risk, but human findings do not; or, if no adequate human studies have been done, animal findings show no risk. The drug is excreted in the breast milk; therefore, caution should be used when breast-feeding.

OTHER BRAND NAMES: Zantac 75 (over-the-counter)

OTHER DRUGS IN THE SAME THERAPEUTIC CLASS: Axid, Pepcid, and Tagamet

IMPORTANT INFORMATION TO REMEMBER: Always complete the full course of therapy, and take the drug only as directed. Individuals may take antacids occasionally for heartburn or temporary flare-ups, but antacids should be taken at least one hour before or two hours after taking the drug. Individuals using the effervescent tablets or granules must dissolve them in water before taking them. The drug is now available over-the-counter (OTC) without a prescription in a 75-mg tablet as Zantac 75.

BRAND NAME: Zarontin

GENERIC NAME: ethosuximide

GENERIC FORM AVAILABLE: No

THERAPEUTIC CLASS: Succinamide antiepileptic

DOSAGE FORMS: 250-mg capsules and 250 mg/5 mL syrup

MAIN USES: Epilepsy and seizures

USUAL DOSE: 250 mg to 1000 mg per day in single or divided doses. Doses for children may be less.

AVERAGE PRICE: $105.43 for 250-mg capsules

SIDE EFFECTS: Most common: Stevens-Johnson syndrome (aching joints and muscles, redness and blistering of the skin, and unusual tiredness or weakness) systemic lupus erythematosus (skin rash, itching, swollen glands, sore throat, fever, and muscle pain), loss of appetite, clumsiness, unsteadiness, dizziness, drowsiness, headache, hiccups, nausea, vomiting, and stomach pain. Less common: irritability, unusual tiredness or weakness, aggressiveness, depression, nightmares, and difficulty in concentrating.

DRUG INTERACTIONS: The drug may decrease the blood levels of Haldol. Haldol may increase the frequency of seizures. The drug may interact with other seizure medications. Dosage adjustments may be necessary. Central nervous system (CNS) depression may be increased when used with alcohol, anxiety medications, and narcotic painkillers.

ALLERGIES: Individuals allergic to ethosuximide or any of its derivatives should discuss this with their doctor or pharmacist before using this drug.

PREGNANCY/BREAST-FEEDING: Category D—Positive evidence of risk. Human studies show risk to the fetus. Nevertheless, potential benefits may possibly outweigh the potential risk. This drug should not be taken by nursing mothers.

OTHER BRAND NAMES: None

OTHER DRUGS IN THE SAME THERAPEUTIC CLASS: Celontin

IMPORTANT INFORMATION TO REMEMBER: This drug may cause drowsiness. Individuals should use caution when driving, operating machinery, or performing any task where mental alertness is required. Alcohol, anxiety medications, and narcotic painkillers may intensify the drowsiness effect of the drug. Avoid drinking alcohol while taking this drug. Only take the drug exactly as directed by your physician. Do not discontinue taking the drug without first consulting your physician. Also, do not increase the dose without first consulting with your physician. Before taking over-the-counter medications, consult your doctor or pharmacist. Report any of the signs and symptoms of Stevens-Johnson syndrome or systemic lupus erythematosus (see "Side Effects" section) to your physician immediately.

BRAND NAME: Zaroxolyn

GENERIC NAME: metolazone

GENERIC FORM AVAILABLE: No

THERAPEUTIC CLASS: Diuretic (water pill)

DOSAGE FORMS: 2.5-mg, 5-mg, and 10-mg tablets

MAIN USES: Swelling and water retention due to congestive heart failure, kidney or liver disease, and high blood pressure

USUAL DOSE: 2.5 mg to 5 mg once daily

AVERAGE PRICE: $62.41 for 2.5 mg; $70.96 for 5 mg; and $87.91 for 10 mg

SIDE EFFECTS: Most common: low potassium, dry mouth, muscle cramps, increased thirst, weakness, nausea, and vomiting. Less common: loss of appetite, constipation, diarrhea, decreased sexual ability, high blood sugar, dizziness, and increased sensitivity to sunburn.

DRUG INTERACTIONS: The drug may increase the toxic effects of Eskalith and Lithobid. The drug may decrease the effects of Coumadin. The drug may require dosage adjustments to some gout and diabetes medications. The drug may cause extremely large volumes of fluid and electrolytes to be lost if used with Lasix or Bumex.

ALLERGIES: Individuals allergic to metolazone or any of its derivatives should discuss this with their doctor or pharmacist before using this drug.

PREGNANCY/BREAST-FEEDING: Category B—No evidence of risk in humans. Either animal findings show risk, but human findings do not; or, if no adequate human studies have been done, animal findings show no risk. The drug is excreted in the breast milk; therefore, caution should be used when breast-feeding.

OTHER BRAND NAMES: Diulo and Mykrox

OTHER DRUGS IN THE SAME THERAPEUTIC CLASS: Diulo and Mykrox

IMPORTANT INFORMATION TO REMEMBER: If the drug is to be taken once daily, take it in the morning due to increased urine output. If stomach upset occurs, take the drug with food or milk. Before taking over-the-counter cold and allergy preparations, consult your doctor or pharmacist—these products may raise your blood pressure. The drug may cause the elimination of potassium from the body. It is therefore a good idea to eat a banana or drink orange, grapefruit, or apple juice every day to replace lost potassium. This drug may also increase the sensitivity of the skin to sunburn in some individuals; therefore, a sunscreen is recommended during periods of prolonged exposure to the sun. Individuals with kidney disease should discuss this with their doctor before taking this drug. Individuals should not switch between Zaroxolyn and the other two brand names (Diulo and Mykrox) without careful adjustments in dose by a physician.

BRAND NAME: **Zebeta**

GENERIC NAME: bisoprolol

GENERIC FORM AVAILABLE: No

THERAPEUTIC CLASS: Cardioselective beta-blocker

DOSAGE FORMS: 5-mg and 10-mg tablets

MAIN USES: High blood pressure

USUAL DOSE: 5 mg to 10 mg once daily

AVERAGE PRICE: $126.15 for 5 mg and $139.58 for 10 mg

SIDE EFFECTS: headache 9%, tiredness 7%, swelling 4%, runny nose 3%, diarrhea 3%, dizziness 3%, depression 2%, nausea 2%, muscle pain 2%, chest pain 1%, trouble breathing 1%, vomiting 1%, dry mouth 1%, and increased sweating 1%.

DRUG INTERACTIONS: The drug may cause additive effects when used with reserpine. The drug may increase the effects of Calan, Cardene, Cardizem, Catapres, Covera-HS, Dilacor XR, DynaCirc, Isoptin, Lanoxin, Norvasc, Plendil, Procardia, Sular, Tiazac, Verelan, and Wytensin. Diabetic medications, insulin, Slo-bid, Theo-Dur, theophylline, Uni-Dur, and Uniphyl dosages may need to be adjusted when taking this drug. The drug may also interfere with glaucoma screening tests.

ALLERGIES: Individuals allergic to bisoprolol or other beta-blockers (such as those listed under "Other Drugs in the Same Therapeutic Class") should discuss this with their doctor or pharmacist before taking this drug.

PREGNANCY/BREAST-FEEDING: Category C—Risk cannot be ruled out. Human studies are lacking, and animal studies are either positive for fetal risk or lacking as well. However, potential benefits may justify the potential risk in using the drug. The drug is excreted in the breast milk; therefore, extreme caution should be used when breast-feeding.

OTHER BRAND NAMES: None

OTHER DRUGS IN THE SAME THERAPEUTIC CLASS: Lopressor, Kerlone, Sectral, Toprol-XL, and Tenormin

IMPORTANT INFORMATION TO REMEMBER: Only take the drug exactly as directed by your physician. Do not discontinue taking the drug without first consulting your physician. This drug may cause some tiredness, especially at first. Individuals should use caution when driving, operating machinery, or performing any task where mental alertness is required. Alcohol, anxiety medications, and narcotic painkillers may intensify the tiredness effect of the drug. Before taking over-the-counter cold and allergy preparations, consult your doctor or pharmacist—these products may raise your blood pressure. This drug may mask the symptoms of low blood sugar in diabetics.

BRAND NAME: Zephrex LA

GENERIC NAME: Combination product containing: pseudoephedrine and guaifenesin

GENERIC FORM AVAILABLE: No

THERAPEUTIC CLASS: Decongestant + expectorant

DOSAGE FORMS: 120-mg pseudoephedrine/600-mg guaifenesin extended-release tablets

MAIN USES: Nasal congestion and cough

USUAL DOSE: one tablet every 12 hours

AVERAGE PRICE: $85.93

SIDE EFFECTS: Most common: none. Less common: drowsiness, nausea, giddiness, dry mouth, blurred vision, pounding heartbeat, flushing, and increased irritability or excitability (especially in children).

DRUG INTERACTIONS: Blocadren, Cartrol, Corgard, Inderal, Kerlone, Levatol, Lopressor, Normodyne, Sectral, Tenormin, Toprol-XL, Trandate, Visken, and Zebeta may increase the effects of the drug. The drug may also reduce the effects of blood-pressure-lowering drugs. Nardil or Parnate may significantly raise blood pressure when taken with this drug.

ALLERGIES: Individuals allergic to pseudoephedrine, guaifenesin, or any of their derivatives should discuss this with their doctor or pharmacist before using this drug.

PREGNANCY/BREAST-FEEDING: Category C—Risk cannot be ruled out. Human studies are lacking, and animal studies are either positive for fetal risk or lacking as well. However, potential benefits may justify the potential risk in using the drug. The drug is excreted in the breast milk; therefore, extreme caution should be used when breast-feeding.

OTHER BRAND NAMES: Ru-Tuss DE

OTHER DRUGS IN THE SAME THERAPEUTIC CLASS: Deconsal II, Duratuss, Entex, Entex LA, Entex PSE, Exgest LA, Guaifed, and Guaifed-PD

IMPORTANT INFORMATION TO REMEMBER: Patients with high blood pressure or heart conditions should consult their doctor before taking this drug. This drug should be taken with plenty of water (eight ounces is preferred). Do not crush or divide tablets—this will destroy the matrix that ensures the delayed release of the drug in the intestines. Swallow the tablets whole. The tablets may, however, be cut in half for easier swallowing. Do not increase the dose without first consulting with your physician.

BRAND NAME: **ZERIT**

GENERIC NAME: stavudine

GENERIC FORM AVAILABLE: No

THERAPEUTIC CLASS: AIDS antiviral

DOSAGE FORMS: 15-mg, 20-mg, 30-mg, and 40-mg capsules

MAIN USES: AIDS

USUAL DOSE: 30 mg to 40 mg every 12 hours

AVERAGE PRICE: $280.00 for 15 mg (60 capsules); $291.20 for 20 mg (60 capsules); $303.80 for 30 mg (60 capsules); and $319.73 for 40 mg (60 capsules)

SIDE EFFECTS: headache 55%, diarrhea 50%, neurological problems (such as clumsiness, or tingling and stinging sensations in the arms, legs, feet, and hands) 40%, chills/fever 38%, nausea/vomiting 35%, muscle pain 35%, rash 33%, weakness 28%, insomnia 26%, stomach pain 26%, nervousness 22%, back pain 20%, sweating 19%, joint pain 19%, general pain 18%, tiredness 17%, trouble breathing 13%, itching 12%, weight loss 10%, appetite changes 10%, allergic reaction 9%, flu-like symptoms 9%, dizziness 9%, chest pain 8%, constipation 7%, conjunctivitis 5%, lymphadenopathy 5%, skin cancer 4%, abnormal vision 3%, urinary problems 3%, pneumonia 3%, confusion 3%, migraine 3%, low blood pressure 3%, ulcerative stomatitis 3%, pelvic pain 2%, high blood pressure 2%, drowsiness 2%, tremor 2%, and pancreatitis 1%. Blood disorders and anemia also occur somewhat frequently.

DRUG INTERACTIONS: There are numerous drugs that can cause peripheral neuropathy (unusual nerve sensations and damage in the arms, legs, fingers, and toes) when taken with this drug. Some of these are: alcohol, Aldomet, Apresoline, Bactrim, Biaxin, cisplatin, Clinoril, Cytovene, dapsone, Depakene, Depakote, Dilantin, diuretics (water pills), Doryx, Dynabac, erythromycin, Eskalith, estrogens, Flagyl, isoniazid, Lasix, Lithobid, Macrobid, Macrodantin, pentamidine, Septra, Sumycin, Vibramycin, and vincristine. Bactrim, probenecid, and Septra may increase the blood levels of the drug. Biaxin may decrease the blood levels of the drug. Before taking any prescription drug, discuss it with your doctor.

ALLERGIES: Individuals allergic to stavudine or any of its derivatives should discuss this with their doctor or pharmacist before using this drug.

PREGNANCY/BREAST-FEEDING: Category C—Risk cannot be ruled out. Human studies are lacking, and animal studies are either positive for fetal risk or lacking as well. However, potential benefits may justify the potential risk in using the drug. The drug is excreted in the breast milk; therefore, extreme caution should be used when breast-feeding.

OTHER BRAND NAMES: None

OTHER DRUGS IN THE SAME THERAPEUTIC CLASS: Epivir, HIVID, Retrovir, and Videx

IMPORTANT INFORMATION TO REMEMBER: If stomach upset occurs, take the drug with food or milk. Also, take the drug at even intervals around the clock (if two times a day, take every 12 hours). Only take the drug exactly as directed by your physician. Do not stop taking the drug without first consulting with your doctor. It is important to have regular blood and liver function tests while taking this drug. Before taking any prescription or over-the-counter (OTC) drugs, consult your doctor or pharmacist.

BRAND NAME: Zestoretic

GENERIC NAME: Combination product containing: lisinopril and hydrochlorothiazide

See individual entries for Zestril and HydroDIURIL

BRAND NAME: Zestril

GENERIC NAME: lisinopril

GENERIC FORM AVAILABLE: No

THERAPEUTIC CLASS: ACE inhibitor

DOSAGE FORMS: 2.5-mg, 5-mg, 10-mg, 20-mg, and 40-mg tablets

MAIN USES: High blood pressure and heart failure

USUAL DOSE: 5 mg to 40 mg once daily

AVERAGE PRICE: $73.50 for 2.5 mg; $108.06 for 5 mg; $116.48 for 10 mg; $121.80 for 20 mg; and $177.91 for 40 mg

SIDE EFFECTS: headache 6%, dizziness 5%, cough 4%, diarrhea 3%, tiredness 3%, nausea 2%, weakness 1%, chest pain 1%, vomiting 1%, muscle cramps 1%, decreased sex drive 1%, rash 1%, and impotence 1%.

DRUG INTERACTIONS: May decrease the absorption of the antibiotic Sumycin or other tetracycline antibiotics. High potassium levels may occur when used together with Dyrenium and Aldactone, and potassium supplements such as Micro-K, K-Dur, Klor-Con, K-Lyte, and Slow-K. Patients on water pills, especially those recently started on a water pill, may experience low blood pressure. The drug may also increase the toxic effects of Eskalith and Lithobid, especially when taken with a water pill.

ALLERGIES: Individuals allergic to lisinopril, Prinivil, or other ACE inhibitors (such as those listed under "Other Drugs in the Same Therapeutic Class") should discuss this with their doctor or pharmacist before using this drug.

PREGNANCY/BREAST-FEEDING: Category C (first trimester)—Risk cannot be ruled out. Human studies are lacking, and animal studies are either positive for fetal risk or lacking as well. However, potential benefis may justify the potential risk in using the drug. Category D (second and third trimesters)—Positive evidence of risk. Human studies show risk to the fetus. Nevertheless, potential benefits may possibly outweigh the potential risk. This drug should not be taken by nursing mothers.

OTHER BRAND NAMES: Prinivil

OTHER DRUGS IN THE SAME THERAPEUTIC CLASS: Accupril, Altace, Capoten, Lotensin, Mavik, Monopril, Prinivil, Univasc, and Vasotec

IMPORTANT INFORMATION TO REMEMBER: Take this drug regularly and exactly as directed by your physician. Do not stop taking Zestril unless otherwise directed by your doctor. Avoid salt substitutes containing potassium. Before taking over-the-counter cold and allergy preparations, consult your doctor or pharmacist—these products may raise your blood pressure. If you experience swelling of the face, lips, or tongue or difficulty in breathing, contact your doctor immediately.

BRAND NAME: Ziac

GENERIC NAME: Combination product containing: bisoprolol and hydrochlorothiazide

See individual entries for Zebeta and HydroDIURIL

BRAND NAME: Zithromax

GENERIC NAME: azithromycin

GENERIC FORM AVAILABLE: No

THERAPEUTIC CLASS: Macrolide antibiotic

DOSAGE FORMS: 250-mg tablets and 600-mg tablets

MAIN USES: Bacterial infections

USUAL DOSE: 500 mg as a single dose on the first day, followed by 250 mg once daily for four more days

AVERAGE PRICE: $45.97 for 250 mg (five capsules); and $95.25 for 600 mg (five tablets)

SIDE EFFECTS: diarrhea 5%, loose stools 5%, nausea 3%, and stomach pain 3%.

DRUG INTERACTIONS: Antacids may decrease the absorption of the drug.

ALLERGIES: Individuals allergic to azithromycin or other macrolide antibiotics (such as those listed under "Other Drugs in the Same Therapeutic Class") should discuss this with their doctor or pharmacist before taking this drug.

PREGNANCY/BREAST-FEEDING: Category B—No evidence of risk in humans. Either animal findings show risk, but human findings do not; or, if no adequate human studies have been done, animal findings show no risk. It is not known whether the drug is excreted in the breast milk; therefore, caution should be used when breast-feeding.

OTHER BRAND NAMES: None

OTHER DRUGS IN THE SAME THERAPEUTIC CLASS: Biaxin, Dynabac, E-Mycin, E.E.S., ERYC, EryPed, ERY-TAB, Ilosone, PCE, and TAO

IMPORTANT INFORMATION TO REMEMBER: It's best to take the drug on an empty stomach—one hour before meals or two hours after meals—if possible. Also, take the drug at the same time every day. Take the drug until all the medication prescribed is gone; otherwise the infection may return. If severe diarrhea occurs while taking this drug, notify your doctor immediately. Do not take antacids within one hour of taking this drug.

BRAND NAME: Zocor

GENERIC NAME: simvastatin

GENERIC FORM AVAILABLE: No

THERAPEUTIC CLASS: Cholesterol-lowering agent

DOSAGE FORMS: 5-mg, 10-mg, 20-mg, and 40-mg tablets

MAIN USES: High cholesterol

USUAL DOSE: 5 mg to 40 mg once daily in the evening

AVERAGE PRICE: $249.41 for 5 mg; $273.42 for 10 mg; and $495.46 for 20 mg; and $495.46 for 40 mg

SIDE EFFECTS: headache 4%, stomach pain 3%, constipation 2%, weakness 2%, diarrhea 2%, gas 2%, and nausea 1%.

DRUG INTERACTIONS: Sandimmune, Lopid, and niacin may cause kidney problems when taken with this drug. Tagamet, Prilosec, and Zantac may increase the blood levels of the drug. The drug may increase the effects of Coumadin. Lopid and the drug, when taken together, may increase the risk of developing rhabdomyolysis (destruction and death of muscle tissue). Symptoms are muscle pain and dark, red-brown colored urine.

ALLERGIES: Individuals allergic to simvastatin, Lescol, Mevacor, Pravachol, or any of their derivatives should discuss this with their doctor or pharmacist before using this drug.

PREGNANCY/BREAST-FEEDING: Category X—Should not be used during pregnancy. Studies in animals and/or humans have shown fetal abnormalities and birth defects. The risks associated with using this drug clearly outweigh the benefits. This drug should never be used by someone who is pregnant or trying to become pregnant. Also, women should never breast-feed while using this drug.

OTHER BRAND NAMES: None

OTHER DRUGS IN THE SAME THERAPEUTIC CLASS: Lescol, Lipitor, Mevacor, and Pravachol

IMPORTANT INFORMATION TO REMEMBER: The drug may be taken with food or milk if stomach upset occurs. Only take the drug exactly as directed by your physician. It is also important to follow the prescribed low cholesterol diet. Report any sign of unexplained muscle pain or tenderness to your doctor, especially if it is accompanied by tiredness or fever.

BRAND NAME: Zofran

GENERIC NAME: ondansetron

GENERIC FORM AVAILABLE: No

THERAPEUTIC CLASS: Antinausea

DOSAGE FORMS: 4-mg and 8-mg tablets

MAIN USES: Prevention of chemotherapy-induced nausea

USUAL DOSE: 4 mg to 8 mg three times daily

AVERAGE PRICE: $47.13 for 4 mg (three tablets) and $78.55 for 8 mg (three tablets)

SIDE EFFECTS: headache 21%–23%, constipation 5%–7%, stomach pain 4%–5%, weakness 2%–3%, dry mouth 1%–2%, rash 1%, and possibly some drowsiness.

DRUG INTERACTIONS: None of any clinical significance

ALLERGIES: Individuals allergic to ondansetron or any of its derivatives should discuss this with their doctor or pharmacist before using this drug.

PREGNANCY/BREAST-FEEDING: Category B—No evidence of risk in humans. Either animal findings show risk, but human findings do not; or, if no adequate human studies have been done, animal findings show no risk. The drug is excreted in the breast milk; therefore, extreme caution should be used when breast-feeding.

OTHER BRAND NAMES: None

OTHER DRUGS IN THE SAME THERAPEUTIC CLASS: Kytril

IMPORTANT INFORMATION TO REMEMBER: This drug may cause some drowsiness. Individuals should use caution when driving, operating machinery, or performing any task where mental alertness is required. Alcohol, anxiety medications, and narcotic painkillers may intensify the drowsiness effect of the drug. Only take the drug exactly as directed by your physician and do not increase the dose without first consulting your physician.

BRAND NAME: Zoloft

GENERIC NAME: sertraline

GENERIC FORM AVAILABLE: No

THERAPEUTIC CLASS: Serotonin reuptake inhibitor antidepressant

DOSAGE FORMS: 50-mg and 100-mg tablets

MAIN USES: Depression and obsessive-compulsive disorder

USUAL DOSE: 50 mg to 200 mg once daily

AVERAGE PRICE: $282.99 for 50 mg and $306.46 for 100 mg

SIDE EFFECTS: nausea 26%, headache 20%, diarrhea 18%, dry mouth 16%, insomnia 16%, sexual dysfunction (males) 16%, drowsiness 13%, dizziness 12%, tremor 11%, tiredness 11%, increased sweating 8%, constipation 8%, agitation 6%, abnormal vision 4%, pounding heartbeat 4%, vomiting 4%, nervousness 3%, gas 3%, appetite changes 3%, urinary disorders 2%, yawning 2%, sexual dysfunction (females) 2%, stomach pain 2%, muscle pain 2%, hot flashes 2%, rash 2%, fever 2%, back pain 2%, increased appetite 1%, twitching 1%, impaired concentration 1%, menstrual disorders 1%, and taste changes 1%.

DRUG INTERACTIONS: The drug may increase the blood levels of Orinase, Tagamet, and Valium. The drug, when taken with Coumadin, may increase the chance of bleeding. The drug should not be used with tryptophan, because tryptophan can be metabolized to serotonin and too much serotonin may cause severe side effects. The drug should not be taken within 14 days of taking Nardil or Parnate. Central nervous system (CNS) depression may be increased when used with alcohol, narcotic painkillers, or other anxiety medications. The drug may increase the blood levels of other drugs used to treat depression. The drug may increase the blood levels of Dilantin.

ALLERGIES: Individuals allergic to sertraline or any of its derivatives should discuss this with their doctor or pharmacist before using this drug.

PREGNANCY/BREAST-FEEDING: Category B—No evidence of risk in humans. Either animal findings show risk, but human findings do not; or, if no adequate human studies have been done, animal findings show no risk. It is not known whether the drug is excreted in the breast milk; therefore, caution should be used when breast-feeding.

OTHER BRAND NAMES: None

OTHER DRUGS IN THE SAME THERAPEUTIC CLASS: Luvox, Paxil, and Prozac

IMPORTANT INFORMATION TO REMEMBER: Only take the drug exactly as directed by your physician. Do not discontinue taking the drug without first consulting your physician. The drug may require two to four weeks of use before improvement may be noticed. This drug may cause some drowsiness. Individuals should use caution when driving, operating machinery, or performing any task where mental alertness is required. Alcohol, anxiety medications, and narcotic painkillers may intensify the drowsiness effect of the drug.

BRAND NAME: Zovirax

GENERIC NAME: acyclovir

GENERIC FORM AVAILABLE: Yes

THERAPEUTIC CLASS: Antiviral

DOSAGE FORMS: 200-mg capsules; 400-mg and 800-mg tablets; 5.0% ointment; and 200 mg/5 mL suspension

MAIN USES: Genital herpes, shingles, chickenpox, and herpes cold sores

USUAL DOSE: 200 mg to 800 mg every four hours (five times daily) while awake. Doses for chickenpox may be less.

AVERAGE PRICE: $143.38 for 200 mg; $278.26 for 400 mg; $541.07 for 800 mg; and $52.46 for 5.0% ointment (15 g)

SIDE EFFECTS: nausea 5%–8%, diarrhea, 2%, headache 2%, rash 2%, and vomiting 1%.

DRUG INTERACTIONS: Probenecid may increase the blood levels of the drug.

ALLERGIES: Individuals allergic to acyclovir, Cytovene, Famvir, Valtrex, or any of their derivatives should discuss this with their doctor or pharmacist before using this drug.

PREGNANCY/BREAST-FEEDING: Category C—Risk cannot be ruled out. Human studies are lacking, and animal studies are either positive for fetal risk or lacking as well. However, potential benefits may justify the potential risk in using the drug. The drug is excreted in the breast milk; therefore, extreme caution should be used when breast-feeding.

OTHER BRAND NAMES: None

OTHER DRUGS IN THE SAME THERAPEUTIC CLASS: Cytovene, Denavir, Famvir, and Valtrex

IMPORTANT INFORMATION TO REMEMBER: Only take the drug exactly as directed by your physician. If stomach upset occurs, take the drug with food or milk. Also, take the drug at even intervals around the clock (if five times a day, take every four hours while awake). Take the drug for the full course of therapy; otherwise the infection may return. The drug should be started at the first sign of shingles or genital herpes in order to be most effective. If the drug is used for genital herpes, avoid sexual intercourse when sores or lesions are present.

BRAND NAME: Zydone

GENERIC NAME: Combination product containing: hydrocodone bitartrate and acetaminophen

See entry for Vicodin

BRAND NAME: Zyflo

GENERIC NAME: zileuton

GENERIC FORM AVAILABLE: No

THERAPEUTIC CLASS: Asthma controller

DOSAGE FORMS: 600-mg tablets

MAIN USES: Asthma and {other breathing disorders}

USUAL DOSE: 600 mg four times daily

AVERAGE PRICE: $76.82

SIDE EFFECTS: headache 25%, general pain 8%, stomach pain 5%, nausea 5%–8%, weakness 4%, accidental injury 3%, muscle pain 3%, chest pain 1%, dizziness 1%, fever 1%, gas 1%, neck pain 1%, nervousness 1%, drowsiness 1%, itching 1%, vaginal infections 1%, and vomiting 1%.

DRUG INTERACTIONS: The drug may increase the blood levels of Inderal, Seldane, Seldane-D, Slo-bid, Theo-Dur, theophylline, Uni-Dur, and Uniphyl.

ALLERGIES: Individuals allergic to zileuton or any of its derivatives should discuss this with their doctor or pharmacist before using this drug.

PREGNANCY/BREAST-FEEDING: Category C—Risk cannot be ruled out. Human studies are lacking, and animal studies are either positive for fetal risk or lacking as well. However, potential benefits may justify the potential risk in using the drug. It is not known whether the drug is excreted in the breast milk; therefore, caution should be used when breast-feeding.

OTHER BRAND NAME: None

OTHER DRUGS IN THE SAME THERAPEUTIC CLASS: Accolate

IMPORTANT INFORMATION TO REMEMBER: The drug is not intended to provide immediately relief of a bronchospasm, shortness of breath, or an asthma attack; it is used only for prevention of attacks. To receive the full benefits of the drug, use it on a regular basis as a maintenance medication. The drug may take two to four weeks before noticeable benefits may be seen. Never exceed the prescribed dosage unless directed to do so by a doctor.

BRAND NAME: Zyloprim

GENERIC NAME: allopurinol

GENERIC FORM AVAILABLE: Yes

THERAPEUTIC CLASS: Anti-gout

DOSAGE FORMS: 100-mg and 300-mg tablets

MAIN USES: Gout and renal calculi

USUAL DOSE: 100 mg to 300 mg daily

AVERAGE PRICE: $28.51 (B)/$13.43 (G) for 100 mg and $80.83 (B)/$36.56 (G) for 300 mg

SIDE EFFECTS: Most common: allergic reaction and skin rash. Less common: diarrhea, drowsiness, headache, indigestion, nausea, vomiting, chills, fever, muscle aches and pains, and unusual hair loss.

DRUG INTERACTIONS: The drug may increase the effectiveness of Coumadin. The drug may increase the blood levels of Imuran and Purinethol.

ALLERGIES: Individuals allergic to allopurinol or any of its derivatives should discuss this with their doctor or pharmacist before using this drug.

PREGNANCY/BREAST-FEEDING: Category C—Risk cannot be ruled out. Human studies are lacking, and animal studies are either positive for fetal risk or lacking as well. However, potential benefits may justify the potential risk in using the drug. The drug is excreted in the breast milk; therefore, extreme caution should be used when breast-feeding.

OTHER BRAND NAMES: Lopurin

OTHER DRUGS IN THE SAME THERAPEUTIC CLASS: Lopurin

IMPORTANT INFORMATION TO REMEMBER: The medication is to help prevent gout attacks; therefore, compliance with therapy is essential. The drug may take one or more weeks to reach maximum effectiveness. The drug does not relieve acute attacks. If stomach upset occurs, take the drug with food or milk. The drug should be taken with large amounts of water during the day to prevent kidney stone formation. This drug may cause some limited drowsiness. Individuals should use caution when driving, operating machinery, or performing any task where mental alertness is required.

BRAND NAME: Zyrtec

GENERIC NAME: cetirizine

GENERIC FORM AVAILABLE: No

THERAPEUTIC CLASS: Nonsedating antihistamine

DOSAGE FORMS: 5-mg and 10-mg tablets and 1 mg/mL syrup

MAIN USES: Allergies

USUAL DOSE: 5 mg to 10 mg daily as needed

AVERAGE PRICE: $221.90 for 5 mg and 10 mg

SIDE EFFECTS: slight drowsiness 11%–14%, slight fatigue 6%, dry mouth 5%, pharyngitis 2%, and dizziness 2%.

DRUG INTERACTIONS: Nizoral may increase the blood levels of the drug.

ALLERGIES: Individuals allergic to cetirizine or any of its derivatives should discuss this with their doctor or pharmacist before using this drug.

PREGNANCY/BREAST-FEEDING: Category B—No evidence of risk in humans. Either animal findings show risk, but human findings do not; or, if no adequate human studies have been done, animal findings show no risk. The drug is excreted in the breast milk; therefore, extreme caution should be used when breast-feeding.

OTHER BRAND NAMES: None

OTHER DRUGS IN THE SAME THERAPEUTIC CLASS: Allegra, Claritin, Hismanal, and Seldane

IMPORTANT INFORMATION TO REMEMBER: Do not take the drug more frequently than every 24 hours. Unless otherwise directed by a physician, take the drug only as needed for relief of allergies. This drug may cause some limited drowsiness. Individuals should use caution when driving, operating machinery, or performing any task where mental alertness is required.

GENERIC TO BRAND-NAME CROSS REFERENCE

Generic	Brand	Page Number
A		
acarbose	Precose	527
acebutolol	Sectral	586
acetaminophen / codeine	Tylenol #2, Tylenol #3, Tylenol #4	679
acetazolamide	Diamox	176
acyclovir	Zovirax	740
adapalene	Differin	179
albuterol	Proventil	545
alclometasone	Aclovate	5
alendronate	Fosamax	258
allopurinol	Zyloprim	742
alprazolam	Xanax	724
amantadine	Symmetrel	621
amcinonide	Cyclocort	142
amiloride	Midamor	396
amiloride/hydrochlorothiazide	Moduretic	402
amiodarone	Cordarone	129
amitriptyline	Elavil	211
amlodipine	Norvasc	463
ammonium lactate	Lac-Hydrin	328
amoxapine	Asendin	45
amoxicillin	Amoxil	27

Generic	*Brand*	*Page Number*
amphetamine	Adderall	8
ampicillin	Omnipen	471
anastrozole	Arimidex	39
antipyrine	Auralgan	54
apraclonidine	Iopidine	305
astemizole	Hismanal	276
atenolol	Tenormin	637
atenolol/chlorthalidone	Tenoretic	637
auranofin	Ridaura	569
azathioprine	Imuran	297
azithromycin	Zithromax	735

B

B-C w/folic acid	Berocca	71
baclofen	Lioresal	346
beclomethasone dipropionate	Beconase, Vancenase	63, 694
benazepril	Lotensin	363
benzonatate	Tessalon	639
benzoyl peroxide	Benzac, Benzagel, Desquam-X	59, 169
benztropine	Cogentin	118
bepridil	Vascor	700
betamethasone dipropionate	Diprosone, Diprolene	188
betamethasone valerate	Valisone	693
betaxolol	Betoptic, Kerlone	74, 319
bethanechol	Urecholine	687
bicalutamide	Casodex	97
biperiden	Akineton	12
bismuth/metronidazole/ tetracycline	Helidac	273
bisoprolol	Zebeta	730
bitolterol	Tornalate	660
brimonidine	Alphagan	21
bromocriptine	Parlodel	492
budesonide	Rhinocort	567
bumetanide	Bumex	83
bupropion	Wellbutrin	719
buspirone	BuSpar	84
butabarbital sodium	Butisol	85

Generic	Brand	Page Number
butalbital/acetaminophen/ caffeine	Fioricet	246
butalbital compound	Fiorinal	247
butoconazole	Femstat	245

C

Generic	Brand	Page Number
calcipotriene	Dovonex	198
calcitonin--salmon	Miacalcin	392
calcitriol	Rocaltrol	577
captopril	Capoten	89
carbachol	Isopto Carbachol	310
carbamazepine	Tegretol	632
carbidopa/levodopa	Sinemet	599
carisoprodol	Soma	607
carteolol	Cartrol, Ocupress	96, 468
cefaclor	Ceclor	101
cefadroxil	Duricef	201
cefixime	Suprax	618
cefpodoxime	Vantin	698
cefprozil	Cefzil	104
ceftibuten	Cedax	102
cefuroxime	Ceftin	103
cephalexin	Keflex	316
cetirizine	Zyrtec	743
chlorambucil	Leukeran	338
chlordiazepoxide	Librium	343
chlordiazepoxide/amitriptyline	Limbitrol	345
chloroquine	Aralen	38
chlorothiazide	Diuril	192
chlorpromazine	Thorazine	643
chlorpropamide	Diabinese	175
chlorthalidone	Hygroton	287
chlorzoxazone 500	Parafon Forte DSC	491
cholestyramine	Questran	552
ciclopirox	Loprox	359
cimetidine	Tagamet	626
ciprofloxacin	Cipro, Ciloxan	109, 110
cisapride	Propulsid	541
clarithromycin	Biaxin	75

Generic	Brand	Page Number
clindamycin	Cleocin T	112
clindex	Librax	341
clobetasol	Temovate	635
clofibrate	Atromid-S	49
clomiphene	Serophene	596
clomipramine	Anafranil	28
clonazepam	Klonopin	320
clonidine	Catapres	99
clorazepate	Tranxene	664
clotrimazole	Lotrimin	365
clozapine	Clozaril	117
colestipol	Colestid	123
contrin	Trinsicon	672
cromolyn sodium	Intal, Nasalcrom	303, 427
crotamiton	Eurax	237
cyclobenzaprine	Flexeril	250
cyclophosphamide	Cytoxan	147
cyproheptadine	Periactin	508

D

danazol	Danocrine	150
dantrolene	Dantrium	x
decongestant S.R.	Naldecon	420
desipramine	Norpramin	461
desmopressin	DDAVP	154
desonide	DesOwen	168
desoximetasone	Topicort	657
dexamethasone	Decadron	155
dexchlorpheniramine maleate T.R.	Polaramine Repetabs	
diazepam	Valium	692
diclofenac sodium	Voltaren	717
diclofenac potassium	Cataflam	98
dicyclomine	Bentyl	68
didanosine	Videx	710
diflorasone	Florone, Psorcon	253, 549
diflunisal	Dolobid	193
digoxin	Lanoxin	331
diltiazem	Cardizem	93

Generic	Brand	Page Number
diphenhydramine	Benadryl	66
dipivefrin	Propine	540
dipyridamole	Persantine	511
disopyramide	Norpace	459
disulfiram	Antabuse	33
divalproex sodium	Depakote	165
dorzolamide	Trusopt	676
doxazosin	Cardura	94
doxepin	Sinequan	601
doxycycline	Vibramycin	707
dronabinol	Marinol	371

E

econazole	Spectazole	609
enalapril	Vasotec	701
enoxacin	Penetrex	502
epoetin alfa	Epogen, Procrit	222, 538
ergoloid mesylates	Hydergine	282
ergotamine	Cafergot	86
erythromycin	E-Mycin	217
erythromycin estolate	Ilosone	292
erythromycin ethylsuccinate	E.E.S.	209
erythromycin ethylsuccinate/sulfisoxazole	Pediazole	500
erythromycin stearate	Erythromycin	228
estradiol	Estraderm, Climara	231, 114
estrogens, conjugated	Premarin	529
ethosuximide	Zarontin	727
etidronate (diphosphonate)	Didronel	178
etodolac	Lodine	351
etretinate	Tegison	631

F

famciclovir	Famvir	240
famotidine	Pepcid	504
felbamate	Felbatol	242
felodipine	Plendil	520
fenoprofen	Nalfon	421

Generic	Brand	Page Number
K		
K-G elixir	KAON-CL10	315
ketoconazole	Nizoral	448
ketoprofen	Orudis	482
ketorolac	Acular, Toradol	7, 658
L		
labetalol	Normodyne	456
lactulose	Cephulac	105
lactulose	Chronulac	108
lamivudine	Epivir	220
lamotrigine	Lamictal	329
lansoprazole	Prevacid	531
latanoprost	Xalatan	723
levobunolol	Betagan	72
levocabastine	Livostin	350
levodopa	Larodopa	334
levonorgestrel	Nordette	452
levothyroxine	Synthroid	625
lindane	Kwell	326
liothyronine	Cytomel	144
lisinopril	Prinivil, Zestril	534, 734
lithium	Eskalith	229
lodoxamide	Alomide	20
lomefloxacin	Maxaquin	375
lonox	Lomotil	354
loperamide	Imodium	296
loracarbef	Lorabid	360
loratadine	Claritin	111
lorazepam	Ativan	48
losartan	Cozaar	137
lovastatin	Mevacor	390
M		
maprotiline	Ludiomil	367
mebendazole	Vermox	705
meclizine	Antivert	35
meclocycline	Meclan	x

Generic	Brand	Page Number
meclofenamate	Meclomen	380
medroxyprogesterone	Provera	546
mefenamic acid	Ponstel	525
mefloquine	Lariam	333
megestrol	Megace	382
melphalan	Alkeran	18
meperidine	Demerol	161
mephenytoin	Mesantoin	385
mephobarbital	Mebaral	379
mesalamine	Asacol, Pentasa, Rowasa	44, 503, 580
mesoridazine	Serentil	594
metaproterenol	Alupent	24
metaproterenol	Metaprel	388
metaxalone	Skelaxin	602
metformin	Glucophage	263
methazolamide	Neptazane	435
methenamine	Hiprex	275
methocarbamol	Robaxin	576
methotrexate	Rheumatrex	566
methyclothiazide	Enduron	218
methyldopa	Aldomet	16
methyldopa/ hydrochlorothiazide	Aldoril	17
methylene blue	Urised	687
methylergonovine	Methergine	388
methylphenidate	Ritalin	574
methylprednisolone	Medrol	381
metipranolol	OptiPranolol	472
metoclopramide	Reglan	557
metolazone	Zaroxolyn	728
metoprolol tartrate	Lopressor	357
metronidazole	Flagyl, MetroGel	249, 389
mexiletine	Mexitil	391
miconazole	Monistat	404
minocycline	Minocin	400
minoxidil	Rogaine, Loniten	578, 355
misoprostol	Cytotec	145
moexipril	Univasc	685

Generic	Brand	Page Number
oxycodone/acetaminophen	Percocet	505
oxycodone/aspirin	Percodan	506

P

Generic	Brand	Page Number
pancrealipase E.C.	Pancrease MT	489
papaverine S.R.	Pavabid	494
paroxetine	Paxil	495
pemoline	Cylert	143
penbutolol	Levatol	339
penciclovir	Denavir	164
penicillin V potassium	Veetids	703
pentazocine/naloxone	Talwin Nx	628
pentoxifylline	Trental	665
pergolide	Permax	510
perphenazine	Trilafon	667
perphenazine/amitriptyline	Etrafon 2-25	236
perphenazine/amitriptyline	Triavil	666
phenazopyridine	Pyridium	551
phenelzine	Nardil	424
phenobarbital	Phenobarbital	515
phenobarbital/ergotamine/ belladonna	Bellergal-S	64
phenoxybenzamine	Dibenzyline	177
phenytoin	Dilantin	183
pindolol	Visken	712
pirbuterol	Maxair	373
piroxicam	Feldene	243
podofilox	Condylox	128
polymyxin B/bacitracin/ neomycin	Neosporin	434
potassium bicarbonate	K-Lyte	324
potassium chloride E.R.	Slow-K	606
pravastatin	Pravachol	526
prazosin	Minipress	398
prednisone	Deltasone	159
prenatal/folic acid	Stuartnatal Plus	612
primidone	Mysoline	418
probenecid	Benemid	67
probenecid/colchicine	ColBENEMID	120

Generic	*Brand*	*Page Number*
S		
salmeterol	Serevent	595
salsalate	Disalcid	189
saquinavir	Invirase	304
selegiline	Eldepryl	212
selenium	Selsun Blue	589
silver sulfadiazine	Silvadene	598
simvastatin	Zocor	736
sodium pentobarbital	Nembutal	432
spironolactone	Aldactone	14
spironolactone/ hydrochlorothiazide	Aldactazide	13
stavudine	Zerit	732
sucralfate	Carafate	91
sulfadoxine	Fansidar	241
sulfamethoxazole	Gantanol	260
sulfamethoxazole/ trimethoprim	Bactrim, Bactrim DS	60
sulfamethoxazole/ trimethoprim	Septra, Septra DS	591
sulfasalazine	Azulfidine	59
sulfisoxazole	Gantrisin	260
sulindac	Clinoril	115
sumatriptan	Imitrex	295
T		
tacrine	Cognex	119
tamoxifen	Nolvadex	451
temazepam	Restoril	561
terazosin	Hytrin	290
terbinafine	Lamisil	330
terbutaline	Brethine	77
terconazole	Terazol	638
terfenadine	Seldane	589
tetracycline	Sumycin	617
theophylline (anhydrous) E.R.	Slo-bid, Slo-Phyllin, Theo-Dur, Uniphyl	603, 605, 642, 684
thiethylperazine	Torecan	659

Generic	Brand	Page Number
V		
valacyclovir	Valtrex	693
valproic acid	Depakene	165
vancomycin	Vancocin	697
venlafaxine	Effexor	210
verapamil	Calan, Covera-HS, Verelan	88, 135, 704
W		
warfarin	Coumadin	134
Y		
yohimbine	Yocon	725
Z		
zafirlukast	Accolate	1
zalcitabine	HIVID	277
zidovudine	Retrovir	563
zolpidem	Ambien	25

GUIDELINES FOR SAFE DRUG USE

- Store all medications in a dry, safe place.
- Keep all medications in the container they come in. Don't mix medicines in a single bottle.
- If you see more than one doctor, make sure they all know about the medications you are taking, prescription and nonprescription.
- Ask your doctor and pharmacist to clearly explain how to take the drug.
- Be sure to ask about any drug interactions with food, alcoholic beverages, and other medications.
- Take the medication only as directed. Don't take any less or any extra medicine without talking to your doctor or pharmacist.
- Report any unusual symptoms or reactions you have while taking the medicine.
- Do not save any unused medicine. Dispose of it by flushing it down the toilet and throw away the bottle.
- Keep all medicines out of the reach of children.
- Don't share your medicine with anyone, and don't use any prescription medicine unless it has been specifically prescribed for you.
- Don't take any medication after its expiration date.
- If you are pregnant, think you are pregnant, or are breast-feeding, tell your doctor before taking any medication.
- Keep a list of all your prescription records.

QUESTIONS FOR YOUR DOCTOR AND PHARMACIST

- What is the brand name of the medicine?
- Is there a generic form available?
- How much does the drug usually cost?
- How does the drug work?
- How often should I take it, and when?
- What should I do if I miss a dose?
- Should I avoid taking this drug with certain foods, alcoholic beverages, or other medications?
- For how long should I take the drug?
- Should I continue to take the drug if I start feeling better?
- Can I refill the prescription when it runs out? How many times?
- What are the side effects of the drug? How common are they?
- How should I store the drug?

NUTRITION GUIDES BY ED BLONZ, PH.D.

☐YOUR PERSONAL NUTRITIONIST: FIBER AND FAT COUNTER

Here is the only guide to fiber that also includes calorie and fat-gram counts. Nutrition expert Dr.
Ed Blonz tells you everything you have to know about the remarkable gifts of fiber. How much you
need to keep healthy, and how to easily include the right amount in your daily diet.

(184874—$3.99)

☐YOUR PERSONAL NUTRITIONIST: ANTIOXIDANT COUNTER

Antioxidant vitamins, found in certain nutrient-rich foods, help your body guard against health
threats you can't control—like air pollution, water pollution, a deteriorating ozone, and food additives. Nutrition expert Dr. Ed Blonz supplies the fat, calorie, and antioxidant vitamin contents of
over 3,000 common and brand-name foods.

(184882—$3.99)

☐YOUR PERSONAL NUTRITIONIST: CALCIUM AND OTHER MINERALS COUNTER

Most Americans—especially women—just don't include enough calcium and other minerals in
their daily diet. These essential nutrients offer the best protection from brittle bones, anemia, and
fatigue. Nutrition expert Dr. Ed Blonz supplies the fat, calorie, and mineral contents of over 3,000
common and popular brand-name foods.

(188802—$3.99)

☐YOUR PERSONAL NUTRITIONIST: FOOD ADDITIVES

To help you make wise choices about the foods you buy, nutrition expert Dr. Ed Blonz brings you
the facts about more than 300 natural and artificial chemical additives that are used in bakery
items, canned foods, boxed foods, dairy, and meat products. (188810—$3.99)

Prices slightly higher in Canada

Payable in U.S. funds only. No cash/COD accepted. Postage & handling: U.S./CAN. $2.75 for
one book, $1.00 for each additional, not to exceed $6.75; Int'l $5.00 for one book, $1.00 each
additional. We accept Visa, Amex, MC ($10.00 min.), checks ($15.00 fee for returned checks)
and money orders. Call 800-788-6262 or 201-933-9292, fax 201-896-8569; refer to ad #BLONZ

Penguin Putnam Inc.   **Bill my:** ☐Visa ☐MasterCard ☐Amex_____(expires)
P.O. Box 12289, Dept. B   Card#_____
Newark, NJ 07101-5289   Signature_____
Please allow 4-6 weeks for delivery.
Foreign and Canadian delivery 6-8 weeks.

Bill to:

Name_____
address_____City_____
ate/ZIP_____
time Phone#_____

to:

_____   Book Total $_____
_____   Applicable Sales Tax $_____
_____   Postage & Handling $_____
_____   Total Amount Due $_____

This offer subject to change without notice.

PENGUIN PUTNAM
──────────────────── online

Your Internet gateway to a virtual environment with hundreds of entertaining and enlightening books from Penguin Putnam Inc.

While you're there get the latest buzz on the best authors and books around—

Tom Clancy, Patricia Cornwell, W.E.B. Griffin, Nora Roberts, William Gibson, Robin Cook, Brian Jacques, Catherine Coulter, Stephen King, Jacquelyn Mitchard and many more!

PenguinPutnam Online is located at
http://www.penguinputnam.com

PENGUIN PUTNAM
NEWS

Every month you'll get an inside look at our upcoming books and new features on our site. This is an ongoing effort on our part to provide you with the most interesting and up-to-date information about our books and authors.

Subscribe to Penguin Putnam News at
http://www.penguinputnam.com/ClubPPI